RSSDI Diabetes Update 2019

Research Society for the Study of Diabetes in India

Celebrating 50 Years
Passion, Quality and Innovation in Healthcare Publishing

RSSDI Diabetes Update 2019

Editor-in-Chief

Banshi Saboo MD PhD FRCP MNAMS
Fellow American College of Endocrinology (FACE)
Fellow International College of Nutrition (FICN - Canada)
Diabetologist, Endocrine & Metabolic Physician
Hon. Diabetologist H. E. The Governor of Gujarat
Scientific Chairman: RSSDI 2019

Co-ordinator

Hardik Chandarana
Founder & CEO
Rx Events, Ahmedabad

Foreword

Siddharth N Shah

JAYPEE

JAYPEE BROTHERS MEDICAL PUBLISHERS
The Health Sciences Publisher
New Delhi | London

Jaypee Brothers Medical Publishers (P) Ltd

Headquarters
Jaypee Brothers Medical Publishers (P) Ltd
4838/24, Ansari Road, Daryaganj
New Delhi 110 002, India
Phone: +91-11-43574357
Fax: +91-11-43574314
Email: jaypee@jaypeebrothers.com

Overseas Office
J.P. Medical Ltd
83 Victoria Street, London
SW1H 0HW (UK)
Phone: +44 20 3170 8910
Fax: +44 (0)20 3008 6180
Email: info@jpmedpub.com

Website: www.jaypeebrothers.com
Website: www.jaypeedigital.com

Inquiries for bulk sales may be solicited at: jaypee@jaypeebrothers.com

RSSDI Diabetes Update–2019/**Banshi Saboo, Hardik Chandarana**

First Edition: **2020**

ISBN: 978-93-89587-12-8

Printed at Sanat Printers

RSSDI Executive Committee

Patrons

Hemraj B Chandalia

C Munichhoodappa

Ashok K Das

Binode K Sahay

OP Gupta

V Seshiah

President

Rajeev Chawla

President Elect

Banshi Saboo

Immediate Past President

PV Rao

Vice Presidents

Vijay Paniker

Ch. Vasanth Kumar

Secretary

B M Makkar

Joint Secretary

Rakesh Sahay

Treasurer

Jayanta Kumar Panda

Executive Committee

Anuj Maheshwari

Sunil Gupta

Vijay Viswanathan

Sanjay Agarwal

Sanjay Kalra

KR Narasimha Setty

CR Anand Moses

Sujoy Ghosh

Co-opted

Jayaprakashsai Jana

Jothydev Kesavadev

Shalini Jaggi

Organizing Committee: RSSDI 2019

Organizing Chairman

KK Pareek

Scientific Chairman

Banshi Saboo

Organizing Secretary

Prakash Keshwani

Chief Patron

Sudhir Bhandari

Chief Coordinator

CL Nawal

Treasurer

Puneet Saxena

Contributors

Editor-in-Chief

Banshi Saboo MD PhD FRCP MNAMS
Fellow American College of Endocrinology (FACE)
Fellow International College of Nutrition (FICN - Canada)
Diabetologist, Endocrine & Metabolic Physician
Hon. Diabetologist H. E. The Governor of Gujarat
Scientific Chairman: RSSDI 2019

Co-Ordinator

Hardik Chandarana
Founder & CEO
Rx Events, Ahmedabad

CONTRIBUTING AUTHORS

A Muruganathan MBBS MD
Governor American College of Physicians India Chapter
Department of General Medicine, AG Hospital
Tirupur, Tamil Nadu, India

A Nanditha MD
Director, Dr. A Ramachandran's Diabetes Hospital
Chennai, Tami Nadu, India

Aastha Chawla MD DVL
Resident
Department of Skin, VD and Leprosy
Sardar Patel Medical College
Bikaner, Rajasthan, India

Abdul Hamid Zargar
MD DM (Endocrinology)
Center for Diabetes and Endocrine Care
National Highway Gulshan Nagar, Srinagar, Jammu & Kashmir
Former:
Member Medical Council of India
Past-President, Endocrine Society of India
Member Institute Body AIIMS, New Delhi
Chairman, Department of Endocrinology
Director & Ex-Officio Secretary to Government
Sheri-Kashmir Institute of Medical Sciences
Srinagar, Kashmir, India

AG Unnikrishnan MD DM (Endocrinology) DNB MNAMS
CEO and Chief Endocrinologist
Chellaram Diabetes Institute
Pune, Maharashtra, India

Ajay Kumar MD
Director
Diabetes Care and Research Centre
GCIB, Patna, India

Ajay Shah MBBS MD DM CCST
Senior Consultant and Head
Department of Endocrinology
Santoka Durlabhji Memorial Hospital
Jaipur, Rajasthan, India

Alok Gupta
Consultant Physician
Diabetologist
Diabetes Research & Education Center
Gorakhpur, Uttar Pradesh, India

Amit Gupta
DNB (Int Med), FRCP (Edin, Glasg), FACP (USA), DFID, Dip Diabetes (Cardiff UK), F Diab, FGSI, MNAMS, FIMSA, FIACM
Director
Promhex Multispeciality Hospital
Greater Noida, Uttar Pradesh, India

Anil Kumar Virmani
MD DRM FICP FIACM FACP
Consultant Physician
Viru's Diabetic Center
Jamshedpur, Jharkhand, India

Anil Samaria MBBS MD
Senior Professor
Department of Medicine
Jawaharlal Nehru Medical College
Ajmer, Rajasthan, India

Anuj Maheshwari
MD FICP FIACM FACP FACE FRCP (London)
Professor and Head
Department of General Medicine
Babu Banarasi Das University
Lucknow, Uttar Pradesh, India

Aravinda Jagadeesha MBBS MD MRCP FRCP FRCP FRCP(Glasgow)
Chairman & Chief Diabetologist
Dr Aravind's Diabetes Center, Basaveshwarangara
Bengaluru, Karnataka, India

Arun Shankar
MBBS RSSDI (DIAB) CCEBDM (PHFI)
Medical Director & Senior Consultant Diabetologist
Jothydev's Diabetes & Research Center
JDC Junction, Mudavanmugal
Trivandrum, Kerala, India

Arvind Gupta
MD FACE FICP FRSSDI F Diab India
Director and Consultant Physician
Internal Medicine and Diabetes
Jaipur Diabetes Research Center
Jaipur, Rajasthan, India

Asha N Shah MD
Professor of Medicine
GCS Medical College
Ex.Professor & HOD Medicine
BJ Medical College & Civil Hospital
Ahmedabad, Gujarat, India

Ashish Sewaram Dengra MBBS MD (Medicine Diploma Diabetes (UK) FIACM Fellow Diabetes India C Diabetology (Mumbai)
Director, Mahi Diabetes,Thyroid Care & Research Center
Consultant Diabetologist
Jabalpur Hospital & Research Center
Jabalpur, India

Ashok K Taneja MD DIP CARD FRCP (UK) FACP (USA) FICP FIAE FDI FAPSC (Taiwan)
Medical Director
Taneja Heart–Diabetes Center
Gurugram, Haryana, India

Ashu Rastogi MBBS MD DM
Assistant Professor
Department of Endocrinology and Metabolism, Postgraduate Institute of Medical Education and Research
Chandigarh, Punjab, India

Ashutosh Chaturvedi
MD (Medicine) Certified in Diabetology (Chennai)
Consultant Physician & Diabetologist
Maxwell Multispeciality Hospital & Jain Chest Care Center
Jaipur, Rajasthan, India

Awadhesh Kumar Singh
MD (Medicine) DM (Endocrinology)
Senior Consultant Endocrinologist
GD Hospital and Diabetes Institute
Kolkata, West Bengal, India

Banshi Saboo MD PhD FRCP MNAMS
Fellow American College of Endocrinology (FACE)
Fellow International College of Nutrition (FICN - Canada)
Diabetologist, Endocrine & Metabolic Physician
Hon. Diabetologist H. E. The Governor of Gujarat
Scientific Chairman: RSSDI 2019

Bharat Panigrahy
MD FICP FACP EULAR Certified in Rheumatology & Pediatric Rheumatology
Senior Consultant in Internal Medicine & Rheumatology
Care Hospital Group
Bhubaneswar, Odisha, India

Bhargav Sosale BE (NTU)
Vice President, Software Design
Remidio Innovative Solutions Pvt Ltd
Bengaluru, Karnataka, India

Bhavana Sosale MBBS MD MRCP (Glasgow) FRCP (Edinburgh)
Diabetologist, Diacon Hospital
Bengaluru, Karnataka, India

Chakrapani M MD
Professor, Department of Medicine
Kasturba Medical College, Mangalore
Manipal Academy of Higher Education
Manipal, India

Chandar Mohan Batra MBBS MD (Medicine) DCH DNB (Endocrinology)
Senior Consultant and Endocrinologist
Indraprastha Apollo Hospital
New Delhi, India

Chandrasekhar Valupadas MD
Professor
Department of General Medicine
Kakatiya Medical College
Mahatma Gandhi Memorial Hospital
Warangal, Telangana, India

CL Nawal MD FICP FACP (USA) FRSSDI
Professor and Head
Department of Medicine
Sawai Man Singh Medical College and Hospital
Jaipur, Rajasthan, India

Dharmendra Panchal MD
Diabetologist and Endocrinologist
Diabetes Care & Hormone Clinic
Sabarmati, Ahmedabad, India
Visiting Endocrinologist
Gujarat Cancer and Research Institute

Dheeraj Kapoor MD DM
Head, Department of Endocrinology
Artemis Hospital
Gurugram, Haryana, India

Edward J Boyko MD MPH
Staff Physician, VA Puget Sound, and Professor, Department of Medicine
University of Washington
Washington, USA

Girish C Verma MD FICP FISC FIAE FIACM
Fellow Diabetes India
Senior Consultant Physician & Diabetologist
Senior Professor of Medicine
Principal & Controller
Government Medical College, Kota
Founder Secretary
RSSDI- Rajasthan Chapter Chairman
Rajasthan Chapter of API (2017-2018)

Girish Mathur MD (Medicine)
FICP FIACM FACP (USA) FRCP (Glasgow)
Vice Dean, Indian College of Physicians (ICP)
Consultant Physician
Kota, Rajasthan, India

Hemraj B Chandalia MD FACP
Director, Endocrinology
Diabetes and Metabolism, Jaslok Hospital and Research Centre, Mumbai
Director, Diabetes Endocrine Nutrition Management and Research Centre
Mumbai, Maharashtra, India

Jagdeep Chugh MD FICP
Senior Consultant
Satyam Medical Center
Gujranwala Town & Fortis Hospital
New Delhi, India

Jalees Fatima MBBS MD FICP FACP (USA) FRSSDI
Professor and Head
Department of Medicine
Era's Lucknow Medical College
Lucknow, Uttar Pradesh, India

Jay Chordia MBBS MD DM
Consultant Endocrinologist
Dr Jay's Diabetes and Hormone Care Center
Udaipur, Rajasthan, India

Jothydev Kesavadev MD FRCP (London, Glasgow, Edinburgh) FACP FACE FRSSDI
Managing Director
Jothydev's Diabetes Research Centres
Kerala, India

Jotideb Mukhopadhyay MBBS MD
Professor
Institute of Postgraduate Medical Education and Research
Seth Sukhlal Karnani Memorial Hospital
Kolkata, West Bengal, India

Jugal Kishor Sharma MD (Med) FICP FRCP (London, Edin & Glasg) FACP(USA) FACE (USA) FRSSDI FIMSA FIACM FGSI FISH
Fellow Diabetes India
Medical Director, Central Delhi Diabetes Center, New Delhi, India

Kiran Shah MBBS MB FCPS (Medicine) Dip Diabetology
Diabetologist, Grant Medical College & Sir JJ Group of Hospitals
Diabetes & Thyroid Care Center
Aditya Jyot Eye Hospital Pvt Ltd
Mumbai, Maharashtra, India

Mangesh Tiwaskar MBBS MD FRCP (London/Ireland/Glasgow) FACP FICP FGSI
Consultant Physician and Diabetologist
Shilpa Medical Center
Mumbai, Maharashtra, India

Manohar KN MD DNB FRCP (Edinburgh) FRCP (Glasgow) FEAC
Consultant Physician & Diabetologist
Manipal Hospital
Examiner - MRCP UK - PACES
Principal Investigator - Clinisearch
Medical Director - GT Foundation
Chairman - DISHA CMEs
Secretary KRSSDI 2018-21
Chairman Reception Committee APICON 2018
Organizing Secretary - KRSSDI 2017

Manoj Chawla
MBBS Diabetology FRCP(Edin) FRSSDI
Consultant Diabetologist and Director
Lina Diabetes Care and Mumbai Diabetes Research Center
Mumbai, Maharashtra, India
Hon. Daibetologist
Asian Heart Institute
SL Raheja Fortis Hospital
BSES MG Hospital
Mumbai, Maharashtra, India

Manoj Saluja MD
Senior Professor
Department of Medicine
Government Medical College
Kota, Rajasthan, India

Meena Chhabra MD (Medicine)
GMC (Bhopal) Diploma in Diabetes from Middlesex University
Senior Consultant Medicine and Diabetes
Specialist Dr Meena Chhabra's Diabetes Clinic
Visiting Consultant
Department of Medicine
Sir Ganga Ram Hospital
New Delhi, India

Meenaxi Sharda MD DCH FICP FIAE
Senior Professor
Department of Medicine
Head of Department
Department of Geriatric Medicine
Government Medical College
Kota, Rajasthan, India

Minal Mohit MBBS MD (Internal Medicine) FDE FPAE FACP (US) FICN (UK) FIACM FDI
Consultant and Head
Department of Endocrinology
Manipal Hospital
Jaipur, Rajasthan, India

Naresh Kanumilli MD
Community Diabetes Consultant-Manchester University Foundation Trust
Clinical Champion- Diabetes UK
Clinical Network Lead for Diabetes-Greater Manchester
Diabetes Research Lead- Greater Manchester Clinical Research Network
PCDS-Committee Member
Northenden Group Practice
489, Palatine Road
Northenden, Manchester

NK Agrawal MBBS MD DM (Endocrinology)
Department of Endocrinology and Metabolism
Institute of Medical Sciences
Banaras Hindu University
Varanasi, Uttar Pradesh, India

NK Singh MD FICP
Director
Diabetes and Heart Research Center
Dhanbad, Jharkhand, India
Chairman, RSSDI
Jharkhand, India

Parimal Swamy MD
Consultant Physician and Chief of Diabetes Care
Jabalpur Hospital & Research Center
Director Apollo Diabetes & Asthma Care Center
Jabalpur, Madhya Pradesh, India

Pratap P Jethwani MD (Medicine)
Postgraduate Diploma in Diabetes (Cardiff, UK)
Fellow-Diabetes India, Fellow-RSSDI
Ex-Tutor- Leicester University (UK) & BMJ Learning
Consultant Diabetes Specialist
Jethwani Hospital
Rajkot, Gujarat, India

Puneet Rijhwani
MBBS MD FRCP (Edin) FICP
Professor and Head
Mahatma Gandhi University of Medical Sciences and Technology
Jaipur, Rajasthan, India

Puneet Saxena MD FICP FRCP FGSI FIACM FRSSDI Fellow Diabetes India
Senior Professor and Unit Head
Department of Medicine
SMS Medical College and Hospital
Jaipur, Rajasthan, India

Purvi Chawla
MBBS MS (Pharm Sci, USA) PG Dipl Diabetol (UK)
Consultant Diabetologist and Director of Clinical Research
Lina Diabetes Care and Mumbai Diabetes Research Centre
Mumbai, Maharashtra, India

RM Anjana MD PhD
Diabetologist and Joint Managing Director
Madras Diabetes Research Foundation
Chennai, Tamil Nadu, India

Raj Kumar Lalwani MBBS MD (Med)
GDDC-Diploma Diabetes (Australia) FIMSA FDI
Senior Consultant Diabetologist
PG Medical Center and National Heart Institute
New Delhi, India

Rajesh Rajput MD DM (Endocrinology) FRCP (Edin) FACE (USA) FICP FIACM FISH FIMSA
Senior Professor and Head
Department of Endocrinology
Postgraduate Institute of Medical Sciences
Rohtak, Haryana, India

Rajeev Chawla MD FRSSDI FACP (USA) FRCP UK (Edin) FACE (USA)
Senior Consultant Diabetologist & Director
North Delhi Diabetes Center
New Delhi, India

Rajnish Saxena
MBBS PGCDM DIP. Diabetology
Director and Diabetologist
Saxena Diabetes & Foot Care Center
Ajmer, Rajasthan, India

Rakesh M Parikh FACE FRCP FCPS MBBS Dip Diabetology
Consultant Diabetologist, Diabecity
Jaipur, Rajasthan, India

Ramesh Kumar Goenka MD FICP FRSSDI
Consultant Physician and Diabetologist
Sunshine Hospital, Bhubaneswar
Associate Professor
Department of Medicine,
Kalinga Institute of Medical Sciences
Bhubaneswar
Consultant Physician & Diabetologist
Satayu Diabetes Care and Research Center
Bhubaneswar, Odisha, India

Ranjit Unnikrishnan
MD FRCP (Lond, Glasg and Edin) FACP FICP
Vice-Chairman
Dr Mohan's Diabetes Specialities Center
Chennai, Tamil Nadu, India

Rohit Kapoor MBBS MD
Medical Director and Head of Department
Endocrinology & Medicine-Care Well Heart & Superspeciality Hospital
Amritsar, Punjab, India

S Arulrhaj MD FRCP (Glassgow)
National President Elect
API Head Acute Medicine
Sundaram Arulrhaj Hospitals & Research Foundation
Tuticorin, Tamil Nadu, India

Sailesh Lodha MD DM FACE
Head, Department of Diabetes and Endocrine Sciences, Eternal Hospital
Jaipur, Rajasthan, India

Sambit Das MD (Medicine)
DM (Endocrinology)
Senior Consultant Endocrinologist
Apollo Center for Obesity, Diabetes and Endocrinology (ACODE) and Sugar Clinics
Apollo Hospitals
Associate Professor
Department of Endocrinology
Hi-Tech Medical College and Hospital
Bhubaneswar, Odisha, India

Sandeep Rai MBBS DNB.MNAMS PGDHS FRCP
Professor and Unit Head
Postgraduate Department of Medicine and Diabetology
Mahatma Gandhi Mission Institute of Health Sciences
Navi Mumbai, Maharashtra, India

Sandeep Tak MD
Senior Professor
Department of Medicine
Sampoornanand Medical College
Jodhpur, Rajasthan, India

Sanjay Agarwal MD FACE
Director, Aegle Clinic-Diabetes Care Head
Department of Medicine, Ruby Hall Clinic
Pune, Maharashtra India
Senior Consultant in Diabetes and Medicine, Jehangir Hospital
Pune, Maharashtra, India

Sanjeeb Kakati MD
Professor and Head
Department of Medicine
Assam Medical College
Dibrugarh, Assam, India

Sanjeev Gulati MD DMRE DFID
Assistant Professor of Medicine
Chirayu Medical College
Director, Sarvottam Hospital
Bhopal, Madhya Pradesh, India

Sanjiv Shah MD
Consultant
Apollo Sugar Clinic
Mumbai, Maharashtra, India

Saumik Datta MD DM FICP
Associate Professor
Department of General Medicine
Calcutta National Medical College
Kolkata, West Bengal, India

Shalini Jaggi Dip Diab (UK) Dip Endo (UK)
FRSSDI FRCP (London, Glas, Edin) FACE (USA)
Consultant Diabetologist and Head
Dr Mohans' Diabetes Specialities Center
New Delhi, India

Sharad Kumar MD DN DNB (Endocrinology)
Professor
Era's Lucknow Medical College
Lucknow, Uttar Pradesh, India

Shashi Panicker MD MSc
Academic Fellow
Department of Medicine
Mahatma Gandhi University of Medical Sciences and Technology
Jaipur, Rajasthan, India
Tutor, Department of Diabetes and Metabolic Diseases
University of South Wales
Cardiff, UK

Shriram V Kulkarni MD (Med) FACP (USA)
FICP FGSI FACM FDI Director
Center for Diabetes, Thyroid, Obesity & Adolescent Research
Navi Mumbai, Maharashtra, India

Sidhartha Das
MD FRCP (GLASG) FRCP (Edin) FRCP (London)
Senior Consultant in Medicine & Diabetes
Formerly Head, PG Department of Medicine & Dean and Principal SCB Medical College & Hospital
Cuttack, Odisha, India

SS Dariya MD (Internal Medicine)
FDI FGSI PGDGM
Consultant, Physician
SMS Hospital
Jaipur, Rajasthan, India

Sunil Kumar Kota MD DNB
Chief Consultant Diabetologist and Endocrinologist
Diabetes and Endocare Clinic
Berhampur, Odisha, India

Supratik Bhattacharyya
MD MRCP (UK) FACP MS FRCP
Director, Skin, Diabetes & Endocrine Center, Naihati
Consultant Endocrinologist
AMRI Hospital, Salt Lake & Apollo Clinic
Kolkata, West Bengal, India

Suraj Prakash Sondhi MD
Director
Omnibus Healthcare India Private Limited
Meerut, Uttar Pradesh, India
Guest Faculty
Department of Medicine
Subharti Medical College
Meerut, Uttar Pradesh, India

Swati Srivastava MBBS MD FRCPE FICP
FIDM FDI ADHA
Consultant Diabetologist and Metabolic Physician
Professor, Unit Head, In Charge Consultant Thyroid clinic,
SMS Medical College and Hospitals, Jaipur
Fellow in Diabetes, Trained in Endocrinology Tech & Applications
Member AACE, Endocrine Society USA,
Executive committee member Rajasthan ICP, Rajasthan API, Rajasthan RSSDI
Organizing Committee member, RSSDI 2019, Diabetes India 2019
Organizing secretary, Midterm IPF conference July 2019
Member Research Review Board, SMS Medical College, Jaipur

Tvisha K Parikh MBBS
Sports Physician
Sir HN Reliance Foundation Hospital
Mumbai, Maharashtra, India

Urman A Dhruv MD
Director
Department of Internal
Medicine and Diabetes
HCG Hospitals
Ahmedabad, Gujarat, India

Vijay P Panikar MD FCPS DNB
Consultant
Department of Diabetes
Endocrine and Metabolism
Lilavati Hospital
Mumbai, Maharashtra, India

Vinod Mittal MD FRSSDI FICP FCAM FCCP FGSI FIAMS FDIFACP (USA)
Sr. Consultant Diabetologist and Head
Center for Diabetes and Metabolic Diseases
Delhi Heart & Lung Institute
Sr. Visiting Consultant
Sir Ganga Ram Hospital
Director, Delhi Diabetes Care Centre
New Delhi, India

Vitull K Gupta MD FAPI FCSI FACP FIACM
Consultant, Kishori Ram Hospital and
Diabetes Care Center
Bathinda, Punjab, India

Yashasvi Gautam MD FICP FIACM
Senior Consultant Physician
Treasurer—RSSDI Rajasthan Chapter
Past President—Associate Physicians of India, Kota Chapter (2008-2010)
Past Treasurer—Indian Medical Association Kota Chapter (2017-2018)
Life Member—API, RSSDI, ISN, IMA, IACM
Honorary Sr. Consultant Physician
Sudha Hospital
Kota, Rajasthan, India
Jaiswal Hospital
Kota, Rajasthan, India

Foreword

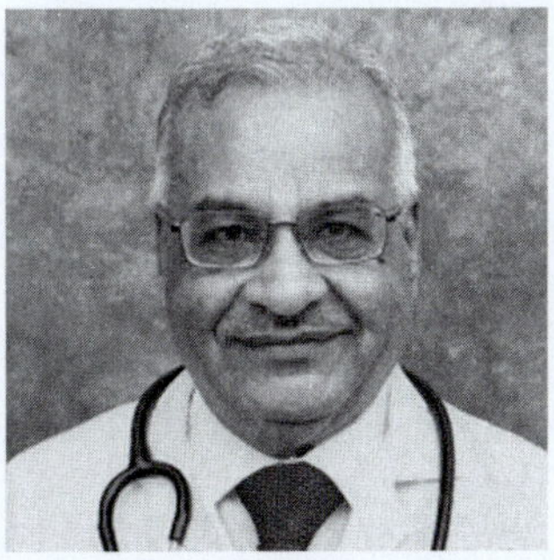

Diabetes Mellitus contributes a significant burden to the global population. There are multiple comorbidities present along with this deadly disease, which in turn complicates therapy and management. While Type 1 diabetes and other types account for 2–5% of all cases of diabetes, type 2 diabetes remains by far the most common form of diabetes and has attained epidemic proportions worldwide. As per the recent International Diabetes Federation (IDF) data, 415 million people in the world are suffering from diabetes and these numbers are expected to rise to 642 million by 2040. It is also estimated that in every 6 second, a person dies due to diabetes or its complications.

Also, diabetes, today, is a major concern of society as well as health sector. Various studies have shown that Type 2 Diabetes is a preventable disorder, or at least, it can be delayed. There are definite risk factors of Type 2 Diabetes Mellitus (T2DM) and by simple questionnaire, we can identify high-risk population. Prevention of T2DM is a major threat to public health for South Asians, particularly for India.

The three major comorbidities in Type 2 Diabetes are Hypertension, Dyslipidemia, and Obesity. Further associations include Smoking and Physical Inactivity and complications include Cardiovascular Disease, Cerebrovascular Disease, and Chronic Kidney Disease, which may coexist as part of the Diabetic Disease Spectrum or may result as a complication of long-standing diabetes.

It is evidently proven that early diagnosis and screening of diabetes help in preventing complications of diabetes and, therefore, the healthcare professionals need to be trained in diabetes management and prevention.

I congratulate Research Society for the Study of Diabetes in India (RSSDI), particularly Dr Banshi Saboo, for coming out with RSSDI Update–2019. I am sure it will help healthcare professionals to upgrade their knowledge about management and prevention of diabetes as well as related complications. The contents of this book are designed to appropriately keep the need of the time in mind and contain all the topics from diagnosis to pathophysiology to management and prevention as well.

I have immense pleasure to write this foreword and I am sure it will be a useful book for postgraduates, physicians, and delegates at large.

Siddharth N Shah
Chairman API House
Mumbai, Maharashtra, India

Preface

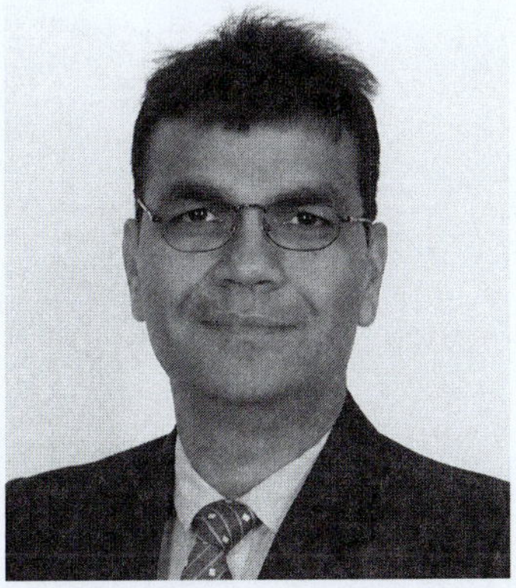

Diabetes mellitus is an important and formidable disease or disease affecting mankind. Its spread has much increased recently and its expression has undergone various modifications with societal, economic, and cultural development.

Research Society for the Study of Diabetes in India—RSSDI, founded in 1972, is committed to increase the standards of diabetes care in India by educating healthcare professionals across the country. RSSDI Update is an integral part of capacity building during its annual conference to be distributed to all attending delegates across the country.

Dissemination of knowledge through book is a popular way of transmission of knowledge since ancient time. I am sure this book will be helpful to the readers in enhancing their practice and improving day-to-day practice as it covers a wide range of topics extending from the epidemiology to pathophysiology, screening, diagnosis, management, latest randomized controlled trials and studies, and their translation into evidence-based practice. It also covers topics like latest advancements in diabetes, reversal of diabetes, technological advancements etc. Every effort has been made to match the standards of previous RSSDI update books.

I am thankful to all the speakers and faculties of RSSDI 2019 who so kindly transformed their scientific presentations into chapters at our request. Compiling everything in one book has been a herculean task managed by a well-coordinated team effort, sifting through the manuscripts, editing, and finalizing them to their current form to bring out all the scientific discussions at the conference into this compact yet comprehensive book.

At this juncture, I would like to mention very personal loss to me while compiling this book. We have lost Dr SM Sadikot (Immediate Past President—IDF and President—Diabetes India), which is a big loss to the Diabetes World in India and internationally.

My gratitude and thanks to President and Secretary of RSSDI, Scientific Committee Members, Local Organizing Committee as well as all contributors and my editing and publishing team who raced against time to successfully bring out this update well in time to reach your hands.

Happy Reading!!!

Banshi Saboo

Acknowledgments

Rajeev Chawla
President, RSSDI

BM Makkar
Secretary, RSSDI

Scientific Committee

Anuj Maheshwari
JJ Mukherjee
Manoj Chawla
Neeta Deshpande
RM Anjana
Sanjay Kalra
Arvind Gupta
Jothydev Kesavadev
Mithun Bhartia
Pratap Jethwani
Sanjay Agarwal
Sujoy Ghosh

Chief Advisor

Shashank Joshi

Local Organizing Committee

Sudhir Bhandari
Chief Patron

KK Pareek
Org. Chairman

CL Nawal
Chief Coordinator

Prakash Keswani
Org. Secretary

Puneet Saxena
Treasurer

Coordinators

Hardik Chandarana | Stuti Gupta | Gaurav Solanki | Isha Agrawal

Jaypee Brothers

Jitendar P Vij | MS Mani | Shashikumar Shambhoo | Richa Saxena | Himani Pandey | Tamali Deb

Special Thanks

Dia Care Team

Contents

Section 3: Diagnosis and Classification

Section 4: Lifestyle Modification

Section 5: Therapeutics

Section 6: Guidelines

Section 7: Diabetes and Complications

Plate 1

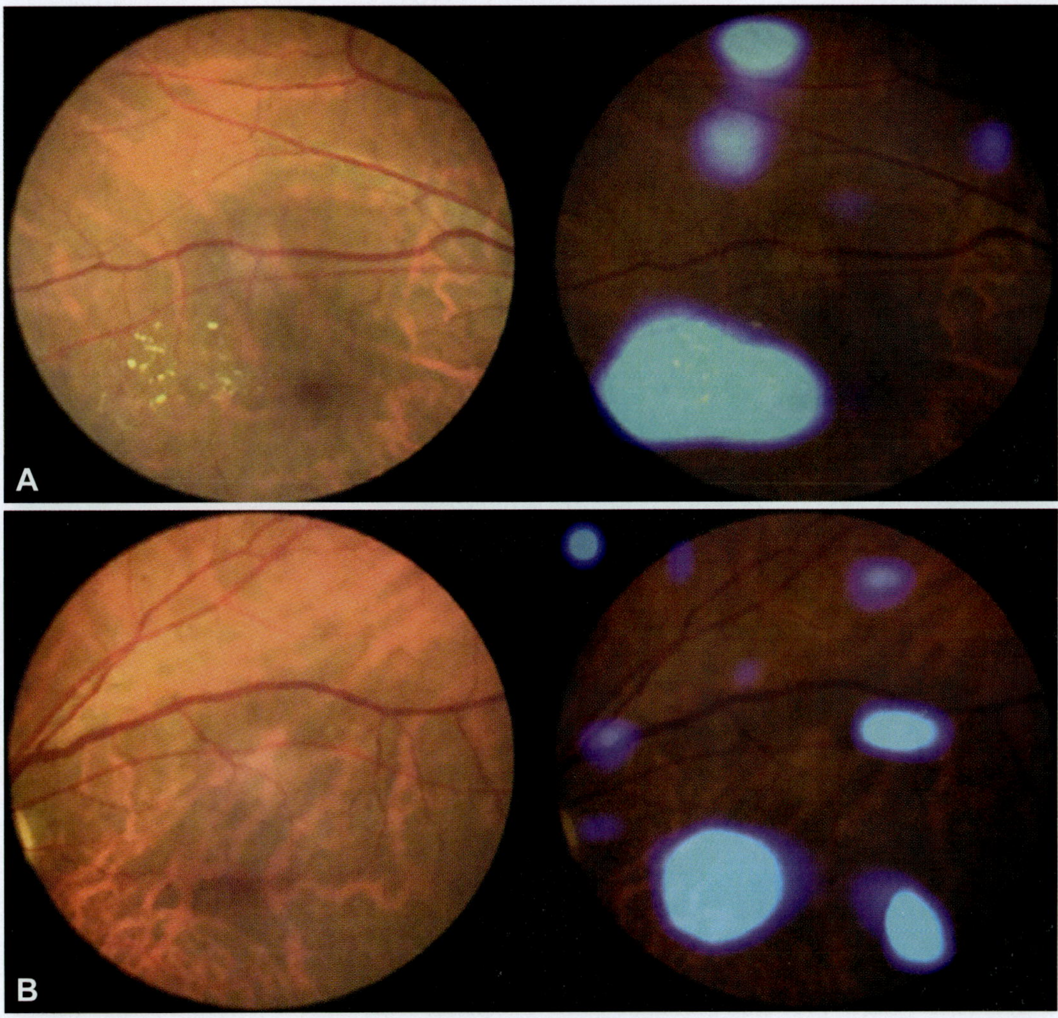

Result: Signs of retinopathy detected. Examples of lesions are highlighted confidence 99%

Figures 2A and B An example of the PDF report generated by the Medios AI in an individual with diabetic retinopathy. ***(Chapter 4)***

(*Source*: Medios AI.)

Plate 2

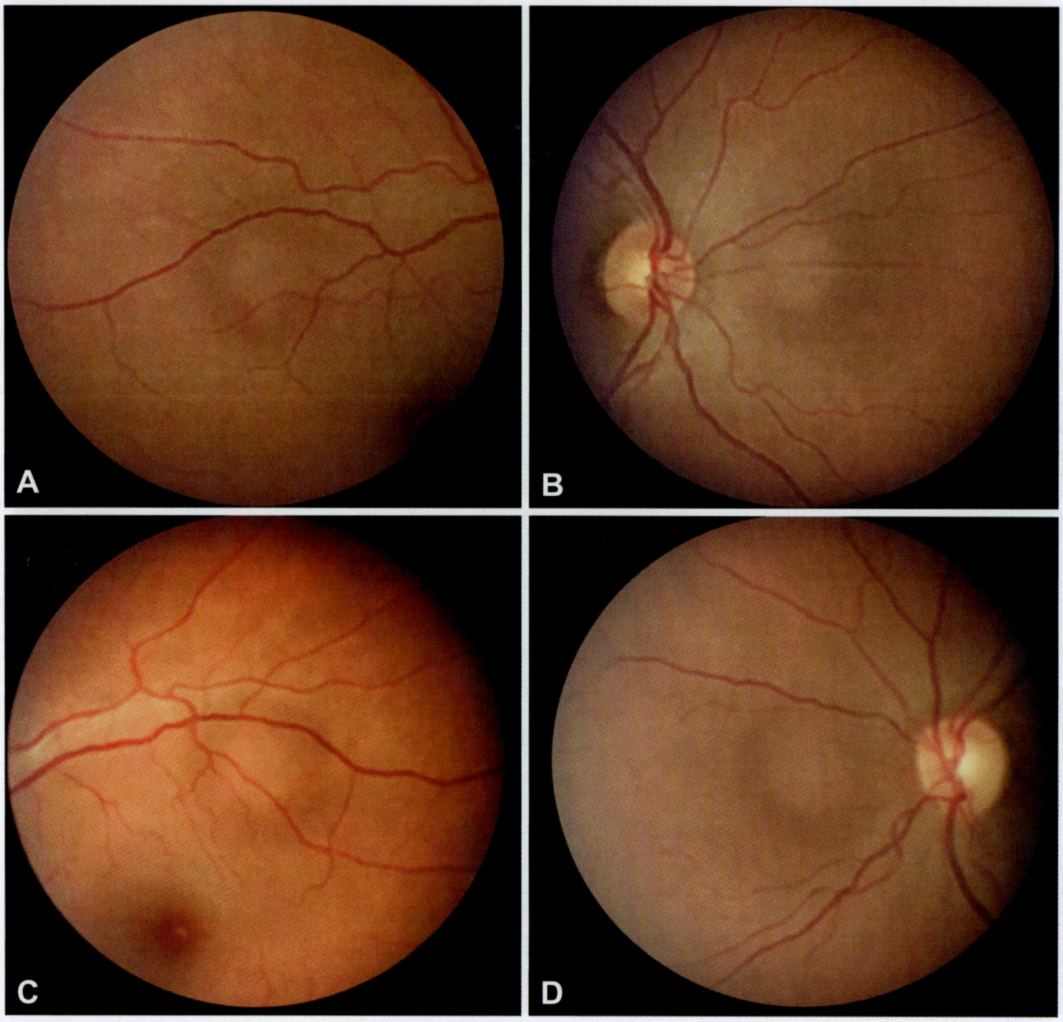

Figures 3A to D An example of the PDF report generated by the Medios AI in an individual without diabetic retinopathy. ***(Chapter 4)***

(*Source*: Medios AI.)

Plate 3

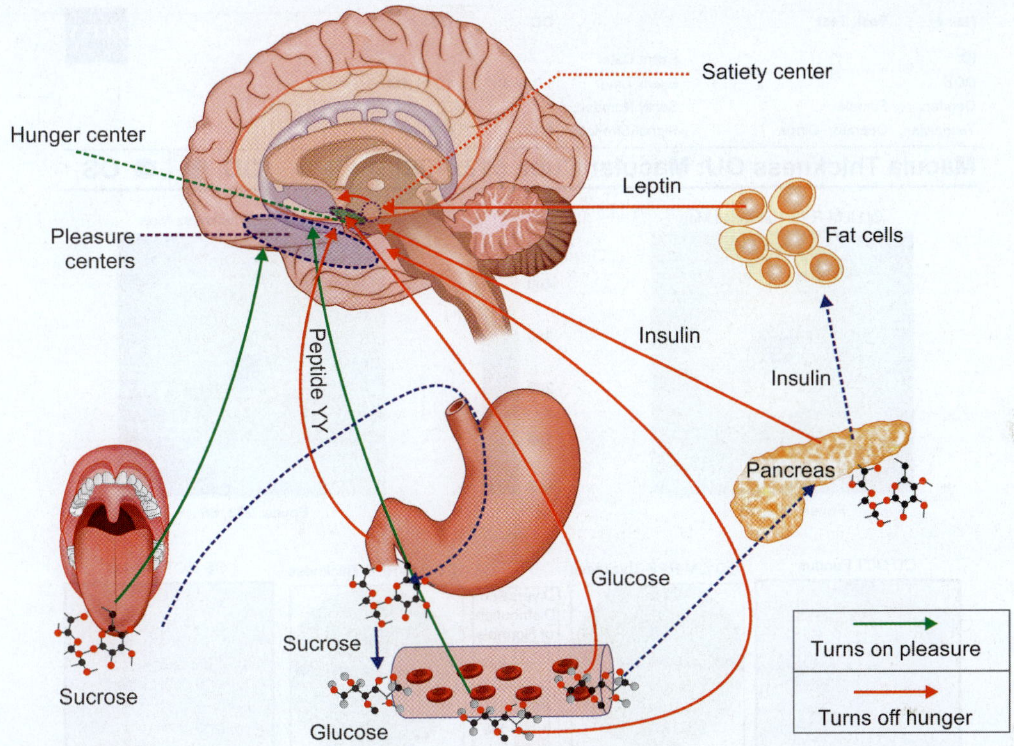

Figure 1 Sucrose ingestion leads to activation of pleasure centers in brain and the calorie inflow also activates multiple gastrointestinal (GI) negative feedback signals to hypothalamus to decrease hunger sensation, while artificial sweetener ingestion also results in activation of pleasure sensation but is followed by no calorie inflow and therefore, there is no feedback inhibition of hunger sensation from GI signals to hypothalamus, leading to increase in food intake and weight gain. ***(Chapter 21)***

(*Source*: Gabymichel, Blaus B, Haggstrom M, et al. Medical gallery of Mikael Haggstrom. Wiki Journal of Medicine. 2014;1(2).)

Plate 4

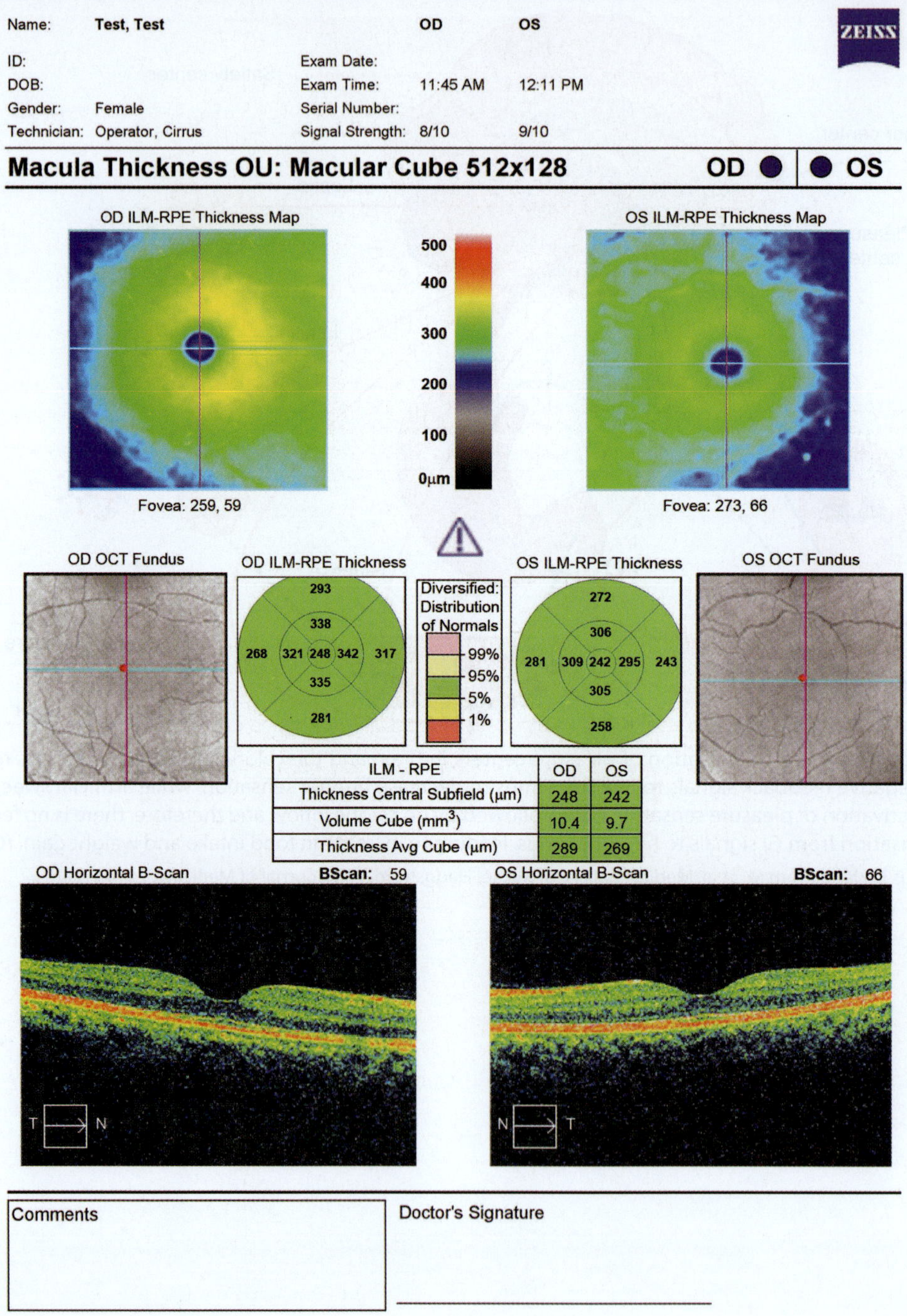

Figure 1 Standard report from Zeiss Cirrus HD OCT device. ***(Chapter 75)***

Plate 5

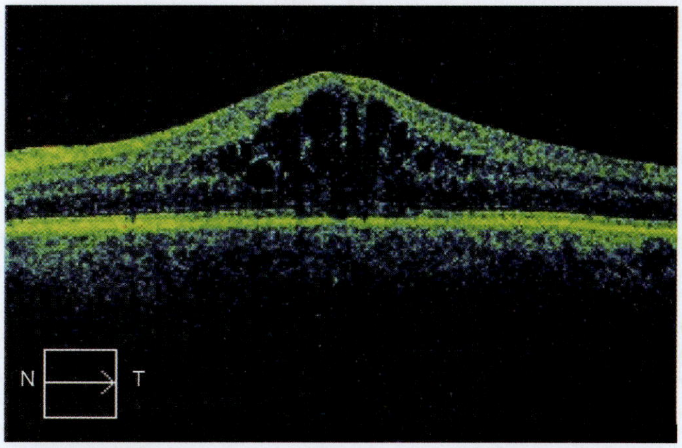

Figure 6 Cystoid macular edema. ***(Chapter 75)***

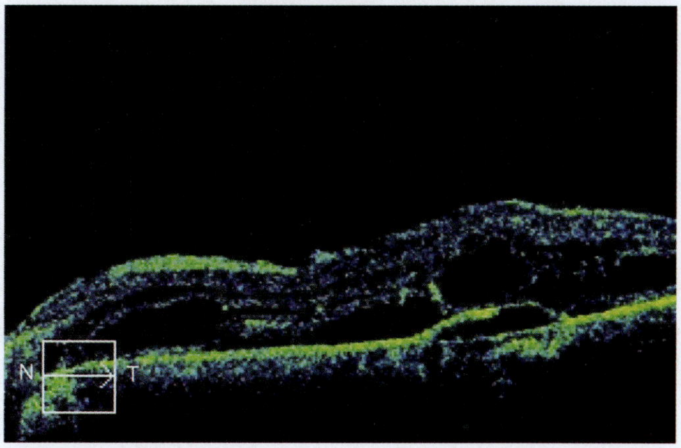

Figure 7 Sponge-like retinal swelling + CME/serous foveal detachment. ***(Chapter 75)***

Plate 6

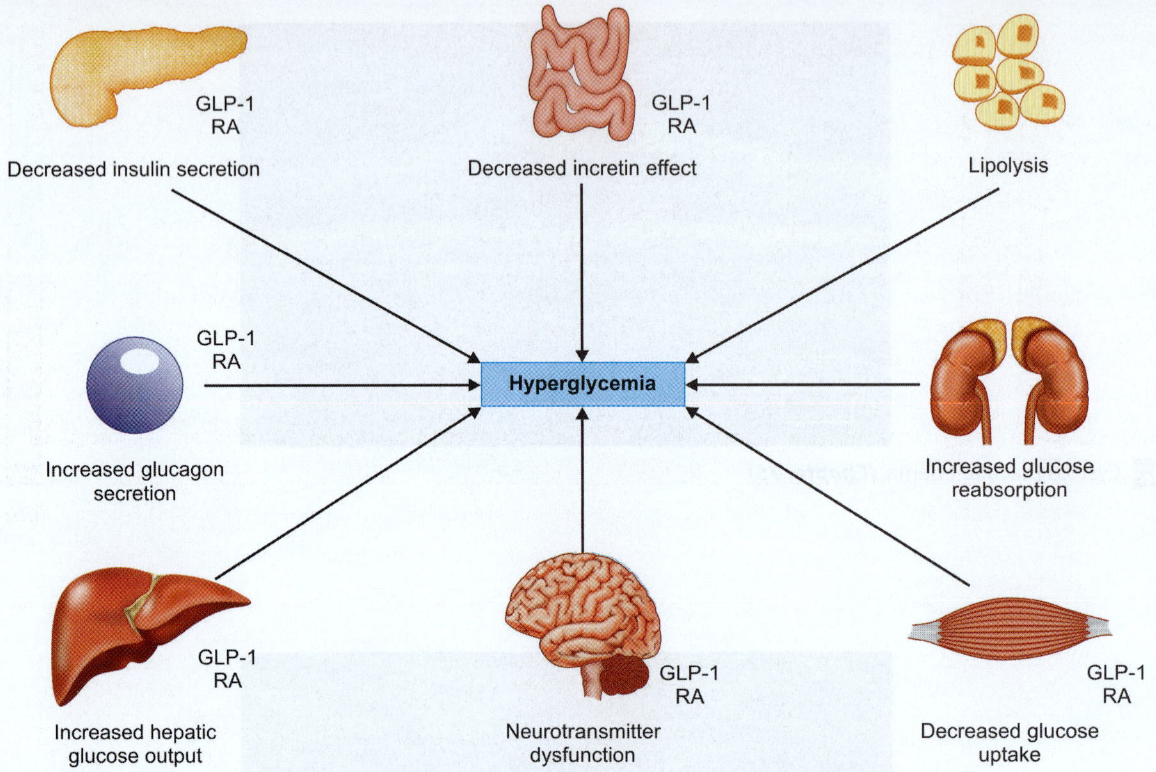

Figure 1 Addressing pathophysiological defects of type 2 diabetes with GLP-1 RA. ***(Chapter 82)***

(*Source*: DeFronzo RA. From the triumvirate to the ominous octet: a new paradigm for the treatment of type 2 diabetes mellitus. Diabetes. 2009;58:773-95.)

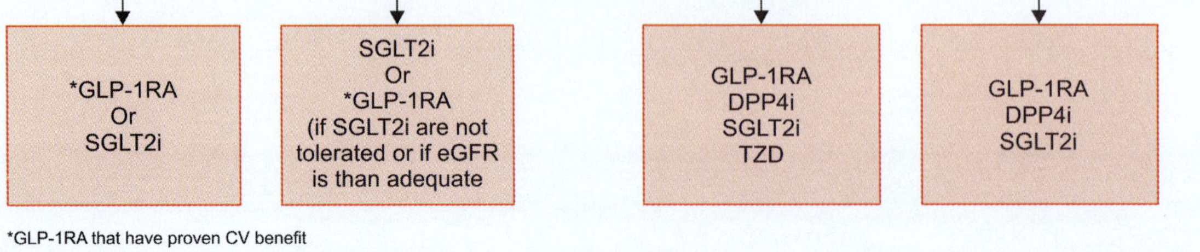

Flowchart 1 ADA/EASD approach to management of uncontrolled type 2 diabetes. (ASCVD: atherosclerotic cardiovascular disease; CKD: chronic kidney disease; DPP4i: dipeptidyl peptidase 4 inhibitors; eGFR: estimated glomerular filtration rate; GLP-1 RA: glucagon like peptide receptor agonists; HF: heart failure; SGLT2i: sodium glucose co-transporter 2 inhibitors; TZD: thlazolidinediones. ***(Chapter 82)***

(*Source*: American Diabetes Association. 9. Pharmacologic Approaches to Glycemic Treatment: Standards of Medical Care in Diabetes-2019. Diabetes Care. 2019;42:S90-102.)

Plate 7

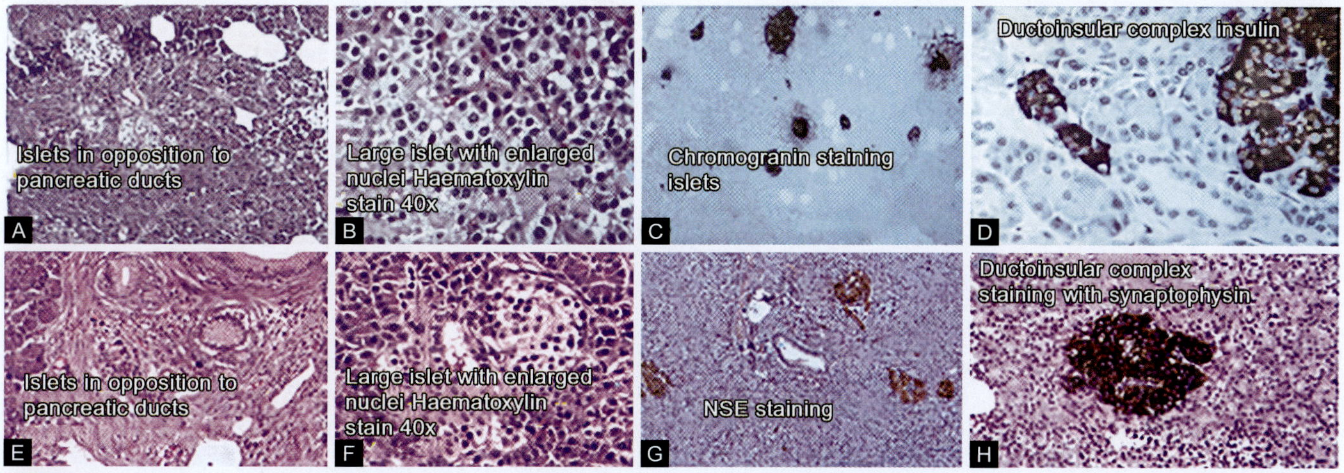

Figure 1 HPE findings of 2 patients showing histopathological features of NIPHS, (A to D) Patient 1; (E to H) Patient 2. ***(Chapter 60)***

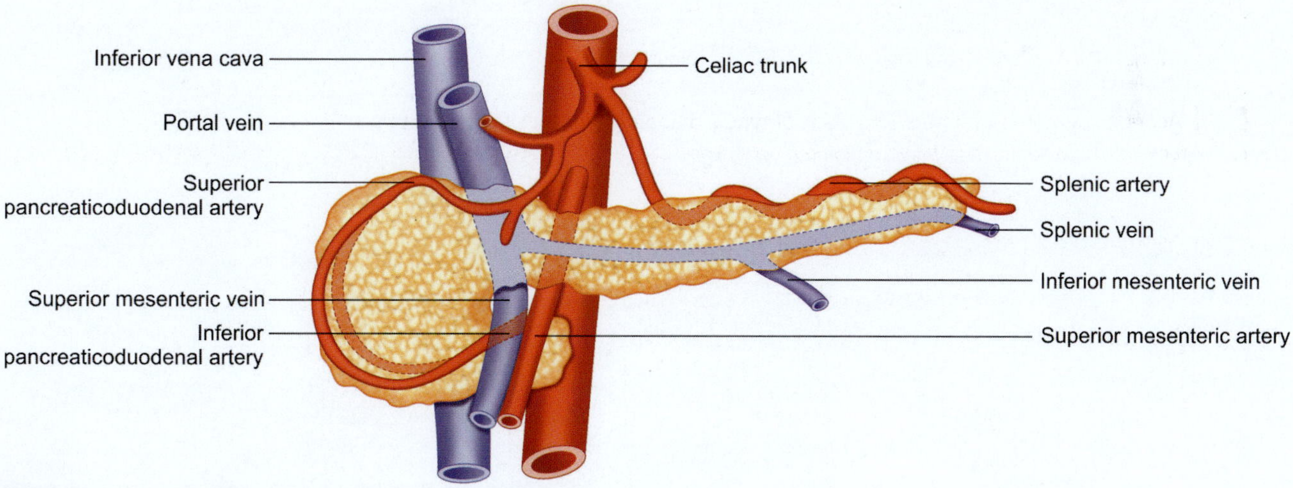

Figure 2 Arterial supply of the pancreas. ***(Chapter 60)***

1

SECTION

Epidemiology

1

CHAPTER

Opportunistic Screening: How Feasible it is in Rural Setting?

Chakrapani M, Nitish Mathur, Unnikrishnan B

INTRODUCTION

Screening is defined by the World Health Organization (WHO) as "services for the presumptive identification of unrecognized disease in an apparently healthy, asymptomatic population by means of tests, examinations or other procedures that can be applied rapidly and easily....."[1] Screening is important for diseases where metabolic and organ complications develop much before symptoms manifest. Screening not only involves early diagnosis, but also a comprehensive plan for a full evaluation, education and management plan.[1] It can either be population screening or opportunistic screening. While population screening is ideal, it involves a huge expenditure and may not be cost effective. Opportunistic screening is the process wherein screening of the individual for a disease is done whenever the person comes in contact with the healthcare system. Growing epidemic of diabetes and other noncommunicable diseases (NCDs) in India can be controlled by a systematic opportunistic screening.[2] National Program for Prevention and Control of Cancer, Diabetes, Cardiovascular Diseases and Stroke (NPCDCS) is an ambitious program of the Government of India which involves opportunistic screening for diabetes, hypertension and common cancers,[2] by providing promotive, preventive, curative, and supportive services in an integrated manner. Implementing this program in rural India is quite a challenge.

NEED FOR OPPORTUNISTIC SCREENING

Opportunistic screening for diabetes is extremely crucial because there is a long period of time before the clinical presentation and target-organ damages are seen at the time of diagnosis itself. Large proportions of diabetic patients have complications at diagnosis since they were asymptomatic for a long period of time.[3] Average hemoglobin A1c (HbA1c) at the time of diagnosis was 9.2, even in newly diagnosed young diabetic patients.[4] Diabetic retinopathy, neuropathy, nephropathy, and ischemic heart disease were noted in 5.1%, 13.2%, 0.9%, and 0.7% of these newly diagnosed young diabetic patients.[4] Interventions done at the earliest stage of the disease are much more cost-effective than interventions done later. In United Kingdom Prospective Diabetes Study (UKPDS), lower blood sugar at diagnosis was associated with lesser long-term micro- and macrovascular complications.[5] Overall cost is less with opportunistic screening for sugar, blood pressure (BP) and lipids done together as a package.[6] In India, half of those identified with diabetes were not aware of their disease.[7] In a recent large observational study, it was noted that 40% of the mortalities are due to cardiovascular causes and modifiable risk factors accounted for 70% cardiovascular deaths.[8,9] Modifying a few simple risk factors in the population can have huge overall gains.[10] Hence, opportunistic screening is required.

Diabetes is a very common condition and the prevalence is rising. Prevalence of diabetes in India was 7.3% and the prevalence of prediabetes was 10.3%.[7] Diabetes is no more considered a mild-chronic disease, because 60% of mortality in India are due to NCDs, overtaking deaths due to trauma and infectious diseases.[2]

IMPORTANCE OF SCREENING IN RURAL POPULATION

Diabetes management and prevention programs traditionally did not focus on rural areas since it was that burden of diabetes is less in rural areas. In a recent large study, prevalence in urban areas was 11.2% and in rural areas it was 5.2%. However, since 70% of Indian population is in rural areas, burden of diabetes in rural areas is at least equal to the burden of diabetes in urban areas.[7] Interestingly, the prevalence of prediabetes was 10.3% and was similar among rural and urban population.[7] There is an increasing trend of diabetes among economically weaker sections of India. Studies done with opportunistic screening have shown that about 40% of the individuals above the age of 30 years have a random glucose of more than 140 mg% even in rural areas.[11] Higher cardiovascular deaths (40%) are observed in low-income countries compared to lower cardiovascular deaths (23%) in high-income countries in spite of having lesser number of risk factors.[9] These complications are compounded in rural areas where ignorance of the disease, socio-political, cultural, and economic factors affect their lifestyle behaviors[12] and a prolonged asymptomatic phase leads to a significant cardiovascular burden among rural population.

COMPREHENSIVE NONCOMMUNICABLE DISEASE SCREENING AND PREVENTION PROGRAM OF THE GOVERNMENT

Government of India has rolled out an ambitious project to contain the damages of NCDs by reinforcing the concept of early detection and effective and affordable management. All individuals above the age of 30 years are to be screened for diabetes by glucometer with opportunistic screening at all the levels of health care including subcenters, by trained paramedical staff.[2] As per the program, anyone with glucometer general random blood sugar (GRBS) of 140 or above with a glucometer testing will be given a referral card for a formal venous blood examination in a fasting state to confirm diabetes mellitus at a suitable healthcare level which is generally community health center or district laboratory. All such patients diagnosed with diabetes are to be evaluated thoroughly and treated according to the protocol. It is unethical to screen the population of individuals for a particular disease unless there is a detailed plan of action for subsequent management of the condition. This program is a comprehensive one wherein protocols for diagnosis, follow-up treatment and management of complications are built in. But there are a lot of logistical challenges that need to be addressed in rural settings.

A major challenge is the high dropout rate after the initial glucometer screening. In the rural areas, dropouts are higher because of various logistical reasons including the need for traveling to distant higher center and the need for fasting blood sample. It has been seen that in the rural areas only about 60% of the individuals referred for the next level complete the process even when the government is providing it free of cost.[11] But innovative approaches involving technology can solve this issue. When reminders using mobile phones were used, conversion rate significantly went up to nearly about 80% and this led to a significantly more number of subjects being diagnosed with diabetes and prediabetes.[11] Involvement of private institutions and nongovernmental organizations (NGOs) and innovative use of technology can improve the yield of this program.

The HOPE 4 study showed that community-based interventions are highly effective in reducing the burden of NCDs, especially in rural areas.[13] However, in India, non-physician health workers were not as effective as their counterparts in other third world countries in community level interventions for NCD. Compared to 90% concordance of their assessment with physicians, Indian health workers could reach up to 30% concordance only. Outsourcing specific tasks to private players like educating the paramedical staff in the rural areas can be a viable option. Previous experience in NCD prevention has confirmed that packaged and bundled intervention consisting of paramedical workers doing screening and risk assessment, innovative use of information technology (IT), lifestyle counseling at or near their home, free supply of medicines and overall supervision by physicians was very effective at the community level.[14]

OUR EXPERIENCE AT DAKSHINA KANNADA DISTRICT, KARNATAKA

Involvement of the private institutions is also important in the implementation of the program. Our institution was involved in one such activity and experience in this program confirmed the potential of the public–private initiatives. The project consisted of two components: (1) Training healthcare workers in integrated preventive activities and (2) Second level laboratory screening of high-risk individuals of 30 years and above and GRBS >140. The project lasted for about 6 months and was implemented in 2015 in the district of *Dakshina* Kannada, Karnataka. Department of Community Medicine took up the initiative of training 1,690 healthcare workers across the district which involved structured and comprehensive modular training.

Following the training program, laboratory workup for opportunistic screening was undertaken. About 6,060 individuals underwent confirmatory test after the initial screening test. Instead of a patient coming to the district laboratory which generally is far away from the remote rural areas in the villages, arrangements were made for sample collection from the Public Health Center (PHC) itself. The success of the program was mainly because of the active participation of the coordinator, whose involvement and commitment was crucial. Seventy percent of the initially screened individuals were diagnosed with newly detected diabetes mellitus.

SOME OF THE CHALLENGES THAT WE ENCOUNTERED

Transporting the blood samples without centrifugation often leads to hemolysis. Centrifuge was installed at the site of blood collection to separate the serum. But erratic power supply and unscheduled power failures in the villages lead to failure of the centrifugation resulting in difficulty in proper processing of the sample. This challenge was overcome by using gel vacutainers. Paramedical personnel in the villages were not accustomed to drawing blood with vacutainers. They were drawing blood samples with syringes only.

The fasting sample was not truly fasting. For many villagers, fasting would imply not eating solid breakfast. Having a liquid diet was still fasting in their belief. Proper education of the public would improve the situation.

Poor network connectivity with the remote areas results in slower and delayed reporting from the central laboratory back to the individuals.

Another interesting challenge was name. Unique identification numbers have to be generated to avoid the common problem of name similarities.

The samples were supposed to be transported through public transport system and received at the central laboratory for processing. Poor transport network, cancellation of the scheduled trips and diversion from the scheduled routes were other issues that had to be tackled.

Previous studies have also observed such logistic issues. Installing centrifuge at primary level, point-of-care HbA1c measurement with random samples and outsourcing venous blood testing to private contractors at PHC were some of the recommendations.[11]

Overall experience was very gratifying because good number of asymptomatic lean diabetics were identified who otherwise would have continued with their abnormal lifestyle behaviors before being diagnosed. General awareness regarding this NCD was generated by this program. Moreover, training large number of healthcare workers resulted in capacity building for scaling up of the activities.

Opportunistic screening should not be seen as one-off event. It has to be part of comprehensive screening, diagnosis, follow-up and treatment plan including all NCDs since most of them are interrelated. Public–private partnership is a crucial element in implementing this program. Instead of organizing isolated, one-time events, public institutions and private partners should integrate their activities with the existing framework of comprehensive plan.

CONCLUSION

Opportunistic screening for diabetes is extremely important for rural India. It is very much feasible if the existing program of the government of India is implemented with the help of private partners, voluntary organizations and NGOs. Technology and improved logistics will be required for the successful implementation.

REFERENCES

1. World Health Organization. (2017). Screening. [online]. Available from www.who.int/cancer/prevention/diagnosis-screening/screening/en/. [Last accessed on September, 2019].
2. Directorate General of Health Services, Ministry of Health and Family Welfare, Government of India. National Programme for Prevention and Control of Cancer, Diabetes, Cardiovascular Diseases and Stroke (NPCDCS), Operational Guidelines (Revised: 2013-17). [online]. Available from mohfw.gov.in/sites/default/files/OperationalGuidelinesofNPCDCS%28 Revised-2013-17%29.pdf. [Last accessed on September, 2019].
3. Kahn R, Alperin P, Eddy D, et al. Age at initiation and frequency of screening to detect type 2 diabetes: a cost-effectiveness analysis. Lancet. 2010;375(9723):1365-74.
4. Sosale B, Sosale A, Mohan A, et al. Cardiovascular risk factors, micro- and macrovascular complications at diagnosis in patients with young onset type 2 diabetes in India: CINDI 2. Indian J Endocrinol Metab. 2016;20(1):114-8.
5. Colagiuri S, Cull CA, Holman RR, et al. Are lower fasting plasma glucose levels at diagnosis of type 2 diabetes associated with improved outcomes?: U.K. prospective diabetes study 61. Diabetes Care. 2002;25(8):1410-7.
6. Rutten G. Screening for type 2 diabetes-where are we now? Lancet. 2010;375(9723):1324-6.
7. Anjana RM, Deepa M, Pradeepa R, et al. Prevalence of diabetes and prediabetes in 15 states of India: results from the ICMR–INDIAB population-based cross-sectional study. Lancet Diab Endocrinol. 2017;5(8):585-96.
8. Yusuf S, Joseph P, Rangarajan S, et al. Modifiable risk factors, cardiovascular disease, and mortality in 155 722 individuals from 21

high-income, middle-income, and low-income countries (PURE): a prospective cohort study. Lancet. 2019. pii: S0140-6736(19)32008-2.

9. Dagenais GR, Leong DP, Rangarajan S, et al. Variations in common diseases, hospital admissions, and deaths in middle-aged adults in 21 countries from five continents (PURE): a prospective cohort study. Lancet. 2019. pii: S0140-6736(19)32007-0.
10. Read SH, Wild SH. Prevention of premature cardiovascular death worldwide. Lancet. 2019. pii: S0140-6736(19)32034-3.
11. Kumar S, Shewade HD, Vasudevan K, et al. Effect of mobile reminders on screening yield during opportunistic screening for type 2 diabetes mellitus in a primary health care setting: A randomized trial. Prev Med Reports. 2015;2(2015):640-4.
12. Chow CK, Raju PK, Raju R, et al. The prevalence and management of diabetes in rural India. Diabetes Care. 2006;29(7):1717-8.
13. Schwalm JD, McCready T, Lopez-Jaramillo P, et al. A community-based comprehensive intervention to reduce cardiovascular risk in hypertension (HOPE 4): a cluster-randomised controlled trial. Lancet. 2019. pii: S0140-6736(19)31949-X.
14. Jafar TH, Samad Z, Bloomfield GS. Parallel community solutions for cardiovascular risk reduction. Lancet. 2019. pii: S0140-6736(19)31995-6.

2 CHAPTER Population-based Screening Strategies for Diabetes: Cost-effective or Not?

Rajnish Saxena

INTRODUCTION

Diabetes is one of the main global health problem accounts with highest morbidity and mortality all around the world.[1] In 2012 60% of all deaths in India are due to noncommunicable diseases (NCDs) and cardiovascular disease (CVD) has major contribution among these NCD and diabetes mellitus contribute 2% of all cases.[2] Type 1 diabetes mellitus (T1DM) and type 2 diabetes mellitus (T2DM) patients increasing all around the globe and leading to severe economic burden to both patients as well as country. More than 80% of T2DM patients are from low- and middle-income countries, under developed and developing country including India 82.2 million people are diabetic and 29.1 million with prediabetes in Southeast Asia.

DIAGNOSIS OF DIABETES MELLITUS

The diabetes mellitus is a metabolic disorder that is characterized by presence of chronic hyperglycemia along with disturbances of carbohydrate, fat, and protein metabolism, which results from defects in insulin secretion, insulin action, or both.[3]

The current diagnostic criteria of diabetes are given in Table 1.

The risk categories for future development of diabetes and CVD are impaired glucose tolerance (IGT), and impaired fasting glycemia (IFG). An individual who falls into the category of IFG on fasting result may also have IGT on the 2-hour value or, indeed, diabetes. When an individual falls into two different categories, the more severe one is applicable.

BURDEN OF DIABETES

The global burden of disease in the year 2017 is about 425 million people had diabetes and numbers are projected to increase by 45% and reach 625 million in the year 2045, among these at present 325 million are of working age group, i.e. 20–64 years of age and they also expected to reach to 438 million in the year 2045.[4]

TABLE 1: Diagnostic criteria of diabetes.[1,3]

If one or more criteria are present, diagnosis of diabetes confirmed	If both of the following criteria are present, diagnosis of IGT is confirmed	If both of the following criteria are present, diagnosis of IFG is confirmatory
FPG ≥126 mg /dL (7.0 mmol/ L)	FPG < 126 mg/dL (7.0 mmol/L)	FPG 110–125 mg/dL (6.1–6.9 mmol/L)
or		
2 Hour after taking 75 gm glucose Plasma glucose ≥200 mg/dL (11.1 mmol/L)	2 hour after taking 75 gm glucose Plasma glucose ≥ 140–200 mg/dL (≥ 7.8–< 11.1 mmol/L)	2 hour after taking 75 gm glucose Plasma glucose <140 mg/dL (< 7.8 mmol/L)
or		
A random plasma glucose >200 mg/dL (11.1 mmol/L or HbA1c ≥ 6.5 %)		

(FPG: fasting plasma glucose; IFG: impaired fasting glycemia; IGT: impaired glucose tolerance)

TABLE 2: Top ten countries with maximum number of diabetics in 2017 and expected diabetics in 2045 (20–79 people).[1]

Rank in 2017	Name of country	Number of people with diabetes	Rank in 2045	Name of country	Number of people with diabetes
1	China	114.4 million	1	India	134.3 million
2	India	72.9 million	2	China	119.8 million
3	United States	30.2 million	3	United States	35.6 million
4	Brazil	12.5 million	4	Mexico	21.8 million
5	Mexico	12.0 million	5	Brazil	20.3 million
6	Indonesia	10.3 million	6	Egypt	16.7 million
7	Russian Federation	8.5 million	7	Indonesia	16.7 million
8	Egypt	8.2 million	8	Pakistan	16.1 million
9	Germany	7.5 million	9	Bangladesh	13.7 million
10	Pakistan	7.5 million	10	Turkey	11.2 million

It has been estimated that globally as many as 212.4 million people or half (50.0%) of all people 20–79 years with diabetes are unaware of their disease. In the year 2017, China, India and United States have largest number of diabetics 114 million, 72.9 million and 30.2 million respectively. The number of diabetes population in India estimated to reach 134.3 million largest among all countries creates a major health problem for country resources. China and United States will be estimated to 119.8 and 35.6 million (Table 2). Maximum other countries in the list of top ten diabetes population are from developing countries. So screening of population for preventing diabetes progression has very important role.

Global estimates of the burden of IFG and IGT are not available, but the number of people with IGT is likely to be even greater than the number with diabetes.[5,6] IGT and IFG are now sometimes referred to as "prediabetes".

Countries with undiagnosed diabetes population: There is not a single country that has diagnosed every person having diabetes. Africa, which is a continent including many low-income countries with wide rural areas, has proportion of undiagnosed diabetes to be 69.2%, which is likely because of and low prioritization of diabetes screening and limited resources. Nearly 37.3% of individuals with diabetes have not been diagnosed even in high-income countries. Worldwide, out of total undiagnosed diabetes cases, 84.5% are in low- and middle-income countries.

The largest numbers of people who have undiagnosed diabetes are the similar countries who have largest number of people having diabetes; China, India, and the United States are on the top rank (Tables 3 and 4).

In the developing world, the diabetes epidemic is accelerating, with a growing proportion of individuals affected in younger age groups. Latest reports mention T2DM to be diagnosed among children and adolescents.[7-9]

TABLE 3: People with diabetes (20–79 years) who are undiagnosed per region—2017.[1]

S.No.	Different regions according to IDF	Number of undiagnosed diabetes patients	% of undiagnosed individuals
1	Africa	10.7	69.2%
2	South East Asia	47.2	57.6%
3	Western Pacific	85.9	54.1%
4	Middle East and North Africa	19.0	49.0%
5	South and Central America	10.4	40.0%
6	Europe	22.0	37.9%
7	North America and Caribbean	17.3	37.6%

(IDF: International Diabetes Federation)

TABLE 4: Undiagnosed diabetics according to economic point of view (20–79 years) in the year 2017.[1,3]

Countries according to income	Number of undiagnosed diabetes	Undiagnosed diabetes %
Higher income	32.9 million	37.3%
Middle income	170.5 million	52.5%
Low income	9 million	76.5%

This may lead to increase in the burden of chronic diabetic complications globally.

In India difference in prevalence is there according to regional and social variation. Usually urban population 7.3% and rural population 3.1% population suffer from diabetes mellitus.[10] In south India, prevalence is much more than the other part of India.

According to ICMR India diabetes (ICMRINDIAB) study maximum number of patients in Tamil Nadu 10.4% to lowest in Bihar with 4.3%. Chandigarh is leading among the metro cities, with 13.6% of population having diabetes.[11]

SCREENING

Screening of Population

Screening is very important for early detection and delaying the onset of disease. We can diagnose the prediabetic condition early and prevent or delay progression to diabetes and also prevent cardiovascular events. There are several potential approaches to screening for diabetes:

- *Screening the entire population*: It is very difficult and almost not possible in large population.
- *Screening of elective or targeted group*: It is done among a subgroup of peoples who have already been recognized as at relatively high risk in association with age, bodyweight, ethnicity, etc.
- *Opportunistic screening*: It is performed at the time when people are attended by health care providers (HCPs), for a reason other than particular disease.

Advantage of Screening of Diabetes

World Health Organization (WHO) and International Diabetes Federation (IDF) advocate the screening because:

- A long, latent, asymptomatic period is present during which condition can be detected.[12,13]
- A significant percentage of people who have T2DM are undiagnosed.
- A significant percentage of new referred cases of T2DM already show evidence of the microvascular complications related to diabetes.
- The prevalence of T2DM rising worldwide.
- The long-term complications of T2DM are very troublesome.
- Evidence supports the efficacy of blood pressure control,[14] blood lipid control,[15,16] and intensive blood glucose control in type 2 diabetes and accumulating evidence that treatment of dyslipidemia (e.g. lowering LDL cholesterol[17]) and hypertension can lead to prevention of CVD in individuals having type 2 diabetes.

Benefits of Early Detection of Type 2 Diabetes

- Increased quality of life and/or life span that may be because of decrease in the frequency and severity of immediate effects of diabetes or the delay or prevention of its long-term complications.
- Any savings or redistribution of healthcare resources that may be feasible due to decreased amounts of care needed for complications of diabetes (decreased hospital admissions and lengths of stay, etc.).

Several evidences regarding the impact of interventions in IGT show that interventions directed at decreasing weight and increasing physical activity and the use of certain pharmacological agents have proved efficient in delaying or decreasing the transition to diabetes in those having IGT.

ECONOMICS OF HEALTH CARE BURDEN

In India, nearly 85–95% of the cost of health care is borne by individuals and their families from their own income. Direct expenditure consumes 27–34% of household income of rural and urban poor population.

In case of middle and higher income group population, in rural area 8–12.6% and in urban area 4.8–16.9% of income is spend toward diabetes care.

According to results of large community-based survey, cost of diabetes in India (CODI), ambulatory care constitute 65% cost. While cost of hospitalization is 35% therapy cost 31%, and specific antidiabetic drug cost constitute to 17%. Ambulatory care consisting of doctor's visit and monitoring constitute 34% cost.[18]

- *Direct cost of diabetes management*: It includes hospital-related costs, laboratory cost, transportation to hospital, drug cost, food and monitoring cost, and the cost incurred toward inpatient care.

  Long-term monitoring care include drug cost toward more than half of the total disease cost.[19,20]

  The average annual direct cost toward ambulatory diabetes care among middle and higher income group was more than ₹ 6,212 in the year 2005 out of which half was drug cost. Another study from Indian capital city Delhi Diabetes Community (DEDICOM) study, it was about ₹ 14,508.[20]
- *Indirect cost for diabetes management*: It includes loss of income associated with morbidity, mortality and

disability. Due to illness patient remain absent from job. Sometimes due to some complications patient can develop permanent disability and mortality also.

According to one North India study, management is higher for those who attended private sector healthcare centers it was about 19,552 while it was very less from government setup, i.e. ₹ 1,204.[12]

- *Socioeconomical burden or cost of diabetes*: More than 5 year education of patient cost about ₹ 2,810 while less than 5 year was about ₹ 400.[19,20]
- *Cost of management of complication*: Properly managed diabetes reduced the chances of hospitalization of patient, ultimately it decrease the economic burden for family and community. It also improves the quality of life of patient. So many studies highlighted the direct relation between timely diagnosis of disease and there complication and ultimately reduction in economic burden.

  In a Chennai-based cost study, it was reported that total cost for patients without complications was ₹ 4,493 in comparison with ₹ 14,691.75 for patients with complications.

  Highest costs were incurred by the foot complications; patients having foot complications spent four times more as compared to patients without foot involvement.

  Patients with renal disease, retinal, and cardiovascular complications spent three times more as compared to patients who had no complications.

  Similarly consultation and hospitalization cost for these patients are also high. It is ₹ 5,256 compared without complications is ₹ 1,083 almost five times high. Treatment cost for these patients also increases with duration of diabetes, presence of complications, hospitalization, insulin therapy, antibiotics, etc. It also increased if surgery is required. The cost of therapy is also high in urban area is we compare with rural settings.

  According to one South East Asia and sub Sahara African study different diabetes related interventions studies includes neuropathy screening and preventive foot care, intensive glycemic control, retinopathy screening and photocoagulation studies alone or combination of all in the studies. Retinopathy screening and photocoagulation was the most cost-effective interventions saved 1891 days per million population and with an annual per capita cost of 0.32 dollars ($) and average cost-effective ratio of 170. When standard glycemic control was included with retinopathy screening and photocoagulation studies then per capita cost increased to 1.14 $ and cost-effective ratio to 512 but saved 2233 days per million population. If standard glycemic control is replaced by intensive glycemic control then per capita cost increased to 2.11 $ and saved 2319 days per million population annually, so overall it is cost-effective.[16]

CONCLUSION

- The topic of screening of T2DM is significant with respect to health of every individual, day-to-day clinical practice, and public health policy.
- In spite of scarcity of direct evidence, early detection is already taking place by screening both by inviting peoples from general population for screening and, opportunistically, when people who seem to be at high risk of developing diabetes attend for health care (generally primary health care) for other purposes.
- There is direct evidence that the incidence of diabetes can be decreased among people at high risk of developing T2DM in the future who may be recognized because of activities directed toward detection of diabetes.
- If screening seems to be useful, the most significant *epidemiological considerations* that determine whether to screen in any given population will be (1) prevalence of undiagnosed T2DM in the population and (2) degree to which T2DM is related to risk of CVD, specific complications of diabetes, and other significant health outcomes in that population. So it is cost-effective in long term because of reduced chances of complication.

REFERENCES

1. International Diabetes Federation. (2017). IDF Diabetes Atlas 2014. [online] Available from http://www.idf.org/diabetesatlas [Last accessed September, 2019].
2. World Health Organization. (2014). Noncommunicable diseases country profile 2014. [online] Available from http://apps.whoint/iris/bitstream/10665/128038/9789241507509_eng.pdf [Last accessed September, 2019].
3. World Health Organization. Definition, Diagnosis and Classification of Diabetes Mellitus and its Complications. Report of a WHO Consultation. Geneva: World Health Organization; 1999.
4. Sadikot SM, Nigam A, Das S, et al. The burden of diabetes and impaired glucose tolerance in India using the WHO 1999 criteria: prevalence of diabetes in India study (PODIS). Diabetes Res Clin Pract. 2004;66(3):301-7.
5. Wild S, Roglic G, Sicree R, et al. Global burden of diabetes mellitus in the year 2000. Global Burden of Disease. Geneva: WHO; 2003.
6. King H, Rewers M. Global estimates for prevalence of diabetes mellitus and impaired glucose tolerance in adults. Diabetes Care. 1993;16:157-77.
7. Rosenbloom AL, Joe JR, Young RS, et al. Emerging epidemic of type 2 diabetes in youth. Diabetes Care. 1999;22:345-54.

8. Dabelea D, Hanson RL, Bennett PH, et al. Increasing prevalence of type II diabetes in American Indian children. Diabetologia. 1998;41: 904-10.
9. Kitagawa T, Owada M, Urakami T, et al. Increased incidence of non-insulin dependent diabetes mellitus among Japanese school children correlates with an increased intake of animal protein and fat. Clin Paediatr (Phila). 1998;37:111-5.
10. Mohan V, Mathur P, Deepa R, et al. Urban rural differences in prevalence of self-reported diabetes in India—the WHO-ICMR Indian NCD risk factor surveillance. Diabetes Res Clin Pract. 2008;80(1):159-68.
11. Anjana RM, Pradeepa R, Deepa M, et al. Prevalence of Diabetes and prediabetes (IFG and/or IGT) in urban and rural India: phase 1 results of the Indian Council of Medical Research-INDiaDIABetes (ICMR-INDIAB) Study. Diabetologia. 2011;54(12):3022-7.
12. Ramachandran A, Snehalatha C, Yamuna A, et al. Insulin resistance and clustering of cardiometabolic risk factors in urban teenagers in southern India. Diabetes Care. 2007;30:1828-33.
13. Ramachandran A, Snehalatha C, Shetty AS, et al. Derivation and validation of diabetes risk score for urban Asian Indians. Diabetes Res Clin Pract. 2005;70:63-70.
14. Ramachandran A, Snehalatha C, Kapur A, et al. High prevalence of diabetes and impaired glucose tolerance in India: National Urban Diabetes Survey. Diabetologia. 2001;44:1094-101.
15. Kumpatla S, Kothadan H, Thakur S. The cost of treating long term diabetic complications in a developing country: a study from India. J Assoc Physicians India. 2013;61(2):102-9.
16. Otegon M, Lim S, Chisholm D, et al. Cost effectiveness of strategies to combat cardiovascular disease, diabetes, and tobacco use in sub Saharan Africa and South East Asia: Mathematical modeling study. BMJ 2012;344:e607.
17. Mohan V, Deepa R, Deepa M, et al. A simplified Indian Diabetes Risk Score for screening for undiagnosed diabetes subjects. J Assoc Physician India. 2005:53:759-63.
18. Kapur A. Economic analysis ao diabetes care. Indian J Med Res. 2007;125(3);473-82.
19. Grover S, Avasthi A, Bhansali A, et al. Cost of ambulatory care of diabetes mellitus; a study from north India. Postgraduate Med J. 2005;81(956);391-5.
20. Kumar A, Nagpal J, Bhartia A, Direct cost of ambulatory care of type 2 diabetes in middle and high income group population of Delhi: the DEDICOM survey. J Assoc Physicians India. 2008;56:667-74.

3 CHAPTER Role of Risk Scores to Identify High-risk Population: Global and Indian

Arun Shankar

INTRODUCTION

High-risk patient, according to American Diabetes Association (ADA), is the one who is overweight or obese (BMI ≥ 25 kg/m^2 or ≥ 23 kg/m^2) and has one or more additional risk factors such as family history of diabetes, history of gestational diabetes, high-risk race or ethnicity.[1] International Diabetes Federation (IDF) has proposed strategy for diabetes prevention in high-risk population involving following approaches—identification of high-risk individuals, evaluation of risk, and interventions for prevention.[1] Lifestyle interventions, namely physical activity and diet, can prevent or delay the onset of diabetes among high-risk populations.[1,2] Evidence also suggests reduction of diabetes risk by 58% with lifestyle modifications in people with impaired glucose control.[1] Approximately, 50% of people with diabetes remain undetected and has already developed complications at the time of diagnosis.[3] Since, diabetes is characterized by a long-latent asymptomatic stage of approximately 7 years before diagnosis; it qualifies for early screening to predict the risk of diabetes.[3]

DEMAND FOR EFFECTIVE SCREENING TOOL

Undiagnosed diabetes is a serious phenomenon since people at high-risk remain untreated and the disease advance to manifest severe diabetes-associated complications.[4] Global prevalence of undiagnosed diabetes is estimated to be between 24.1% and 75.1%. Interestingly, the Diabetes Epidemiology: Collaborative Analysis of Diagnostic Criteria in Asia (DECODA) studies have demonstrated that for each diagnosed case of diabetes, there are 1.6 undiagnosed cases of diabetes.[4]

Evaluation of blood glucose has been used as a screening tool for identifying individuals at high-risk for diabetes.[5] However, a controversy exists if fasting glucose is sufficient or an oral glucose tolerance test is also a need for detection of asymptomatic diabetes. Along with being an invasive procedure, blood glucose screening is a costly and time-consuming method. In addition, it only estimates current glycemic status and is susceptible to wide variation.[5]

An effective primary prevention approach would be to identify high-risk individuals even before impaired glucose control sets in, i.e. in a normoglycemic state.[5] Thus, the strategy would be to prevent the transition of normoglycemic state to impaired glucose state and lastly, prevent diabetes occurrence.[5]

RISK SCORES FOR IDENTIFICATION OF HIGH-RISK DIABETES POPULATION

A risk score is a prognostic tool expected to accurately identify individuals at absolute risk and may or may not provide accurate risk estimation.[6] A number of risk scores have been developed which are based on noninvasive measures or questionnaire and show good discriminatory ability (Table 1). The components of these risk scores are mainly, nonmodifiable risk factors such as age and family history, high body mass index and waist circumferences, high blood pressure, and medication use. In addition, the risk scores may also include biochemical measures such as lipid and plasma glucose levels, consumption of fruits and vegetables, measures of glucose, and insulin control (homeostasis model assessment and measures of insulin secretion and resistance from oral glucose tolerance tests), novel biomarkers (C-reactive protein and

TABLE 1: Various risk scores and their variables.

Sl. no.	Risk score	Study population	Variables in the risk score
1.	Atherosclerosis Risk in Communities Study Diabetes Risk Score, United States	Atherosclerosis Risk in Communities study, United States	Age, ethnicity, parental history, systolic BP, waist circumference, height, fasting glucose, triglycerides, HDL cholesterol
2.	Cambridge Diabetes Risk Score, United Kingdom	Population from general practices, United Kingdom	Age, sex, BMI, smoking status, corticosteroid use, antihypertensive use, family history
3.	Finnish Diabetes Risk Score, Finland	FINRISK, Finland	Age, BMI, waist circumference, antihypertensive use, previous diabetes, physical activity, fruit and vegetables intake
4.	Framingham Offspring Diabetes Risk Score, United States	Framingham Offspring Study, United States	Age, sex, parental history, BMI, waist circumference, fasting glucose, HDL cholesterol, triglycerides, hypertension
5.	German Diabetes Risk Score, Germany	EPIC-Potsdam, Germany	Age, waist circumference, height, hypertension, physical activity, smoking, and consumption of whole-grain bread, red meat, coffee, moderate alcohol
6.	Prospective Cardiovascular Munster Diabetes Risk Score, Germany	Prospective Cardiovascular Munster Study, Germany	Age, BMI, fasting glucose, HDL cholesterol, family history, hypertension
7.	Rancho Bernardo Diabetes Risk Score, United States	Rancho Bernardo Study, United States	Model for predicting persons with 2-hour glucose ≥140 mg/dL: sex, age ≥ 70 years, triglycerides ≥ 150 mg/dL, fasting glucose
8.	San Antonio Diabetes Risk Score, United States	San Antonio Heart Study, United States	Age, sex, ethnicity, BMI, family history, systolic BP, HDL cholesterol, fasting glucose + 2-hour glucose

(BMI: body mass index; BP: blood pressure; HDL: high-density lipoprotein)

(*Source*: Adapted from Buijsse B et al. Risk assessment tools for identifying individuals at risk of developing type 2 diabetes. Epidemiol Rev. 2011;33:46-62.)

plasma adiponectin concentrations), genetic information (multiple single nucleotide polymorphisms).[6]

A good risk score is the one that demonstrates accurate estimation of a person's risk for developing diabetes.[7] Also, it should be able to distinguish between high-risk and low-risk population. The prediction is expected to match closely with what was observed on performance. Also, it should exhibit good performance when implemented on a new population.[7]

Indian Diabetes Risk Score

Indian diabetes risk score (IDRS) by the Madras Diabetes Research Foundation (MDRS) has been derived from a large epidemiological study, Chennai Urban Rural Epidemiological Study (CURES), conducted on a representative population of Chennai.[4,8]

Features of Indian Diabetes Risk Score

Indian diabetes risk score is based on four modifiable risk factors—(1) age, (2) abdominal obesity, (3) family history of diabetes, and (4) physical activity. American Diabetic Association also recommends these risk factors. The IDRS categories and scoring for each of the risk factor are given in the Table 2.[8]

Methodology of Indian Diabetes Risk Score Factors

A simple questionnaire and one anthropometric measurement (waist circumference) is utilized for obtaining information on the modifiable risk factors included in IDRS.[8] The questions are:

- What is your age?
- Do you have a family history of diabetes? If yes, does your father, mother, or both have diabetes?
- Do you exercise regularly?
- How physically demanding is your work (occupation)?

Sensitivity and Specificity of Indian Diabetes Risk Score

Indian diabetes risk score demonstrates optimal sensitivity and specificity in detecting high-risk diabetes population, particularly for the score of 60 and above.[4]

TABLE 2: Indian diabetes risk score (IDRS) scoring of risk factors.

Modifiable risk factor	Category		Scoring
Age	<35 years		0
	35–49 years		20
	≥50 years		30
Abdominal obesity (waist circumference)	Males	Females	–
	≥90–99 cm	≥80–89 cm	10
	≥100 cm	≥90 cm	20
	Others	Others	0
Family history of diabetes	No history		0
	If, one parent is diabetic		10
	If, both parents are diabetic		20
Physical activity	Leisure time exercise and physically demanding occupational work		0
	Either exercise or physically demanding work		20
	Others		30
Total score	Minimum score		0
	Maximum score		100

(*Source*: Adapted from: Mohan V et al. A simplified Indian Diabetes Risk Score for screening for undiagnosed diabetic subjects. J Assoc Physicians India. 2005;53:759-63.)

- Sensitivity and specificity of IDRS for a score of ≥60 is 72.5% and 60.1%, respectively.[4,8]
- The positive and negative predictive value were estimated to be 17.0% and 95.1%, respectively.[4,8]
- The accuracy of the score was estimated to be 61.3%.[4,8]

In an urban setting (sample size of 155), IDRS predicted the risk of diabetes with sensitivity of 95.12% and specificity of 28.9% in individuals with score of 60 and above.[4]

Merits of Indian Diabetes Risk Score

- It is derived from a large representative sample of India with similar demographics to the rest of population.[4,8]
- Simple, safe, noninvasive and inexpensive measures are used.[4,8]
- Indian diabetes risk score is based on four simple easily obtainable risk factors.[4,8]
- It is easily applicable and can be effectively performed to detect very high-risk population.[4,8]

Importantly, IDRS takes into consideration the severity of the risk factors and thus, represent a simplified and cost-effective method, which can be effectively employed for mass screening purpose among undiagnosed diabetic patients in Indian population.[8]

IMPORTANCE OF SCREENING FOR DIABETES

The main purpose of screening is to differentiate an asymptomatic person at high risk of developing diabetes from the person at low risk for diabetes.[9] ADA recommends screening all people of age ≥ 45 years or BMI ≥25 kg/m^2 and an additional risk factor every 3 years using A1c, fasting plasma glucose, or oral glucose tolerance tests.[2,9,10] The criteria for screening in asymptomatic population[3] are:

- Significant burden of the disease
- Known natural history of the disease
- Known preclinical or asymptomatic stage during which the disease can be diagnosed
- Superior benefit from treatment after early detection than delayed treatment
- Availability of acceptable and reliable tests to detect the preclinical stage of disease
- Cost-effectiveness of screening and treatment along with availability of facilities and resources to treat newly diagnosed cases.
- Screening will be a systematic ongoing process and not merely an isolated one-time effort.

The need for screening for diabetes is brought by the following facts of the disease:[9,11]

- Growing incidence of diabetes
- Long latent asymptomatic period before symptomatic diagnosis
- High-undiagnosed cases
- Presence of microvascular complications in a newly diagnosed patient.

APPLICATION AND SIGNIFICANCE OF RISK SCORES IN CLINICAL PRACTICE

According to IDF, 66% of Indian population is unaware of their diabetic status.[3] The primary factors for widespread diabetes incidence involve lifestyle changes including dietary changes and low physical activity, genetic predisposition, urbanization and globalization.[3] ICMR-INDIAB study revealed that approximately, 43.2% of the people are aware of the condition called diabetes. In addition, knowledge of the fact that diabetes could be prevented was present in 56.3% and 63.4% of general and diabetic population, respectively. CURES study reported that only 25% are unaware of diabetes.[3] Moreover, global estimates of undiagnosed diabetes in adults vary between 24.1% and 75.1% across different regions of the world.[4] The Diabetes Epidemiology: Collaborative Analysis of Diagnostic Criteria in Asia (DECODA) studies showed that there are 1.6 cases undiagnosed for every known case of diabetes in the community.[4]

Given the critical scenario of no diagnosis, late diagnosis, and inadequate management on diagnosis, there is high risk for development of microvascular (coronary artery disease, cerebrovascular disease, and/or peripheral vascular disease) as well as micro-vascular complications (retinopathy, nephropathy, and neuropathy) with disease progression.[3] Also, due to poor healthcare, infection, and chronic kidney failure contribute majorly to diabetes-associated mortality, which is estimated to be 55% in individuals of age < 60 years and 27% in people < 50 years of age.[3] In low- and middle-income countries, studies have estimated the pooled prevalence of diabetes-associated complications to be 5.6% over a 25-year period.[3]

Indian diabetes risk score has demonstrated to be more effective, accurate, and highly cost-effective screening method for undiagnosed patients with diabetes. It allows detection of a considerable proportion of people along with effective reduction of overall cost when used before an oral glucose tolerance test.[3] For screening diabetes, it is essential that the risk assessment tool used is "population specific", thus aiding in tools are effective in exposing the real burden of disease.[4] Also, since there are ethnic differences in the risk factors for diabetes, it becomes necessary to determine and implement ethnic specific scores.[8]

Diabetes screening for detecting high-risk population allows for timely diagnosis and adequate treatment facilities, thus, increasing quality of life-years over a time.[4] Screening in undiagnosed population gives the advantage of primary as well as secondary prevention of events on disease progression.[4] Screening would help in diagnosing cases, which would have been otherwise missed. Also, screening would reduce the associated treatment costs in high-risk population.[10]

CONCLUSION

The undiagnosed diabetes is very dangerous as unaware individuals of their disease status are left untreated and end up with dreadful complications. There is a need for effective and efficient diabetes screening strategies along with the development of primary preventive strategies. A cost-effective screening tool to detect undiagnosed diabetes is the one which accurate risk assessment using low-cost methods. Screening using risk score is simple, safe, and cost-efficient method, which significantly reduces the number and cost of invasive glucose tests at the screening phase. Besides identification of high-risk population, the purpose of risk score is to spread awareness of the modifiable risk factors and healthy lifestyle. Implementation of risk scores have the capability to detect undiagnosed cases which would have been probably missed and significantly reduce treatment-related costs.

REFERENCES

1. Galaviz KI, Narayan KMV, Lobelo F, et al. Lifestyle and the prevention of type 2 diabetes: A status report. Am J Lifestyle Med. 2015;12(1):4-20.
2. Gilmer TP, O'Connor PJ. The growing importance of diabetes screening. Diabetes Care. 2010;33(7):1695-7.
3. Joshi SR. Diabetes care in India. Ann Glob Health. 2015;81(6):830-8.
4. Dudeja P, Singh G, Gadekar T, et al. Performance of Indian Diabetes Risk Score (IDRS) as screening tool for diabetes in an urban slum. Med J Armed Forces India. 2017;73(2):123-8.
5. Lindström J, Tuomilehto J. The diabetes risk score: a practical tool to predict type 2 diabetes risk. Diabetes Care. 2003;26(3):725-31.
6. Buijsse B, Simmons RK, Griffin SJ, et al. Risk assessment tools for identifying individuals at risk of developing type 2 diabetes. Epidemiol Rev. 2011;33:46-62.
7. Noble D, Mathur R, Dent T, et al. Risk models and scores for type 2 diabetes: systematic review. BMJ. 2011;343:d7163.
8. Mohan V, Deepa R, Deepa M, et al. A simplified Indian Diabetes Risk Score for screening for undiagnosed diabetic subjects. J Assoc Physicians India. 2005;53:759-63.
9. Martinez-Millana A, Argente-Pla M, Valdivieso Martinez B, et al. Driving type 2 diabetes risk scores into clinical practice: Performance analysis in hospital settings. J Clin Med. 2019;8(1). pii: E107.
10. Chatterjee R, Narayan KM, Lipscomb J, et al. Screening for diabetes and prediabetes should be cost-saving in patients at high risk. Diabetes Care. 2013;36(7):1981-7.
11. Julka S, Goyal R, Sharma R. Screening for diabetes in high risk a passé. Indian J Endocrinol Metab. 2014;18(6):872.

4 CHAPTER Screening for Diabetic Retinopathy—Need of an Hour

Bhargav Sosale, Bhavana Sosale

INTRODUCTION

India has close to 73 million individuals with diabetes.[1] Microvascular and macrovascular complications of diabetes lead to morbidity and mortality and increase cost of care. The goals of treatment of diabetes include prevention of complications or reduction in the progression of complications in those with preexisting complications.

Many individuals with diabetes remain undiagnosed as the disease is asymptomatic in the initial stages. Hence, complications may be present even at the time of diagnosis of diabetes. Screening for complications from 'day 1' is of paramount importance.[2]

Diabetic retinopathy (DR) is a microvascular complication of diabetes. It is a leading cause of blindness across the world in individuals with type 1 diabetes mellitus (T1DM) and type 2 diabetes mellitus (T2DM). The risk factors for development of DR include duration of diabetes, degree of glycemic control, smoking, hypertension, and dyslipidemia.

Prolonged hyperglycemia leads to various pathophysiological pathways such as sorbitol pathway, accumulation of end glycosylation products, protein C activation and microvascular occlusion, impairment in vascular signaling pathways, production of reactive-oxygen species, renin-angiotensin aldosterone system upregulation and finally results in a common pathway that causes hypoxia and end-organ ischemia.[3]

RATIONALE FOR EARLY SCREENING

Studies such as Chronic Complications in Newly Diagnosed patients with type 2 diabetes in India (CINDI), CINDI 2, and the Chennai Urban Rural Epidemiology Study (CURES) have estimated the proportion of individuals with micro- and macrovascular complications at diagnosis in India. CINDI included 4,600 individuals newly diagnosed with T2DM, and CINDI 2 included 1,500 individuals with new-onset T2DM under the age of 40 years, also known as young-onset diabetes (YOD). CINDI 1, CINDI 2, and CURES reported the proportion of individuals with DR at the time of diagnosis of diabetes as 6%, 5% and 5%, respectively.[4–6]

SCREENING METHODS

Man, or Machine?

A dilated comprehensive retinal examination should be performed by an ophthalmologist to screen for DR.[2] Only about half the individuals when referred visit the retina specialist for an evaluation. Travel time, distance, and pupil dilatation are challenges to screening.

High-quality retinal imaging can be considered as an alternative to remotely screen patients in areas without access to a retinal specialist. Ideally, retinal photographs must be taken and stored at each examination. Challenges with telemedicine include Internet access, availability of a fundus camera, and accessibility of a retina specialist to read the image.

Artificial intelligence (AI) algorithms for screening for DR have also been developed over the past few years. IDx, Eyenuk, and Remidio Innovations Solutions Pvt. Ltd. are some of the tech companies working in this arena. These algorithms use big data and advances in machine learning and neural networks to recognize normal and abnormal patterns in the retinal images and produce an output of a healthy or an unhealthy image. Artificial intelligence algorithms have been trained and validated for the detection of referable DR (more than mild nonproliferative DR).

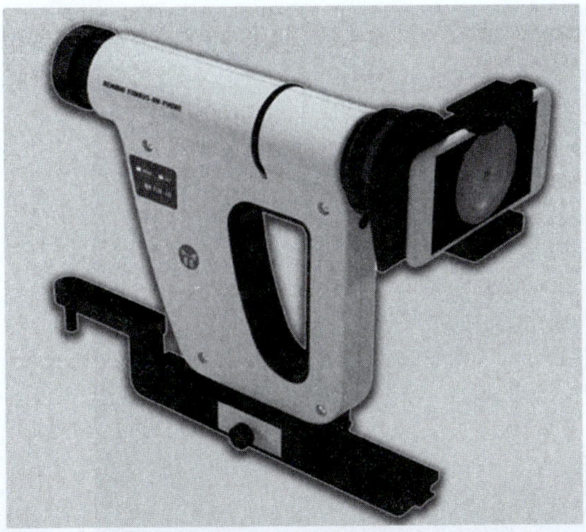

Figure 1 The Remidio NM fundus-on-phone camera.

Most AI algorithms work on cloud-based platforms where the image uploaded online is analyzed by the software and a report is generated. Studies report the sensitivity of IDx-DR and Eyenuk in the diagnosis of DR as 87% and 95.8%, respectively.[7,8] These systems work with a traditional large, expensive table-top fundus camera. The cost of equipment and the need for high-speed Internet are challenges. The only exception is the portable Medios AI with the Remidio Fundus on Phone (FOP) which works completely offline.

The AI algorithm developed by Medios Technologies, a subsidiary of Remidio, is a novel system and a first of its kind in the field of DR.

The AI is integrated into a portable smartphone-based fundus camera, called the Remidio non-mydriatic (NM) FOP, and works offline (Fig. 1). This cost-effective, small camera produces images comparable with Topcon and Zeiss and has been validated in clinical studies.[9] The AI produces a binary report of DR versus no DR in a few seconds after the retinal image is captured (Figs. 2A and B and 3A to D). The AI in a landmark study by Natarajan et al. demonstrated a sensitivity and specificity of 100% and 88.4%, respectively, in the diagnosis of referable DR (more than moderate nonproliferative DR).[10] The AI has been validated with both mydriatic and nonmydriatic images (SMART STUDY).

WHEN SHOULD WE SCREEN PATIENTS FOR DIABETIC RETINOPATHY?

Individuals with T1DM should undergo screening within 5 years after the onset of diabetes or at age > 10 years or the onset of puberty (whichever is earlier).[2] Individuals with T2DM should undergo screening at the time of diagnosis of diabetes. Women with preexisting diabetes who are planning pregnancy should be screened prior to conception or in the first trimester. Subsequent monitoring every trimester may be indicated if retinopathy if present.

HOW OFTEN SHOULD THE RETINAL EXAMINATION BE REPEATED?

Individuals with no evidence of DR can be screened annually.[2] The presence of retinopathy necessitates more frequent monitoring (every 3–6 months based on the severity of disease). Monitoring intervals post laser or after vitrectomy or treatment of maculopathy can vary from monthly to every 4–6 months after stabilization.

ARTIFICIAL INTELLIGENCE AND DIABETIC RETINOPATHY SCREENING

There is a large scope for the use of AI algorithms for DR diagnosis. These technologies can create a significant public health impact as they can make DR screening scalable.

The biggest challenge to screening today is the lack of ophthalmologists in urban, rural, and semiurban areas. Making such technology accessible can aid general practitioners, family physicians, and health-care workers at the most basic levels of care in screening for DR. Early diagnosis at the grassroot level can prevent blindness by ensuring early referral and treatment.

The Medios AI with the Remidio FOP has been validated with nonmydriatic and mydriatic images. The ability to screen without mydriasis reduces screening time. Elderly individuals or those with small pupils (<3 mm) can still be screened after dilatation with a drop of tropicamide. The use of the equipment requires no technical skill, and anyone can be trained to use such devices and capture retinal images for diagnosis. This was also seen in the study reported in JAMA Ophthalmology, where minimally trained health-care workers used this device to screen for DR in community-based health- care dispensaries.[10]

WHO SHOULD SCREEN?

Clinical practice recommendations recommend screening by an ophthalmologist. The number of individuals with diabetes greatly surpasses the number of ophthalmologists.[11] Studies have also shown that intergrader difference and clinical training play a big role in diagnosis and grading of DR. Studies comparing retinal

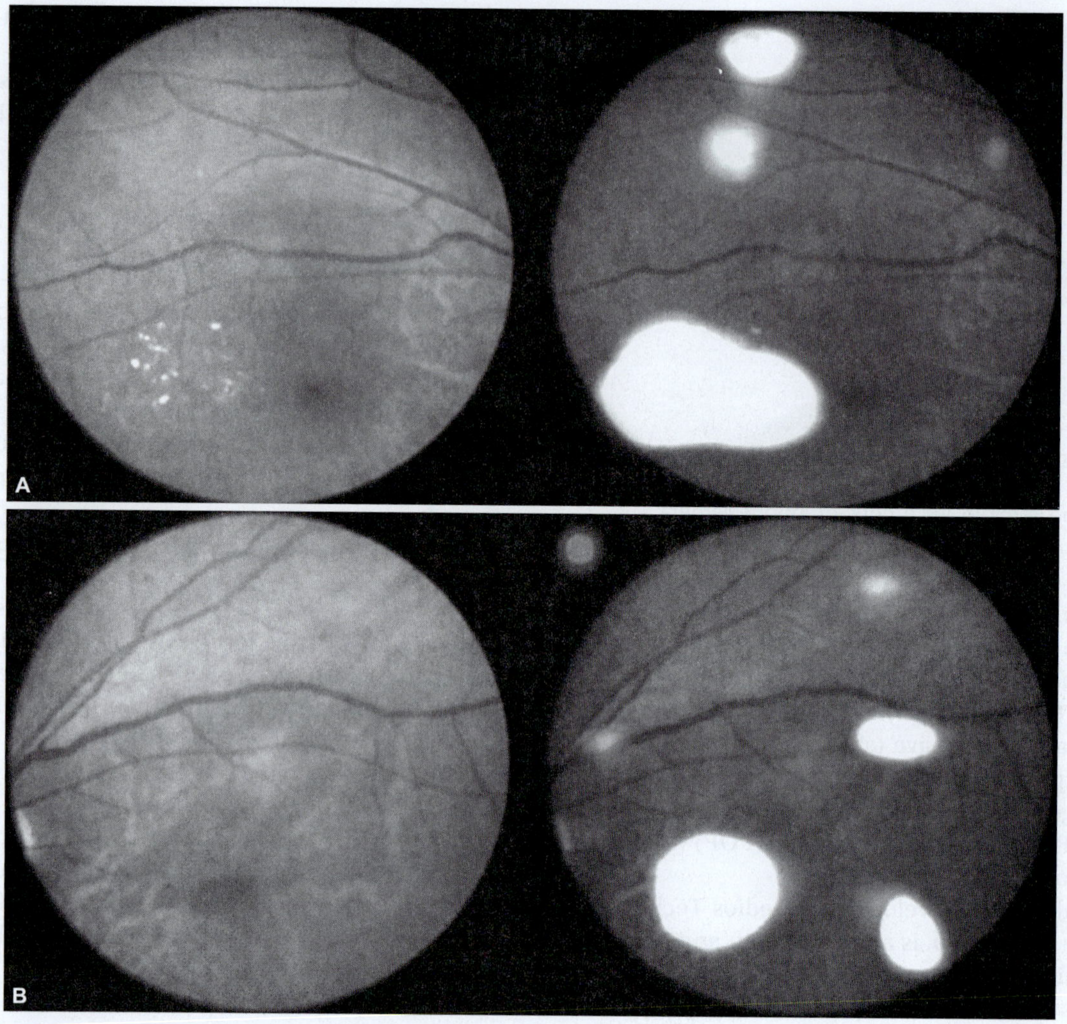

Result: Signs of retinopathy detected. Examples of lesions are highlighted.
Confidence: 99%

Figures 2A and B An example of the PDF report generated by the Medios AI in an individual with diabetic retinopathy. *(For color version see color plate No. 1)*

(*Source*: Medios AI.)

specialists, general ophthalmologists, and optometrists have observed a greater precision when patients are screened by a retina specialist > general ophthalmologist > ophthalmic nurses.[12] If only retinal specialists were to screen for DR, the entire burden of screening a country would rest on the retina specialists.

We need to move from a 'treatment focused' health-care system toward a 'prevention focused' health-care system and large-scale screening programs are the need of the hour.

It is thus imperative for all health-care workers, nurses, doctors, family physicians, general practitioners, diabetologists, endocrinologists, ophthalmologists, and retina specialists to take care on the challenge of screening. Artificial intelligence can help achieve this and make screening accessible and affordable to those who need it most.

Screening for DR using AI algorithms is a paradigm shift in diabetes care. Artificial intelligence can help every physician and health-care worker prevent blindness by ensuring early screening for detection of DR.

CONCLUSION

Screening for DR is the need of the hour. Technology and AI can aid all doctors and health-care workers in

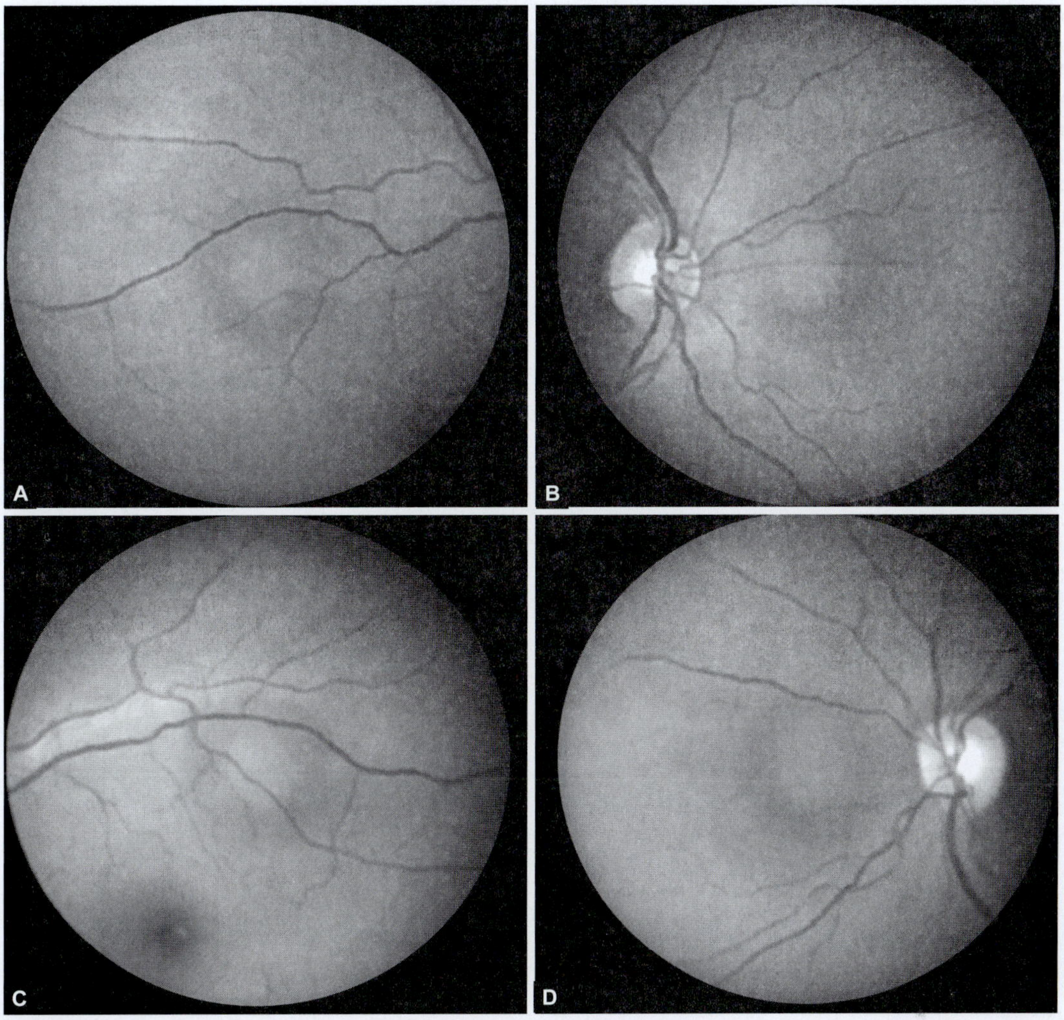

Result: No signs of retinopathy detected. Re-examine after 6 months.
Confidence: 87%

Figures 3A to D An example of the PDF report generated by the Medios AI in an individual without diabetic retinopathy.
(*Source*: Medios AI.) ***(For color version see color plate No. 2)***

solving public health problems on a large scale. Use of novel technologies like the Medios AI with the low-cost portable Remidio NM FOP can help scale DR screening and prevent blindness even in resource-limited settings with no Internet or electricity.

It is time for man to work with the machine. Recent advances indicate a turning point in diabetes care, the time when the physician can focus on prevention of blindness.

REFERENCES

1. International Diabetes Federation. (2017). IDF DIABETES ATLAS – ACROSS THE GLOBE 2017. [online]. Available from www.diabetesatlas.org/across-the-globe.html. [Last accessed on September, 2019].
2. American Diabetes Association. Microvascular complications and foot care Sec 10 in Standards of Medical Care in Diabetes 2017. Diabetes Care. 2017;40(Suppl. 1):S88-98.
3. Rask-Madsen C, King G. Vascular complication of diabetes: mechanisms of injury and protective factors. Cell Metab. 2013;17(1):20-33.
4. Sosale A, Prasanna Kumar KM, Sadikot SM, et al. Chronic complications in newly diagnosed patients with type 2 diabetes mellitus in India. Indian J Endocrinol Metab. 2014;18:355-60.
5. Sosale B, Sosale AR, Mohan AR, et al. Cardiovascular risk factors, micro and macrovascular complications at diagnosis in patients with young onset type 2 Diabetes in India: CINDI 2. Indian J Endocr Metab. 2016;20:114-18.
6. Rema M, Premkumar S, Anitha B, et al. Prevalence of diabetic retinopathy in urban India: The Chennai Urban, Rural Epidemiology Study (CURES) eye study, I. Invest Ophthalmol Vis Sci. 2005;46(7):2328-33.
7. Abramoff MD, Lavin PT, Birch M, et al. Pivotal trial of an autonomous AI-based diagnostic system for detection of diabetic retinopathy in primary care offices. NPJ Digital Med. 2018;1:39.

8. Rajalakshmi R, Subashini R, Anjana RM, et al. Automated diabetic retinopathy detection in smartphone-based fundus photography using artificial intelligence. Eye (Lond). 2018;32(6):1138.
9. Rajalakshmi R, Arulmalar S, Usha M, et al. Validation of smartphone based retinal photography for diabetic retinopathy screening. PloS One. 2015;10(9):e0138-285.
10. Natarajan S, Jain A, Krishnan R, et al. Diagnostic accuracy of community-based diabetic retinopathy screening with an offline artificial intelligence system on a smartphone. JAMA Ophthalmol. 2019. doi:10.1001/JAMAOphthalmol.2019.2923. [Epub ahead of print]
11. Sosale AR. Screening for Diabetic Retinopathy – is the use of artificial intelligence and cost-effective fundus imaging the answer? Int J Diabetes Dev Ctries. 2019;39(1):1-3.
12. Ruamviboonsuk P, Teerasuwanajak K, Tiensuwan M, et al. Interobserver agreement in the interpretation of single-field digital fundus images for diabetic retinopathy screening. Ophthalmology. 2006;113(5):826-32.

2 SECTION Pathophysiology and Metabolism

5 CHAPTER Inflammation and Diabetes

Anil Samaria, Meenakshi

INTRODUCTION

Diabetes, a multifaceted metabolic disorder, results from absolute or relative insulin deficiency or resistance to its action. The body glucose levels are affected and the main diagnostic features are impaired glucose tolerance and hyperglycemia. Diabetes-associated chronic hyperglycemia can result in dysfunction or failure of end organs including retina, kidneys, heart, and blood vessels.[1,2]

The World Health Organization (WHO) published the first global report on diabetes in 2016, which revealed that 422 million adults were living with diabetes. This shows a four-fold increase since 1980 and an estimated rise to 552 million is expected by 2030.[3] The risk factors such as insufficient physical activity, energy-rich diet, sedentary lifestyle, and following western culture have increased the prevalence of diabetes. Diabetes can be classified into type 1 (T1DM) and type 2 (T2DM). The unmodifiable risk factors for T2DM are genetic predisposition, ageing, and ethnicity or modifiable factors are obesity, unhealthy diet, physical inactivity, and smoking. Increased evidence show that inflammatory pathways are the principal, common pathogenetic mediators in the natural course of diabetes under the stimulus of above-mentioned risk factors.[3]

Over a century ago, high doses of sodium salicylate administered to diabetic patients or people suspected with diabetes caused decreased glycosuria in them. This was probably the first association between inflammation and diabetes. A landmark study was conducted in 1993 by Hotamisiligil et al. in animal models to correlate inflammation with diabetes. The study revealed the role of tumor necrosis factor-alpha (TNF-alpha) with regards to obesity and diabetes, especially insulin resistance. Elevated concentration levels of circulating inflammatory markers and mediators, and acute phase reactants including fibrinogen, C-reactive protein, interleukin (IL)-6, plasminogen activator inhibitor-1, sialic acid, and white cells revealed the association of inflammation with obesity and T2DM. In the target cells, chronically activated pro-inflammatory pathways contribute to obesity, insulin resistance, and related metabolic disorders.[4]

TYPE 1 DIABETES AND INFLAMMATION

Destruction of insulin-producing pancreatic beta cells characterizes T1DM, an autoimmune disorder. Type 1 diabetes mellitus is heterogeneous with regards to its onset age, autoimmune response, and effectiveness of treatment. The significant heterogeneity seen in T1DM in regard to the age of onset, severity of autoimmune response and efficacy of therapy. T1DM pathogenesis involves both humoral and cellular immunities. Although the initial event is still not known, predisposition related theories remain applicable, which states that environmental trigger factors in early life like nutrition, infections, and chemicals are able to activate self-targeting immune cascades.[5]

Inflammatory Infiltrates in Type 1 Diabetes

The theories suggest that the insulitis is cell inflammation during the course of T1DM caused by humoral and cell-mediated autoimmune destruction of beta cell and pancreatic islets. Defective Regulatory T cells (Tregs) are seen in T1DM. Evidences from studies conducted in animal models demonstrate the role of CD4+ and

CD8+ T cells (effector T-cells/Teff) in targeting beta-cell autoantigens and related peptide epitopes, thus leading to T1DM. Adoptive T-cell transfer models have demonstrated the ability of T-cell subtypes to induce destructive peri-islet inflammatory infiltrate and overt diabetes. Initially, immune B cells (CD20+) were found to closely align with migrating CD8+ T cells following different patterns, either high or low rate of infiltration in islet. . The profile of these cells changes as the disease progresses. Macrophages, with their ability to secrete cytokines like Interleukin 1 beta (IL-1beta) and TNF-alpha, are vital inflammatory mediators and produce reactive oxygen species (ROS).[6] T1DM may also occur due to the presence of excess lymphocytes and neutrophils in the surrounding pancreatic exocrine tissue.

Inflammatory Mediators and Type 1 Diabetes Mellitus

In T1DM, the inflammation of pancreatic beta cells may probably be due to synergistic action of the involved cytokines, interferon gamma (IFN-gamma) and innate inflammatory cytokines, TNF-alpha, and IL-1beta. Upregulation of inducible nitric oxide synthase (iNOS) happens due to the combined action of these inflammatory molecules, thus producing nitric oxide (NO). Beta-cell destruction is also caused due to Reactive Oxygen Species (ROS). The inflammatory environment response is affected by the specific gene-guided modulation of beta-cell apoptosis, induces by IFN-gamma and modulated by PTPN2 gene.[7] Pancreatic beta-cell death may occur through multiple pathways. A vicious cycle is created by the disruptive effects of inflammatory and autoimmune-mediated pancreatic islet attack. The initial cytokine stress may persist causing metabolic stress and more loss in beta-cell function (Fig. 1).[8]

Various Anti-inflammatory Trials on Type 1 Diabetes[9,10]

Refer to Table 1.

TYPE 2 DIABETES AND INFLAMMATION

There is insulin resistance initially compensated by insulin hypersecretion in beta cells in patients at risk of T2DM. When the disorder is diagnosed, unable to cope up due to pancreatic functional reserve, beta cells eventually do not secrete enough insulin. The degree of beta-cell dysfunction and insulin resistance can vary among different people.[11]

Contribution of Adipose Tissue and Obesity in Type 2DM

Overeating and insufficient physical activity are pathologically linked with a cluster of diseases encompassing metabolic syndrome and obesity. The relation between development of diabetes and obesity and the role of adipose tissue are well known.

Systemic insulin resistance may occur due to fat accumulation in liver (steatosis) and muscles. Accumulation of fat in subcutaneous tissues as well as in liver, pancreas, muscles and pericardium is due to high calorie intake and insufficient physical activity. Tissue insulin resistance is increased due to this fat accumulation. Likewise, beta-cell dysfunction is due to pancreatic fat accumulation. Steatosis, commonly associated with obesity, results in fasting hyperglycemia due to reduced hepatic insulin sensitivity.[12,13]

Two major inflammatory pathways, namely, stress-activated Jun N-terminal kinases (JNK) and the transcription factor NF-kappa B are activated and accompanied by subacute chronic inflammation.

Peripheral insulin resistance and glucose homeostasis are associated with the brown adipose tissue (BAT) which also plays a significant role in energy regulation. On the other hand, white adipose tissue (WAT) and particularly, visceral WAT (tissues around the trunk, upper body or abdomen) seems to be the major source of inflammatory markers which produce cytokines. Chronic low-grade inflammation is triggered systemically and locally by the macrophages and immune cells (B and T cells) infiltrating the adipose tissue and producing more cytokines and chemokines. Adipokines refer to a group of bioactive substances like IL-1, IL-6, IL-10, TNF-alpha, chemokines, leptin, adiponectin, angiotensinogen, resistin, monocyte chemoattractant protein and serum amyloid protein. Adipokines amplify the inflammatory state which is caused by the production of pro-inflammatory cytokines. In obese subjects, additional inflammatory responses are stimulated by adipokines, which promote obesity-induced metabolic and cardiovascular diseases.[14]

Gut Microbiota in Type 2 Diabetes and Inflammation

The gut microbiome varies between obese and lean subjects. Diet and metabolism influence the composition of gut microbiome and vice versa. There exists a two-way relationship between the gut microbiome and immune function with regard to host's energy. The interaction

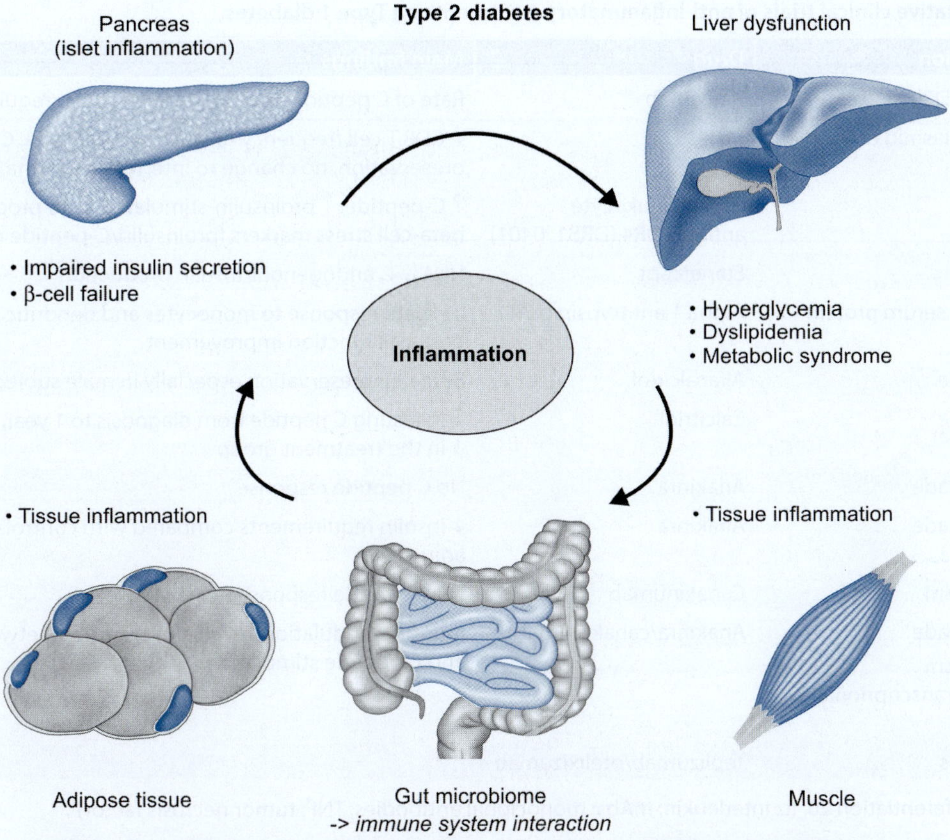

Activation of several immune cells are involved in pancreatic beta-cell death through a variety of inflammatory cytokines. Regulatory T cells are defective in this autoimmune disease, while effector T-cells (Teff) participate in the development of type 1 diabetes targeting several beta-cell autoantigens and related peptide epitopes. The profile of immune B cells also changes during disease progression and macrophages are also critical mediators of islet inflammation due to their direct toxicity on beta-cells by reactive oxygen species. Dendritic cells, natural killer cells and natural killer T cells may have a partial role in the process.

Figure 1 Inflammatory mediators in Type 1 diabetes.

between the gut microbiome products and the immune system can cause a low-grade inflammation by inducing tissue metabolic modifications; these changes influence adipogenesis and/or insulin resistance and mark the onset of obesity and diabetes, respectively. The microbial products of the altered gut floral composition including lipopolysaccharide (LPS), metabolites, and short-chain fatty acid (SCFAs) can directly and indirectly affect the immune cells in the gut.[15,16]

- Low-grade inflammation may be caused by LPS, which is mediated by induced cytokines from the immune cells and adipocytes.
- Gene expression of human monocytes can be modulated and pro-inflammatory cytokine and chemokine production can be reduced by SCFAs. They also suppress the inflammatory T-cell function by promoting regulatory T-cell generation in multiple ways. The release of IFN-gamma inducible protein 10 (IP-10) into human colonic sub-epithelial myofibroblasts is blocked by SCFAs, thus acting systemically and locally on immune cells and intestinal tissue cells, respectively (Fig. 2).

Inflammation in Pancreatic Beta-cell Failure and Type 2 Diabetes

Apart from the individual etiologies, the common pathway of pathogenesis for both types of diabetes appears to be the inflammation of the pancreatic beta cell, islets of Langerhans (insulitis). The autoinflammatory process results in the reduction of both beta cell number and function. The already "stressed" beta cells seem to stimulate local inflammation

TABLE 1: Representative clinical trials of anti-inflammatory treatments on Type 1 diabetes.

Mechanism of action	Drug	Main findings
Monoclonal anti-CD20 antibody	Rituximab	Rate of C peptide decline ↓, lower insulin requirements, HbA ↓
Engineered DNA plasmid encoding proinsulin	BHT-3021	↓ CD8 T cell frequency reactive to proinsulin, C peptide preservation, no change to interferon-gamma, IL-4, IL-10
Proinsulin peptide	Human leukocyte antigen-DR4 (DRB1*0401)	↑ C-peptide, ↑ proinsulin-stimulated IL-10 production, favorable beta-cell stress markers (proinsulin/C-peptide ratio)
TNF-antagonism	Etanercept	HbA_{1c} ↓, endogenous insulin production ↑
Anti-inflammatory serum protein	Alpha 1 antitrypsin (AAT)	IL-1beta response to monocytes and dendritic monocytes ↓, beta-cell function improvement
Vitamin D analogue	Alfacalcidol	Beta-cell preservation especially in male subjects
Vitamin D analogue	Calcitriol	↑ in fasting C peptide from diagnosis to 1 year, daily insulin dose ↓ in the treatment group
IL-1 receptor blockade	Anakinra	No C peptide response
IL-1 receptor blockade	Anakinra	↓ insulin requirements compared with controls, ↓ insulin dose adjusted
IL-1 beta antagonism	Canakinumab	No C peptide response
IL-1 receptor blockade IL-1 beta antagonism (plasma-induced transcriptional meta-analysis)	Anakinra/canakinumab	Immunomodulation/reverse relationship between inflammation and C peptide stimulation
ALPHAti-CD3 mAbs	Teplizumab/otelixizumab	

(CD20: cluster of differentiation 20; IL: interleukin; mAbs: monoclonal antibodies; TNF: tumor necrosis factor)

and alter the balance between beta cell mass and function in genetically predisposed subjects. The role of macrophages in the inflammation of the islet cells has been discussed earlier. Factors such as amyloid polypeptide, free fatty acids (FFAs) and endocannabinoids stimulate the islet macrophages to secrete IL-1 beta within the islets. The initially secreted IL-1beta regulates its production in pancreatic beta cells by autostimulation. This process, while increasing nitric oxide production, also decreases ATP concentration in the mitochondria, thus causing further beta-cell dysfunction and reduced insulin secretion. Production of ROS and other pro-inflammatory cytokines and chemokines in the beta cells is enhanced by the oxidative stress; it distorts blood flow thus destroying their function.

Beta-cell dysfunction was also caused by activated IL-1beta signaling pathway in the islets of numerous T2DM models. The decline in function of beta cells has also been attributed to islet autoimmunity as the T2DM progresses.

However, it has been assumed that induced apoptosis in the inflamed pancreatic beta cells produce hyperglycemia initially. Apoptosis is induced by IL-6 and other inflammatory cytokines, which are the pathogenic markers that predict the disease progression. A relationship between obesity, insulitis, and diabetes is also created by overproduction of TNF-alpha in the adipose tissue. It causes increased insulin resistance in peripheral tissues by feeding the inflammation and beta-cell death in pancreatic islets. The incidence and progression of T2DM is more influenced by immune system activation; adipose tissue inflammation involves adaptive and innate immunity. There is a switching of macrophage phenotype from mostly anti-inflammatory M2-type to predominantly pro-inflammatory M1-type which plays a crucial role in the initiation and amplification of insulitis. Nevertheless, studies reveal that macrophage infiltration in adipose tissue follows recruitment of B cells and T cells.[17]

Other organs like liver, skeletal muscles, and neural system affect the metabolic homeostasis and inflammatory state in T2DM.

Diabetes Mellitus Treatments and Inflammation

Non-pharmacological therapies, such as lifestyle interventions and pharmacological and bariatric surgical

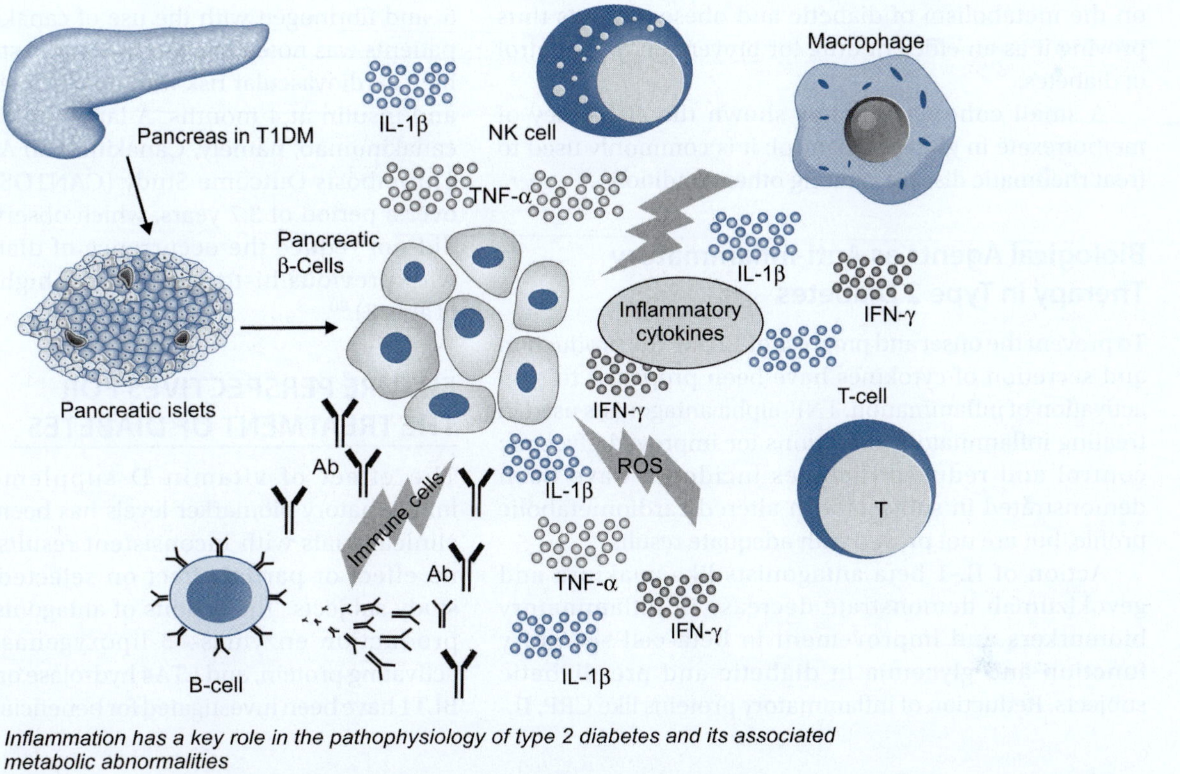

Figure 2 The vicious cycle of inflammation in various target organs in Type 2 diabetes.

approaches for weight loss, appear to reduce inflammation assessed as circulating CRP and IL-6 concentrations, and improves cardiovascular and all-cause mortality.

The primary mechanism of action of insulin and other antidiabetic agents involves intrinsic anti-inflammatory effects associated with inflammatory marker reduction. Inflammation reduces as NF-kappa B activity in peripheral blood mononuclear cells is decreased by the action of insulin.

- *Metformin*: The anti-inflammatory action of metformin seems independent of glycemia. In addition to its metabolic effects, the action of the drug is predominantly on the immune cells and vascular tissues.
- *Dipeptidyl peptidase-4 inhibitors (DPP-4) and glucagon-like peptide-1 (GLP-1) receptor agonists*: Apart from antidiabetic properties, intrinsic anti-inflammatory properties are also found in DPP-4 inhibitors and GLP-1 receptor agonists. Yet, their influence on reduction of inflammation, diabetes and cardiovascular efficiency remain vague.
- *Thiazolidinediones*: Binding of thiazolidinediones and activation to the peroxisome proliferator-activated receptor gamma (PPAR gamma) appears to influence transrepression of NF-kappa B and reduced expression of NF-kappa B targets, thus causing anti-inflammatory actions.
- *Sodium-glucose cotransporter-2 inhibitors (SGLT2 inhibitors)*: SGLT2 inhibitors are newer drugs that increase renal excretion of glucose. There may be improvement in the circulating biomarkers of inflammation as demonstrated by the preliminary study in humans; nevertheless, more evidence is required to prove their action.[18]

Anti-inflammatory Drugs in Type 2 Diabetes

Numerous studies have supported the use of anti-inflammatory treatment targeting the anti-inflammatory pathway for cardiometabolic diseases in the last decade. For instance, salicylates, especially aspirin, have been used in CVD prevention to manage thrombosis and in rheumatoid diseases for a long time.[19] Over a century ago, there were reports that salicylates are the first class of drugs to reduce glucose levels in diabetic subjects. Studies have revealed the positive action of salicylate products on the metabolism of diabetic and obese patients thus proving it as an efficient drug for prevention and control of diabetes.

A small cohort study has shown the efficiency of methotrexate in glycemic control; it is commonly used to treat rheumatic diseases among other conditions.

Biological Agents as Anti-inflammatory Therapy in Type 2 Diabetes

To prevent the onset and progress of T2DM, the production and secretion of cytokines have been proposed to stop activation of inflammation. TNF-alpha antagonists used in treating inflammatory conditions for improved glycemic control and reduced diabetes incidence have been demonstrated in subjects with altered cardiometabolic profile, but are not proved with adequate results.

Action of IL-1 beta antagonists like anakinra and gevokizumab demonstrate decrease in inflammatory biomarkers and improvement in beta-cell secretory function and glycemia in diabetic and pre-diabetic subjects. Reduction of inflammatory proteins like CRP, IL-6, and fibrinogen with the use of canakinumab in T2DM patients was noted in a study. But the study also revealed high cardiovascular risk with no effect on HbA1c, glucose, and insulin at 4 months. A large randomized trial with canakinumab, namely, Canakinumab Anti-inflammatory Thrombosis Outcome Study (CANTOS) was conducted over a period of 3.7 years, which observed that the drug did not reduce the occurrence of diabetes in patients with previous history of MI and high-sensitivity CRP (Table 2).[20]

FUTURE PERSPECTIVES FOR THE TREATMENT OF DIABETES

The effect of vitamin D supplements on serum inflammatory biomarker levels has been studied through clinical trials with inconsistent results. There is either no effect or partial effect on selected markers in the study subjects. The actions of antagonists of leukotriene production enzymes—5-lipoxygenase (5-LO), 5-LO-activating protein, and LTA4 hydrolase or receptor binding BLT1 have been investigated for beneficial cardiometabolic

TABLE 2: Representative clinical trials of anti-inflammatory treatments on Type 2 Diabetes—metabolic profile.

Mechanism of action	Drug	Main findings
IL-1 receptor blockade	Anakinra	HbA1c, leukocyle ↓, CRP ↓ insulin secretion ↑
IL-1 receptor blockade	Anakinra	Sustained CRP ↓, insulin secretion ↑, insulin requirement ↓
IL-1 receptor blockade	Anakinra	Insulin sensitivity ↑
IL-1 receptor blockade	Anakinra	Insulin secretion ↑ (first-phase insulin secretion improved)
IL-1 receptor blockade	Anakinra	Insulin secretion ↑
IL-1 beta antagonism	Gevokizumab	HbA1c ↓, CRP ↓, insulin secretion ↑
IL-1 beta antagonism	Canakinumab	Insulin secretion ↑, CRP ↓
IL-1 beta antagonism	Canakinumab	CRP ↓, HbA1c ↓,insulin secretion ↑ (not statistically significant)
IL-1 beta antagonism	Canakinumab	Significant CRP and IL-6 ↓, 6 month HbA1c ↓, but not consistent Hba1c ↓ long-term
Il-1 beta antagonism	Canakinumab	CRP ↓, fibrinogen ↓, IL-6 ↓, no effect on HbA1c, glucose and insulin levels
IL-1 beta antagonism	LY2189102	HbA1c ↓, CRP ↓, insulin secretion ↑
IKKbeta-NF-kappaB inhibition	Salsalate	FBG ↓, CRP ↓, insulin sensitivity ↑, adiponectin ↑
IKKbeta-NF-kappaB inhibition	Salsalate	FBG ↓, CRP ↓, adiponectin ↑
IKKbeta-NF-kappaB inhibition	Salsalate	FBG ↓, insulin ↑, CRP ↓
IKKbeta-NF-kappaB inhibition	Salsalate	HbA1c ↓, FBG ↓, triglyceride ↓, adiponectin ↑

Contd...

Contd...

Mechanism of action	Drug	Main findings
IKKbeta-NF-kappaB inhibition	Salsalate	HbA1c ↓, FBG ↓, insulin secretion ↑, triglyceride ↓
IKKbeta-NF-kappaB inhibition	Salsalate	FBG ↓, adiponectin ↑
IKKbeta-NF-kappaB inhibition	Salsalate	HbA1c ↓, FBG ↓, triglyceride ↓, leukocyte ↓, uric acid ↓, adiponectin ↓
TNF antagonism	CDP571	No effect on insulin sensitivity
TNF antagonism	Single dose of soluble TNF receptor-Fc fusion protein (Ro 45-2081)	No effect on insulin sensitivity
TNF antagonism	Soluble TNF receptor-Fc fusion protein etanercept	CRP ↓, adiponectin ↑, LDL ↓, no effect on insulin sensitivity
TNF antagonism	Soluble TNF receptor-Fc fusion protein etanercept	CRP ↓, insulin secretion ↑, no effect on insulin sensitivity
TNF antagonism	Soluble TNF receptor-Fc fusion protein etanercept	FBG ↓
TNF antagonism	Infliximab	Fasting glucose improvement, ratio of high molecular weight to total adiponectin ↑, sICAM-1 ↑, no effect on CRP
Decrease in TNF and IL-1 beta levels by an unknown mechanism of action	Diacerein	HbA1c ↓, FBG ↓, insulin secretion ↑
DHFR inhibitor—antimetabolite	Low-dose methotrexate	No effects on CRP, IL-1 beta or IL-6
DHFR inhibitor (DMARD)—combination with sulphasalazine glycocorticosteroids/ hydroxychloroquine	Methotrexate	HbA1c ↓

(CRP: C-reactive protein; DHFR: dihydrofolate reductase inhibitor; FBG: fasting blood glucose; IKKbeta: ikappaB kinase-beta; IL: interleukin; mAbs: monoclonal antibodies; NF-kappaB: nuclear factor-kappaB; sICAM-1: soluble intercellular adhesion molecule-1; TNF: tumor necrosis factor)

results; results are yet to be reported though. The action of JNK and toll-like receptors (TLRs) are being studied for their potential to target cholinergic pathways and immune modulating. Several other methods to modulate the human gut microbiome and evaluate anti-inflammatory diet effects are still under study.[1]

CONCLUSION

The research on prevention and management approaches of diabetes has become imperative due to its rising prevalence. The proven establishment of relationship between diabetes and inflammation has made researchers identify strategies that target inflammatory pathways prevent or control diabetes and its complications.

Till now, all the immunotherapeutic trials for human T1DM have always focused on patients well after the adaptive immune response to beta cell islets have been established, that is, after clinical onset of diabetes. These approaches are preserve only remaining beta-cell function. Actual cure can be possible only when the lost beta cell mass with autoimmune processes are replaced simultaneously. The primary trials with anti-inflammatory and immunomodulatory medications are promising in T1DM cases as it is an immunological response rather than a metabolic disorder. A key to permanent treatment could probably be the use of stem cells to regenerate the lost beta cells in addition to anti-inflammatory and immunomodulatory strategies. Extensive reviews regarding the treatment of T1DM and T2DM suggest that suppression of various inflammatory response pathways at the same time should be focused in future research rather than focusing on one pathway at a time.

REFERENCES

1. Tsalamandris S, Antonopoulos AS, Oikonomou E, et al. The role of inflammation in diabetes: Current concepts and future perspectives. ECR-Volume 14 Issue 1 Spring. 2019;50-9.
2. Inzucchi SE. Diagnosis of diabetes. N Engl J Med. 2013;368:193.
3. Whiting DR, Guariguata L, Weil C, Shaw J. IDF diabetes atlas: global estimates of the prevalence of diabetes for 2011 and 2030. Diabetes Res Clin Pract. 2011;94:311-21.
4. Marques-Vidal P, Schmid R, Bochud M, et al. Adipocytokines, hepatic and inflammatory biomarkers and incidence of type 2 diabetes. the CoLaus study. PLoS One. 2012;7:e51768.
5. Atkinson MA, Eisenbarth GS. Type 1 diabetes: new perspectives on disease pathogenesis and treatment. Lancet. 2001;358:221-9.
6. Willcox A, Richardson SJ, Bone AJ, et al. Analysis of islet inflammation in human type 1 diabetes. Clin Exp Immunol. 2009;155:173-81.
7. Moore F, Colli ML, Cnop M, et al. PTPN2, a candidate gene for type 1 diabetes, modulates interferon-gamma-induced pancreatic beta-cell apoptosis. Diabetes. 2009;58:1283-91.
8. Pirot P, Eizirik DL, Cardozo AK. Interferon-gamma potentiates endoplasmic reticulum stress-induced death by reducing pancreatic beta cell defence mechanisms. Diabetologia. 2006;49:1229-36.
9. Pescovitz MD, Greenbaum CJ, Krause-Steinrauf H, et al. Rituximab, B-lymphocyte depletion, and preservation of beta-cell function. N Engl J Med. 2009;361:2143-52.
10. Moran A, Bundy B, Becker DJ, et al. Interleukin-1 antagonism in type 1 diabetes of recent onset: two multicentre, randomised, double-blind, placebo-controlled trials. Lancet. 2013;381:1905-15.
11. Tabák AG, Jokela M, Akbaraly TN, et al. Trajectories of glycaemia, insulin sensitivity, and insulin secretion before diagnosis of type 2 diabetes: an analysis from the Whitehall II study. Lancet. 2009;373:2215-21.
12. DeFronzo RA. Pathogenesis of type 2 diabetes mellitus. Med Clin North Am. 2004;88:787–835, ix.
13. Sattar N, Gill JM. Type 2 diabetes as a disease of ectopic fat? BMC Med. 2014;12:123.
14. Nikolajczyk BS, Jagannathan-Bogdan M, Shin H, Gyurko R. State of the union between metabolism and the immune system in type 2 diabetes. Genes Immun. 2011;12:239-50.
15. Nastasi C, Candela M, Bonefeld CM, et al. The effect of short-chain fatty acids on human monocyte-derived dendritic cells. Sci Rep. 2015;5:16148.
16. Arpaia N, Campbell C, Fan X, et al. Metabolites produced by commensal bacteria promote peripheral regulatory T-cell generation. Nature. 2013;504:451–5.
17. Ehses JA, Perren A, Eppler E, et al. Increased number of islet-associated macrophages in type 2 diabetes. Diabetes. 2007;56:2356-70.
18. Drucker DJ, Nauck MA. The incretin system: glucagon-like peptide-1 receptor agonists and dipeptidyl peptidase-4 inhibitors in type 2 diabetes. Lancet. 2006;368:1696-705.
19. Guirguis-Blake JM, Evans CV, Senger CA, et al. Aspirin for the primary prevention of cardiovascular events: a systematic evidence review for the U.S. Preventive Services Task Force. Ann Intern Med. 2016;164:804-13.
20. Ridker PM, Howard CP, Walter V, et al. Effects of interleukin-1beta inhibition with canakinumab on hemoglobin A1c, lipids, C-reactive protein, interleukin-6, and fibrinogen: a phase IIb randomized, placebo-controlled trial. Circulation. 2012;126:2739-48.

6 CHAPTER Gut Microbiota and Diabetes

Alok Gupta, Rupesh Singh Yadav, Amit Sagar

INTRODUCTION

Gut microbiota is a system itself with a lot of dynamicity which is incorporated in gut in a way that influences the normal function, immunity, metabolism and geneticity not only in the gut but also other systems of the body. Microbiota are implicated in autism, psychiatric disorder, multiple sclerosis harmful bacterial infections, autoimmune diseases and cancer. Recent research indicates its role in metabolic diseases and diabetes also.

HUMAN INTESTINAL MICROBIOTA

It is an organ in itself, like many of the organ system in our body. In terms of absolute mass, it is small but in terms of number, it is quite large. It accounts for as many as 100 trillions of microorganisms (10 times the human cells). In terms of amount of genetic information, microbiota is diverse, most of the genetic process going on in our body is in fact microbial and it is not just bacterial as we thought of. There are archaeas, fungi, and millions and trillions of viruses, all of which are taking part in forming microbiota. So there are >1,800 genera and >15,000–36,000 species by rRNA sequencing. Not all of these species are found in any single human being but everybody harbors on an average of 100–150 species, which is dominated by mainly three bacterial phyla-Firmicutes (64%) are gram-positive and Bacteroidetes (23%) are gram-negative and Actinobacteria are gram-positive. Dominated by three genera—Bacteroides, Prevotella, and Ruminococcus, which are independent of age, gender, ethnicity, or body mass index (BMI).[1] As much as 99% of our microbiota is anaerobic, fastidious, therefore, it is tedious to culture them and these cannot be grown in isolation as they require specific conducive conditions which are difficult to meet in laboratories. The establishment of gut microbiota is dependent on the mode of delivery, with effect from this point, gut microbiota remains quite stable, although minor changes can be there. Babies delivered normally are dominated by Lactobacilli, Prevotella, and Atopobium. Whereas those delivered by C-section have microbiota that of maternal skin community like *Staphylococcus*. Prevotella is related with carbohydrate and simple sugars while bacteroides enterotypes is associated with animal proteins, amino acids, and saturated fats. Bacterial communities at a particular body site have more similarity among different subjects than in the same subject but at different body sites,[2] although there is also considerable inter-individual variability.

INTESTINAL MICROBIOTA AS ORGAN

Microbiota can be viewed as an organ because of various functions and interplay of vast chemical, immunological and genetical signals which are unique to different individuals. It measures about 1.5 kg. Metabolic activity rivals to that of liver indicating the vast biochemical reactions going on in this microbial world. Immune system and GI system do not mature, unless there is intense diversified eubiotic microbiota. Normal development of some other organs also do not take place without the gut microbiota, like myelination of CNS is also related to complex interactions between gut, gut microbiota and brain (some of these interactions are mediated through vagus nerve), but we do not really have a full grasp of such interplay. Everything from mouth to anus is the external world and throughout our life our gut microbiota modulates immune system and is responsible

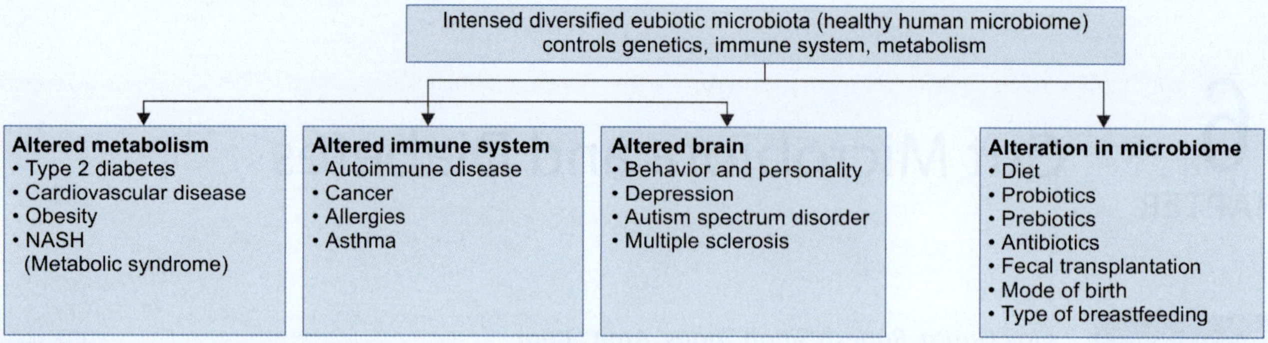

Flowchart 1 Physiology of gut microbiome, alterations, and related diseases.

for colonization resistance, that is, if we do not have our normal commensal flora we are open to opportunistic and pathogenic organism. Gut microbiota modulates metabolism, so it is very important in terms of glucose-insulin metabolism, weight metabolism, and there is a clear-cut role although we fully do not understand the link between the gut microbiota and dysbiosis and the risk of obesity and metabolic diseases like type 2 diabetes mellitus.

PATHOPHYSIOLOGY AND METABOLISM

Microbiota have diverse action or influence in human body ranging from immune response, enzymatic response, metaboli response and even genetic influence over the body, depicted in Flowchart 1.

TRANSFER OF MATERNAL MICROBIOTA

The microbiota is so important that it is not only just humus but it is important aspect of biology in general, in that all living creatures are in symbiosis with microbial organisms and we are living in symbiosis to lot of them and it is important for our health that human body is exposed to these human microorganism, which we get from our mothers. Newborn is exposed to as soon he comes out through birth canal and will have a different gut microbiota than those born through C-section. There is wonderful system that developed whereby a mother can transfer her gut microbiota to her baby through breast milk, mediated by dendritic cells or immune cells present in the gut and transfer microbiota to lymphocytes, travel via lymphatics to the breast milk to her baby finally. On an average there is transfer of 200–1,000 CFU/mL of breast milk, *Bifidobacterium*, and other species of Lactobacilli, Streptococcus, and Staphylococcus, some women who do not pass, may have dysbiotic microbiota. The microbiota is wired into all aspects of our biology. It can dictate host physiology. It controls (1) metabolism/obesity which is linked to type 2 diabetes, cardiovascular disease, and metabolic syndrome; (2) immune system which is linked to autoimmune disease, cancer and allergies; and (3) brain/behavior/personality which is linked to depression, autism spectrum disorders and multiple sclerosis. Unlike our human genome, our microbiome is malleable which gives us the extensive scope of future researches in clinical medicine and other fields. The many microbiota derived digested products have nearly similar structural configurations as our most of antibiotics have in general and these are constantly going into the blood streams and influencing our biology.

ROLE OF DIET IN MICROBIOTA

The diet definitely has a role to play in fact what we eat will decide the composition our gut flora. Since most of microbe mainly reside in our distal ileum and colon so to feed them our food should be such that it reaches up to these sites where most of them live. If we do not eat proper and sufficient food our microbes will soon become hungry and they will start eating our mucus linings and will come closer and closer to our own cells which leading to aberrant immune interactions and giving rise to many diseases. Our ancestors use to have daily intake of 100–150 g fibers per day, the recommended daily intake of dietary fiber is nearly 35 g and only the 15 g is taken by most of us daily. And the more diversity of fibers we eat, the more diverse would be our microbiome which is crucial for better health. Cotillard et al. in their 2013 study, with some dietary interventions (1,200 kcal women and 1,500 kcal men, 35% protein, 25% lipid, 44% low-glycemic index carbohydrates and enrichment in soluble fibers), showed an improvement in clinical measures in terms of decreased adiposity, improved insulin sensitivity, decreased triglycerides, decreased inflammation (highly sensitive C-reactive protein).

GUT MICROBIOTA AND DIABETES

Following mechanisms are postulated depending on the studies done in mice and human beings:

1. Increased energy harvest from the diet
2. Chronic low-grade endotoxemia
3. Regulation of tissue fatty acid composition
4. Modulation of gut-derived peptide secretion.

RELATIONSHIP BETWEEN MICROBIOTA AND TYPE 1 DIABETES

The involvement of microbiota in type 1 diabetes development in animals was first proposed in 1987.[3] A recent Finnish human study compared the microbiome of four children with type 1 diabetes with aged and HLA-DQ matched control children demonstrated reduction in stability and diversity of fecal microbiota among children in the 1st year of life who successively develop type 1 diabetes.[4]

"PERFECT STORM" FOR TYPE 1 DIABETES

It is now increasingly apparent that the nexus of the intestinal barrier, the composition of intestinal microbiota, and the mucosal immune system play a significant role in the development of various allergic and autoimmune diseases. In type 1 diabetes, evidence for synergism among "leaky" intestinal mucosal barrier, altered mucosal immunity, and aberrant intestinal microbiota that contributes in pathogenesis of disorder has started to emerge Table 1.[4]

The mechanisms by which the microbiota can precipitate type 1 diabetes in susceptible individuals are associated with changes in intestinal permeability and intestinal immunity modifications. In the health state, the intestinal epithelium helps to prevent the commensal and pathogenic bacteria as well as food antigens, to induce systemic immune response.[5] In type 1 diabetes, the development of a more permeable intestinal barrier (a key component to human defense mechanisms) may be attributable to metabolites of gut microbiota, as much as to any direct action of microbes themselves. Children with type 1 diabetes have low numbers of Bifidobacteria, which are lactate-producing microorganisms.[4] Butyrate, a short-chain fatty acid, is derived from lactate and is a potent anti-inflammatory agent promoting gut barrier function by ensuring tight junctions between epithelial cells. Its relative deficiency may contribute to the increased intestinal permeability seen in children developing type 1 diabetes.[6] Intestinal immunity is significantly impaired in type 1 diabetes. Activation of immune responses, with generation of autoreactive T cells, may occur due to bacterial cell component (autoantigenic mimics) in the microbiota. Mechanisms that mediate such immune

TABLE 1: Important studies related to microbiota and type-1 DM.

Studies	Result
Kuitunen et al.[16], Sapone et al.[17], Secondulfo et al.[18]	Shows altered gut permeability towards lactulose and mannitol in type 1 diabetes
Bosi et al.[19]	In prediabetics with ß-cell autoimmunity, altered gut permeability to lactulose and mannitol in type 1 diabetes
Secondulfo et al.[18]	Showed the change in micro-villi and inter-villous space in type 1 diabetes
Sapone et al.[17]	Showed the change in tight junctions in type 1 diabetes
Savilahti et al.[20], Westerholm-Ormio et al.[21]	Highlighted intestinal inflammation in biopsy specimen in children with type 1 diabetes
Auricchio et al.[22]	Activation of intestinal immunity and T-cells against gliadin
Bister et al.[23]	Showed increased inflammation in children with type 1 diabetes and positive anti-transglutaminase antibodies
Oikarinen et al.[24]	Demonstrated increased infection rate of enterovirus in type 1 diabetes
Tiittanen et al.[25]	Failure of regulatory T-cell activation, despite innate immunity activation in type 1 diabetes

changes may include activation of Toll-like receptors (proteins that play a key role in immune systems) by gut bacteria themselves or through G-protein-coupled receptor (GPCR) stimulation by bacterial metabolites.[7] In addition, gut bacteria-derived pathogen-associated molecular patterns (PAMPs) can induce inflammation and lead to beta-cells destruction by inflammatory cytokines. Lastly bacteria that permeate a "leaky" intestine may cause further inflammation and beta-cells destruction.

RELATIONSHIP BETWEEN THE MICROBIOTA AND TYPE 2 DIABETES

The microbiota may influence human metabolism through a number of mechanisms. Lipopolysaccharides (LPS) from the capsule of gram-negative bacilli activate inflammatory signaling pathways, via Toll-like receptor 4, resulting in inflammation and diminishing insulin sensitivity.[8] High-fat diets can have an effect on the microbiota; these diets can lead to increased levels of LPS either through increase in epithelial permeability or increased uptake in chylomicrons from intestinal epithelium itself.[9] Also there are microbiota which counter favorably, the adverse effects on insulin sensitivity and inflammation of β-cells. Short-chain fatty acids (e.g. acetate, propionate, butyrate) that originate from bacterial fermentation of the insoluble dietary fiber in bowel can bind to GPR41 and GPR43.[10] This leads to decreased inflammation in immune cells; whereas, in the L-cells as well as the digestive tract, it results in increase in secretion of peptide YY (PYY) and glucagon-like peptide 1 (GLP1) and improvement in insulin sensitivity.[11] In mucosal cells lining the colon, the short-chain fatty acid butyrate exerts vital impacts as an energy substrate; whereas, propionate and acetate increase hepatic lipogenesis and gluconeogenesis. Additionally, deconjugated bile acids can be metabolized to secondary bile acids by bacteria.[12] Secondary bile acids bind to the GPCR TGR5 that results in increase in production of GLP-1 from L-cells and enhancement in energy expenditure in muscles that leads to additional enhancements in insulin sensitivity. Latest evidence that links the microbiota to type 2 diabetes recommends that alterations in gut microbiota (that is termed as dysbiosis) can result in epithelial leakage and dysfunction. Increase in intestinal permeability leads to absorption of large molecules from bowel and, successively, to immune dysfunction, low-grade inflammation, and changes in lipid and glucose metabolism through signaling changes. These changes associate for increasing insulin resistance and increase the likelihood of development of type 2 diabetes.[13]

GUT MICROBIOTA AND ORAL HYPOGLYCEMIC AGENTS

Antidiabetic drugs has its main effect on composition of microbiome, chiefly enhancing the short-chain fatty acid (SCFA)—resulting in production of bacteria, which are responsible for weight loss and suppression of inflammation. Type 2 diabetes, like outcomes of obesity, leads in induction of dysbiosis principally by decreasing butyrate-producing bacteria and Akkermansia muciniphila, which is presently considered as a biomarker for the glucose intolerance. Evidences are now suggestive of that intestinal microbiota and SCFAs exert positive effects on oral hypoglycemic agents (OHAs) in type 2 diabetes. Gut microbiota may dampen the side effects cause by OHAs by binding and transforming a wide spectrum of bioactive substances.

METFORMIN AND GUT MICROBIOTA

Metformin increase SCFA bacteria which secrete acetate, propionate, butyrate, which act on L-cells to increase GLP1/GLP2 and metformin also increase Akkermansia muciniphila which act on goblet cells to decrease LPS, metabolic endotoxemia, due to which there is an increase adiponectin expression, enhanced insulin sensitivity, and pancreatic β-cells proliferation. It was reported that metformin enhance life span of Caenorhabditis elegans cocultured with *Escherichia coli* by causing an alteration in microbial folate and methionine metabolism. These interactions among gut microbiota and metformin may have a contribution in the metformin's pleiotropic effects. Gut microbiota can represent as a new approach for alleviating adverse effects of metformin and thus improve patient compliance.

Antibiotics and Gut Microbiota

The association between gut microbiota and antibiotics therapy has earned much interest. In the early years of life, it is found that the use of antibiotics has been demonstrated to disturb healthy microbiota, along with adverse metabolic effects; whereas, other studies observed that antibiotics results in moving disturbed microbiota to healthier state (i.e. in opposite direction). However, it is debated that the microbiota of very early infant is especially susceptible to microbial perturbations following antibiotic therapy.[14]

MICROBIOTA IN FUTURE CLINICAL PRACTICE

Improvement in understanding of the relationship among microbiota and development of type 1 diabetes, type 2 diabetes, and obesity points toward potential beneficial methods for preventing or ameliorating these disease states. It is suggested by latest evidence that alterations in the microbiota enhance the risk of development of type 1 diabetes via reduction in bacterial diversity, leakage in gut barriers, and enhancement in inflammation. Several intervention comprising early administration of antibiotic targeting gram-negative bacteria; modification in diet consisting use of prebiotics; metabolites like butyrate, propionate, and acetate; and transplantation of microbiota have been demonstrated to modulate development of type 1 diabetes among animal models. It still needs to be observed that how effective these strategies are among human beings. Transplanting donor microbiota into intestine of people having recurrent *Clostridium difficile* infection is a well-known and successful therapy. By using the similar technique, an improvement in insulin sensitivity has been noted when the microbiota of insulin-sensitive people, having low BMIs, are transplanted into the obese people with metabolic syndrome. It remains to be demonstrated how useful this pioneering technique can be in the future and is not without its conceptual challenge for those who receive donor transplants.[15]

CONCLUSION

Any significant change in bacterial diversity may affect the gut fermentation profile, gut wall permeability, and mucosal and systemic immunity. Alteration in microbiota may trigger mechanisms responsible for oxidative stress, endotoxemia, obesity, and hyperglycemia. Many studies in mice have shown the role of microbiota in possible causative factor in metabolic syndrome and diabetes. Some dietary interventions have also shown the conceptual change in understanding the relationship of diabetes with intestinal microbial world. However there is little published work that characterizes the microbiome and metagenomics of diabetes as well as modification of the course of disease through microbiota interventions. It is clear, therefore, that the changes in the microbiome may have substantial effects on host metabolism but it is too early to predict the future interventions.

REFERENCES

1. Benson AK, Kelly SA, Legge R, et al. Individuality in gut microbiota composition is a complex polygenic trait shaped by multiple environmental and host genetic factors. Proc Natl Acad Sci U S A. 2010;107(44):18933-8.
2. Fukuda S, Suzuki Y, Murai M, et al. Isolation of a novel strain of Butyrivibrio fibrisolvens that isomerizes linoleic acid to conjugated linoleic acid without hydrogenation, and its utilization as a probiotic for animals. J Appl Microbiol. 2006;100:787-94.
3. Brown CT, Davis-Richardson AG, Giongo A, et al. Gut microbiome metagenomics analysis suggests a functional model for the development of autoimmunity for type 1 diabetes. PLoS One. 2011;6(10):e25792.
4. Kostic AD, Gevers D, Siljander H, et al. The dynamics of the human infant gut microbiome in development and in progression toward type 1 diabetes. Cell Host Microbe. 2015;17(2):260-73.
5. Mazmanian SK, Liu CH, Tzianabos AO, et al. An immunomodulatory molecule of symbiotic bacteria directs maturation of the host immune system. Cell. 2005;122(1):107-18.
6. Hague A, Elder DJ, Hicks DJ, et al. Apoptosis in colorectal tumour cells: induction by the short chain fatty acids butyrate, propionate and acetate and by the bile salt deoxycholate. Int J Cancer. 1995;60:400-6.
7. Round JL, Lee SM, Li J, et al. The Toll-like receptor 2 pathway establishes colonization by a commensal of the human microbiota. Science. 2011;332(6032):974-7.
8. Cani PD, Neyrinck AM, Fava F, et al. Selective increases of bifidobacteria in gut microflora improves high-fat diet-induced diabetes in mice through a mechanism associated with endotoxemia. Diabetologia. 2007;50:2374-83.
9. Hildebrandt MA, Hoffmann C, Sherrill–Mix SA, et al. High-fat diet determines the composition of the murine gut microbiome independently of obesity. 2009;137:1716-24. e2.
10. Marietta EV, Gomez AM, Yeoman C, et al. Low incidence of spontaneous type 1 diabetes in non-obese diabetic mice raised on gluten-free diets is associated with changes in the intestinal microbiome. PLoS One. 2013;8(11):e78687.
11. Tolhurst G, Heffron H, Lam YS, et al. Short-chain fatty acids stimulate glucagon-like peptide-1 secretion via the G-protein-coupled receptor FFAR2. Diabetes. 2012;61:364-71.
12. Levin MC, Borén J. The extracellular matrix protein MAGP1 is a key regulator of adipose tissue remodeling during obesity. Diabetes. 2014;63:1858-9.
13. Kristensen NB, Bryrup T, Allin KH, et al. Alterations in fecal microbiota composition by probiotic supplementation in healthy adults: a systematic review of randomized controlled trials. Genome Medicine. 2016;8:52.
14. Ley RE, Bäckhed F, Turnbaugh P, et al. Obesity alters gut microbial ecology. Proc Natl Acad Sci U S A. 2005;102(31):11070-5.
15. Vrieze A, Van Nood E, Holleman F, et al. Transfer of intestinal microbiota from lean donors increases insulin sensitivity in individuals with metabolic syndrome. Gastroenterology. 2012;143:913-6. e917.
16. Kuitunen M, Saukkonen T, Ilonen J, et al. Intestinal permeability to mannitol and lactulose in children with type 1 diabetes with the HLA-DQB1*02 allele. Autoimmunity. 2002;35:365-8.
17. Sapone A, de Magistris L, Pietzak M, et al. Zonulin upregulation is associated with increased gut permeability in subjects with type 1 diabetes and their relatives. Diabetes. 2006;55:1443-9.
18. Secondulfo M, Iafusco D, Carratù R, et al. Ultrastructural mucosal alterations and increased intestinal permeability in non-celiac, type 1 diabetic patients. Dig Liver Dis. 2004;36:35-45.

19. Bosi E, Molteni L, Radaelli MG, et al. Increased intestinal permeability precedes clinical onset of type 1 diabetes. Diabetologia. 2006;49:2824-7.
20. Savilahti E, Ormälä T, Saukkonen T, et al. Jejuna of patients with insulin-dependent diabetes mellitus (IDDM) show signs of immune activation. Clin Exp Immunol. 1999;116:70-7.
21. Westerholm-Ormio M, Vaarala O, Pihkala P, et al. Immunologic activity in the small intestinal mucosa of pediatric patients with type 1 diabetes. Diabetes. 2003;52:2287-95.
22. Auricchio R, Paparo F, Maglio M, et al. In vitro–deranged intestinal immune response to gliadin in type 1 diabetes. Diabetes. 2004;53:1680-3.
23. Bister V, Kolho KL, Karikoski R, et al. Metalloelastase (MMP-12) is upregulated in the gut of pediatric patients with potential celiac disease and in type 1 diabetes. Scand J Gastroenterol. 2005;40:1413-22.
24. Oikarinen M, Tauriainen S, Honkanen T, et al. Detection of enteroviruses in the intestine of type 1 diabetic patients. Clin Exp Immunol. 2008;151:71-5.
25. Tiittanen M, Westerholm-Ormio M, Verkasalo M, et al. Infiltration of Foxp3 expressing cells in jejunal mucosa in celiac disease but not in type 1 diabetes. Clin Exp Immunol. 2008;152:498-507.

7 CHAPTER Beta-Cell Dysfunction: Proposed Mechanisms

Sandeep Tak

INTRODUCTION

Type 2 diabetes mellitus (T2DM) is an epidemic in progression in developing countries although it seems to have plateaued in developed countries. Environmental factors such as sedentary lifestyle, obesity, and unhealthy diet are the main reason. Multiple genetic factors also predispose to T2DM. Inability of beta-cells to maintain insulin levels to control glycemia and overcome insulin resistance (IR) is the main pathophysiological abnormality. Increased hepatic gluconeogenesis, increased glucose reabsorption from kidney, increased lipolysis, and inflammation also play an important role in the pathogenesis of T2DM. Other hormonal abnormalities including increased glucagon secretion, decreased incretin effect, increased leptin, and decreased adiponectin also contribute. However, the beta-cell dysfunction and failure remain the core abnormality in T2DM.

THE BETA CELL

The pancreatic islet was first described by Paul Langerhans in 1869 as "a network of cells, almost perfect in homogeneity and structure, arranged in groups, scattered between acinar cells of the pancreas."[1] The islet is a very complex "mini-organ" in pancreas. Five types of highly specialized endocrine cells are found in the pancreatic islet, viz., alpha cells produce glucagon; beta-cells produce insulin; delta cells produce somatostatin; PP cells produce pancreatic polypeptide, and epsilon cells produce ghrelin. Islets are highly vascular, surrounded by fenestrated endothelial cells. Beta-cells are the predominant cell type in human islet, accounting for 60–70% of islet cells. The main function of beta-cells is to secrete and regulate insulin secretion in response to stimuli. The main stimuli for insulin release are glucose which binds to glucose transporter on beta-cells. Incretin receptors are also present on beta-cells.

Entry of glucose into the beta-cell via glucose transporters leads to a glucose phosphorylation by glucokinase and the closure of potassium-ion channels that leads to membrane depolarization. Membrane depolarization leads to opening of voltage-gated calcium channel in influx of calcium and increased calcium ion induces degranulation and insulin secretion[2] (Fig. 1). Other receptors such as G-protein coupled receptors and effect of amino acids and fatty acids on beta-cells are not fully understood. Probably there is a role of vitamin D activating enzymes and receptors within the beta-cell.

Hyperinsulinemia in response to IR is the first stage of T2DM development. However, IR remains stable throughout the course of disease if left untreated but there is a gradual decline in insulin production. Once the insulin levels fall below the critical level, the patient develops diabetes. Therefore, it is basically a failure of beta-cells to compensate for IR for a long period of time in a subset of individuals that lead to development of T2DM. Increased beta-cell apoptosis and reduced beta-cell mass may be the main reason for beta-cells dysfunction and failure.

Functional defects in the beta-cells in T2DM are well characterized. The loss of first-phase insulin secretion is an early defect.[3] It is also associated with the loss of oscillations in insulin secretion.[4] In fact, loss of oscillatory secretion of insulin is the first abnormality and even found in nondiabetic relatives of subjects with T2DM.[5] Another mechanism involves inefficient conversion of the pro-insulin into insulin, resulting in a 4–5 times increase in pro-insulin levels in the beta-cells of patients with T2DM.[6]

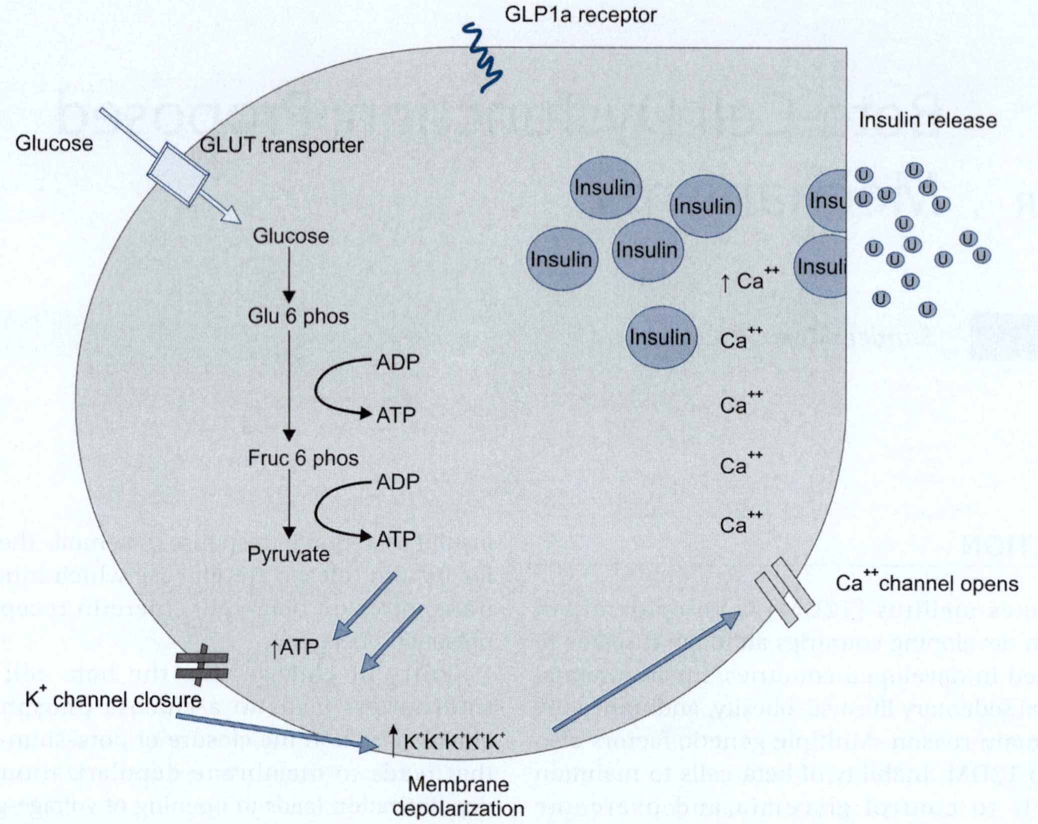

(ADP: adenosine diphosphate; ATP: adenosine triphosphate; GLP-1α: glucagon-like peptide 1α)

Figure 1 Mechanism of insulin secretion from beta-cell.

Incretin system defects may also lead to beta-cell dysfunction.[7] Glucagon-like peptide 1 (GLP-1) and glucose-dependent insulinotropic polypeptide (GIP) are the incretin hormones, released after meal ingestion, and stimulate insulin secretion in a glucose-dependent manner. Incretins increase the expression of *PDX-1* gene, which is important for beta-cell proliferation. They also increase expression of *GLUT2* and *glucokinase* genes, responsible for insulin release. Incretin receptors are downregulated in subjects with T2DM.[8] This may lead to impaired incretin-induced insulin secretion. Type 2 diabetics also have increased activity of DPP4 enzymes. Nondiabetic relatives of those with diabetes and people with impaired glucose tolerance may also display defects in the incretin system.

Gene expression defects are also associated with beta-cell dysfunction and failure. Transcription factors like hypoxia-inducible factor (HIF)-1α[9] and *ARNT*[10] proteins play a vital role in insulin secretion. HIF-1α and ARNT have significantly less expression in the pancreatic islets of T2DM subjects as compared to nondiabetics. Knockout mice lacking the genes for these proteins in beta-cells develop impaired glucose tolerance and diabetes.[11]

Genome-wide association studies (GWAS) and human genome-sequencing project have led to a plethora of data on the possible genetic background of various diseases including T2DM. The transcription factor 7-like 2 (TCF7L2) is most strongly linked to T2DM. TCF7L2 has important effects on beta-cell proliferation and incretin-related insulin secretion and glucose-induced insulin secretion.[12] Twenty percent of the population has polymorphism in TCF7L2 and this can be a reason why only a small subset of patients with IR develops T2DM.[13]

PROPOSED MECHANISMS OF BETA-CELLS FAILURE

Normally diabetes onset is associated with reduced beta-cell mass, but patients may have almost normal beta-cell mass with impaired insulin secretion. Therefore, it is functional beta-cell mass that is more important than absolute beta-cell mass. Important factors that

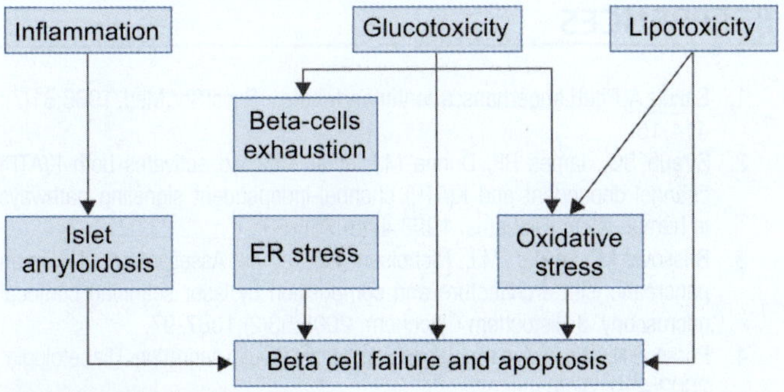

(ER: endoplasmic reticulum)

Flowchart 1 Proposed mechanisms of beta-cells dysfunction.

lead to beta-cell dysfunction are glucotoxicity and lipotoxicity. They lead to increased oxidative stress and endoplasmic reticulum (ER) stress. Inflammation and amyloid deposition are other important mechanisms that may induce beta-cell dysfunction and death. Probably, a combination of multiple mechanisms may ultimately lead to beta-cell dysfunction (Flowchart 1).

Glucotoxicity: Glucose is the main regulator of insulin secretion, and chronic hyperglycemia is associated with impaired beta-cell function and impaired insulin secretion.[14] This is called glucotoxicity, and normalization of the glucose level in subjects with T2DM has a positive impact on beta-cell function.[15] Chronic glucotoxicity may lead to altered gene expression that results in functional defects in beta-cells. This is also termed "beta cell de-differentiation."[16] It is also associated with altered beta-cell signaling and architecture. High glucose levels activate the Fas-FLIP pathway, which results in greater beta-cell differentiation and proliferation. However, in chronic hyperglycemia, this adaptive pathway may eventually fail resulting in early apoptosis as well as reduced functional beta-cell mass.[10]

Lipotoxicity: Fewer than 12% of obese hyperlipidemic human subjects become diabetic.[17] This suggests that lipotoxicity may be just one of the factors in the development of beta-cell failure in T2DM. The exact mechanism of so-called lipotoxicity is not clear. Probably, effects of specific fatty acids on beta-cells depend on the degree of fatty-acid saturation and length of carbon chain. Saturated fatty acids with long carbon chain-like palmitic acid or stearic acid are cytotoxic and can induce beta-cells apoptosis whereas mono- or poly-unsaturated fatty acids have protective effect on beta-cells.

Islet inflammation: The basic markers of inflammation, such as the white blood cells count and C-reactive protein, are elevated in patients with T2DM and in those at risk of diabetes. Chronic low-grade inflammation in pancreas and, in particular, in pancreatic islet can cause beta-cell dysfunction and beta-cell apoptosis. Subjects with T2DM have significant macrophage infiltration the islets of prior to beta-cell apoptosis.[18] The islets cells respond to metabolic stress. Hyperglycemia and exposure to fatty acids lead to increased expression of cytokines, particularly interleukin-1 beta (IL-1β). Long-term expression of this cytokine may result in the production of reactive oxygen species (ROS), inflammation, and eventually beta-cell apoptosis.[10] Use of anti-inflammatory therapies, such as IL-1 receptor antagonist[19] or nonsteroidal anti-inflammatory drugs, results in small improvements in beta-cell function independent of an effect on IR suggesting the role of inflammation in beta-cell dysfunction.

Beta-cell exhaustion: It is postulated that a prolonged period of IR with hyperinsulinism leads to depletion of available insulin granules, thereby reducing the insulin secretion.[20] However, beta-cell exhaustion is unlikely to be the sole pathogenic mechanism. It may play an important role in a multifactorial setting. Studies have examined the benefits of "beta-cell rest" strategies. When inhibitors of insulin secretion, such as diazoxide or somatostatin, were given to subjects with diabetes, paradoxical improvement in beta-cell function was observed following a period of "rest."[21]

In a randomized controlled trial with early intensive insulin therapy in newly diagnosed T2DM patients, with the aim to provide rest to beta-cells, it was observed that beta-cell function was maintained better and better glycemic remission was achieved as compared to oral hypoglycemic agents for at least 1 year after diagnosis.[22] This has led to the discussion of the therapeutic implications of beta-cell failure and the possibility of reversing this complex process. Although highly controversial, the use of certain sulfonylureas such as glibenclamide has been linked to beta-cell death, while there is evidence that incretin-based therapy and insulin replacement increase beta-cell mass in mice and have a positive effect on function.[23]

Hormones: Leptin is a hormone secreted by adipocytes and its main action is to control appetite. Leptin levels are elevated in T2DM. Persistent and significantly high level of leptin impairs insulin secretion[24] and may induce beta-cell death. Conversely, adiponectin, which is also secreted from adipose tissue, has anti-inflammatory and insulin-sensitizing effect. Its secretion is downregulated in T2DM.

Islet amyloid: Deposition of amyloid in islet has long been postulated to be the reason for beta-cell death in

T2DM. Its precise role and mechanism are not certain. More than 90% of type 2 diabetic subjects have amyloid deposits in at least one islet compared to 12% of age-matched nondiabetic in a postmortem study.[25] Amylin is a peptide co-stored with insulin in beta-cells and its misfolding leads to deposition of amyloid fibrils. Insulin resistance is associated with increased production of pro-insulin and pro-amylin, and this may be the first step in development of islet amyloid. But it is still unclear whether amyloidosis is the cause of beta-cell failure or an end-result of several distinct processes including hyperinsulinemia.

Endoplasmic reticulum stress: The ER is an organelle in the cell that is responsible for protein handling and packaging. Beta-cells are highly specialized secretory cells and IR and diabetes put additional demand on beta-cells. Fast and rapid turnover of proteins and insulin may put ER under severe stress.[26] Morphologically, ER stress is characterized by ER swelling as proteins accumulate. ER stress may be mediated by genetic or environmental factors. Mutations in pro-insulin gene in mice lead to morphological evidence of ER stress and subsequent diabetes.[20] Exposure of islets to high-glucose levels, cytokines, and fatty acids may also lead to signs of ER stress.

Oxidative stress: Mitochondrial metabolism of high glucose levels leads to overproduction of ROS and subsequent oxidative stress. This may result in beta-cell dysfunction or apoptosis.[20] Glutathione is an important antioxidant produced in body, and overexpression of glutathione peroxidase in beta-cells protects cells from oxidative damage and improved beta-cell mass. In a study, marked improvement in insulin secretion was observed following 24 hours of exposure to glutathione in human subjects with T2DM.[27]

CONCLUSION

Beta-cell dysfunction and failure in response to increasing demand because of ongoing IR play a main role in the pathogenesis of T2DM. Other factors responsible for beta-cell failure includes inflammation, ER stress, effects of hormones and most importantly genetic susceptibility. It has long been postulated that almost 50% beta-cells are lost at the time of diagnosis of diabetes but this view is now actively contested. In fact there are evidences to suggests that early intervention may improve or even reverse beta-cell dysfunction. More basic research in complex mechanisms of beta-cell failure may provide more therapeutic options and may one day help in realizing the dream of inducing remission in T2DM.

REFERENCES

1. Sakula A. Paul Langerhans: a centenary tribute. J Royal Soc Med. 1988;81(7): 414-15.
2. Straub SG, James RF, Dunne MJ, et al. Glucose activates both K(ATP) channel-dependent and K(ATP) channel-independent signaling pathways in human islets. Diabetes. 1998;47(5):758-63.
3. Brissova M, Fowler MJ, Nicholson WE, et al. Assessment of human pancreatic islet architecture and composition by laser scanning confocal microscopy. J Histochem Cytochem. 2005;53(2):1087-97.
4. Porkson N. The in vivo regulation of pulsatile insulin secretion. Diabetologia. 2002;45(1):3-20.
5. O'Rahilly S, Turner RC, Matthews DR. Impaired pulsatile secretion of insulin in relatives of patients with non-insulin-dependent diabetes. New Engl J Med. 1988;318(19):1225-30.
6. Kahn SE, Halban PA. Release of incompletely processed pro-insulin is the cause of the disproportionate pro-insulinemia of NIDDM. Diabetes. 1997;46(1):1725-32.
7. Perley MJ, Kipnis DM. Plasma insulin responses to oral and intravenous glucose: studies in normal and diabetic subjects. J Clin Invest. 1967;46(12):1954-62.
8. Shu L, Matveyenko AV, Kerr-Conte J, et al. Decreased TCF7L2 protein levels in type 2 diabetes mellitus correlate with downregulation of GIP- and GLP-1 receptors and impaired beta-cell function. Human Mol Gen. 2009;18(13):2388-99.
9. Gunton JE, Kulkarni RN, Yim S, et al. Loss of ARNT/ HIF1β mediates altered gene expression and pancreatic-islet dysfunction in human type 2 diabetes cell. Cell Metab. 2005;122:337-49.
10. Gunton JE, Kulkarni RN, Yim S, et al. Loss of ARNT/ HIF1β mediates altered gene expression and pancreatic-islet dysfunction in human type 2 diabetes cell. Cell Metab. 2005;122:337-49.
11. Faerch K, Vaag A, Holst JJ, et al. Impaired fasting glycaemia vs impaired glucose tolerance: similar impairment of pancreatic alpha and beta-cell function but differential roles of incretin hormones and insulin action. Diabetologia. 2008;51(5):853-61.
12. da Silva Xavier G, Loder MK, McDonald A, et al. TCF7L2 regulates late events in insulin secretion from pancreatic islet beta-cells. Diabetes. 2009;58(4):894-905.
13. Grant SFA, Thorleifsson G, Reynisdottir I, et al. Variant of transcription factor 7-like 2 (TCF7L2) gene confers risk of type 2 diabetes. Nat Gen. 2006;38:320-23.
14. Unger RH, Grundy S. Hyperglycaemia as an inducer as well as a consequence of impaired islet cell function and insulin resistance: implications for the management of diabetes. Diabetologia. 1985;28:119-21.
15. Turner RC, McCarthy ST, Holman RR, et al. Beta-cell function improved by supplementing basal insulin secretion in mild diabetes. Br Med J. 1976;1:1252-54.
16. Leahy JL, Cooper HE, Deal DA, et al. Chronic hyperglycaemia is associated with impaired glucose influence on insulin secretion: a study in normal rats using chronic in vivo glucose infusion. J Clin Invest. 1986;77: 908-15.
17. Agren G, Narbro K, Naslund, et al. Long-term effects of weight loss on pharmaceutical costs in obese subjects: a report from the SOS intervention study. Int J Obes Relat Metab Dis. 2002;26:184-92.
18. Ehses JA, Perren A, Eppler E, et al. Increased number of islet associated macrophages in type 2 diabetes. Diabetes. 2007;56:2356-70.
19. Larsen CM, Faulenbach M, Vaag A, et al. Interleukin-1receptor antagonist in type 2 diabetes mellitus. New Engl J Med. 2007;356: 1517-26.

20. Baetens D, Malaisse-Lagae F, Perrelet A, et al. Endocrine pancreas: three-dimensional reconstruction shows two types of islets of Langerhans. Science. 1979;206(4424):1323-25.
21. Greenwood RH, Mahler RF, Hales CN. Improvement in insulin secretion in diabetes after diazoxide. Lancet. 1976;1:444-7.
22. Weng J, Li Y, Xu W, et al. Effect of intensive insulin therapy on beta-cell function and glycaemic control in patients with newly diagnosed type 2 diabetes: a multicentre randomised parallel-group trial. Lancet. 2008;371:1753-60.
23. Leahy JL, Hirsch IB, Peterson KA, et al. Targeting beta-cell function early in the course of therapy for type 2 diabetes mellitus. J Clin Endocrinol Metab. 2010;95:4206-16.
24. Kieffer TJ, Habener JF. The adipoinsular axis: effects of leptin on pancreatic beta-cells. Am J Physiol Endocrinol Metab. 2000;278:E1-14.
25. Rocken C, Linke RP, Saeger W. Immunohistology of islet amyloid polypeptide in diabetes mellitus: semi-quantitative studies in a post-mortem series. Virch Arch Pathol Anat Histopathol. 1992;421: 339-44.
26. Laybutt DR, Preston AM, Akerfeldt MC, et al. Endoplasmic reticulum stress contributes to beta-cell apoptosis in type 2 diabetes. Diabetologia. 2007;50:752-63.
27. Del Guerra S, Lupi R, Marselli L, et al. Functional and molecular defects of pancreatic islets in human type 2 diabetes. Diabetes. 2005;54: 727-35.

CHAPTER 8 Role of Alpha Cells in Diabetes Pathophysiology

Saumik Datta

INTRODUCTION

Serum blood glucose concentration is an effect of crucial interplay of different hormones coming from pancreatic as well as extrapancreatic sources. *Islets of Langerhans* were discovered in 1869 by German anatomist Paul Langerhans. Almost 3 million islets are distributed throughout pancreas of a healthy adult. Islet cells are equipped with five types of cells. Because of most sophisticated and well-regulated intercellular network, dysfunction of one islet cell type renders other cells incapable of a normal response to their normal stimuli.

ALPHA CELLS PHYSIOLOGY

However, there are definite interspecies variation in the relative proportion of different cells as well as inter cells orientation.

In Rodent islets, beta cells are localized predominantly in the center of the islet, surrounded by alpha, delta, and other cell types. Human islets display random distribution of alpha, beta, and delta cells throughout the islet.

Alpha cells in human are producing glucagon. They share 30–45% of total islet cells in humans. Human alpha cells are arranged with L-, T-, and P/Q-type calcium channels.

Adenosine triphosphate (ATP)-sensitive potassium channels is principal actor in coupling of glucose and glucagon. Closure of these channels leads to membrane depolarization, inactivation of sodium channels, and ultimately reduced calcium-mediated exocytosis of glucagon. At low-glucose levels, the intracellular ATP/adenosine diphosphate (ADP) ratio is low. ATP-sensitive potassium channels generate a membrane potential of approximately –60 mV. This leads to opening of low-voltage-activated T-type calcium channels. Subsequently, membrane depolarization occurs to the extent that sodium channels and high-voltage-activated N-type calcium channels are activated. As a consequence, calcium-induced glucagon secretion takes place. However, Rorsman and colleagues have worked with α cells after exposure to a suppressive concentration of glucose (6 m). Electrical activity of alpha cells in high-glucose environment altered in such a way that action potentials occurred at a higher frequency and lower amplitude.[1] This is responsible for reduction of P/Q-type calcium-channel activity, which subsequently inhibited glucagon secretion.

Beta cells are producing insulin and amylin. They are 50–60% in human islets. Delta cells are responsible for somatostatin production and less than 10% of islet cells in adult human being are marked as delta cells. Epsilon cells which is very less in number, produces ghrelin (<1%). PP cells are secreting pancreatic polypeptide. In human islets, alpha and beta cells are found in close relationship with each other throughout the cluster. So, it is very much expected that they will work in orchestrated way in health and happiness. That rhythm will be lost in morbid conditions.

Glucose activates beta cells but inhibits alpha cells. Glucagon activates alpha cells, which in turn, activate beta cells and delta cells. Somatostatin exerts inhibitory effect on alpha cells and beta cells.

Glucagon is well recognized as the counter-regulatory hormone to insulin. It stimulates hepatic glycogenolysis, gluconeogenesis, fatty-acid oxidation and ketogenesis. The main stimulus for glucagon release from alpha cells is low blood glucose levels. Apart from this, amino acids such as L-arginine stimulate secretion of this polypeptide hormone.

Activation of autonomic nervous system and gastric inhibitory polypeptide also can stimulate glucagon secretion. In contrast, high glucose levels, insulin, somatostatin, amylin and glucagon-like peptide 1 (GLP-1) are principal suppressors of glucagon release.

ALPHA CELLS IN TYPE 2 DIABETES MELLITUS

For a long time it was thought that pathology related to β cells is principally responsible for diabetes mellitus. The United Kingdom Prospective Diabetes Study (UKPDS) has shown us that almost 50% of β cells are lost at the time of diagnosis. But, it is now clear that the pathology is not limited to β cells only. But, α cells are also insulted in similar way. In fasting state, healthy human being secretes insulin every 10–15 minutes. This regular pulse is lost not only in diabetes as well as in their nondiabetic relatives also. Abnormal secretion of islet amyloid polypeptide is also noticed frequently. But, in addition to that, increased glucagon secretion has also been noted in fasting state. When fasting insulin, glucagon and glucose were taken into consideration it was found that insulin level is inappropriately low in respect to glucose level. At the same time, Serum glucagon level is elevated.[2] This may be due to altered paracrine regulation.[3] Other authorities are in favor of direct influences of substrates. Fasting hyperglucagonemia is observed in some but not all type 2 diabetes mellitus (T2DM) patients with moderate glycemic control.[4,5]

Insulin resistance at the level of liver is due to improper insulin signaling. But, elevated glucagon has also definite role in elevation of fasting blood sugar level. Baron et al. found that inhibition of glucagon secretion by somatostatin reduced 50% of the hepatic glucose output.[6] Glucagon accounts possibly for 40–50% of basal hepatic glucose output.[7]

So, similar to β-cell malfunction in this bihormonal disorder, there are a number of characteristic dysfunctions in α-cell.

Beta-cells in pancreatic islets of a diabetic person are going to decrease. But, α-cell mass remains similar to that of nondiabetic individuals. It leads to relative increase in ratio of α-cells to β cells in islets. Some, but not all, type 2 diabetic patients have increased fasting glucagon levels. That can be even 50% greater than nondiabetic subjects.[8] At the same time, some of type 2 diabetic persons show apparent α-cell dysfunction without any major changes of their islet cell composition. Matsuda et al. proposed that diabetic patients had enhanced sensitivity of hepatic glucose production to glucagon.[9]

Paradoxical glucagon response to meal is also not uncommon in people with T2DM. Elevated glucagon levels following a carbohydrate meal leads to postprandial hyperglycemia.

After meal, hepatic glucose output is suppressed abruptly in normal individuals. But, this change is not noticed and it remains at near fasting levels in diabetic subjects. This deviation from normal physiology, failure of glucagon suppression after food, contributes to the postprandial hyperglycemia. Post-meal hyperglucagonemia is responsible for as much as 50% of the pathological increase in plasma-glucose excursions following oral glucose intake in T2DM people.[10] Glucagon secretion is under control of insulin. In diabetes, with either dysfunction or loss of β cells from islet, inhibitory control of insulin on α cells is lost leading to postprandial hyperglucagonemia. However, this α cells dysfunction is possibly more prominent in elderly persons. K_{ATP}-channels similar to β-cells are also active in α cells. Increased α-cell K_{ATP}-channel activity may be one important issue behind this aberrant behavior of α cells.

ALPHA CELLS IN TYPE 1 DIABETES MELLITUS

Let us look into the alpha cells in type 1 diabetes mellitus (T1DM). Type 1 diabetes mellitus is characterized by selective loss of β-cell mass. However, Unger and colleagues proposed that glucagon hypersecretion is the major culprit in T1D-associated hyperglycemia.[11]

Alpha cells in humans and nonobese diabetic mice and streptozotocin (STZ)-treated mice and rats, become hypertrophic and hyperplastic.[12–14] Alpha and beta cells of the islet share a common embryonic origin. They are able to transdifferentiate into other type of cells.[15] That may also explain change in mass of α cells to some extent, apart from loss of influence of β cells on α cells.

We should also remember that alpha cell undergoes significant functional changes.

Type 1 diabetes is a progressive disease. During the prediabetic state, the β cells are selectively destroyed, and the alpha cells undergo expansion. However, because β cells can compensate for cell loss by increasing insulin secretion, patients remain asymptomatic. Serum insulin levels and glucose levels and glucagon release remain relatively normal. The stimulus-secretion coupling of the α cells remain intact during this prediabetes period.

Following loss of 80% of the β-cell mass in islets, patient becomes overtly diabetic. The expanded α-cell mass is uninhibited by insulin. They secrete aberrantly high levels of glucagon. Insulin-to-glucagon ratio is markedly reduced. Even after successful initiation of treatment, this phase is still often characterized by hyperglucagonemia and post-meal hyperglycemia. After 10 or more years, α-cell mass is not further affected. But, stimulus-secretion coupling is inefficient enough leading to a loss of adequate counter-regulation, and potentially life-threatening hypoglycemia.

These abnormal behaviors could be further influenced by the relative resistance of alpha cells to glucose toxicity, lipotoxicity and inflammatory cytokines.[16,17] β-cell viability and secretory function are negatively influenced by high glucose, lipids and inflammatory cytokines. But, α-cell mass and glucagon secretion are enhanced in the presence of these factors.[16,17] Concentration response curve of the effect of glucose on α cells is bell-shaped.[18] Low-glucose stimulates glucagon release, and moderately high-glucose levels inhibit glucagon secretion, very-high-glucose concentrations can increase glucagon release from α cells. Thus, extreme hyperglycemia could lead to aberrant glucagon secretion initiating a vicious cycle, in which very-high-glucose increases glucagon release.

Failure of counter-regulation in response to hypoglycemia is very important issue. Hypoglycemia unawareness is a common condition with increased duration of disease as well as in the background of recurrent hypoglycemia. Up to 40% of patients with diabetes suffer from some level of hypoglycemia unawareness. Normal signs of hypoglycemia are not recognized. Patient may land up with dangerously low-plasma glucose levels. Hypoglycemia unawareness is due to blunted hormonal responses to hypoglycemia. In particular, glucagon secretion is impaired. Insufficient glucagon secretion is associated with intact glucagon production. Coupling of extracellular glucose concentration to glucagon secretion is impaired. For example, reduced release of neuronostatin may lead to impaired glucagon secretion.[19] Alternatively, decreased expression glucagon receptor and neuronostatin receptor can desensitize the α cells to these positive secretory signals.

CONCLUSION

So, there is enough evidence in literature that though β-cell pathology is occupying the center of the stage, we cannot keep α cells out of the theater. α cells undergo hypertrophy and hyperplasia. It also displays number of dysfunction.

Owing to α-cell dysfunction, there is oversecretion when it is not needed and poor production when it is needed. GLP-1 receptor agonists and DPP-IV inhibitors can neutralize this unfriendly behavior to some extent. But, definitely we are in need of some agent which can neutralize α-cell pathology more aggressively.

REFERENCES

1. Zhang Q, Ramracheya R, Lahmann C, et al. Role of K_{ATP} channels in glucose-regulated glucagon secretion and impaired counter regulation in type 2 diabetes. Cell Metab. 2013;18(2013):871-82.
2. Avogaro A, Crepaldi C, Miola M, et al. High blood ketone body concentration in type 2 non-insulin dependent diabetic patients. J Endocrinol Invest. 1996;19:99-105.
3. Maruyama H, Hisatomi A, Orci L, et al. Insulin within islets is a physiologic glucagon release inhibitor. J Clin Invest. 1984:74:2296-9.
4. Unger RH, Aguilar-Parada E, Muller WA, et al. Studies of pancreatic alpha cell function in normal and diabetic subjects. J Clin Invest. 1970;49:837-48.
5. Reaven GM, Chen YD, Golay A, et al. Documentation of hyperglucagonemia throughout the day in non-obese and obese patients with noninsulin-dependent diabetes mellitus. J Clin Endocrinol Metab. 1987;64:106-10.
6. Baron AD, Schaeffer L, Shragg P, et al. Role of hyperglucagonemia in maintenance of increased rates of hepatic glucose output in type II diabetics. Diabetes. 1987;36:274-83.7.
7. Gelling RW, Du XQ, Dichmann DS, et al. Lower blood glucose, hyperglucagonemia, and pancreatic alpha cell hyperplasia in glucagon receptor knockout mice. Proc Natl Acad Sci U S A. 2003;100:1438-43.
8. Reaven GM, Chen YD, Golay A, et al. Documentation of hyperglucagonemia throughout the day in non-obese and obese patients with noninsulin-dependent diabetes mellitus. J Clin Endocrinol Metab. 1987;64:106-10.
9. Matsuda M, Defronzo RA, Glass L, et al. Glucagon dose-response curve for hepatic glucose production and glucose disposal in type 2 diabetic patients and normal individuals. Metabolism. 2002;51:1111-9.
10. Dinneen S, Alzaid A, Turk D, et al. Failure of glucagon suppression contributes to postprandial hyperglycaemia in IDDM. Diabetologia. 1995;38:337-43.
11. Unger RH, Cherrington AD. Glucagonocentric restructuring of diabetes: a pathophysiologic and therapeutic makeover. J Clin Invest. 2012;122:4-12.
12. Gomez Dumm CL, Console GM, Luna GC, et al. Quantitative immunohistochemical changes in the endocrine pancreas of nonobese diabetic (NOD) mice. Pancreas. 1995;11:396-401.
13. Orci L, Baetens D, Rufener C, et al. Hypertrophy and hyperplasia of somatostatin-containing D-cellsin diabetes. Proc Natl Acad Sci U S A. 1976;73:1338-42.
14. Plesner A, Ten Holder JT, Verchere CB. Islet remodeling in female mice with spontaneous autoimmune and streptozotocin-induced diabetes. PLoS One. 2014;9:e102843.
15. Spijker HS, Ravelli RB, Mommaas-Kienhuis RM, et al. Conversion of mature human beta-cells into glucagon-producing alpha-cells. Diabetes. 2013;62:2471-80.
16. Vasu S, Moffett RC, McClenaghan NH, et al. Differential molecular and cellular responses of GLP-1 secreting L-cells and pancreatic alpha cells to glucotoxicity and lipotoxicity. Exp Cell Res. 2015;336:100-8.
17. Vasu S, Moffett RC, McClenaghan NH, et al. Responses of GLP1-secreting L cells to cytotoxicity resemble pancreatic beta-cells but not alpha-cells. J Mol Endocrinol. 2015;54:91-104.
18. Salvatori AS, Elrick MM, Samson WK, et al. Neuronostatin inhibits glucose-stimulated insulin secretion via direct action on the pancreatic alpha-cell. Am J Physiol Endocrinol Metab. 2014;306:E1257-63.
19. Samson WK, Stein LM, Elrick M, et al. Hypoglycemia unawareness prevention: targeting glucagon production. Physiol Behav. 2016;162:147-50.

9 CHAPTER Physical Inactivity and Diabetes Mellitus

Jagdeep Chugh

INTRODUCTION

Diabetes has reached epidemic proportion worldwide and is associated with a large economic burden, increased risk of cardiovascular disease, and premature mortality. Hyperglycemia is the hallmark clinical manifestation of diabetes and evolves through a multifactorial etiology of genetic, environmental, and behavioral factors.[1]

For decades, exercise has been considered a cornerstone of diabetes management, along with diet and medication. However, high-quality evidence on the importance of exercise and fitness in diabetes was lacking till recently.[2] A cluster-randomized study found that diet alone, exercise alone, and combined diet and exercise were equally effective in reducing the progression from impaired glucose tolerance (IGT) to diabetes. Most proximal behavioral cause of insulin resistance is physical inactivity. Several streams of scientific research have demonstrated a role for physical inactivity in the etiology and causation of diabetes and its related morbidity. The mechanisms that underlie these protective effects likely include the regulations of body weight, the reduction of adiposity, insulin resistance, blood pressure, dyslipidemia, and inflammation, and the enhancement of insulin sensitivity, glucose tolerance, and fibrinolytic and endothelial functions. Physical inactivity has been linked to many potential risk factors for diabetes and its cardiovascular sequel, that researches have not yet fully disentangled the more important and the less important pathways by which exercise lowers disease risk.[3] Centers for Disease Control and Prevention and the American College of Sports Medicine have jointly published recommendations that adults should indulge in moderate physical exercise for at least 30 minutes per day preferably all days of week.[4]

Here we will just discuss about physical inactivity, related problems, especially in context of diabetes, leaving aside drug and dietary management of diabetes. We will discuss about causes, care, and probable solutions.

PHYSICAL INACTIVITY

Physical activity is defined as any body movement that requires energy expenditure. An important distinction to make that physical activity refers to a behavior, specifically a body movement that occurs from skeletal muscle contraction and results in increased energy expenditure above resting metabolic rate.[5]

Physical activity should not be confused with exercise, which is a part of physical activity that is planned, structured, repetitive, and purposeful. Physical activity includes exercise and other activities, which involve bodily movements and are done routinely as a part of playing, occupational working, household work, daily movement, and leisure time activities.[5]

Physical inactivity is due to lack of movements:
- Physical inactivity tends to increase with age.
- Women are more physically inactive as compared to men.
- Hispanic and black adults are physically more active as compared to non-Hispanic white adults.

Many studies show that 21st century generation is getting too sedentary due to:
- Increased use of technology.
- Increased use of automobiles.

Problems Associated with Physical Inactivity

Physical inactivity leads to multiple risk factors and this leads to chronic metabolic disorders like diabetes mellitus and cardiovascular diseases. It is the leading cause of major noncommunicable diseases and is one of the most modifiable and preventable risk factor for these pathologies.

Diabetes and Physical Inactivity

Physical inactivity increases the risk of type 2 diabetes mellitus (DM) by 7%. During physical activity, whole-body oxygen consumption increases. To meet its energy needs, skeletal muscles increases its own stores of glucagon and triglycerides, and free fatty acids (FFAs) derived from the breakdown of adipose tissue, triglycerides, and glucose released from liver. A decrease in plasma insulin and the presence of glucagon appears to be necessary for the early increase in hepatic glucose production during physical activity; and during prolonged exercise, increase in plasma glucose and catecholamine appears to play a key.[6]

Diabetes due to physical inactivity may be due to:

- Increased weight gain.
- Link between physical inactivity and obesity is well established. It is estimated that for every 1 kg increase in weight, the prevalence of diabetes increases by 1%.
- Physical inactivity is associated with increased insulin resistance and poor glycemic control.
- Physical inactivity increases visceral fat. The excessive FFAs, released by adipose tissues, lead to a decrease in insulin sensitivity of muscles fat and liver, which is followed by raised glucose level, insulin resistance, and type 2 diabetes. The dangerous hormones secreted by these adipose tissues lead to *metabolic syndrome* and its consequences.
- In a few studies, it has been shown that constipation is associated with decreased physical activity; it indirectly leads to increase in sugar levels because of stasis of food and further increased absorption of food from gut.

Cardiovascular System

These patients develop high blood pressure and other cardiovascular problems. When we do not exercise, the heart function starts deteriorating and cardiovascular fitness deteriorates and atherosclerosis of arteries and heart vessels can develop.

Anxiety

Physical inactivity can cause anxiety and/or depression. These patients have low sense of *well-being and low motivation, due to which they are not willing to move.*

Cancers

Physical inactivity increases the risk of certain cancers especially colon cancer and breast cancers.

Intestinal Effect

Constipation is a very common in patients with physical inactivity. Exercise causes increased motility and proper digestion of food, which helps in body getting rid of excreta.

Gallstones are common in patients with decreased physical activity.

Muscle Atrophy and Joint Problems

Physical inactivity causes muscle wasting, and the muscles become lean and thin. As a result of above the metabolism is disturbed and the fats start depositing around atrophied muscles and the person gains weight. Physical inactivity causes joint stiffness and may cause arthralgias also. It is further worsened by atrophied muscles and gradually increasing fats and weight.

Back stiffness and low back pain is also very common in physically inactive patients.

Physical inactivity increases the risk of fall in such patients due to multifactorial reasons. Routine physical activity, especially weight-bearing and impact exercise, prevents bone loss associated with ageing.

Mortality

Many premature deaths are related to physical inactivity, directly or indirectly. It has been identified as the fourth leading risk factor for global mortality (6% of deaths globally).[7]

Causes of Physical Inactivity

Physical inactivity is a complex physical–social–cultural–economic problem. So it requires a population based multispectral, multidisciplinary and culturally relevant approach. Before we proceed further and advice the patients regarding bodily movements, we should try to *identify* the causes of low physical inactivity:

- *Age*: Old and frail patients
- *Immobility*: Fracture/joint problems/arthritis/neuropathies, etc.
- *Technical*: Persons living in high-rise buildings without lift to come down.
- Obesity ←→ physical inactivity
- *Depressed patients*: Generally are not willing to move
- *Medication*: Antidepressants, sedatives, antihistaminics, etc.
- Alcoholics and night birds
- No park or club or walking stretch near the house
- Unstable cardiac patients
- Bronchial asthma patients
- Extreme hot and cold weathers
- Too busy with family or children, etc.
- Students preparing for competitive exams
- Excessive addiction to mobile, laptop, and TVs
- People from poor socio-economic strata, who get less time and opportunities for activity.
- Patients with retinopathy and visual problems
- Pregnant and nursing mothers.

Governmental solutions to the problem of physical inactivity:

- There should be *progressive* government policies to increase physical activity.
- There should be parks, safe cycle paths, pavements, and pedestrian zones. There should be enough *free* outdoor sports centers.
- High-quality physical education and competitive sports should be a part of curriculum and should be compulsory in all schools and beyond.
- There should be enough options for physical activity for persons with disability and less resource.
- Government of India is pushing for *yoga*. Free yoga classes and camps are everywhere. Yoga is very good both for the body and soul.
- Government is installing free, open gymnasiums in many parts of country, which will help in long way.

Medical Solutions

As an internist, our duty is to identify and treat the root cause of physical inactivity and encourage physical activity. We must spend some quality time with the patient and pinpoint the cause rather than advising them to take "10,000" steps per day.

POINTS TO BE REMEMBERED AND QUOTED

- Any activity helps
- Moderate physical activity brings health benefits.
- Make it personal
- Slow and steady wins the race
- Always keep in mind that *"Rolling stones gather no mass"*. So keep moving any part of your body, anywhere, and anytime.
- Physical inactivity at times is just a mental block and it just needs some push from an expert and the scenario changes.

Before beginning an exercise program one should check for following:

- Have had a heart attack?
- Have a family history of heart-related problems before age of 55 years?
- Have heart, lung, liver or kidney disease?
- Feel pain in chest or joints or breathlessness during physical activity?
- Have high blood pressure, high cholesterol, *unstable* diabetes, arthritis, osteoporosis or asthma?
- Have had joint replacement surgery recently?
- Have an untreated joint or muscle injury, or persistent symptoms of a joint or muscle injury?
- Is there any pregnancy?
- Overweight or morbidly obese?
- Taking medication for any chronic condition?
- Excessive smoking or alcoholism?
- Unsure of health status?

SOLUTIONS

Here focus will be on the role of physical activity in the prevention of type 2 diabetes:

- Old, frail, and visually challenged patients can go to the park in wheelchair.
- Some domestic help should be there to assist. They must use sticks or other devices for support and confidence.
- Patient with fracture/arthritis can do limited exercise, may be at home or in bed. The person can exercise with joints which are not involved. They can take the help of physiotherapist or domestic help. Use proper fitting corsets. Take a safe painkiller before exercise which minimizes the agony.
- The persons who cannot climb down can go to rooftop or walk in their homes.

- Obesity should be tackled by exercise, medication, or diet therapy. It is again a big topic and cannot be discussed here.
- Depressed patients should be counseled or given mood elevators.
- Antihistamines and sedatives should be reduced and given some other remedies.
- Person taking excessive alcohol daily and going for late night party should be counseled and convinced.
- Patient with limited cardiac reserve and bronchial asthma should be properly evaluated, and some safe and limited options should be given. They can take tablet Sorbitrate or cardiac medicines before exercise. Asthma patient can take nebulizer or inhaler pump before exercise.
- In extreme weather conditions, the patients should exercise at home or do some yoga.
- The patients should be encouraged to spare some time from daily routine for their recreation and exercise. They should be told about the benefits of physical activity.
- The bookworms should be encouraged to exercise as it increases the circulation to body and brain and decreases the boredom. If they have limited time, then a few minutes of skipping is good for brain and body.
- Change to comfortable and acceptable mode of exercise—jog-run-walk-swim-cycle-yoga-gym-play, whichever suits the patient. *Just do it.*
- For lonely person, encourage for group walks. Many parts in India are having laughter clubs. There is some physical activity along with that daily laughing classes, this elevates the mood and improves oxygen of lungs and body.
- Encourage hobbies. In every person, there is some hidden hobby and there is some physical activity in each hobby. Dancing is a very good hobby.
- The patients should be encouraged to do their daily chores like gardening, marketing, going and buying milk, vegetables, etc., cleaning the home, opening the door, etc. Use steps rather than lift.
- Pursue to go "*offline*" and switch to "*on life*".
- Early to bed and early to rise, should be encouraged.
- Take public transport rather than own vehicle. One can take cycle or walk to office or market.
- Use "Apps" in mobile to measures the daily steps in high-tech clients.

CONCLUSION

Physical inactivity can initiate and accelerate the pathogenesis of diabetes, and subsequent morbidity and mortality. Conversely, regular physical activity can retard the progression from one stage to another, and it may even reverse process.[1]

So, patients should be encouraged to engage in regular physical activity and reduce sedentary lifestyle, indulge in activities to promote health, psychological well-being, and a healthy body weight. Achieve physical fitness by including cardiovascular conditioning, stretching exercise for flexibility, and endurance.

REFERENCES

1. LaMonte MJ, Blair SN, Church TS. Physical Activity and diabetes prevention. J App Physiol (1985). 2005;99(3):1205-13.
2. Sigal RJ, Kenny GP, Wasserman DH,et al. Physical activity/Exercise and Type 2 Diabetes. Diabetes care. 2004;27(10):2518-39.
3. Bassuk SS, Manson JE. Epidemiological evidence for the role of physical activity in reducing risk of type 2 diabetes and cardiovascular disease. J Appl Physiol. 1985;99(3):1193-204.
4. Centers for Disease Control and Prevention. Surgeon General's report on physical activity and health. JAMA. 1996;276(2):522.
5. https:/www.who.int/dietphysicalactivity/pa/en/.
6. American Diabetes Association. Physical Activity/Exercise and Diabetes. Diabetes care. 2004;27(supl1):s58-62.
7. https://www.ncbi.nlm.nih.gov/books/NBK305049/.

10 CHAPTER Dietary Components as Etiological Factors in Type 2 Diabetes

Sharad Kumar

INTRODUCTION

Diabetes: A Global Emergency

Type 2 diabetes accounts for most of the cases of diabetes mellitus encountered world over. It is the fourth or may be the fifth leading cause of death in most developed countries, and there is ample evidence that it has reached epidemic proportions in many developing and newly industrialized economies.[1] As per International Diabetes Federation (IDF), type 2 diabetes mellitus (T2DM) is a growing problem and costs to society are very high and worse are in fact escalating further.[2]

Indian Scenario—Rapid Nutritional Transition

Currently India is undergoing a rapid nutritional transition, with adoption of a diet having an excess of calories, saturated fats, including excessive trans-fats, simple sugars, and salt, coupled with a low intake of fiber. Such dietary transition in association with a sedentary lifestyle has led to an increase in obesity and diet-related several noncommunicable diseases such as T2DM, predominantly in urban, but also in rural areas.[3] According to IDF 2017, India is home to the second largest number of persons living with diabetes worldwide. With an estimated 72.9 million people already suffering from diabetes in India, diabetes has become a major health care problem in India.

DIET AS A CAUSATIVE FACTOR IN TYPE 2 DIABETES MELLITUS

Relation between Diet and Type 2 Diabetes Mellitus

The role of diet in the etiology of T2DM is most significant, as it starts affecting the chance of developing diabetes even in an unborn child. The nutritional status of the mother affects the body mass index of the offspring, and therefore his or her chances of developing diabetes later is a well-documented fact.

As is widely known, consumption of dietary fats, refined food grains, and sugar, in excessive amounts, has effects on the development of obesity and consequently diabetes.[4] One of the widely quoted proofs of the fact is the observation that there was a decline in diabetes-related mortality during the First and the Second World Wars, due to food shortage and famines in the involved countries such as Germany and other European countries. However, there was no change in diabetes-related mortality rate in countries without any shortage of food during the same time period.[5]

We can say that a diabetic patient's dietary practices, as also of others, are by and large influenced by cultural backgrounds. Consequently, an association between dietary knowledge and dietary practices among all T2DM patients is noted. It can be observed that there is a significant influence of diet in the lifestyle of a person, causing obesity and thus contributing to the genesis of various metabolic diseases. For example, persons who consume high-fat diet develop an increased risk of cardiovascular disease (CVD), more so, if they are already diabetic.[6] Further, the trend of skipping breakfast which has dramatically increased, especially over the past 10 years, in everyone, i.e. children, adolescents, and adults, is a significant contributor of developing obesity. This apparently paradoxical observation is supported with a significant body of evidences that skipping breakfast is related to overweight body structure and other health issues including increased chances of developing diabetes in later life.[7] This habit is often found in association with or as a cause of frequent eating or snacking with mostly calorie-dense and often unhealthy snacks, which also contributes in increasing the body weight and risk of metabolic diseases.[8] Consequently, this western dietary pattern consisting of an increased consumption of processed red meat, fried snacks, dairy products, refined grains, and a variety of sweets and desserts leads to a total intake of excessive calories which is associated with an increased risk of T2DM risk.[9]

> A diet high in fat, calories, and refined grains increases your risk of diabetes,
> BUT
> A poor quality of diet can also lead to obesity, a risk factor for diabetes, and other health problems.

The concept of *glycemic index* (GI) is an indicator of the postprandial blood glucose rise after consuming a particular carbohydrate-containing food, compared with the same quantity of a reference food, such as white bread or glucose (better to compare with glucose, a more standard substance). The *glycemic load* represents both the quality and the quantity of the carbohydrates consumed, meaning the amount of carbohydrate consumed as well as the GI of that carbohydrate.[10] The post-meal glucose excursion depends upon this glycemic load and if it is excessive, it may contribute to β-cell exhaustion as an immediate response and to development of obesity, if consumed over a long period, again contributing to insulin resistance and subsequent development of diabetes. Consumption of refined grains, desserts, fast foods, and lot of empty calories in the form of fruit juices and alcohol has demonstrated a direct correlation with subsequent development of β-cell exhaustion and possible development of T2DM.[11]

Thus a diet high in fat, calories, and cholesterol increases one's risk of developing diabetes as well as chances of related vascular complications. Further, the portion size also matters because how much one eats is just as important as what one eats. A very large quantity of relatively healthy food stuffs can also contribute to obesity and therefore to related complications.

Role of High-fat Diets in Type 2 Diabetes Mellitus

There is a worldwide notion that high-fat diets are associated with impaired insulin action. There have been reports and studies that support the same.[12] Saturated fats, in particular, seem to have the most detrimental effects as revealed by many animal studies. On the basis of this information as well as being aware of the risks of cardiovascular diseases associated with high saturated fat intake, several organizations in the US including American Diabetes Association, American Heart Association, and US Department of Agriculture recommend Americans to restrict their fat intake up to 30% of calories and opt for food that are low in saturated fats. Moreover, it is probable that high-fat diets promote weight gain, which then leads to insulin resistance and its metabolic consequences. There is a large body of evidence that supports this widely held view.[13] Several other evidences of the fact that obesity has a significant role in the development of diabetes and related sequel are now widely accepted. This indicates that any diet or habit that induces obesity will consequently promote the onset of diabetes as well.[14] Insulin action, body weight control, and probably onset of diabetes may be highly influenced by the amount and type of the fat in the diet considering the significance of fats in fuel and energy metabolism.[15]

Major Types of Fats in Relation to Insulin Resistance and Type 2 Diabetes

Obesity is a risk as well as a consequence of insulin resistance and thus an important determining factor of Type 2 diabetes.[16] There is a chance that several dietary fatty acids could affect insulin resistance, independent of obesity. The composition of fatty acids in the cell membranes mediates the influence of fatty acids in the dietary intake.[16] Studies reveal that insulin sensitivity appears to directly affect the fatty acid composition of the phospholipids in various skeletal muscle cell membranes. A specific fatty acid profile of cell membranes could influence insulin action through alterations in insulin receptor binding or affinity and influencing ion permeability and cell signaling.[17]

Types of Dietary Fat and Risk of Type 2 Diabetes

Observational studies and widely available data suggest a potential beneficial effect of polyunsaturated dietary fat and a potential adverse effect of saturated fat in Type 2 diabetes, although the total dietary fat does not appear to predict the risk of Type 2 diabetes. In addition, some studies had evaluated insulin resistance, which is also influenced by chronic insulin demand. This may be getting generated by excessive calories being consumed, but it still remains a conjecture. In addition, an important issue is of the presence of several confounding factors in diet, such as presence or absence of fiber, other nutrients, and type of heating and reheating, which are also likely to influence its metabolic consequences.

Fatty acids such as eicosapentaenoic acid (EPA) and docosahexaenoic acid (DHA), which have long N3 chains (Omega-3 fatty acids), are abundantly found in fish and fish oil in high concentrations.[18] Because the intake of fish oil could directly influence the fatty acid composition of membrane phospholipids, it is recommended that a higher intake of such oils could be beneficial for insulin sensitivity.

Partial hydrogenation of vegetable or fish oils solidifies them and causes the formation of trans-fatty acids. Metabolic studies reveal that trans-fatty acids increase serum LDL cholesterol concentration and decrease HDL cholesterol concentration as compared to cis-unsaturated fatty acids.[19] It has been observed that desaturase enzyme activity is inhibited by trans-fats. This observation has led to the hypothesis that trans-fat could also affect insulin sensitivity because indices of delta-5-desaturase activity were noticed with lower insulin sensitivity. The fact therefore becomes strongly predictive that consumption of trans-fats is potentially diabetogenic.

Role of Dietary Carbohydrate in Type 2 Diabetes Mellitus

Based on chemical structure, carbohydrates are grouped as simple and complex. It is believed that rapid post-prandial sugar increase is caused due to rapid digestion and absorption of simple sugars. Based on this belief, most dietary studies recommend replacing the simple carbohydrates or sugars in the diet with complex carbohydrates or starches. Simple sugars, because they provide only empty calories, contribute to insulin resistance as an immediate response as compared to complex carbohydrates which have also other nutrients besides fiber and therefore produce a gradual surge in blood glucose. These empty calories of simple sugars do not give satiety, therefore encouraging overeating and further contributing to the future onset of obesity and diabetes.

Voluntary energy intake increases after consumption of high-GI meals because of the less satiety associated with such carbohydrates as compared to complex carbohydrates with low-GI meals.[20] Excess energy consumption is promoted by continuous intake of high-GI diets, thus causing weight gain. This may lead to the onset of diabetes or to the maintenance of excess weight gain, especially in susceptible people (e.g. sedentary or overweight subjects).[20]

MYTHS REGARDING DIET AND DIABETES

Reduce Sugar

There is no evidence that restriction of sugar helps in preventing development of diabetes or leads to rise in plasma glucose significantly. A moderate amount of free sugar (up to 50 g/day) is permitted by European Association for the Study of Diabetes (EASD) as well as by others.[21]

Reduce Carbohydrates

An important source of calories is carbohydrates, which should be allowed in permitted quantities. The overemphasis to reduce them does not appear to be useful in preventing development or control of diabetes, and hence carbohydrate-rich foods such as rice and potatoes can be allowed within their quota of calories as long as the diet remains well balanced.[21]

Fruits

Most fruits have low GI and a plenty of fiber. Their juice containing fructose does not raise plasma glucose significantly, and there is no reason therefore to recommend that fruits be restricted by those who want to prevent or control diabetes.[21]

Dietary Restrictions

Most people (72%) believe that diet restrictions are a must for preventing or controlling diabetes. The fact remains that a healthy, well-balanced diet, in an ideal body weight person is what is actually only required.[22]

Sweet Foods

Another myth is about sweet food items in the diet. About 79.7% doctors recommend restrictions in sweet food items such as cake, *jalebi*, and sweet biscuits to their diabetic patients.[23] However, there seems to be no scientific reason to restrict these items as long as their calorie content is within the recommended quota of their daily diet. Because of these unwarranted restrictions, a lot of anxiety and guilt feeling is created amongst the diabetic patients and their families, affecting their quality of life as well as mental health.[23]

CONCLUSION

It is generally agreed that dietary modification is an important means of preventing Type 2 diabetes. The epidemic of diabetes can be contained by containing the epidemic of obesity. The objective can be best met by emphasizing the necessity of achieving and maintaining the ideal body weight, right from the time of pregnancy. Besides counting the calories, the type of calories should also be watched. In general, refined food grains, juices, and trans-fat should be avoided; saturated fats and simple sugars be reduced; and ample quantity of fiber be included in all the meals. On the basis of clinical goals for each individual, individualizing percent of calories from fats and carbohydrates is recommended nowadays instead of a low-fat, high-carbohydrate diet for diabetic patients or for people who want to prevent the onset of diabetes.

REFERENCES

1. Steyn NP, Mann J, Bennett PH, et al. Diet, nutrition and the prevention of type 2 diabetes. Public Health Nutr. 2004;7(1A):147-65.
2. IDF Diabetes Atlas: Global estimates of diabetes prevalence for 2017 and projections for 2045. Diabetes Res Clin Pract. 2018;138:271-81.
3. Misra A, Sharma R, Gulati S, et al. Consensus dietary guidelines for healthy living and prevention of obesity, the metabolic syndrome, diabetes, and related disorders in Asian Indians. Diabetes Technol Ther. 2011;13(6):683-94.
4. Rippe, JM, Theodore JA. Sugars, obesity, and cardiovascular disease: Results from recent randomized control trials. Eur J Nutr. 2016;55:45-53.
5. Lumey LH, Van Poppel FW. The Dutch famine of 1944-45: Mortality and morbidity in past and present generations. Soc Hist Med. 1994;7:229-46.
6. Persell SD, Keating NL, Landrum MB, et al. Relationship of diabetes-specific knowledge to self-management activities, ambulatory preventive care, and metabolic outcomes. Prev Med. 2004;39:746-52.
7. Siega-Riz AM, Popkin BM, Carson T. Trends in breakfast consumption for children in the United States from 1965-1991. Am J Clin Nutr. 1998;67:748S-56.
8. McCrory MA, Campbell WW. Effects of eating frequency, snacking, and breakfast skipping on energy regulation: Symposium overview. J Nutr. 2011;141:144-7.
9. van Dam RM, Rimm EB, Willett WC, et al. Dietary patterns and risk for Type 2 diabetes mellitus in U.S. men. Ann Intern Med. 2002;136:201-9.
10. de Munter JS, Hu FB, Spiegelman D, et al. Whole grain, bran, and germ intake and risk of Type 2 diabetes: A prospective cohort study and systematic review. PLoS Med. 2007;4:e261.
11. Joosten MM, Chiuve SE, Mukamal KJ, et al. Changes in alcohol consumption and subsequent risk of Type 2 diabetes in men. Diabetes. 2011;60:74-9.
12. Paniagua JA. Nutrition, insulin resistance and dysfunctional adipose tissue determine the different components of metabolic syndrome. World J Diabetes. 2016;7(19):483-514.
13. Tuomilehto J, Lindstrom J, Eriksson JG, et al. Finnish Diabetes Prevention Study Group: Prevention of type 2 diabetes mellitus by changes in lifestyle among subjects with impaired glucose tolerance. N Engl J Med. 2001;344:1343-50.
14. Diabetes Prevention Program Research Group. Long-term effects of lifestyle intervention or metformin on diabetes development and microvascular complications over 15-year follow-up: the Diabetes Prevention Program Outcomes Study. Lancet Diab Endocrinol. 2015;3(11):866-75.
15. van Dam RM, Willett WC, Rimm EB, et al. Dietary fat and meat intake in relation to risk of type 2 diabetes in men. Diabetes Care. 2002;25:417-424.
16. Reaven GM. Role of insulin resistance in human disease. Diabetes. 1998;37:1595-607.
17. Vessby B. Dietary fat and insulin action in humans. Br J Nutr. 2000;83:591-6.
18. Storlien LH, Jenkins AB, Chisholm DJ, et al. Influence of dietary fat composition on development of insulin resistance in rats. Relationship to muscle triglyceride and omega-3 fatty acids in muscle phospholipid. Diabetes. 1991;40:280-9.
19. Ascherio A, Katan MB, Zock PL, et al. Trans fatty acids and coronary heart disease. N Engl J Med. 1999;340:1994-8.
20. Ludwig DS. Dietary glycemic index and obesity. J Nutr. 2000;130: 280S-283S.
21. Toeller M. Lifestyle Issues: Diet. In: Holt RI, Cockram C, Flyvbjerg A, Goldstein BJ, (Eds). Textbook of Diabetes. Chichester: John Wiley & Sons; 2010.
22. Kumar S, Kiran MD. Patient knowledge of diabetes—Is there a need to spend more time with the patient? Int J Med Sci Diagn Res. 2019;3:31-6.
23. Kumar S, Abhyankar M, Malabade R. Knowledge, attitude and awareness of diabetes nutrition in physicians. Curr Res Diabetes Obes J. 2019;9(4): 555769.

11 CHAPTER

Insulin Resistance, Pathogenic Mechanism behind Acute and Chronic Complications

Sidhartha Das, Saroj K Tripathy

INTRODUCTION

More than 80 hormones known to be present in human body activate cyclic adenosine monophosphate (cAMP) for their actions but few like insulin along with atrial natriuretic peptide (ANP), brain-type natriuretic peptide (BNP) and nitric oxide are unique as they act by activating cyclic guanosine monophosphate (cGMP). The major metabolic fuel for the cells in the human body is glucose. Entry of glucose into the cells (barring the tissues of vital organs) is mediated by insulin. Insulin is an anabolic hormone, though mainly responsible for glucose homeostasis, is protean and has got widespread other actions as well. These include lipogenesis, protein synthesis, regulation of various genes in insulin responsive cells, anti-apoptotic functions and anti-inflammatory functions.[1] Insulin also has mitogenic activity and helps in protection of endothelium and mitochondrial functions. Effects of insulin are mainly of two types, i.e. metabolic plus anti-apoptotic and nonmetabolic in nature.[2] The metabolic and anti-apoptotic effects of insulin are mediated through signaling pathways involving insulin receptor substrate (IRS) protein, phosphorylation and activation of genes responsible for regulation of phosphatidyl inositol-3 kinase (PI-3K), protein kinase B (AKT), molecular target of rapamycin (mTOR) and P70S6 kinase.[2] The nonmetabolic, proliferative and mitogenic effects are mediated by Ras, Raf and mitogen-activated protein kinase (Erk1/Erk2). Insulin acts on adipose tissue, skeletal muscles and cardiac muscles in a stimulatory or inhibitory manner.[2] So insulin as a hormone is not only essential for glucose homeostasis but also involved in a wide range of different metabolic and nonmetabolic functions.

UNDERSTANDING INSULIN RESISTANCE (FIG. 1)

The hormone insulin acts by binding to insulin receptors of the cells for glucose entry. When either the cells have less number of insulin receptors or become unresponsive to insulin action after insulin binds to its receptors (post-receptor defect), it is referred to as insulin resistance (IR) to overcome this IR, the pancreatic β cells secrete more insulin for similar biological effect causing hyperinsulinemia.[2] A stage comes when the pancreatic β cells cannot cope with this anymore and the spectrum of hyperglycemic states like impaired glucose tolerance (IGT), prediabetes and diabetes mellitus (DM) ensues. Insulin resistance has been defined as "resistance to the metabolic effects of insulin, i.e. its suppressive effects on endogenous glucose production, stimulatory effects on glucose uptake in peripheral tissue especially peripheral muscles, glycogen synthesis and inhibitory effect of insulin on adipose tissue." Insulin resistance is of two types, i.e. type A (defect in insulin signaling pathways) and type B (autoantibodies-directed against insulin receptors).[2]

Though our knowledge of acute and chronic complication in diabetes and prediabetes is enormous, IR is fast emerging as the common soil where various maladies have their root. Starting from clustering with conventional risk factors of cardiovascular disease (CVD), IR is also proven to be associated with nontraditional risk factors of CVD as well. Insulin resistance has been incriminated in metabolic syndrome, polycystic ovarian syndrome (PCOS), sexual dysfunction, gestational diabetes mellitus (GDM), fetal developmental abnormalities and perinatal morbidity.[3] IR is being increasingly recognized as a chronic low-level inflammatory state and is pro-atherosclerotic.[3]

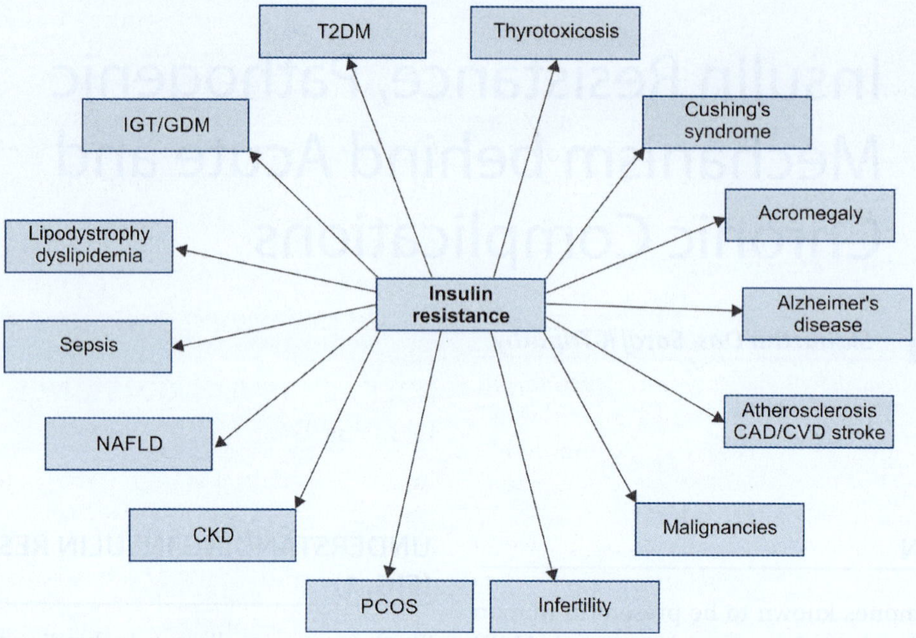

(CAD: coronary artery disease; CKD: chronic kidney disease; CVD: cardiovascular disease; GDM: gestational diabetes mellitus; IGT: impaired glucose tolerance; NAFLD: nonalcoholic fatty liver disease; PCOS: polycystic ovarian syndrome; T2DM: type 2 diabetes mellitus)

Figure 1 Understanding insulin resistance (IR).

FACTORS BEHIND INSULIN RESISTANCE

Insulin resistance has been found to be more common in Latino, African-Americans, Native Americans and Asian Americans. People with family history of diabetes are more prone to develop IR. Aging, ethnicity, increase in abdominal (visceral) fat, lack of exercise, smoking, lack of sleep and presence of acanthosis nigricans have been associated with IR. Genetics also plays a major role in development of IR and numbers of genetic linkages have been incriminated in IR development. Derangements in insulin-signaling pathways and process of glucose uptake and metabolism involving numerous proteins causes development of IR.[2] Hence, candidate genes that can potentially influence insulin action is legion, anyone of which can have variants influencing insulin sensitivity and resistance.[2] Common genetic variations resulting in IR involves fatty acid-binding protein 2 (FAB2), β_3-adrenergic receptor (B-3AR), insulin receptor substrate 1 (IRS-1), angiotensin-converting enzyme (ACE), lipoprotein lipase and tumor necrosis factor-alpha (TNF-α).[2]

How we Diagnose Insulin Resistance?

Homeostasis assessment model (HOMA) developed by Matthew and coworkers has been revalidated as a reliable method to assess IR by just utilizing single fasting plasma glucose (FPG) and corresponding fasting insulin level.[4]

Homeostasis assessment model insulin resistance (HOMA-IR) is used for assessment of IR whereas HOMA-B is used for assessment of β-cell function. HOMA-IR has been shown to exactly mirror the IR values obtained by the euglycemic glucose clamp technique in the assessment of insulin sensitivity.[5] The calculation for HOMA-IR and HOMA-B is given below:

$$\text{HOMA-IR} = \frac{\text{FSI (mu/L)} \times \text{FPG (mmol/L)}}{22.5}$$

$$\text{HOMA-B} = \frac{360 \times \text{Fasting insulin (mU/mL)}}{[\text{FPG (mg/dL)} - 63]}$$

Homeostasis assessment model insulin resistance score of 1 is ideal and HOMA-IR more than 2 is taken as insulin resistance. HOMA-IR score of more than 1 implies less than 100% insulin sensitivity and suggests initiation of IR. Different studies have revealed IR score less than 2 to be normal. A study by Das et al. has revealed HOMA-IR value of less than 2 to be normal value of IR in Indian people.[3] HOMA-IR score of 2.06 ± 0.14 was also found by Bonora et al. in nondiabetic populations.[5]

In HOMA-B calculation normal β-cell function is assumed to be 100% in normal population and β-cell dysfunction is detected by discrepancy in this.[4]

The importance of IR in acute and chronic complication of diabetic subjects is well known but the role of IR in other diseases is fast emerging as an important entity.

ROLE OF INSULIN RESISTANCE IN ATHEROSCLEROTIC DISEASES LIKE CARDIOVASCULAR DISEASE AND STROKE

Insulin is anti-atherogenic by its action on fat metabolism by inhibiting adipocyte lipolysis and stimulating lipogenesis by acting on different enzymes like triglyceride lipase, pyruvate dehydrogenase, FA synthetize and by promoting nonesterified free-fatty acid (NEFA) reesterification.[6] So naturally IR promotes atherosclerosis. Insulin resistance clusters with several traditional risk factors several [DM, hypertension (HTN), increase in very-low-density lipoprotein (VLDL), triglycerides (TG) and decrease in high-density lipoprotein (HDL)] and nontraditional risk factors (markers of coagulation, systemic proatherosclerotic chronic low inflammatory state, subclinical vascular disease, dysregulated adipokine signaling and oxidative stress) for CVD.[1] The relationship of IR with atherosclerosis and inflammation is not a mere association but has been proven to be causative. Regarding the presence of inflammation in IR studies have revealed positive correlation between IR and acute-phase reactants like high-sensitivity C-reactive protein (*hs*-CRP) which can be used as predictors of outcome and risk for future CV events in CAD patients.

In a study by S Das and SN Routray, et al. IR was also found even in normoglycemic angiographically established CAD patients.[7] They observed HOMA-IR more than 2.5 in 90% of diabetic patients, 78% in IGT patients and 40% in normoglycemic patients with CAD suggesting IR as the probable culprit for high incidence of CAD in India.[7] Not only established diabetic patients have more risk for cerebrovascular accidents (CVA) people with IR but also have more thrombotic CVA and peripheral arterial diseases (PAD).

ROLE OF INSULIN RESISTANCE IN CHRONIC KIDNEY DISEASES

It has been seen that even in patients of early stages of chronic kidney disease (CKD) there is peripheral resistance to insulin and IR has been positively correlated with the rate of progression of CKD.[8] High IR has been documented in many studies in CKD irrespective of their diabetic status. Uremia exerts inhibitory effect on insulin secretion by β cells.[8] β-cell dysfunction has been documented in CKD patients when compared with controls by various studies. Significant increase in IR and β-cell dysfunction in CKD is clearly associated with accelerated atherosclerosis.[9,10] HOMA-IR values positively correlates with CIMT (carotid intima-media thickening), a marker of atherosclerosis among both diabetic and nondiabetic subjects as well.

ROLE OF INSULIN RESISTANCE IN LIVER DISEASES

Insulin resistance has been incriminated in various liver diseases like nonalcoholic fatty liver disease (NAFLD), simple steatosis, nonalcoholic steatohepatitis (NASH) and cirrhosis of liver.[11] A study by S Das, SP Singh, et al. (2010) has revealed that IR was significantly higher in Grade III-NASH patients as compared to Grade I NASH patients irrespective of their glycemic status.[11] Other Indian studies have also documented increase IR in NAFLD patients.[12] The association of IR with NAFLD who have some features of metabolic syndrome (MS) as well, suggests NAFLD may be the liver component of MS.[6,13] Various other studies have established positive correlation between values of IR and necroinflammatory changes in the liver.

ROLE OF INSULIN RESISTANCE IN MATERNAL AND CHILD HEALTH

Nowadays epidemic of diabetes and atherosclerotic diseases in adults is attributed to undernutrition and IR in their fetal life.[14] Undernutrition in utero gives rise to maladaptation, metabolic dysfunction in liver, changes in the structures of heart, blood vessels and kidney, resetting of pituitary-adrenal-growth hormone-insulin axis and also changes in the pancreas. Insulin does not cross the placental barrier but the role of IR in fetal metabolism with deleterious effect has been documented.[14] Insulin resistance has been found in both low- and high-birth-weight babies. This U-shaped trend suggests interaction between environmental factors and genetics even in fetal life. Insulin resistance is proven to be the primary pathogenic mechanism behind polycystic ovarian syndrome (PCOS).[15] The development of IR in pregnancy, especially during late pregnancy is attributed to the appearance of many hormones, like placental growth hormone, human placental lactogen, estrogen, progesterone, prolactin, cortisol and TNF-α and they antagonize insulin action and results in IR and GDM. Endothelium dysfunction and low-grade inflammation by IR is considered as the central pathophysiological process in the development of GDM in MS patients. As Indian women have 11-fold increased risk for development of GDM as compared to Caucasian women, looking for IR and glucose intolerance during pregnancy is important. The subfertility in obese women is also now attributed to IR where hypothalamic kisspeptin suppression causes hypogonadism and decreased ovulation.[16]

ROLE OF INSULIN RESISTANCE IN SEPSIS AND MULTIORGAN DYSFUNCTION SYNDROME

In acute inflammatory states and infections IR is also emerging as a major player. In sepsis interplay of clinical, inflammatory, endocrine, hematological and metabolic changes results in organ failure. Profound negative nitrogen balance, acute hyperglycemia and IR play major role in sepsis.[17] Even mild hyperglycemia is potentially harmful by its procoagulant, apoptotic properties compounded by increased risk of infections due to impaired neutrophil function and delayed wound healing.[17] Mortality rises in sepsis due hyperglycemia and IR. A clinical trial conducted by Van den Berg et al. involving adults admitted in intensive care unit (ICU) who were on mechanized ventilation has shown that intensive insulin therapy has reduced overall in hospital mortality by 34%, bloodstream infection by 46%, acute renal failure requiring dialysis by 41%.[18] Hyperglycemia increases the rolling, adhesion and transmigration of leukocytes by upregulating the adhesion molecules such as intercellular cell adhesion molecule 1 (ICAM-1), vascular cell adhesion molecule 1 (VCAM-1) and P and E selectin due to IR. The renal dysfunction in sepsis also contributes to IR. Insulin resistance in sepsis is due to the combined effect of neuroendocrine dysfunction and cytokines. Studies have revealed that β-cell over-exhaustion also occurs in critically-ill patients. Insulin resistance and β-cell function assessment has been found to be a reliable indicator of the severity of sepsis and has a bearing on the mortality of patients with multiorgan dysfunction syndrome (MODS).[17]

ROLE OF INSULIN RESISTANCE IN MALIGNANCIES

Studies have revealed clear association between MS and increased risk of endometrial carcinoma. In the industrialized countries excess weight gain has been associated with endometrial carcinoma as well. Hyperglycemia, IR, and hyperinsulinemia promote growth of cancer cells by elevating the level of free insulin-like growth factor-1 (IGF-1). The lack of anti-apoptotic stimulus in IR promotes invasion of cancer cells and metastasis.

REFERENCES

1. Libby P, Ridker PM, Hansson GK. Inflammation in atherosclerosis: from pathophysiology to practice. J Am Coll Cardiol. 2009;54(23):2129-38.
2. Reaven GM. Role of insulin resistance in human disease. Diabetes. 1988;37(12):1595-607.
3. Das S, Bhoi SK, Baliarsinha AK, et al. Autoimmunity, insulin resistance and beta cell function in subjects with low body weight type 2 diabetes mellitus. Metab Syndr Rel Dis. 2007;5(2):136-41.
4. Matthews DR, Hosker JP, Rudenski AS, et al. Homeostasis model assessment: insulin resistance and β-cell function from fasting plasma glucose and insulin concentrations in man. Diabetologia. 1985;28(7):412-9.
5. Bonora E, Targher G, Alberiche M, et al. Homeostasis model assessment closely mirrors the glucose clamp technique in the assessment of insulin sensitivity: studies in subjects with various degrees of glucose tolerance and insulin sensitivity. Diabetes Care. 2000;23(1):57-63.
6. Das S, Baliarsinha AK. Insulin resistance and dyslipidemia two-way relationship. In: Venkataraman S (Ed). Medicine Update, Volume 14., Mumbai, Maharashtra: The Association of Physician in India; 2004. pp. 100-5.
7. Das S, Das GK, Behera M, et al. Prevalence of metabolic syndrome in angiographically established coronary artery disease patients. South Asian J Prev Cardiol. 2007;11(3):93-9.
8. Fadda GZ, Massry SG. Glucose and insulin metabolism. Metabolism and endocrine disturbances in uremia. In: Massry SG, Glassoek RJ (Eds). Massry and Glassock's Textbook of Clinical Nephrology, 4th revised edition. Philadelphia, PA: Lippincott Williams and Wilkins; 2000. pp. 1390-4.
9. Chen J, Muntner P, Hamm LL, et al. Insulin resistance and risk of chronic kidney disease in nondiabetic US adults. J Am Soc Nephrol. 2003;14(2):469-77.
10. Kobayashi S, Maesato K, Moriya H, et al. Insulin resistance in patients with chronic kidney disease. Am J Kid Dis. 2005;45(2):275-80.
11. Das S, Singh SP, Parida PK, et al. Non-alcoholic fatty liver disease in subjects with type 2 diabetes mellitus and non-diabetics with special reference to insulin resistance and hepatic histopathological changes. Diabetes Metab Syndr Clin Res Rev. 2010;4(4):226-9.
12. Amarapurkar DN, Patel ND. Prevalence of metabolic syndrome in non-diabetic and non-cirrhotic patients with non-alcoholic steatohepatitis. Trop Gastroenterol J Digest Dis Found. 2004;25(3):125-9.
13. Marchesini G, Brizi M, Bianchi G, et al. Nonalcoholic fatty liver disease: a feature of the metabolic syndrome. Diabetes. 2001;50(8):1844-50.
14. Das S, Behera MK, Misra S, et al. β-cell function and insulin resistance in pregnancy and their relation to fetal development. Metab Syndr Relat Dis. 2010;8(1):25-32.
15. Misra S, Parida N, Das S, et al. Effect of metformin in Asian Indian women with polycystic ovarian syndrome. Metab Syndr Relat Dis. 2004;2(3):192-7.
16. Das S, Misra B, Roul L, et al. Insulin resistance and β-cell function as prognostic indicator in multi-organ dysfunction syndrome. Metab Syndr Relat Dis. 2009;7(1):47-51.
17. Awlaqi AA, Alkhayat K, Hammadeh ME. Metabolic syndrome and infertility in woman. Int J Woman's Health Reprod Sci. 2016;4(3):89-95.
18. Van den Berghe G, William A, Herman G. Intensive insulin therapy in medical ICU. N Engl J Med. 2001;345:1359-67.

12 CHAPTER

Do Differences in Body Composition Explain Racial and Ethnic Differences in Type 2 Diabetes Mellitus Risk?

Edward J Boyko

INTRODUCTION

At the very end of the last century, type 2 diabetes mellitus prevalence increased dramatically in high-income countries. Soon afterward, a similar increase was seen in low- and middle-income countries in parallel with economic improvement, which was due to increase in prevalence of overweight and obesity, and lifestyle changes characterized by less physical activity and greater availability of food of higher caloric density. Risk however varied across and within countries; especially notable were racial and ethnic differences.[1] Compared to Caucasians of European ancestry, nearly all other ethnic/racial groups are at higher risk for type 2 diabetes. The identification of the causes of such differences became a high-priority research interest. The most likely explanation was thought to be genetic differences across racial and ethnic groups. However, thorough research on genetic factors has not succeeded in explaining ethnic/racial differences specifically, and in general has not succeeded in explaining more than 10–15% of type 2 diabetes inheritance.[1,2] The identification of causes of such ethnic/racial differences in diabetes risk is still a high-priority research interest, as a solution to this problem may further understanding of the pathophysiology of this disorder and present new options for prevention and/or treatment.

Excess adiposity is a well-recognized risk factor for the development of type 2 diabetes mellitus. A discordance, though, exists between diabetes prevalence and degrees of adiposity across countries. Figure 1 displays prevalence of

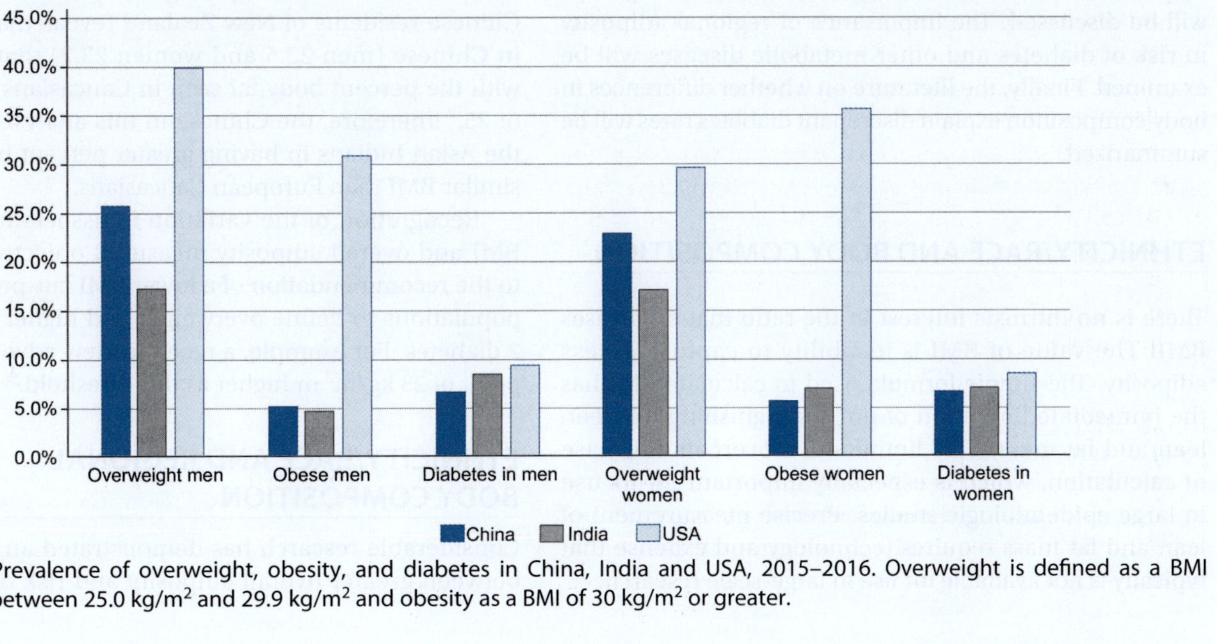

Figure 1 Prevalence of overweight, obesity, and diabetes in China, India and USA, 2015–2016. Overweight is defined as a BMI between 25.0 kg/m^2 and 29.9 kg/m^2 and obesity as a BMI of 30 kg/m^2 or greater.

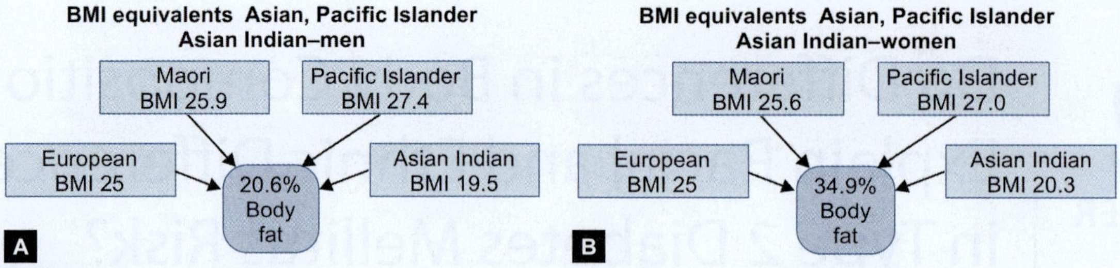

Figures 2A and B BMI equivalents by ethnicity/race at a given body fat proportion as determined by DXA. (A) Men; (B) Women.

overweight and obesity defined as body mass index (BMI) $\geq$25 kg/m^2, <30 kg/m^2, and $\geq$30 kg/m^2, respectively in China, India, and the United States in 2015 from the Global Burden of Disease Study.[3] The prevalence of overweight and obesity in the United States greatly exceeds that seen in China and India. The lowest prevalence of overweight and obesity is seen in India, except for Indian women, whose obesity prevalence is slightly higher than Chinese women. Despite the much lower rates of obesity and overweight in China and India, the prevalence of diabetes in 2015 or 2016 is nearly the same in India as the United States and just slightly lower than India in China.[4-6] These findings suggest several possibilities, such as factors other than body composition driving risk of diabetes in China and India, or that use of BMI as an index of body composition requires different interpretation in South and East Asian populations.

This chapter will address several issues pertinent to the understanding of ethnic/racial differences in diabetes risk in view of these observations. The value of an overall adiposity index and its meaning across ethnic/racial groups will be discussed. The importance of regional adiposity in risk of diabetes and other metabolic diseases will be examined. Finally, the literature on whether differences in body composition explain discrepant diabetes rates will be summarized.

ETHNICITY/RACE AND BODY COMPOSITION

There is no intrinsic interest in the ratio that comprises BMI. The value of BMI is its ability to capture excess adiposity. The simple formula used to calculate BMI has the immediate limitation of not distinguishing between lean and fat mass. This limitation is overcome by ease of calculation, which is especially important for its use in large epidemiologic studies. Precise measurement of lean and fat mass requires technology and expense that typically is not available for use in large-scale research.

When BMI has been studied as a surrogate for fat mass, results clearly demonstrate that its interpretation varies depending on ethnicity/race. Researchers in New Zealand compared BMI to dual-energy X-ray absorptiometry (DXA) measurements of body fat percent across 30–39-year-old European Caucasian, indigenous Maori, South Pacific Islander, and Asian Indian participants.[7] The results for men are shown in Figure 2A. At a BMI of 25, European Caucasians measure a body fat percent of 20.6%. This same body fat percent was associated with a higher BMI in both Maori and Pacific Islanders (25.9–27.4), and a much lower BMI among Asian Indian (19.5). These results demonstrate that Maori and Pacific Islander men are leaner than European Caucasians at a BMI of 25, while Asian Indians would have a much higher body fat percent. Very similar results are seen with regard to the differences in the relationships between BMI and percent body fat by ethnicity/race among women (Fig. 2B), although it should be noted that percent body fat is greater at similar levels of BMI to men for all ethnic/racial groups. A similar comparison conducted among European Caucasian and Chinese residents of New Zealand revealed a lower BMI in Chinese (men 22.5 and women 23.2) that correlated with the percent body fat seen in Caucasians with a BMI of 25.[8] Therefore, the Chinese in this analysis resembled the Asian Indians in having greater percent body fat at a similar BMI than European Caucasians.

Recognition of the variation in association between BMI and overall adiposity measured objectively has led to the recommendation of a lower BMI cut-point in Asian populations to define overweight and higher risk of type 2 diabetes. For example, a recent review advocated a cut-point of 23 kg/m^2 or higher as this threshold.[9]

ETHNICITY/RACE AND REGIONAL BODY COMPOSITION

Considerable research has demonstrated an association between greater overall adiposity and risk of metabolic

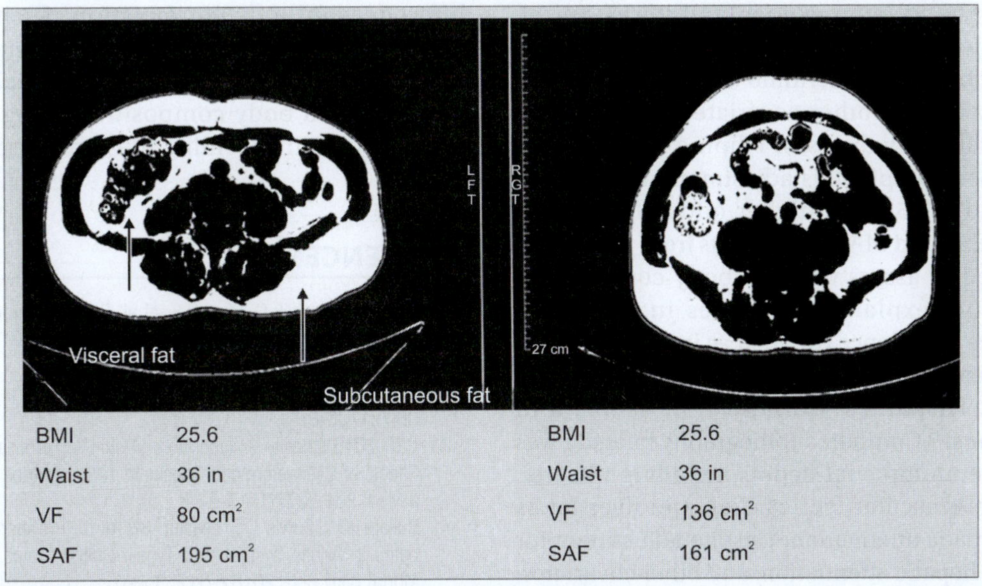

Figure 3 Abdominal CT scans demonstrating cross-sectional visceral and subcutaneous fat areas in two men with identical BMI and waist circumference but discrepant visceral and subcutaneous fat areas.

diseases such as diabetes mellitus. However, it has more recently been recognized that fat distribution also is relevant in the prediction of risk of diabetes and associated conditions, with the visceral fat depot showing a stronger association with conditions such as diabetes and hypertension than the subcutaneous fat depot or overall adiposity.[10,11] Although a correlation exists between fat stored viscerally, and both overall adiposity and surface measurements such as waist circumference and body size, it is well known that considerable differences may exist with regard to size of the visceral fat depot across individuals with similar BMI and waist circumference. Figure 3 demonstrates two such individuals with identical measurements of BMI and waist circumference but substantially different visceral and abdominal subcutaneous fat areas.

Furthermore, size of regional adipose depots have been shown to vary by ethnicity/race.[12] Research comparing visceral fat areas measured at the L4-L5 level using computed tomography in Caucasian American men from Pennsylvania, USA, and Japanese men from Kusatsu, Japan demonstrated higher visceral fat areas in Japanese men for all quartiles of waist circumference and significantly higher areas in quartiles 2 and 3. Further research performed in the USA demonstrated significant ethnic differences among five ethnic groups studied, with Japanese Americans showing the greatest visceral fat area relative to total adiposity (Table 1).[13]

TABLE 1: **Visceral adipose tissue area in Caucasian and Japanese men aged 40–49 years by waist circumference quartile.**

	Visceral fat area	
Waist circumference quartiles (Q1–Q4)	Caucasians (n = 177)	Japanese (n = 239)
Q1 (waist circumference: 68.0–82.8 cm)	47.6 cm²	52.9 cm²
Q2 (waist circumference: 82.9–88.9 cm)	70.2 cm²	84.8 cm²
Q3 (waist circumference: 89.0–96.8 cm)	85.5 cm²	101.7 cm²
Q4 (waist circumference: 96.9–114.3 cm)	117.8 cm²	120.3 cm²

DO DIFFERENCES IN BODY FAT DISTRIBUTION EXPLAIN RACIAL AND ETHNIC DIFFERENCES IN DIABETES RISK?

Given that body composition varies by ethnicity, a potential explanation for the noted differences in risk of diabetes mellitus and other associated disorders by ethnicity/race is differing distribution of body fat. This question has been addressed to date in only two studies to my knowledge. Araneta and Barrett-Connor explored differences in diabetes risk and visceral adiposity measured using computed tomography in 181 Filipino, 193 African-American, and 196 Caucasian women.[14] Filipino women were noted to have significantly higher visceral fat area than Caucasian women despite similar BMI and waist circumference. Diabetes prevalence was highest among the Filipino women and lowest in the Caucasian women. A multivariable logistic regression analysis was performed to determine whether adjustment for visceral fat area and other covariates mediated the greater probability of diabetes in Filipino compared to Caucasian women. Despite this adjustment, the Filipino women still had a 7.51-fold higher odds of diabetes. Similarly, the MESA and MASALA cohorts from the United States were used to assess whether body composition differences could explain differences in abnormal glucose tolerance prevalence (defined as impaired fasting glucose or diabetes mellitus) in South Asians compared to Caucasians, Hispanics, Chinese-Americans, and African-Americans.[15] Computed tomography imaging was used to measure multiple fat depots including visceral, abdominal, intermuscular, pericardial, and liver fat as measured by hepatic attenuation. Despite adjustment for these fat depots, hepatic attenuation, and other covariates, a significantly higher prevalence of abnormal glucose tolerance persisted in South Asians compared to the four other ethnic groups. These results argue against differences in body composition explaining ethnic/racial differences in diabetes prevalence. The main limitation of the research conducted by Araneta et al. and Flowers et al. is its cross-sectional design, which does not permit assessment of temporal sequence. Longitudinal research is needed to establish whether changes in fat depot sizes precede or follow the development of diabetes mellitus.

CONCLUSION

Important ethnic/racial differences exist regarding the risk of developing type 2 diabetes mellitus. Multiple explanations for such differences have been explored. A better understanding of the factors driving these differences in risk could potentially lead to better understanding of the pathogenesis of type 2 diabetes and such knowledge might lead to improvements in treatments and/or prevention strategies. Body composition clearly varies by ethnicity/race. Research performed to date though has not demonstrated that these ethnic/racial body composition differences explain or mediate the differences in diabetes risk by ethnicity/race. Clearly missing from research performed is a prospective investigation of whether ethnic and racial differences continue to be associated with a higher risk of diabetes mellitus after adjusting for differences in body composition. Such research may take years to conduct, but the possibility exists that an existing cohort study that enrolled multiple ethnic groups and measured body composition using imaging might be a shortcut in providing these necessary longitudinal findings.

REFERENCES

1. Golden SH, Yajnik C, Phatak S, et al. Racial/ethnic differences in the burden of type 2 diabetes over the life course: a focus on the USA and India. Diabetologia. 2019;62(10):1751-60.
2. Florez JC. Mining the Genome for Therapeutic Targets. Diabetes. 2017; 66(7):1770-8.
3. GBD 2015 Obesity Collaborators, Afshin A, Forouzanfar MH, et al. Health Effects of Overweight and Obesity in 195 Countries over 25 Years. N Engl J Med. 2017;377(1):13-27.
4. Bullard KM, Cowie CC, Lessem SE, et al. Prevalence of Diagnosed Diabetes in Adults by Diabetes Type—United States, 2016. MMWR Morb Mortal Wkly Rep. 2018;67(12):359-61.
5. India State-Level Disease Burden Initiative Diabetes C. The increasing burden of diabetes and variations among the states of India: the Global Burden of Disease Study 1990-2016. Lancet Glob Health. 2018;6(12): e1352-62.
6. Liu M, Liu SW, Wang LJ, et al. Burden of diabetes, hyperglycaemia in China from to 2016: Findings from the 1990 to 2016, global burden of disease study. Diabetes Metab. 2019;45(3):286-93.
7. Rush EC, Freitas I, Plank LD. Body size, body composition and fat distribution: comparative analysis of European, Maori, Pacific Island and Asian Indian adults. Br J Nutr. 2009;102(4):632-41.
8. Wen JY, Rush EC, Plank LD. Assessment of obesity in New Zealand Chinese: a comparative analysis of adults aged 30-39 years from five ethnic groups. NZ Med J. 2010;123(1327):87-98.
9. Hsu WC, Araneta MR, Kanaya AM, et al. BMI cut points to identify at-risk Asian Americans for type 2 diabetes screening. Diabetes Care. 2015; 38(1):150-8.
10. Boyko EJ, Fujimoto WY, Leonetti DL,et al. Visceral adiposity and risk of type 2 diabetes: a prospective study among Japanese Americans. Diabetes Care. 2000;23(4):465-71.
11. Hayashi T, Boyko EJ, Leonetti DL, et al. Visceral adiposity is an independent predictor of incident hypertension in Japanese Americans. Ann Intern Med. 2004;140(12):992-1000.
12. Lear SA, Humphries KH, Kohli S,et al. Visceral adipose tissue accumulation differs according to ethnic background: results of the Multicultural Community Health Assessment Trial (M-CHAT). Am J Clin Nutr. 2007;86(2): 353-9.
13. Lim U, Monroe KR, Buchthal S, et al. Propensity for Intra-abdominal and Hepatic Adiposity Varies Among Ethnic Groups. Gastroenterology. 2019; 156(4):966-75e10.
14. Araneta MR, Barrett-Connor E. Ethnic differences in visceral adipose tissue and type 2 diabetes: Filipino, African-American, and white women. Obes Res. 2005;13(8):1458-65.
15. Flowers E, Lin F, Kandula NR, et al. Body Composition and Diabetes Risk in South Asians: Findings From the MASALA and MESA Studies. Diabetes Care. 2019;42(5):946-53.

13 CHAPTER Could We Have Changed the Drivers of the Diabetes?

CL Nawal, RS Chejara

INTRODUCTION

Diabetes mellitus is a common metabolic disorder characterized by hyperglycemia due to absolute insulin deficiency and/or insulin resistance.[1] Traditional risk factors like sedentary lifestyle, obesity, smoking, and intake of energy-dense food with high-glycemic index are clearly linked with onset of diabetes mellitus. Genetically, no single gene is responsible for development of diabetes but involvement of multiple genes and mutations are identified. Interplay of genetic susceptibility, environmental factors, and lifestyle drive an individual into diabetic status. In recent years, many new risk factors have been identified in individuals that can help physicians to prevent and intervene to delay or prevent the onset of diabetes.[2]

ESTABLISHED DRIVERS OF DIABETES MELLITUS

The role of already established risk factors in prediction and prevention of diabetes (Box 1), obesity is a major risk factor that can drive an individual into diabetic status. Markers such as body mass index (BMI), waist circumference, and waist/hip ratio are closely linked with obesity.

Hyperinsulinemia and insulin resistance increase with weight gain and diminish with weight loss. Metabolic syndrome and insulin resistance syndrome encompass obesity, hypertension, and are strongly associated with development of diabetes. Insulin resistance is more strongly linked to intra-abdominal fat than to fat elsewhere. Despite nearly universal insulin resistance, most obese persons do not develop diabetes; however, obesity is a major risk factor for diabetes. Up to 80% of patients with type 2 diabetes mellitus are obese. Weight loss and exercise, even of modest degree, are associated with increased insulin sensitivity and improved glucose control in diabetes.

Major genes that predispose diabetes are yet to be identified; it is clear that the disease is polygenic. Susceptibility genes or polymorphisms that have been identified may contribute to the risk of type 2 DM include: Calpain-10, Pro12Ala (common) variant of peroxisome proliferator-activated receptor γ, and Glu23Lys variant of the adenosine triphosphate-sensitive potassium channel Kir6.2. Concordance in identical twins: 70–90%, 1% with disease: increased risk both parents with disease: risk approaches 40%. A genetic defect may not manifest itself unless an environmental event or another genetic defect, such as obesity, is superimposed.[1]

Ethnicity and positive family history of diabetes can predict future development of diabetes in offspring. African American, Hispanic American, Native American, Asian American, Pacific Islanders are at increased risk. South East Asian regions, particularly Indians and Chinese, are at more risk as compared to Europeans. India is having leading number of cases in the world and called diabetic capital of the world.[3]

BOX 1 Risk factors for developing diabetes.

- Family history of diabetes
- Obesity
- Race/ethnicity
- Sedentary lifestyle
- Gestational diabetes mellitus and polycystic ovarian syndrome
- Dyslipidemia

INTRAUTERINE PROGRAMMING OF DIABETES MELLITUS TYPE 2

Nutrition

With direct effects of genetic and environmental influences, there is strong evidence to link nutrition during intrauterine life and adult-onset diseases. Hales and Baker proposed that low-birth weight and fetal growth are crude markers of fetal well-being but commonly used. Low-birth weight is considered as a poor fetal nutrition and has been associated with metabolic abnormalities in later life.[4] Dutch Hunger Winter, a famous example of prenatal famine, showed that individuals who are exposed to famine in utero exhibit decreased glucose tolerance around 50 years later as compared with those born years before the famine. They have decreased muscle mass and increased fat mass compared with individuals of normal birth weight. Fat and lean mass both prenatally and postnatally show relationship with in utero exposure with a potential impact on future risk of diabetes type 2.[5]

Infection and Inflammation

Intrauterine infections affect the somatic as well as metabolic development of offspring. Viral infections are associated with poor growth of the fetus and birth defects such as enterovirus infection are associated with development of diabetes type 1. Similarly, inflammation during intrauterine life can alter immune and metabolic pathways. Causal effect of infections and inflammation may be linked through epigenetic reprogramming and changes in metabolism for the development of diabetes.[6,7]

ENDOCRINE DISRUPTORS

Humans are constantly exposed to environmental toxic chemicals through food, water, skin contact, and air pollution. These chemicals are associated with increased risk of endocrine and metabolism-related disorders. They are commonly called as endocrine-disrupting chemicals (EDCs). There is a long list of such toxic compounds including agriculture, chemical industry, food additives, air pollutants, water contaminants, preserved food products, paint and solvents, and medical care products. They contain pesticides, bisphenols, phthalates, polychlorinated phenyls, triclosan, parabens, and many more which have been proven EDCs in many studies.[8]

In the prototype of all EDCs, bisphenol A (BPA) is a common contaminant used in plastic and paper industry. Plastic utensils, water bottles, and toys contain bisphenol compounds. BPA promotes signaling via extranuclear signal transduction pathways including extracellular signal regulated kinase (ERK) and mitogen-activated protein kinase (MAPK). It also binds through estrogen receptor and produces metabolic changes in beta cells of pancreas. It affects the structures and functions of islet cells. Poor development of pancreas and decreased beta cell mass ultimately lead to decreased insulin secretion and development of diabetes mellitus.[9,10] Our recent studies also suggest that mitochondrial dysfunction could be a contributory factor in BPA-induced impairment of beta cell function.[11] Unlike pharmaceutical compounds, which hit specific molecular targets, EDCs affect multiple pathways making the understanding of the complex actions more difficult. Large number of environmental toxicants can work as EDCs.[12-14]

NOVEL BIOCHEMICAL RISK FACTORS FOR TYPE 2 DIABETES

Recently, many novel risk factors and biochemical markers for the prediction of future development of diabetes are being developed. Insight into other pathophysiology mechanisms has shown considerable interest of researchers. No one of them clearly predicts future diabetic risk but their presence may be used in different type of risk-scoring models.[2]

Adipose-derived Predictors of Diabetes

Adiponectin

This hormone is derived from fat cells and it increases insulin sensitivity and lipid clearance. Its insulin-sensitizing effect is attributable due to suppression of hepatic glucose production. As the obesity increases, its level decreases, and it also has anti-inflammatory effects. The role of adiponectin in pathogenesis of diabetes and obesity is better established than prediction of diabetes.[15,16]

Leptin

Leptin is a good biomarker of total fat mass in human. It regulates body weight and is closely associated with insulin resistance and metabolic syndrome. In BRHS study, leptin has found to be associated with risk of diabetes type 2 after adjusting other confounding factors like age, sex, and waist circumference.[15]

PAI-1

This hormone is synthesized by various tissue cells including hepatocytes, endometrium, and adipocytes. Levels increase with obesity. Many cytokines and hormones regulate the genes encoding PAI-1. The risk of diabetes type 2 may be indirectly related to hyperinsulinemia and inflammatory pathways associated with PAI-1.[17]

Hepatic-derived Drivers of Diabetes

ALT and GGT

High levels of alanine aminotransferase (ALT) and γ-glutamyltransferase (GGT) are associated with diabetes mellitus type 2 that is independent of confounding factors including obesity. Elevated levels are found with increased levels of liver fat content and NAFLD. Similarly, increased levels of GGT have strong association with incident diabetes after adjusting confounding variables like BMI.[18,19]

Sex Hormone-binding Globulin

Sex hormone-binding globulin (SHBG) is secreted by hepatocytes and is the main binding protein for circulating sex hormones in serum. Low levels are associated with incident diabetes and insulin resistance.[20]

Ferritin

Ferritin is a nutritional biomarker used for estimation of iron stores. It is also an acute phase reactant. There is positive association with diabetes mellitus type 2. Iron may directly damage the hepatocytes, promote oxidative stress, and impede the suppression of glucose production by insulin due to interplay of multiple diabetes-related factors and serum ferritin. To establish cause and effect relationship, further research is needed.[11]

Insulin-like Growth Factor-1

Insulin-like growth factor (IGF) is required for somatic growth and differentiation since intrauterine life. In adult life, majority of circulating hormone is secreted by hepatocytes and closely regulated by growth hormone influence. Together with insulin, IGF-1 is playing important role in glucose metabolism and homeostasis. In few studies, IGF-1 levels above the median work are associated with a subsequent low risk of insulin resistance and diabetes.[21]

Endothelium-derived Factors

Endothelial dysfunction plays a key role in insulin resistance and diabetes mellitus type 2. There are many endothelium-derived factors like tissue plasminogen activator (tPA), cell adhesion molecule, and von Willebrand's factors. Increased levels of tPA and PAI-1 complex are associated with incident diabetes and endothelial dysfunction. Various cell adhesion molecules like E-selectin and ICAM-1 are associated with increased diabetes risk, even after adjustment for confounding factors such as BMI, HbA1C, C-reactive protein (CRP), and fasting insulin.[22]

Inflammatory Factors

Research has linked inflammatory factors with obesity and diabetes. Early studies has only cross-sectional observation but now they have been followed since a long and found focused on molecular function and its function on metabolism; CRP is basically a hepatic-derived molecule driven by interleukin (IL)-6, a strong inflammatory mediator. CRP levels are also correlating with many other parameters relevant to diabetes. Multiple studies have been conducted and found significant relative risk of the tune of 2.37 (CI 1.57–3.58) compared to those with low CRP even after adjustment for obesity.[23]

Other factors such as acute phase response markers, raised WBC, fibrinogen, sialic acid, and low serum albumin are also linked to diabetes risk. Similarly, nutritional biomarkers like vitamin-C and vitamin-D levels and risk of diabetes are being studied but their direct correlation in cause and effect hypothesis is not established.

MODIFYING THE DRIVERS OF DIABETES

We have learned that there are multiple factors playing role as "drivers of diabetes". Starting from intrauterine life to growth and development of an individual throughout life, a battery of genetic and environmental factors drives them to develop diabetes mellitus. There is involvement of multiple genes and multiple metabolic pathways and their affection by multiple factors making the understanding and prevention of this complex metabolic disorder difficult.

What would have been better, if we could change the drivers of diabetes? Best of the best care throughout the development, away from the malnutrition, without environmental pollutants, perfect balance between energy requirement and expenditure can save us from diabetes.

Diabetes is a lifestyle disorder and prevention of diabetes is successful only when nutrition is balanced with energy intake and expenditure.

American Diabetes Association (ADA) recommends following recommendations for primary prevention in individuals who are at higher risk of developing diabetes:[9]

1. Among individuals at high risk for developing type 2 diabetes, structured programs that emphasize lifestyle changes, which include moderate weight loss (7% body weight) and regular physical activity (150 min/week), with dietary strategies including reduced calories and reduced intake of dietary fat, can reduce the risk for developing diabetes and are therefore recommended.
2. Individuals at high risk for type 2 diabetes should be encouraged to achieve the US Department of Agriculture (USDA) recommendation for dietary fiber (14 g fiber/1,000 kcal) and foods containing whole grains (one-half of grain intake).
3. There is not sufficient and consistent information to conclude that low-glycemic load diets reduce the risk for diabetes. Nevertheless, low-glycemic index foods that are rich in fiber and other important nutrients are to be encouraged.
4. Observational studies report that moderate alcohol intake may reduce the risk for diabetes, but the data do not support recommending alcohol consumption to individuals at risk of diabetes.
5. No nutrition recommendation can be made for preventing type 1 diabetes.
6. Although there are insufficient data at present to warrant any specific recommendations for prevention of type 2 diabetes in youth, it is reasonable to apply approaches demonstrated to be effective in adults, as long as nutritional needs for normal growth and development are maintained.

Clinical trial data from both the Finnish Diabetes Prevention Study and the Diabetes Prevention Program (DPP) in the US strongly support the potential for moderate weight loss to reduce the risk for type 2 diabetes. The lifestyle intervention in both trials emphasized lifestyle changes that included moderate weight loss (7% of body weight) and regular physical activity (150 min/week), with dietary strategies to reduce intake of fat and calories. In the DPP, subjects in the lifestyle intervention group reported dietary fat intakes of <34% of energy at baseline and <28% of energy after 1 year of intervention. A majority of subjects in the lifestyle intervention group met the physical activity goal of 150 min/week of moderate physical activity. In addition to preventing diabetes, the DPP lifestyle intervention improved several CVD risk factors, including dyslipidemia, hypertension, and inflammatory markers.[10,24]

Screening of the individuals for the prevention and early detection of diabetes mellitus, who are at increased risk, is beneficial in reducing the total burden on society. Modifiable risk factors such as obesity, hypertension, and dyslipidemia can be managed early to prevent future appearance of diabetes. Besides traditional risk factors, novel risk factors should be included in calculating risk and prevention of diabetes. Due to complex pathophysiology of this metabolic disorder, attributable risk for a particular risk factor cannot be assigned.

Industrialization and technological advancement is a continuous process of development. Health hazards related to them and their byproducts should be studied in parallel. Environmental pollutants, chemical toxicants, and food additives identified in causing as trigger factors for diabetes should be discouraged to human use or banned permanently. Consumption of high-carbohydrate diet, refined sugars, and low-fiber diet with use of food additives and coloring agents should be discouraged.

CONCLUSION

Obesity and diabetes are increasing in epidemic proportions and increasing the global burden on health resources. Besides traditional risk factors for diabetes mellitus like genes, lifestyle, and behavioral change, impact of intrauterine environment and epigenetics on future risk on adult life is increasingly recognized. Many novel risk factors working as drivers of diabetes including pesticides, bisphenols, polychlorinated biphenyls, phthalates, triclosan, and parabens commonly used by humans have been identified. They can work as EDCs and interfere with metabolic functions. Further longitudinal human studies are required to assign attributable risk for these drivers of diabetes.

REFERENCES

1. Fauci A, Braunwald E, Kasper K, et al. Chapter 338. Harrison's Principal of Internal medicine, 17th edition.
2. Sattar N, Wannamethi SG, Forouuhi NG. Novel biochemical risk factors for type 2 diabetes: pathogenic insights or prediction possibilities? Diabetologia. 2008;51(6):92640.
3. Golden SH, Yajnik C, Phatak S, et al. Racial/ethnic differences in the burden of type 2 diabetes over the life course: a focus on the USA and India. Diabetologia. 2019;62(10):1751-60.
4. Ravelli AC, van der Meulen JH, Michels RP, et al. Glucose tolerance in adults after prenatal exposure to famine. Lancet. 1998;351(9097):173-7.

5. Fernandez-Twinn DS, Hjort L, Novakovic B, et al. Intrauterine programming of obesity and type 2 diabetes. Diabetologia. 2019;62(10):1789-801.
6. Dahlquist GG, Ivarsson S, Lindberg B, et al. Maternal enteroviral infection during pregnancy as a risk factor for childhood IDDM. A population-based case-control study. Diabetes. 1995;44(4):408-13.
7. Allen DW, Kim KW, Rawlinson WD, et al. Maternal virus infections in pregnancy and type 1 diabetes in their offspring: systematic review and meta-analysis of observational studies. Rev Med Virol. 2018;28(3):e1974.
8. Sargis RM, Simmons RA. Environmental neglect: endocrine disruptors as underappreciated but potentially modifiable diabetes risk factors. Diabetologia. 2019;62(10):1811-22.
9. American Diabetes Association, Bantle JP, Wylie-Rosett J, et al. Nutrition Recommendations and Interventions for Diabetes, A position statement of the American Diabetes Association. Diabetes Care. 2008;31 Supl 1: S61-78.
10. Tuomilehto J, Lindstrom J, Eriksson JG, et al. Prevention of type 2 diabetes mellitus by changes in lifestyle among subjects with impaired glucose tolerance. N Engl J Med. 2001;344(18):1343-50.
11. Jiang R, Manson JE, Meigs JB, et al. Body iron stores in relation to risk of type 2 diabetes in apparently healthy women. JAMA. 2004;291(6):711-7.
12. Bansal A, Rashid C, Xin F, et al. Sex- and dose-specific effects of maternal bisphenol A exposure on pancreatic islets of first- and second-generation adult mice offspring. Environ Health Perspect. 2017;125(9):097022.
13. Tiano JP, Mauvais-Jarvis F. Importance of oestrogen receptors to preserve functional beta-cell mass in diabetes. Nat Rev Endocrinol. 2012;8(6): 342-51.
14. Whitehead R, Guan H, Arany E, et al. Prenatal exposure to bisphenol A alters mouse fetal pancreatic morphology and islet composition. Horm Mol Biol Clin Invest. 2016;25(3):171-9.
15. Wannamethee SG, Lowe GD, Rumley A, et al. Adipokines and risk of type 2 diabetes in older men. Diabetes Care. 2007;30(5):1200-5.
16. Daimon M, Oizumi T, Saitoh T, et al. Decreased serum levels of adiponectin are a risk factor for the progression to type 2 diabetes in the Japanese population: the Funagata Study. Diabetes Care. 2003;26(7):2015-20.
17. Davidson M, Zhu J, Lu W, et al. Plasminogen activator inhibitor-1 and the risk of type 2 diabetes mellitus in American Indians: the Strong Heart Study. Diabet Med. 2006;23(10):1158-9.
18. Schindhelm RK, Diamant M, Dekker JM, et al. Alanine aminotransferase as a marker of nonalcoholic fatty liver disease in relation to type 2 diabetes mellitus and cardiovascular disease. Diabetes Metab Res Rev. 2006;22(6):437-43.
19. Wannamethee SG, Shaper AG, Lennon L, et al. Hepatic enzymes, the metabolic syndrome, and the risk of type 2 diabetes in older men. Diabetes Care. 2005;28(12):2913-8.
20. Haffner SM. Sex hormone-binding protein, hyperinsulinemia, insulin resistance and noninsulin-dependent diabetes. Horm Res. 1996;45(3-5):233-7.
21. Sandhu MS, Heald AH, Gibson JM, et al. Circulating concentrations of insulin-like growth factor-I and development of glucose intolerance: a prospective observational study. Lancet. 2002;359(9319):1740-5.
22. Rask-Madsen C, King GL. Mechanisms of disease: endothelial dysfunction in insulin resistance and diabetes. Nat Clin Pract Endocrinol Metab. 2007;3(1):46-56.
23. Dehghan A, Kardys I, de Maat MP, et al. Genetic variation, C-reactive protein levels, and incidence of diabetes. Diabetes. 2007;56(3):872-8.
24. Knowler WC, Barrett-Connor E, Fowler SE, et al. Reduction in the incidence of type 2 diabetes with lifestyle intervention or metformin. N Engl J Med. 2002;346(6):393-403.

CHAPTER 14 Diabetes Reversal

Banshi Saboo, Dharmendra Panchal

INTRODUCTION

Diabetes mellitus type 2 is a chronic silently progressive disorder. Natural history of the disease encompasses various clinical stages starting from normal glycemia to impaired glucose tolerance, impaired fasting hyperglycemia, prediabetes to overt diabetes, and end up in grievous complications. Reversal of diabetes is possible as evident by bariatric surgery, low calorie diet, and low carbohydrate diet. Currently available literature defines reverse journey of diabetes in various ways as remission or reversal or postdiabetes. The postulated mechanism behind reversal of diabetes is weight loss attributable to restriction of food intake. In real world scenario, acceptance for the people with type 2 diabetes for restricted calorie is very low. Also in all studies, durability of reversal is also questioned beyond 1 year and even the available definitions for the reverse journey of diabetes do not define clinical status of the patient across the diabetes journey. We propose the clinical classification of diabetes and its reversal pathway which is more practical and sustainable.

REVERSAL CONCEPT[1,2]

Reversal is defined as a change to an opposite direction, position, or course of action.

Remission is defined as absence of signs and symptoms of the disease. It is evident from the definition that disease can recur at any time in the future.

Cure is defined as restoration of health and no evidence of the disease process.

When apply these definitions in context of type 2 diabetes, reversal is referred as the change in opposite direction of the clinical state of the patient or in underlying disease processes. To say that "type 2 diabetes is reversing" is a statement meaning that there is reversal in clinical state of the patient which may vary from decreased requirement of medicine with maintaining good glycemic control at a point in time to stoppage of diabetes medicines. Though, it does not imply more future prediction, can define a state in the continue journey of diabetes which may lead to remission. So a state of reversal in diabetes is just like a car reversed into a space.

When patient with type 2 diabetes is able to sustain nondiabetic glucose control over a period of time without any medicine, it is called as diabetes in remission considering the risk of future relapse. Although to state cure in context of type 2 diabetes is not reasonable as there is always a chance for relapse but prolonged remission might be operationally considered as cure.

DEFINITIONS

To define reversal or remission in type 2 diabetes, there are two questions need to be answered (Table 1).

1. Level of glycemic threshold to be achieved.
2. Duration minimum to sustain the defined glycemic threshold.

NATURAL HISTORY OF TYPE 2 DIABETES[3–6]

Natural history of the disease encompasses various clinical stages starting from normal glycemia to impaired glucose tolerance, impaired fasting hyperglycemia, and prediabetes to overt diabetes.

Two distinct hallmarks of type 2 Diabetes are insulin resistance and β-cell dysfunction.[7] pathophysiology

TABLE 1: Definitions into diabetes reversal.

Ref.	Terminology	FPG (mg/dL)	HbA1c (%)	Duration	Treatment
ABCD[8]	Remission	<126	<6.5	6 months	No
ADA[1]	Partial remission	100–125	<6.5	1 year	No
ADA[1]	Complete remission	<100	<5.7	1 year	No
ADA[1]	Prolonged remission	<100	<5.7	5 years	No
R Taylor et al.[2]	Post diabetes	<126	<6.5	2 months	No
V Sarathi et al.[9]	Partial reversal	100–125		3 months	No
V Sarathi et al.[9]	Complete reversal	<100		3 months	No

operating behind the development of type 2 diabetes starts with genetic predisposition for insulin resistance, which when triggered by epigenetic factors and positive energy balance leads to fatty liver. Fatty liver becomes established years before the onset of type 2 diabetes. It appears necessary but not sufficient for the development of type 2 diabetes. The subsequent period of years of overexposure of the islets to an elevated plasma triacylglycerol level and a modest increase in the plasma glucose level is necessary to precipitate beta cell decompensation. It is evident that at the diagnosis of type 2 diabetes, β-cell function is typically reduced to 50% of normal by homeostatic model assessment (HOMA) modeling and to a greater extent on dynamic testing. Although it is accepted that increased apoptosis plays a role in decreased β-cell mass over time, apoptosis alone is insufficient to explain the profound islet dysfunction in established type 2 diabetes. Loss of the fully differentiated phenotype is a recently recognized potential mechanism underlying loss of β-cell function in type 2 diabetes. Chronic glucolipotoxicity leads to loss of β-cell transcriptional factors to form dedifferentiated β-cell also known as empty cells, which contribute to impaired β-cell function. β-cell dedifferentiation also enables conversion toward other pancreatic endocrine phenotypes that are less susceptible to nutrient-induced mitochondrial and endoplasmic reticulum stress, a phenomenon known as β-cell to α-cell conversion, which is responsible for aberrant postprandial hyperglucagonemia. Thus muscle insulin resistance determines the rate at which fatty liver progresses, and ectopic fat deposition in the liver and islets underlies the related dynamic defects of hepatic insulin resistance and b β-cell dysfunction (Table 2).

TABLE 2: Steps in pathogenesis of type 2 diabetes.[3]

Natural history	Time scale
Genetic predisposition to insulin resistance	Lifelong
Positive energy balance	Years
Accelerated progression of insulin resistance	Years
Increased hepatic fat and plasma triacylglycerol	Years
Increased hepatic glucose output	Few years
Initial increased plasma glucose	Few years
Glucolipotoxicity	Months to years
Reduced first phase insulin secretion	Months to years
Hyperglycemia	Months
β cell dysfunction and irreversible loss	>2 years

REVERSAL OF TYPE 2 DIABETES

Type 2 diabetes may now be seen as a potentially reversible state associated with longstanding nutrient overload in susceptible individuals. The evidence of this came from various studies of bariatric surgery, very low calorie diet, and low carbohydrate diet therapy in individuals with type 2 diabetes. There are sufficient studies showing that by changing lifestyle dramatically, the control of diabetes can be significantly improved and a significant proportion of patients can either reduce or come off their glucose-lowering therapies (Table 3).

MECHANISM OF REVERSAL OF TYPE 2 DIABETES[3-6]

The first hint that type 2 diabetes was a fully reversible syndrome came from bariatric surgery. Initially, it was postulated that postbariatric surgery beneficial glycemic effect was mediated by increased postmeal Glucagon-like peptide 1 (GLP-1) secretion. However, because GLP-1 has negligible glucose effects in the fasting state and no enteral feeding had preceded the observation of normalized fasting plasma glucose, the concept that a postmeal spike in

TABLE 3: Studies of type 2 diabetes reversal.[6]

Study	Counterpoint[7]	Counterbalance[10]	Direct[11]
Description	Reversal in people diagnosed with type 2 diabetes for less than 4 years	6 months sustained reversal in people diagnosed with type 2 diabetes for up to 23 years	12 months sustained reversal by primary care intervention in people diagnosed with type 2 diabetes for up to 6 years
N	11	29	64
Duration (year)	0–4	0–23 (<4 year-14; >8 year-15)	0-6
Past Treatment	Diet ± metformin	All OAD except TZD	All except insulin
Weight loss (kg)	15·3 (all responders)	*Responders*: 15·8; *Non-responders*: 13·6	*Responders*: 16·2; *Non-responders*: 13·4
Timing of observations after weight loss	Immediately after weight loss	Weeks, then 6 months, after weight loss	2–4 weeks, then 7–8 months, after weight loss
HbA1c	*Baseline*: 7·4%; After weight loss: 6·0	Responders *Baseline*: 7·1% After weight loss: 5·9% Non-responders *Baseline*: 8·4% After weight loss: 7·8%	Responders *Baseline*: 7·4% After weight loss: 5·8% Non-responders *Baseline*: 7·9% After weight loss: 7·6%
Number (%) that achieved non-diabetic status*	11 (100%)	13 (43%)	29 (64%)

Data for the DiRECT substudy are currently available only up to 12 months of follow-up.
*Nondiabetic status defined as HbA1c < 6·1% and fasting plasma glucose < 110 mg/dL.
(HbA1c: glycated hemoglobin; TZD: thiazolidinediones OAD: oral antidiabetic)

GLP-1 concentration could account for the improvement after bariatric surgery is physiologically improbable.[6] It is now known that glycemic benefit is directly in relation to the degree of weight loss rather than allocation to either surgical or medical group. The mechanism behind reversal of diabetes is weight loss attributable to restriction of food intake whether after bariatric surgery or through diet alone, which leads to rapid fall in hepatic and intrapancreatic fat because of decreased export of very low density lipoprotein triglyceride from the liver. Removal of the fat allows re-expression of the insulin gene leading to redifferentiation of β-cells and resumption of acute glucose-mediated insulin secretion. The counterpoint study has enlightened the time course of recovery of β-cell function. After 1 week of calorie restriction, there was no improvement in the first-phase insulin glucose though the fasting plasma glucose was already normalized. This happened due to very rapid return of normal hepatic insulin sensitivity. By 4 weeks into the counterpoint study, a first-phase insulin response could be seen in the group as a whole, and by 8 weeks, this was well within the normal range and significantly improved from baseline. The slow normalization of the first-phase insulin response may be due to slow normalization of total intrapancreatic fat. So, redifferentiation provides an attractive potential underlying mechanism for the recovery of β-cell function after a reduction in islet fat content over the time course. However, muscle insulin resistance remains almost unchanged by weight loss-induced reversal of diabetes. Insulin resistance in muscle is permissive but not determinant in the natural history of type 2 diabetes (Table 4).

TABLE 4: Steps in reversal of type 2 diabetes.[3]

Reverse step	Time scale
Negative energy balance	Days
Reduced hepatic fat	Days
Increased hepatic insulin sensitivity	Days
Improved first phase insulin secretion	Week
Decreased plasma glucose	Weeks
Decreased plasma triacylglycerol	Weeks

NEWER CLINICAL CONCEPT OF DIABETES REVERSAL

As discussed earlier when we say that "type 2 diabetes is reversing" is a statement meaning that there is reversal in clinical state of the patient which may vary from decreased requirement of medicine with maintaining good glycemic control at a point in time to stoppage of diabetes medicines. Current definition of reversal in diabetes fails to define patient's clinical journey with medical management, which encompass vast majority of the patients. The proposed method for diabetes reversal by calorie restriction is not applicable practically to most patients as well as there is always the chance of relapse and if it is not monitored, it may end up into some gravious complications. Hence, we propose that even the person with type 2 diabetes who is able to achieve glycemic target with treatment and if it is possible to maintain glycemic target with gradual reduction in medical treatment along with maintaining good lifestyle should be defined as reversal. This clinical classification can be useful as motivation tool for the patient to adhere the lifestyle therapy to upgrade their state toward remission. Also it can clearly point out their current state of diabetes. To make it simpler, we can classify the currently available diabetes treatment into five groups (Table 5):

1. Insulin secretor (IP)	:	Insulin, SU, and glinides
2. Insulin sensitizer (IS)	:	Metformin, TZD
3. Incretin enhancer (IE)	:	GLP1 Ra, dipeptidyl peptidase-4 inhibitor (DPP4i)
4. Glucose restrictor (GR)	:	Alpha-glucosidase inhibitor (AGI)
5. Glucose excretor (GE)	:	Sodium-glucose cotransporter type 2 inhibitor (SGLT2i)

TABLE 5: Clinical definition of diabetes reversal.

	A1C*	Medication
Control	<7.0	Any
Reversal stage 1	<6.5	IE/IS/GE/GR
Reversal stage 2	<6.5	IS, GE, GR
Reversal stage 3	<6.5	IS
Reversal stage 4	<5.7	IS
Remission	<5.7	No
Prolonged remission	<5.7	No

*At least two HbA1c 3 months apart.

CONCEPT OF PERSONAL FAT[2,6,12]

After weight loss in both Counterbalance and DiRECT, half of those who returned to nondiabetic glucose control still had a body mass index (BMI) > 30 kg/m^2. Thus there is no relevance of an individual's BMI category in achieving and maintaining diabetes reversal. Rather personal threshold permitting safe storage of fat in the subcutaneous compartment is more important. The personal fat threshold concept says that ectopic fat accumulation only occurs when an individual's capacity to store fat safely in the subcutaneous compartment is exceeded. The concept also explains the increased predisposition of some ethnic groups such as South Asians to develop type 2 diabetes at a relatively low BMI.

DURATION OF DIABETES AND REVERSAL[2,12]

The importance of duration of type 2 diabetes since diagnosis is clear from the Counterbalance dataset, with 60% remission in those with duration < 4 years, compared with 21% with duration > 8 years. No patients who had been diagnosed with diabetes for more than 11 years returned to nondiabetic fasting plasma glucose concentrations. The β-cell dysfunction and loss of end-differentiated β-cell phenotype can be restored by substantial weight loss. Thus 2–3 years of type 2 diabetes does not usually produce irreversible β-cell damage while after 10 years onward β-cell dedifferentiation precipitates irreversible loss of insulin secretion unless a substantial decrease in body weight is achieved.

CLUSTERS OF DIABETES MELLITUS[13,14]

A recent study has identified five replicable clusters of adult-onset diabetes with different disease progression and risk of diabetes complications. The five clusters are (Table 6):

1. Severe autoimmune diabetes (SAID),
2. Severe insulin deficient diabetes (SIDD),
3. Severe insulin-resistant diabetes (SIRD),
4. Mild obesity-related diabetes (MOD) and
5. Mild age-related diabetes (MARD)

Based on insulin resistance, it would likely be SIRD, MOD, and MARD that could go into remission.

CONCLUSION

Type 2 diabetes is potentially reversible disorder, provided efforts are done in early stage of the disease (< 2 years)

TABLE 6: Clusters of diabetes.[13,14]

Subgroup	BMI	Metabolic control	Insulin physiology
SAID	Relatively low	Poor	Insulin deficiency
SIDD	Relatively low	Poor	Insulin deficiency
SIRD	High	Fair	Insulin resistance
MOD	High	Fair	Insulin resistance
MARD	Relatively low	Fair	Insulin resistance

(MARD: mild age-related diabetes; MOD: mild obesity-related diabetes; SAID: severe autoimmune diabetes; SIDD: severe insulin deficient diabetes; SIRD: severe insulin-resistant diabetes)

when there is sufficient pancreatic β-cell reserve. Weight loss and calorie restriction are known to induce remission in disease. Redifferentiation of β-cell plays a major role in diabetes reversal. Still, it is very difficult to for the majority of the patients to adopt restricted calorie diet and even if the evidence is strong for remission of diabetes after bariatric surgery, it is unlikely to be advocated at the population level due to the high cost and lack of surgeons well trained to perform bariatric surgeries and there is always possibility of relapse in future if weight is regained. As majority of type 2 diabetes patient are on some medical management and if they are able to maintain the glycemic target, it is advisable to deintensify the therapy with continue effort to improve lifestyle. Clinical staging of the reverse journey in type 2 diabetes is therefore very useful to motivate and guide the patient towards remission. It also helps to formulate realistic achievable goals for type 2 diabetes management based on patient characteristic such as age, duration of disease, comorbidities, etc. we advocate the use of clinical approach for the reversal in diabetes for the better management and achieve the desirable target.

REFERENCES

1. Buse JB, Caprio S, Cefalu WT, et al. How Do We Define Cure of Diabetes? Diabetes Care. 2009;32(11):2133-5.
2. Taylor R, Barnes AC. Can type 2 diabetes be reversed and how can this best be achieved? James Lind Alliance research priority number one. Diabet Med. 2019;36(3):308-15.
3. Taylor R. Pathogenesis of type 2 diabetes: tracing the reverse route from cure to cause. Diabetologia. 2008;51:1781-9.
4. White MG, Shaw JA, Taylor R. Type 2 diabetes: The pathologic basis of reversible b-cell dysfunction. Diabetes Care. 2016;39:2080-8.
5. Lim EL, Hollingsworth KG, Aribisala BS, et al. Reversal of type 2 diabetes: normalisation of beta cell function in association with decreased pancreas and liver triacylglycerol. Diabetologia. 2011;54:2506-14.
6. Taylor R, Al-Mrabeh A, Sattar N. Understanding the mechanisms of reversal of type 2 diabetes. Lancet Diabetes Endocrinol. 2019;7(9):726-36.
7. Taylor R. Type 2 Diabetes: Etiology and reversibility. Diabetes care. 2013;36:1047-55.
8. Nagi D, Hambling C, Taylor R. Remission of Type 2 Diabetes: A Position Statement from the Association of British Clinical Diabetologists (ABCD) and the Primary Care Diabetes Society (PCDS). [online] Available from https://www.researchgate.net/publication/334075558_Remission_of_type_2_diabetes_a_position_statement_from_the_Association_of_British_Clinical_Diabetologists_ABCD_and_the_Primary_Care_Diabetes_Society_PCDS [Last accessed October, 2019].
9. Sarathi V. Reversal of diabetes in newly diagnosed T2DM. J Nat Sci Biol Med. 2017;8(1): 60-1.
10. Steven S, Hollingsworth KG, Al-Mrabeh A, et al. Very low calorie diet and 6 months of weight stability in type 2 diabetes: pathophysiological changes in responders and non-responders. Diabetes Care. 2016;39:158-6.
11. Taylor R, Al-Mrabeh A, Zhyzhneuskaya S, et al. Remission of human type 2 diabetes requires decrease in liver and pancreas fat content but is dependent upon capacity for β cell recovery. Cell Metab. 2018;28:547-56.
12. Taylor R. Calorie restriction for long-term remission of type 2 diabetes. Clin Med. 2019;19(1):37-42.
13. Ang GY. Reversibility of diabetes mellitus: Narrative review of the evidence. World J Diabetes. 2018;9(7):127-31.
14. Ahlqvist E, Storm P, Käräjämäki A, et al. Novel subgroups of adult-onset diabetes and their association with outcomes: a data-driven cluster analysis of six variables. Lancet Diabetes Endocrinol. 2018;6:361-9.

3 SECTION

Diagnosis and Classification

15 CHAPTER

Type 3c Diabetes: A Different Variety

Chandrasekhar Valupadas

INTRODUCTION

Diabetes mellitus (DM) is a heterogeneous disease characterized by hyperglycemia and complications associated with it. It can be caused by multiple pathological defects in multiple organ systems in the body. The *ominous octet* is the term used to describe eight pathological defects which results in hyperglycemia, shown in Figure 1. However, no single defect is said to be causative but more commonly multiple pathologies work in simultaneously. This complexity resulted in confusion for classifying this pandemic disease of the world, though World Health Organization (WHO) oversimplify into four types, type 1 being auto immune, type 2 with insulin resistance, type 3 secondary forms of DM, and type 4 gestational diabetes. Nevertheless, for proper diagnosis and optimal management of diabetes, not only classification of disease but also true understanding of the pathogenesis and organ responsible for disease development is more important. One such disease which comes to discussions these days is

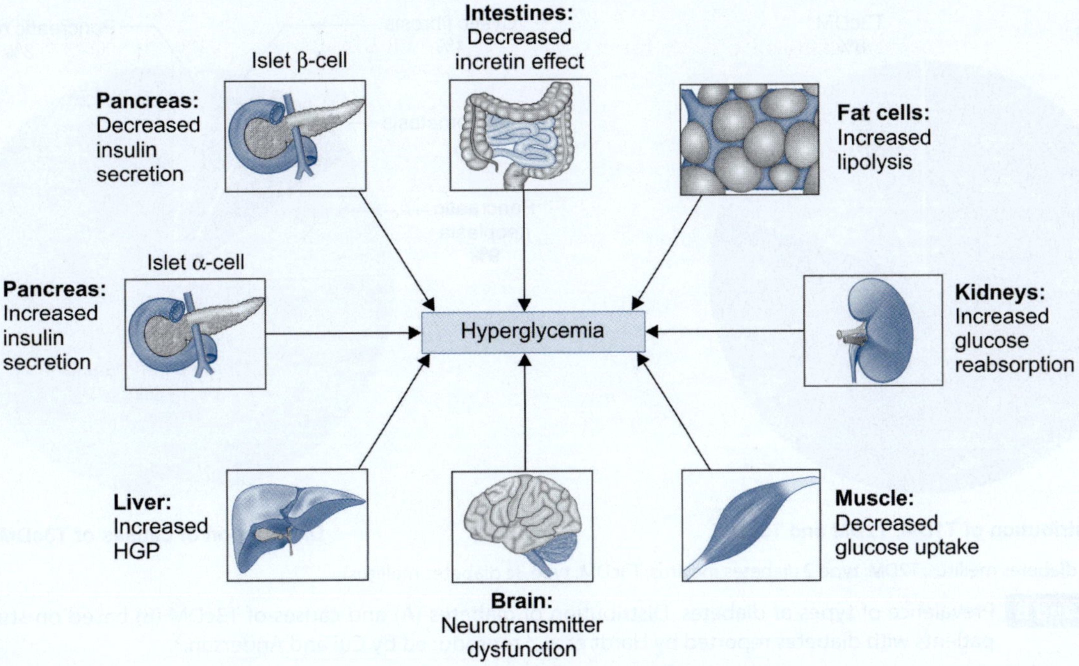

Figure 1 The ominous octet: pathophysiologic abnormalities of type 2 diabetes mellitus.

so called "pancreatogenic diabetes", which is also classified as type 3c diabetes mellitus (T3cDM). This chapter will review its prevalence, pathophysiological aspects, clinical characteristics, diagnostic criteria, and management aspects of T3cDM in contrast with common type 1 diabetes mellitus (T1DM) and type 2 diabetes mellitus (T2DM).

ESTIMATED PREVALENCE

True global prevalence of T3cDM is still not known; however, two possible strategies exist for generating an estimate. First strategy is to evaluate the prevalence of diabetes among patients having pancreatic diseases. Second strategy is to evaluate the prevalence of pancreatic diseases in a cohort comprising diabetic patients. On the basis of some studies, it seems reasonable to assume that the true prevalence of T3cDM is possibly in the range of 1–9% of diabetes patients (Figs. 2A and B).[1–3]

DEFINITION

In history, diabetes that is caused because of diseases related to the exocrine pancreas was defined as pancreatogenous or pancreatogenic diabetes. However, in recent times, WHO and by the American Diabetes Association referred and classified it as T3cDM.[4,5] T3cDM means "diabetes because of impairment in pancreatic endocrine function associated with pancreatic exocrine damage caused because of acute, relapsing and chronic pancreatitis, pancreatic cancer, and cystic fibrosis, pancreatectomy, and hemochromatosis, as well as rare causes like neonatal diabetes caused by pancreatic agenesis". Data on the prevalence of T3cDM is limited.

PATHOPHYSIOLOGY

Pancreas is the organ which collectively works as exocrine and endocrine gland (Fig. 3). Endocrine dysfunction represents deficiency of insulin, glucagon, pancreatic polypeptide (PP), and incretin hormones secreted by islets of Langerhans. There is slight interplay of mechanisms with production of glucagon from alpha-cells and other autocrine hormones from delta-cells. Abnormality of endocrine function results in diabetes. Typically, there is some degree of exocrine dysfunction (i.e. abnormality in the acinar and duct tissue of pancreas) along with malabsorption and maldigestion of nutrients.[3,6,7] The exocrine dysfunction in turn impairs secretion of glucagon-like peptide 1 (GLP-1) and glucose-dependent insulinotropic polypeptide (GIP) causing incretin defect (paracrine actions between pancreas and gut) through enteroinsular axis. With decreased incretin hormones

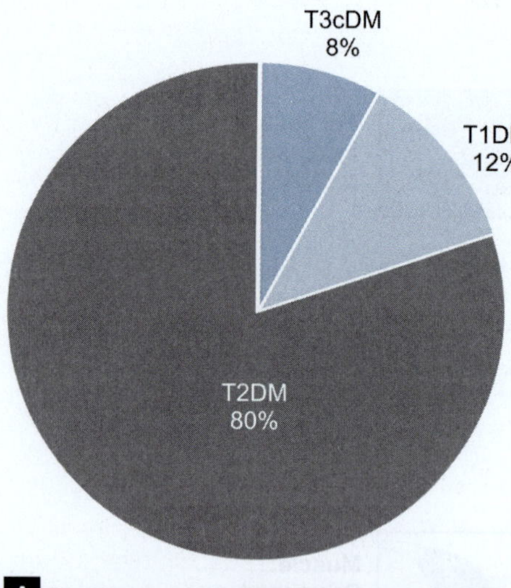

A **Distribution of T1DM, T2DM and T3cDM**

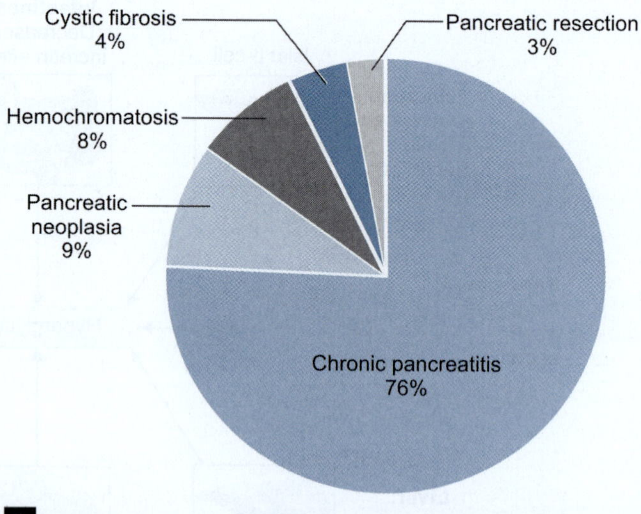

B **Distribution of causes of T3cDM**

(T1DM: type 1 diabetes mellitus; T2DM: type 2 diabetes mellitus; T3cDM: type 3c diabetes mellitus)

Figures 2A and B Prevalence of types of diabetes. Distribution of diabetes (A) and causes of T3cDM (B) based on studies of 1,922 patients with diabetes reported by Hardt et al.,[2] reproduced by Cui and Andersan.[3]

(*Source*: Hardt PD, Brendel MD, Kloer HU, et al. Is pancreatic diabetes (type 3c diabetes) underdiagnosed and misdiagnosed? Diabetes Care. 2008;31:S165-9; Cui Y, Andersen DK. Pancreatogenic diabetes: special considerations for management. Pancreatology. 2011;11:279-94.)

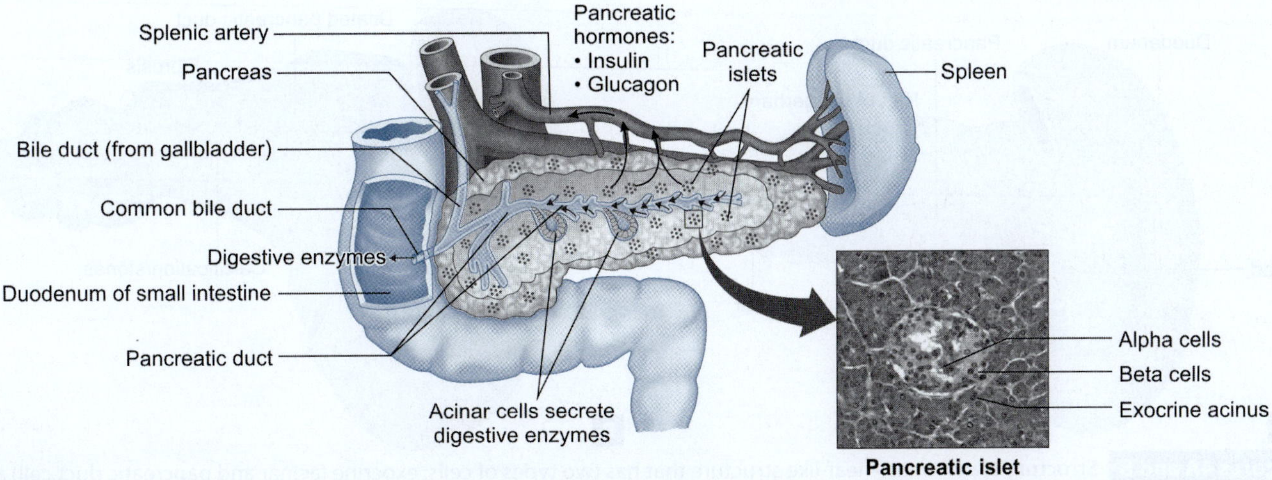

Figure 3 Pancreas. The pancreatic exocrine function involves the acinar cells secreting digestive enzymes that are transported into the small intestine by the pancreatic duct. Its endocrine function involves the secretion of insulin (produced by beta cells) and glucagon (produced by alpha cells) within the pancreatic islets. These two hormones regulate the rate of glucose metabolism in the body. The micrograph reveals pancreatic islets. LM × 760.

(*Source*: Anatomy and Physiology. (2012). The Endocrine System. Chapter 17. The Regents of University of Michigan Medical School 2012. [online] Available from https://opentextbc.ca/anatomyandphysiology/chapter/17-9-the-endocrine-pancreas/. [Last accessed September, 2019].[7])

there is progressive islet failure in T3cDM. Hence oral pancreatic enzyme replacement therapy (PERT) not only improves dyspepsia and steatorrhea but also prevents the further progression of T3cDM.

Interestingly, there is interplay between exocrine and endocrine pancreas because of anatomical proximity though physiologically unrelated. As a direct result of other illnesses affecting exocrine pancreas, such as cystic fibrosis, ductal adenocarcinoma, and pancreatitis, diabetes may also develop. It is essential to notice that T3cDM is not a single entity; it takes place due to a variety of exocrine pancreatic diseases along with variable mechanisms of hyperglycemia. The pathophysiological background of T3cDM varies, although it is categorized as a unified group of secondary diabetes. Pancreatic damage disturbs the complex interplay of digestion, absorption, and utilization of nutrient at the different levels.

Ultimately, pathogenesis of T3cDM is because of decrease in insulin secretion, although insulin sensitivity of the hepatic and peripheral tissue differs.[6,8] Impaired counter-regulation because of poor glucagon secretion; blunted catecholamine response; and impaired hepatic gluconeogenesis activation lead to high glycemic excursions resulting in poor management.[9]

Fibrosis of pancreatic tissue induces insulin deficiency which can be explained by anatomical and physiological interactions between islet cells and acinar tissue (Figs. 4A and B). The common insuloacinar portal circulation (Fig. 5) is reason for exocrine pancreas and is exposed to higher concentrations of islet hormones, which is essential for efficacy of acinar tissue. During parenchymal replacement by fibrous tissue there is ischemic islets atrophy with random survival of some residual functional acini and islets, unlike selective insulinitis and diffuse destruction by autoimmune process in T1DM. Tissue sensitivity to insulin is not overtly impaired in chronic pancreatitis, this is distinctive from T2DM. Beta-cell function inversely regulates alpha-cell function through paracrine mechanisms. During the process of development of T3cDM, glucagon secretion becomes impaired; causing associated "brittle diabetes" in T3cDM. Since PP cells are peripherally placed, there function is diminished in the early course. PP deficiency is responsible for isolated hepatic insulin resistance and is hallmark of T3cDM.

CLINICAL FEATURES

Because exocrine insufficiency is generally present prior to endocrine insufficiency in case of chronic pancreatitis, majority of the patients having T3cDM have a prior history of pancreatitis with abdominal pain, steatorrhea (increase in fat in floating stools) or maldigestion with glucose intolerance and nutritional deficiencies.[8]

Some of the cases present with indigestion and abdominal pain devoid of a prior history of pancreatitis.

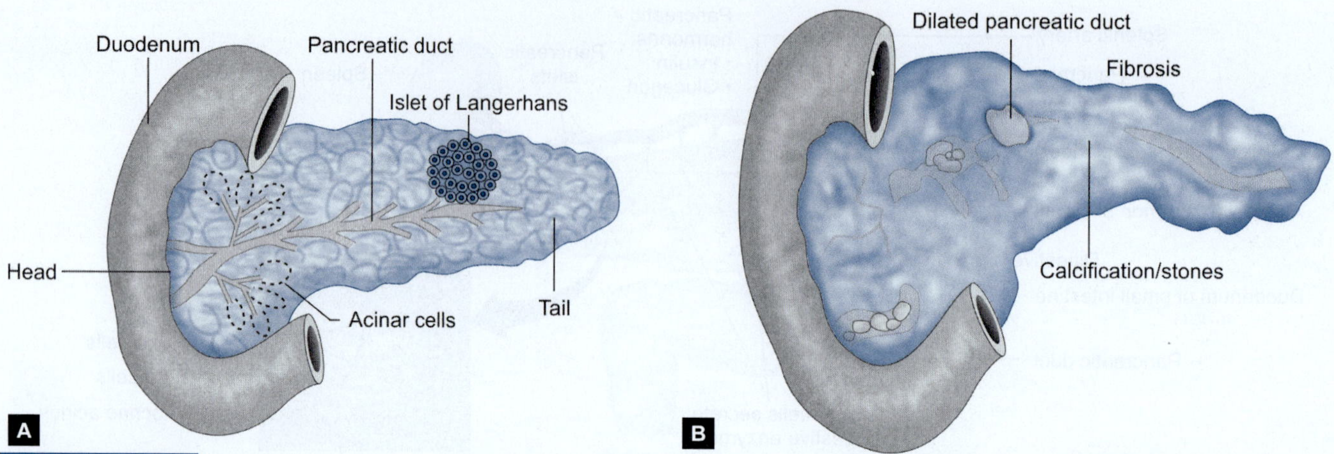

Figures 4A and B Structure of pancreas—leaf-like structure that has two types of cells: exocrine (acinar and pancreatic duct cell) and endocrine (islets of Langerhans) cells (A). The inflammatory process in the pancreas promotes fibrosis (scarring of tissue), calcification or stones and dilated pancreatic duct (B).

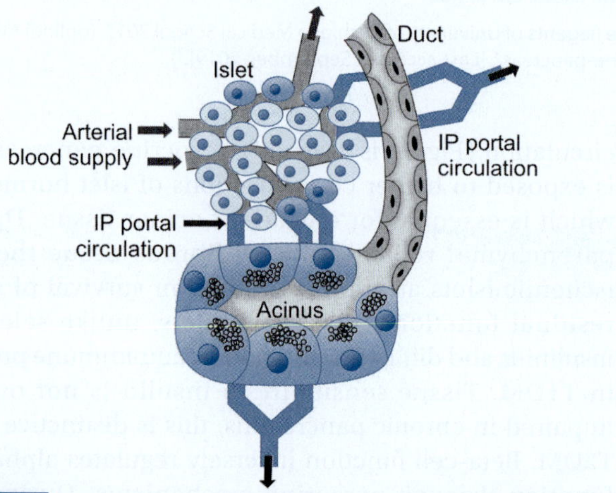

Figure 5 Schematic representation of the islet-acinar-ductal axis. An endocrine islet is shown receiving arterial blood supply. Some of this arterial blood drains into an intrapancreatic (IP) portal circulation that bathes adjacent acinar and ductal cells. The insulin-rich blood supply exerts trophic effects on these cells that are most evident in the acinar cells making up one such acinus. The acinar cells are large and have many enzyme-rich zymogen granules (shown as small circles within each acinar cells).

Infrequently, only glucose intolerance may be visible without any features of pancreatic disease.

In the later stages of the disease, along with progressive loss of islet cells and decrease in glucagon secretion too, progresses to the brittle diabetes that is characterized by marked glycemic lability and recurrent hypoglycemia.[10,11]

The beta-cell deficit is rarely absolute, unlike T1DM, and therefore these patients rarely have diabetic ketoacidosis.

Table 1 explains comparative clinical features of T1DM, T2DM, and T3cDM.

DIAGNOSTIC CRITERIA FOR TYPE 3C DIABETES

There are no diagnostic criteria that are universally accepted for T3cDM. The diagnosis can be made in patients who meet the following three criteria as outlined in Table 2.[12]

However, because of many significant factors, these criteria are limited, comprising overlapping of features with long-standing T1DM and T2DM, low standardization of methods used to determine β-cell function and insulin resistance, lack of published high-quality data, etc.

Complications of Type 3c Diabetes Mellitus

Renal dysfunction, retinopathy, microangiopathic complications, and neuropathy occur as recurrently in T3cDM as in the case of T1DM as well as T2DM. Macrovascular complications are thought to occur less frequently because of chronic malabsorption and commonly occurring undernutrition, but there is a lack of research and long-term studies, as well as incomplete understanding of the risks is present.

MANAGEMENT

As of now there no RCTs data available hence lack of evidence-based guidelines specific to management of T3cDM. However, general measures for the management of any type of DM are also applicable, for example, control

TABLE 1: Clinical features for all forms of diabetes.[8]

	Type 1 diabetes mellitus	Type 2 diabetes mellitus	Type 3c diabetes mellitus		
Associated with	Autoimmunity	Obesity	Cystic fibrosis	Chronic pancreatitis	Pancreatic resection
Age of onset (median)	2nd decade	6th decade	3rd decade	5th decade	Within 5 years of surgery
Hepatic insulin sensitivity	Normal/decreased	Decreased	Unknown	Normal/decreased	Normal/decreased
Pancreatic insufficiency	No	No	Yes	Yes	Yes
Diabetic ketoacidosis	Yes	No	No	No	No
Peripheral insulin sensitivity	Normal/decreased	Decreased	Unknown	Normal	Normal
Hypoglycemic risk	Increased	Normal	Normal or Increased	Normal or Increased	Normal or Increased
Pancreatic polypeptide response	Normal/decreased	Normal/increased	Absent	Decreased or Absent	Absent
Insulin levels	Decreased/absent	Normal/increased	Normal/decreased		
GIP levels	Normal/decreased	Variable	Decreased		
Glucagon levels	Normal/increased	Normal/increased	Normal/decreased		
GLP-1 levels	Normal	Variable	Variable		

(GIP: glucose-dependent insulinotropic polypeptide; GLP-1: glucagon-like peptide 1)

TABLE 2: Diagnostic criteria for type 3c diabetes.[13]

Major criteria (all must be fulfilled)	Major criteria (all must be fulfilled)	Minor criteria
Conceptual	Proposed by Ewald and Bretzel	Proposed by Ewald and Bretzel
i. Presence of diabetes ii. Presence of the exocrine pancreas disease iii. Diabetes, reasonably certain to be secondary to their exocrine pancreatic disease	i. Exocrine pancreatic insufficiency (by monoclonal fecal elastase-1 testing or direct function tests) ii. Consistent pancreatic abnormalities on imaging (endoscopic ultrasound, MRI, or CT scan) iii. Absence of related autoimmune markers of type 1 diabetes	i. Absence of pancreatic polypeptide secretion ii. Impaired β-cell function iii. Absence of insulin resistance iv. Impaired incretin secretion and v. Low serum concentrations of lipid soluble vitamins (A, D, E, or K)

of hyperglycemia to achieve and maintain HbA1c < 7% is the goal for the management of T3cDM as like in patients with T2DM and T1DM.

The condition can be managed by many factors. Table 3 summarizes management approaches for T3cDM.

The various forms of management include the following:

- *Lifestyle modifications*: Pancreatic inflammation is decreased by avoidance of toxins to the body like smoking and alcohol. Intake of diet rich in fiber and consumption of normal amounts of fat may be helpful. Oral pancreatic enzymes can also be given. Sufficient levels of vitamin D should be maintained, which can also decrease symptoms and help in management of the disease in a better way.
- *Nutrition* as mentioned in Table 3
- *Hypoglycemic agents*: Primary defect in T3cDM is insulin deficiency; thus, insulin is drug of choice in many patients. The anabolic effects of insulin are beneficial particularly in malnourished patients. The basal-bolus regimens of T1DM should be adopted and individualize the management. In acutely ill patients continuous subcutaneous infusion (CSCI) or infusion pump therapy may be adopted.

TABLE 3: Principles of management/management strategies for type 3c diabetes in case of chronic pancreatitis.[14]

Principles of management	Management strategies
• Prevent • Hyperglycemia • Hypoglycemia • Malabsorption • Exacerbation of malnutrition • Comorbidities related with diabetes (e.g. renal disease, retinopathy)	• Meal pattern should be with regular with regular starchy carbohydrates • Small, frequent meals should be taken • Meals should not be skipped • Glucose levels should be measured frequently, specifically if on insulin, following physical activity, if on poor diet, and if any hypoglycemic symptoms present • Alcohol should be avoided, smoking cessation • Adequacy of pancreatic enzyme replacement therapy (PERT) should be ensured • Minimize high glycemic index/high-sugar fluids or foods • A diary should be maintained for recording glucose levels, diet, exercise, PERT, at least until maintenance of acceptable glucose control • Routine assessment/monitoring by dietician is recommended

At diagnosis of T3cDM ——→ Escalation of treatment based on A1c levels > 7%				
Lifestyle + Metformin + Pancreatic enzyme Rx	Lifestyle + Metformin + TZD or alpha GI + Pancreatic enzyme Rx	Lifestyle + Metformin + Basal insulin + Pancreatic enzyme Rx	Lifestyle + Metformin + Intensive insulin Rx + Pancreatic enzyme Rx	Lifestyle + Metformin + Intensive insulin Rx + Adjunct Rx + Pancreatic enzyme Rx

(T3cDM: type 3c diabetes mellitus; TZD: thiazolidinediones; GI: gastrointestinal)

Figure 6 Suggested algorithm for managing T3cDM.[3]

In chronic and mild hyperglycemic (HbA1c < 8%) oral hypoglycemic agents (OHA) like metformin can be used. Though gastrointestinal side effects are a concern with metformin, it has favorable action in chronic pancreatitis of reducing the risk of pancreatic cancer. Treatment with secretagogues like sulfonylureas and glinides should be taken with caution. Incretin-based therapy (e.g. GLP-1 analogs and gliptins) and thiazolidinediones are relatively contraindicated. GLP-1 analogs are associated with an elevated frequency of gastrointestinal side effects, symptoms that are commonly experienced by patients with chronic pancreatitis. Both gliptins and GLP-1 analogs have been related with cases of pancreatitis induced by drugs. Incretin-based therapies in pancreatogenic diabetes should be avoided until more data are accessible.

- *Islet cell transplantation*: Islet cell transplantation is considered as definitive treatment in T3cDM, particularly in chronic and recurrent pancreatitis for providing pain relief and recurrent hospitalizations. Since it only prevent T3cDM in chronic pancreatitis patients, it is ineffective in already established disease. Hence prior assessment of functional beta cell mass is mandatory before contemplating islet cell transplantation.

Figure 6 illustrates the suggested algorithm for managing T3cDM.

Promising New Drugs

Pancreatic polypeptide is one of the evolving drugs, which has shown great potential in T3cDM treatment, secondary to chronic pancreatitis. It enhances the expression of insulin receptors in the liver, making it possible to use circulating insulin better and more efficiently. It also increases insulin sensitivity and decreases requirement of insulin in patients with T3cDM.[11]

CONCLUSION

Clinically, T3cDM is an important in view of its treatment challenge as brittle diabetes. Until now it has been underrecognized and poorly managed. Truly, it is a "different variety" of diabetes and there are important knowledge gaps in understanding right from its classification, pathogenesis, clinical features, and management issues. Further research is essential with better collaboration between epidemiologists, physicians, gastroenterologists and endocrinologists to fill these gaps, which is the need of hour in the setting of skyrocketing numbers of T2DM in India (which is masking true prevalence of T3cDM) and high prevalence of "alcohol use disorders" with all types of pancreatitis in India.

REFERENCES

1. Phil AH, Melena DB, Dana KA et al. Type 3c (pancreatogenic) diabetes mellitus secondary to chronic pancreatitis and pancreatic cancer. Lancet Gastroenterol Hepatol. 2016;1:226-37.
2. Hardt PD, Brendel MD, Kloer HU, et al. Is pancreatic diabetes (type 3c diabetes) underdiagnosed and misdiagnosed? Diabetes Care. 2008;31: S165-9.
3. Cui Y, Andersen DK. Pancreatogenic diabetes: special considerations for management. Pancreatology. 2011;11:279-94.
4. World Health Organization. Definition, diagnosis and classification of diabetes mellitus and its complications. Part 1: Diagnosis and classification of diabetes mellitus. Geneva: World Health Organization; 1999. [online] Available from http://apps.who.int/iris/bitstream/10665/66040/1/WHO_NCD_NCS_99.2.pdf. [Last accessed September, 2019].
5. American Diabetes Association. Diagnosis and classification of diabetes mellitus. Diabetes Care. 2014;37(Suppl 1):S81-S90.
6. Whitcomb D. Chronic pancreatitis, type 3c diabetes, and pancreatic cancer risk. JOP. 2014;15:2773.
7. Anatomy and Physiology. (2012). The Endocrine System. Chapter 17. The Regents of University of Michigan Medical School 2012. [online] Available from https://opentextbc.ca/anatomyandphysiology/chapter/17-9-the-endocrine-pancreas/. [Last accessed September, 2019].
8. Gudipaty L, Rickels MR. (2015). Pancreatogenic (type 3c) diabetes. Pancreapedia: Exocrine Pancreas Knowledge Base. [online] Available from http://www.pancreapedia.org/sites/www.pancreapedia.org/files/DOI%20V3.%20formatted%20Type%203c%20DM%20chapter%208-13-15.pdf. [Last accessed September, 2019].
9. Tiengo A, Vigili de Kreutzenberg S, Del Prato S. Diabetes in pancreatitis, pancreatectomy and other pancreatic diseases. In: Ghigo E, Porta M, (Eds). Diabetes Secondary to Endocrine and Pancreatic Disorders. Front Diabetes. Basel: Karger; 2014. pp. 119-43.
10. Murli M, Alok KV, Sathisha UV, et al. Pathogenic mechanisms of pancreatitis. World J Gastrointest Pharmacol Ther 2017;8(1):10-25.
11. Lakshmi Venkataraman. Type 3c (Pancreatogenic) Diabetes. Available from: https://www.medindia.net/patientinfo/type-3c-diabetes.htm.
12. Dana KA, Murray K, Gloria MP, et al. Diabetes, Pancreatogenic Diabetes, and Pancreatic Cancer. American Diabetes Association. Diabetes 2017;66(5):1103-10.
13. Ewald N and Bretzel RG. Diabetes mellitus secondary to pancreatic diseases (Type 3c) - Are we neglecting an important disease? Eur J Intern Med 2013;24:203-06.
14. Duggan SN and Colon KC. A Practical Guide to the Nutritional Management of Chronic Pancreatitis. Nutrition Issues in Gastroenterology; Pract Gastroentero. 2013: series 118.

16 CHAPTER Drug-induced Diabetes

Girish C Verma, Ashee Verma

INTRODUCTION

The use of many drugs at a time is a common phenomenon by the physician due to existence of multiple diseases in a patient (e.g. diabetes mellitus, hypertension and ischemic heart disease present together). Use of various drugs in specialties other than medicine is also a frequent phenomenon in the present era.

A number of toxins, chemical agents, and drugs are known for causing impaired glucose tolerance or secondary forms of diabetes.[1]

Drug-induced diabetes is recognized by American Diabetes Association (ADA) as well as World Health Organization (WHO) as a separate etiological category.[2]

Drug- and toxin-induced diabetes can be defined as new development of hyperglycemic state, which fulfills the definition of diabetes and is due to of intake of a drug.

The following drugs can cause impaired glucose tolerance or can worsen the hyperglycemia in a diabetic patient:[1]

- *Diuretic and antihypertensives*: Thiazides, chlorthalidone, loop diuretics (furosemide, ethacrynic acid, and metolazone), diazoxide, clonidine, and β-adrenergic antagonist.
- *Hormones*: Glucocorticoids, adrenocorticotropic hormone, α-adrenergic agonist, growth hormone, glucagon, oral contraceptives, and progestational agents.
- *Psychoactive agents*: Lithium, opiates, ethanol, phenothiazines, atypical antipsychotics (clozapine, olanzapine)
- *Anticonvulsants*: Dilantin
- *Antineoplastic agents*: Streptozotocin, L-asparaginase, mithramycin
- *Antiprotozoal agents*: Pentamidine
- *Rodenticide*: Pyriminil (Vacor)
- *Antiretroviral agents*: Protease inhibitors (PIs), nucleoside reverse transcriptase inhibitor 3-hydroxy-3-methylglutaryl coenzyme A (HMG-CoA)
- *Reductase inhibitors*: Statins
- *Miscellaneous*: Nicotinic acid, immunosuppressant (cyclosporine, tacrolimus), N-nitrosamines, theophylline.

These offending drugs are grouped according to the mechanism by which they induce diabetes:[2]

- The first group drug—interfering in insulin production and secretion
- The second group—block insulin action
- The third group drugs—those drugs interfering in both insulin secretion and action
- The final group drugs—increasing blood glucose using mechanism independent on insulin's action.

Insulin therapy is considered to be the most efficacious approach in cases where diabetes is caused due to drug and that drug needs to be continued.[2] In the patient of prediabetes, diabetes, or insulin resistance, drug that is assumed to be having adverse effect on blood glucose level should be avoided. It has been reported that some of the agents cause new diabetes in previously nondiabetic people.[2]

- Drugs that cause diabetes by interfering with insulin production and secretion:
  - Beta-receptor antagonists, tacrolimus
  - Pyriminil, didanosine
  - Pentamidine, L-asparaginase
  - Diphenylhydantoin, opiates.
- Drug that cause diabetes by reducing the effective sensitivity of insulin:
  - Glucocorticoids, β-receptor agonist
  - Megestrol acetate, growth hormone
  - Oral contraceptive, protease inhibitors.

- Drugs that act on both insulin secretion and insulin sensitivity:
  - Thiazide diuretics, diazoxide
  - Cyclosporine, atypical antipsychotics (clozapine, olanzapine)
  - Beta-receptor antagonists.
- Treatments that induce diabetes by increasing nutrients flux, increases hepatic glucose output due to enhanced gluconeogenesis:
  - Nicotinic acid
  - Total parenteral nutrition

Common and frequently used drugs which induce diabetes or worsen hyperglycemia are being discussed.

GLUCOCORTICOIDS

In patients with diabetes, glucocorticoids are reported to worsen hyperglycemia, but they can also lead to significantly increased blood glucose and insulin concentration among previously identified normoglycemic individuals when high doses are given (i.e. equivalent to 30 mg/day or more prednisolone).[3] Among 14–28% of the subjects who receive long-term glucocorticoids, impaired glucose tolerance has been reported.[4,5]

Gulliford et al.[6] reported that a large primary care population, which was drawn from 114 family practices, was orally administered with glucocorticoids. The individuals were found to be associated with up to 2% incident cases of diabetes mellitus.

MEGESTROL ACETATE

Megestrol acetate is a progestin steroid that is used for appetite stimulation and weight gain in cachexia associated with acquired immunodeficiency syndrome (AIDS) and cancer. Two case reports exist related to new onset diabetes among patients who had AIDS and were taking 80 mg of megestrol four times daily. The mechanism has not been studied but is probably a combination of steroid-induced decreased sensitivity to insulin and increased caloric intake.[7,8]

ORAL CONTRACEPTIVE

Oral contraceptives increase average glucose concentration among patients with and without diabetes by reducing insulin sensitivity.

In Nurses' Health Study including 121,700 women for > 15 years, current use of oral contraceptive did not enhanced the relative risk (RR) for diabetes (RR = 0.86) and past use conferred a small increase (RR = 1.12), which was not associated with duration or dose of exposure.[9]

DIURETICS

The diabetogenic effect of diuretics particularly high-dose thiazides and chlorthalidone have been well recognized. A 12-years follow-up epidemiological study revealed that the risk of the developing diabetes over the risk in controls was increased three- to fourfold in subject receiving thiazides, five- to sixfold in those receiving β-adrenergic blockers, and 11-fold in subject receiving both drugs.[10] Other large surveys have reported a 40–80% increased risk for initiation of treatment for diabetes with thiazides and with the use of the multiple antihypertensive agents with or without thiazides.[11] Most studies have indicated that the mechanism involved in the increase risk is the insulin secretary defect caused by thiazide diuretics is due to hypokalemia and the defect can be corrected by K^+ replacement.[12,13] Diazoxide, a nondiuretic thiazide, has pronounced inhibitory effects of β-cell as well as peripheral effects.[14,15]

BETA-BLOCKERS

For β-blockers, an inhibitory effect of β-cells secretion would be anticipated. In some cases, propranolol precipitated hyperglycemic, hyperosmolar, nonketotic coma. The diabetogenic effect of β-blockers should not negate the proven benefits of these agents in reducing mortality in patients with known coronary heart disease.[1]

PHENYTOIN

Phenytoin has direct inhibitory effect on β-cell secretion. This effect appears to be dose-related and hyperglycemic nonketotic coma precipitated by phenytoin toxicity has been reported.[1] Diabetes usually resolves when treatment is withdrawn or completed.

PENTAMIDINE

Pentamidine (an antiprotozoal agent) and pyriminil (Vacor) (a rodenticide) resemble streptozotocin and alloxan chemically. An increase in the incidence of diabetes by pentamidine use has been reported. Use of aerosolized pentamidine has minimized the effect of this agent on carbohydrate metabolism. Accidental or intentional injection of pyriminil may result in the development of diabetes with or without ketoacidosis as a result of β-cell destruction.[1]

NICOTINIC ACID

Nicotinic acid in higher dosage causes glucose intolerance by inducing peripheral insulin insensitivity.[1] Nicotinic acid therapy is associated with the increase level of glucose in both diabetic and nondiabetic patients and uncontrolled hyperglycemia is a frequent reason for discontinuing therapy. Mechanism of nicotinic-induced hyperglycemia is an increase in hepatic blood glucose output due to enhanced gluconeogenesis secondary to rebound increase in flow of free fatty acids to liver.

IMMUNOSUPPRESSANTS

By immunosuppressants, an increased incidence of diabetes in transplant recipients receiving cyclosporine has been reported. Direct inhibitory effect of cyclosporine on β-cell and peripheral effect on glucose transport have been implicated. Tacrolimus has also been reported to be associated with an increased incidence of diabetes or worsening of preexisting glucose intolerance.[1] Diabetes mellitus (DM) developed in post-transplant patient in such manner is known post-transplant diabetes mellitus (PTDM).

OPIATES

A hyperglycemic effect of morphine and other opiates has been recognized. In healthy diabetic subject, infusion of β-endorphin resulted in hyperglycemia accompanied by hyperglucagonemia.[1] These results are in keeping with observation of impaired β-cell responsiveness to glucose in the subjects addicted to narcotics.

ALCOHOL

In an epidemiologic survey of more than 12,000 participants followed-up over a period of 3–6 years, an intake of more than three drinks of alcohols per day was associated with a 50% increased risk of diabetes in men, whereas no increase in men or women was seen with the moderate intake, i.e. less than three drinks daily.[16]

ATYPICAL ANTIPSYCHOTICS

Atypical antipsychotics have number of reports showing potential diabetogenic effects particularly clozapine and olanzapine. In one series of 82 patients treated with clozapine over a period of 5 years, 30% were diagnosed with diabetes, most requiring treatment. This may be secondary to the weight gain seen with these agents. The diabetes developed in the manner is labeled as antipsychotic associated diabetes.[1] Severe mental illness and its associated lifestyle changes, by themselves are known to be associated with increased risk for obesity diabetes.

ANTIRETROVIRAL AGENTS

Diabetes is fourfold common in human immunodeficiency virus (HIV) infected man exposed to highly active antiretroviral therapy (HAART) then HIV negative men.[17] Commonly, type 2 diabetes has been observed following HAART therapy. However, recent report showed development of autoimmune diabetes and antiglutamic acid decarboxylase (anti-GAD) antibodies after immune system recovery following HAART therapy which suggest that type 1 diabetes can also arise in this group from treatment.[18]

Protease inhibitors (ritonavir, saquinavir, darunavir) are part of HAART therapy and they have shown to increase insulin resistance by inhibiting glucose transporter type 4 (GLUT4). Therapeutic level of PIs are sufficient to impaired glucose sensing by β-cells thus together with peripheral insulin resistance β-cell dysfunction likely to contribute altered glucose homeostasis.[19] Hyperglycemia resolve in almost all patients when PIs are discontinued.[18] Nucleoside reverse transcriptase inhibitors are another class of anti-HIV drugs associated with diabetes especially when used for longer period. In this group, the risk is highest with stavudine but risk is also significant with zidovudine and didanosine.

STATINS

They are the commonly used drugs which has been purported to cause diabetes. In a meta-analysis of 13 placebo-controlled trials, it was reported that statin used compared to placebo increased the risk of diabetes.[19]

One meta-analysis compared intensive dose of statin use with moderate statin therapy in five trials. It was reported that higher statin dose was associated with the greater risk of developing diabetes. The mechanism behind how statin cause diabetes is still not known. However, it has been advised that these drugs can have an effect on muscles and liver insulin sensitivity that lead to increase in diabetes risk.[20]

In spite of the increased risk of diabetes related to use of statin, risk benefit analysis has revealed the useful nature of statin for cardiovascular disease; this outweighs the risk of diabetes related to use of statin.[21]

There are many more drugs which alter glucose homeostasis already mentioned in the list like β-adrenergic agonist, asparaginase, cyclosporine, tacrolimus, etc.

In the most drugs, hyperglycemia resolves after stopping the drug. There are drugs like tacrolimus, PI, and newer atypical antipsychotic drugs which can cause *de novo* diabetes. Alpha-interferon therapy has been associated with the development of both type 1 and type 2 DM; sometimes associated with ketoacidosis, autoimmune mechanism have been implicated.[22]

As far as treatment is concerned in cases where hyperglycemia is produced by the drug through insulin resistance, thiazolidinediones, and metformin which improves insulin sensitivity may be used as in case of hyperglycemia due to PI. In case of corticosteroid-induced hyperglycemia if the drug is essential to be continued, insulin is the choice.

CONCLUSION

Thus it is mandatory for a physician to know about the diabetogenic effect of various drugs used in the clinical practice so as to have better glucose control in their diabetic patients and avoid unwanted glucose intolerance in nondiabetic patients. However, we have to weigh the advantages and disadvantages of the drug which is being used in a particular clinical condition.

REFERENCES

1. Ganda OP. Secondary form of diabetes. Joslin's Diabetes Mellitus, 14th edition. Boston, Massachusetts: Lippincott Williams and Wilkins; 2011. pp. 477-92.
2. Lohani KK. Drug induced diabetes mellitus. Medicine Update. JAPI. 2010;20:70-3.
3. Pagano G, Caballo-perrin P, Cassoder M, et al. In vivo and in vitro study of mechanism of prednisolone induced insulin resistance in healthy subjects. J Clin Invest. 1983;72:1814-20.
4. Schubert G, Schulz H. Contribution to clinical picture of steroid diabetes. Dtsch Med Wochenschr. 1963;8:1175-88.
5. Lieberman P, Pattesson R, Kunske R. Complication of long term steroid therapy for asthma. J Allergy Clin Immunol. 1972;49:329-36.
6. Guliford MC, Charlton J, Latinovic R. Risk of diabetes associated with prescribed glucocorticoids in a large population. Diabetes Care. 2006;29:2728-9.
7. Henry K, Rathgaber S, Sullivan C, et al. Diabetes mellitus induced by megestrol acetate in a patient with AIDS and cachexia. Ann Intern Med. 1992;116:53-4.
8. Panwalker AP. Hyperglycemia induced by megestrol acetate. Ann Intern Med. 1992;116:878.
9. Rimm E, Manson J, Stamfer M, et al. Oral contraceptive use and the risk of type 2 diabetes in a large population of women. Diabetologia. 1992;35:967-72.
10. Bengtsson C, Blohme G, Lapidus L, et al. Do antihypertensive drug precipitate diabetes? BMJ. 1984;289:1495-7.
11. Gurwitz JH, Bohn RL, Glymn RJ, et al. Antihypertensive drug therapy and the institution of treatment for diabetes mellitus. Ann Intern Med. 1993;118:273-8.
12. Gorden P. Glucose tolerance with hypokalemia: failure of short term potassium depletion in normal subject to reproduce glucose and insulin abnormalities of clinical hypokalemia. Diabetes. 1973;22(7):544-51.
13. Grunfeld C, Chappell DA. Hypokalemia and diabetes mellitus. Am J Med. 1983;75:553-4.
14. Trube G, Rorsman P, Ohno-Shosaku T. Opposite effect of tolbutamide and diazoxide on ATP dependent K^+ channels in mouse pancreatic beta cells. Pflugers Arch. 1986;407:493-9.
15. Mohan LR, Mohan V. Drug induced diabetes mellitus. JAPI. 1997;45: 876-9.
16. Kao WH, Puddy IB, Boland LL, et al. Alcohol consumption and the risk of type 2 diabetes mellitus atherosclerosis in community study. Am J Epidemic. 2001;154:748-75.
17. Defronzo RA, Ferrannini E, Zimmet P, et al. International Textbook of Diabetes Mellitus, 4th edition. Oxford UK: Wiley Blackwell Publication; 2015. pp. 3-16.
18. Kalra S, Kalra B, Agarwal N, et al. Understanding diabetes in patients with HIV/AIDS. Diabetol Metab Syndr. 2011;3:2.
19. Stattar N, Preiss D, Murray HM, et al. Risk of incidence diabetes a collaboration meta-analysis of randomised statin trials. Lancet. 2010;375: 735-42.
20. Preiss D, Seshasai SR, Welsh P, et al. Risk of incident of diabetes with intensive those compared with moderate dost statin therapy a meta-analysis. JAMA. 2011;305:2556-64.
21. Wang KI, Liu CJ, Chao TF, et al. Statins risk of diabetes and implications on outcome in the general population. J Am Col Cardiol. 2012;60:1231-8.
22. Bhatti A, McGarrity TJ, Gabbay R. Diabetic ketoacidosis induced by Alpha interferon and ribavirin treatment in patient with Hepatitis C. Am J Gastroenterol. 2001;96:604-5.

17 CHAPTER Strategies for Reducing Glycemic Index in Indian Cuisine

Parimal Swamy

INTRODUCTION

Consumption of food with high glycemic index/glycemic load (GI/GL) and postprandial hyperglycemia (PPHG) is associated with adverse outcome and complications in diabetes.[1] Similarly high GI/GL diets are implicated in the development and progression of coronary artery disease in non-diabetic subjects.[2] Numerous studies have shown the potential for amelioration of diabetes-related complications by controlling PPHG.[3] Both GI and GL are most important drivers of postprandial glycemic excursion in normal and diabetic subjects,[4] hence their control (reduction) may prove an important intervention for prevention of diabetes-related complications and as a public health enhancing measure.

Traditionally Indians consume high amount of carbohydrates. Despite wide variations in culinary habits, Indians across the nation consume approximately 64% of energy from carbohydrates.[5] The major constituents of dietary carbohydrates are various cereal-based preparations with relatively low amount of vegetables and pulses thus making standard Indian diet a high GI/GL diet.

CONCEPT OF GLYCEMIC INDEX AND GLYCEMIC LOAD

Glycemic index is defined as blood glucose response of a food containing 50 g of available carbohydrate as incremental area under the curve (iAUC) over a period of 2 hours (Table 1).[6] The GI value is expressed as the percentage of ratio of iAUC of test food and 50 g of reference food (usually glucose solution or white bread).

$$GI = (iAUC\ test\ food/iAUC\ reference\ food) \times 100$$

TABLE 1: Glycemic index and food classification.

Glycemic index	Food classification
<55	Low
56–69	Medium
≥70	High

TABLE 2: Glycemic load and food classification.

Glycemic load	Food classification
≤10	Low
11–19	Medium
≥20	High

Glycemic load accounts for the amount of carbohydrate in the food and how each gram of carbohydrate in the food raises blood glucose levels (Table 2).[7]

$$GL = GI \times available\ carbohydrate\ (g)/100$$

Glycemic index compares equal quantities of available carbohydrate in foods and provides a measure of carbohydrate quality whereas GL provides a summary measure of the relative glycemic impact of a "typical" serving of the food.

IMPACT OF GLYCEMIC INDEX AND GLYCEMIC LOAD ON CARDIOMETABOLIC HEALTH

Extent of acute blood sugar excursion after meal mediated by GI and GL of the food is associated with various determinants of cardiometabolic risk.

Post-meal glucose excursion was found to be positively associated with oxidative stress, triglycerides, and C-reactive protein. High GI/GL food leads to endothelial dysfunction as indicated by impaired flow mediated dilatation.[8]

Postprandial glucose excursion even below diabetic range is associated with coronary atherosclerosis progression. A recent meta-analysis has shown strong and probably causal relationship between coronary artery disease and GI/GL.[9]

Reduction in GI/GL of diet is associated with reduction in fat mass and confers cardiovascular risk reduction in young obese individuals.[10] Low GI/GL diet improves glycemic status and glucose variability.[11]

STRATEGIES FOR REDUCTION OF GLYCEMIC INDEX AND GLYCEMIC LOAD

Real world data shows that Indians consume carbohydrate rich diet. Major sources of carbohydrates are cereals, mainly wheat and rice. Traditional staple food articles Indian flat bread (C*hapatti/Roti*) and cooked white rice have high GI, 62 and 73 respectively. India is the second largest producer of potatoes. Potatoes constitute as a major ingredient in various Indian culinary preparations. As GI and GL of potatoes is high (more than 70 and 28 respectively) their inclusion in Indian diet is responsible for adverse glycemic response. Indians also eat dessert (sweets) after major meals. As behavioral science studies show that it is very difficult to change food habits, we will discuss strategies to reduce GI/GL without changing the texture and palatability of food.

Rice

Though there are many varieties of specially cultivated rice claiming to have GI of less than 60 but they lack scientific evidence. Brown rice has a GI of 68 (high medium) and there may be issues of cost and palatability. Special breeding techniques can produce rice with low GI. One such high fiber white rice developed in India has GI of 61 (medium). As this high fiber rice has scientific validation with no palatability issue it can be considered a potential alternative to commercially available white rice.[12] Another method of reducing the GI of white rice is storing cooked parboiled rice for 24 hours at 4°C then reheating it before consumption. This method resulted in better taste, satiety and 1.7 fold less glycemic response as compared to freshly cooked non-parboiled rice.[13]

Indian Flat Bread (*Chapatti/Roti*)

It is common practice in India to mix the powder of pulses/legumes to wheat flour for preparation of *roti/chapatti.* There is scientific evidence of significant reduction of GI of *roti/chapatti* from 63 to 41 after mixing a specific combination of Bengal gram, *methi* (fenugreek) powder and spices to wheat flour.[14] Though it requires some preparation but it is worth the effort as it makes *roti/chapatti* a low GI food.

Potato

Studies show eating new potatoes curbs the glycemic response. Eating boiled potatoes or adding vinegar dressing to cold boiled potatoes also reduces the GI.[15]

Cold storage, reheating and boiling leads to formation of resistant starch and amount of resistant starch is responsible for low GI of cooked food.

Dessert

Indians are fond of eating dessert after meal, during religious occasions and festivals (which are many). Traditionally these desserts are prepared with white sugar or *jaggery* making them a very high GI food articles. As their consumption is frequent and many times socially compelling it is worthwhile to alter their composition to bring down the GI to acceptable level. Though artificial sweetening agents are commonly available their long-term usage is not free of adverse effect. One safe natural alternative is stevia. Stevia has almost 0 (zero) GI and associated with favorable insulin response in non-diabetic subjects. There is a problem of bitter aftertaste with stevia which can be masked with adding little quantity of other naturally occurring sugars.[16]

There are other techniques besides changing the variety of dietary constituents or cooking methods to reduce GI of food-like addition of substances which actively reduce the GI, providing premeal load of fat or protein, changing the sequence of consumption of various foodstuff and using low GI meal strategically.

Functional Food Additive

Various commercial ventures are trying to develop food additive having active GI reducing capabilities. One such product is developed by a Singapore startup. It attracted significant attention as the company secured a major investment from big venture capitalist. It is commercially produced and claims to reduce the GI of rice and wheat products to around 50 (low GI) without changing the taste or texture! It has to be mixed with wheat or rice products (either to flour or while cooking). Company has in-house

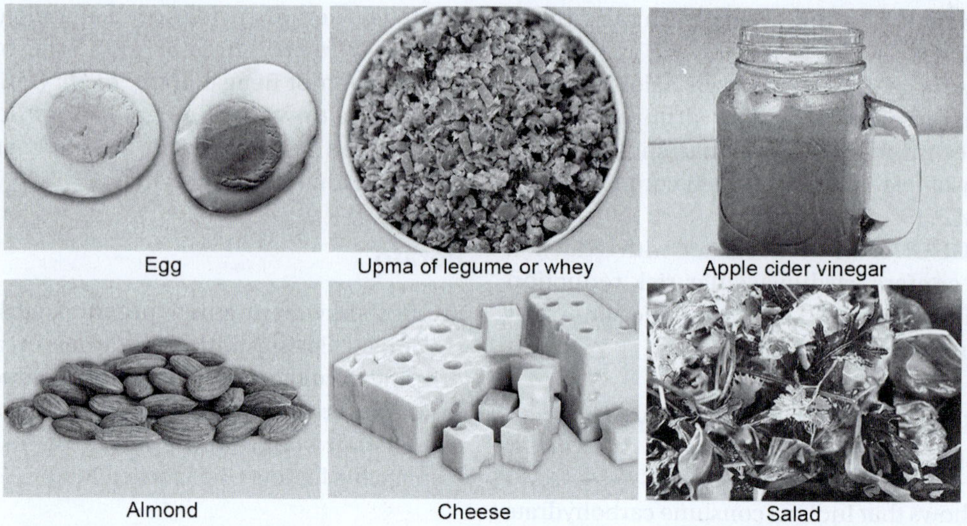

Figure 1 Tasty healthy snack—meal replacement—appetite and GI regulating premeal. (Choose ingredients according to personal and cultural preference).

experimental data but no published trial. It contains a combination of insoluble fiber (70%), soluble fiber (15%), proteins (2%), hydrocolloids (0.5%) and a small amount of various carbohydrate enzyme inhibitors (0.5%).[17]

Addition of Natural Glycemic Index Stabilizer

Trials have shown meaningful reduction of GI and glycemic response by adding almonds, vinegar, modest amount of alcohol (especially wine) and proteins to high carbohydrate diet.[8] Nutritionist and dietitian should come forward and evolve recipes for commonly consumed food article using these ingredients maintaining the traditional taste and texture of end products.

Commercially available protein supplements deserve special mention as they may add nutritional value to protein deficient Indian diet while reducing the GI. There is some data about the different effects of protein from various sources in diabetic subjects. While both whey (dairy) protein and lupine (legume) protein reduce the glycemic excursion, whey stimulates insulin secretion and lupine reduces the glycemic response of meal without significant insulin response. Theoretically whey may be used in insulin deficient and lupine in insulin-resistant patients.[18]

MANIPULATING THE SEQUENCE OF FOOD CONSUMPTION

Fibers in natural food affect the digestion of carbohydrate. Human experiments confirm the beneficial effect of adding raw vegetable and salad on glycemic response. Eating vegetable first leads to significantly lower glycemic excursion of subsequent carbohydrate containing meal in both diabetic and non-diabetic subjects. Similarly a combination of fat and protein preload reduces the glycemic response of the subsequent meal. Preloading with fat and proteins has favorable effect on stomach emptying, beta cell function and incretin secretion.[19]

Second Meal Effect

Second meal effect means the GI of one meal can influence the GI of next meal. Eating foods with low GI and indigestible carbohydrates can reduce glycemic responses of next meal, and can be a very useful intervention for diabetes management. There are several mechanisms responsible for this phenomenon namely, presence of indigestible fibers, production of lactic acid, reduction of free-fatty acids, better insulin action and incretin effect. Low GI meal can favorably influence the blood sugar of next meal taken after 4 hours in diabetic subjects. In non-diabetic subjects low GI dinner can reduce the glycemic excursion of next day breakfast (Fig. 1).[19]

GLYCEMIC INDEX IN THE ERA OF PERSONALIZED MEDICINE

It was realized early after the concept of GI became mainstream that different subjects have different glycemic response to same food (having different GI for same food). With the rise of precision/personalized medicine and machine learning it is now possible to predict individual glycemic response to different food in different subjects. For this anthropometric parameters, dietary history, microbiome properties from stool samples, genotyping and continuous glucose monitoring data are fed to special computer program which can recognize subtle patterns and makes algorithm to predict glycemic response. Once the machine (computer) learns the pattern it is possible to predict glycemic response to specific food and classify food into "good" and "bad" with fecal microbiome sample, anthropometric data, and basic genetic analysis.[20]

CONCLUSION

Various sociocultural and economic factors have made Indian cuisine a high GI diet. Intensive and persistent educational campaign at mass level is required to make people aware about the importance of dietary GI/GL and need to manipulate them to enjoy a healthy life. Health-care providers and dietitian should make a proactive effort to find out ways and educate patients and their families so that eating food remains an enjoyable experience while preserving health-enhancing effect of the cuisine. With the increasing use of continuous glucose monitoring now it is possible to personalize the diet of our patients to some extent. With the availability of functional food and precision medicine we may hope to find out an individualized, tasty and healthy cuisine for our patients.

REFERENCES

1. Hanefeld M, Fischer S, Julius U, et al. Risk factors for myocardial infarction and death in newly detected NIDDM: the Diabetes Intervention Study, 11-year follow-up. Diabetologia. 1996;39:1577-83.
2. Nielson C, Lange T, Hadjokas N. Blood glucose and coronary artery disease in nondiabetic patients. Diabetes Care. 2006;29(5):998-1001.
3. Node K, Inoue T. Postprandial hyperglycemia as an etiological factor in vascular failure. Cardiovasc Diabetol. 2009;8:23.
4. González-Rodríguez M, Pazos-Couselo M, García-López JM, et al. Postprandial glycemic response in a non-diabetic adult population: the effect of nutrients is different between men and women. Nutr Metab. 2019; 16:46.
5. Joshi SR, Bhansali A, Bajaj S, et al. Results from a dietary survey in an Indian T2DM population: a STARCH study. BMJ Open. 2014;4(10).
6. Jenkins D, Wolever T, Barker H, et al. Glycemic index of foods: a physiological basis for carbohydrate exchange. Am J Clin Nutr. 1981;34: 362-6.
7. Salmerón J, Manson JE, Stampfer MJ, et al. Dietary fiber, glycemic load, and risk of non-insulin-dependent diabetes mellitus in women. JAMA. 1997;227:472-7.
8. O'Keefe JH, Gheewala NM, O'Keefe JO. Dietary Strategies for Improving Post-Prandial Glucose, Lipids, Inflammation, and Cardiovascular Health. J Am Coll Cardiol. 2008;51(3):249-55.
9. Livesey G, Livesey H. Coronary Heart Disease and Dietary Carbohydrate, Glycemic Index, and Glycemic Load: Dose-Response Meta-analyses of Prospective Cohort Studies. Mayo Clin Proc Innov Qual Out. 2019;3(1): 52-69.
10. McMillan-Price J, Petocz P, Atkinson F, et al. Comparison of 4 diets of varying glycemic load on weight loss and cardiovascular risk reduction in overweight and obese young adults: a randomized controlled trial. Arch Intern Med. 2006;166(14):1466-75.
11. Henry CJ, Kaur B, Chin Quek RY, et al. A Low Glycaemic Index Diet Incorporating Isomaltulose is Associated with Lower Glycaemic Response and Variability, and Promotes Fat Oxidation in Asians. Nutrients. 2017;9(5). pii: E473.
12. Mohan V, Anjana RM, Gayathri R, et al. Glycemic Index of a Novel High-Fiber White Rice Variety Developed in India—A Randomized Control Trial Study. Diabetes Technol Ther. 2016;18(3):164-70.
13. Lu LW, Venn B, Lu J, et al. Effect of Cold Storage and Reheating of Parboiled Rice on Postprandial Glycaemic Response, Satiety, Palatability and Chewed Particle Size Distribution. Nutrients. 2017;9(5):475. pii: E475.
14. Ankita M, Yenagi NB, Kasturba B. Designing of low glycaemic chapati of dicoccum wheat for the effective management of diabetes. Karnataka J Agric Sci. 2010;23(3):476-9.
15. Leeman M, Ostman E, Björck I. Vinegar dressing and cold storage of potatoes lowers postprandial glycaemic and insulinaemic responses in healthy subjects. Eur J Clin Nutr. 2005;59(11):1266-71.
16. Stephen DA, Corby KM, Hongmei H, et al. Effects of stevia, aspartame, and sucrose on food intake, satiety, and postprandial glucose and insulin levels. Appetite. 2010;55(1):37-43.
17. FPO Driving IP Forward. 2015. [Online] Available from www.freepatentsonline.com/y2019/0029307.html. [Last accessed on September, 2019].
18. Schopen K, Ewald AC, Johannes BW, et al. Short-Term Effects of Lupin vs. Whey Supplementation on Glucose and Insulin Responses to a Standardized Meal in a Randomized Cross-Over Trial. Front Physiol. 2017;8:198.
19. Monnier L, Bonnet F, Colette C. Tailoring nutrient sequence and content to improve glucose tolerance: Why and how to do it? Diabetes Metab. 2016;42:211-4.
20. Noecker C, Borenstein E. Getting Personal about Nutrition. Trends Mol Med. 2016;22(2):83-5.

18 CHAPTER Optimizing Protein Content in Indian Cuisine

Manohar KN, Pariksha Rao, Vijay Kumar K

INTRODUCTION

The concept of the "thin-fat" India is well established. We Indians have less lean mass than the other ethnic groups at the same body fat. This persists even after consideration of differences in age, body size, and lifestyle.[1] This South Asian phenotype of high fat mass and low lean mass accounts for much of the greater levels of insulin and HOMA (homeostasis model assessment) compared with the other ethnic groups, putting Indians at increased risk for insulin resistance and diabetes not only because of a higher fat mass but also because of lower lean mass.[2]

While it can be assumed that such differences reflect evolutionary adaptations to different environments, problems can arise when individuals, shaped by one environment, move to another.[3] Rural India is in a state of flux, such that millions are migrating to an urbanized lifestyle of limited physical activity and calorie-dense nutrition. The result is a rising level of urban obesity, diabetes and heart disease. Interventions that reduce fat mass and increase muscle mass, such as caloric restriction, increased high-quality protein intake and regular exercise can play a pivotal role.[4]

PROTEINS TO THE RESCUE!

The word "protein" is derived from the Greek word "proteios," which means primary or holding first place.

SOURCES OF PROTEIN

All foods except refined sugar, oil, and fats contain protein to varying degree. Some foods contain a high amount of protein and classified as protein rich foods. Examples of such foods are animal foods like meat, eggs, fish, poultry, milk and milk products, pulses, oil seeds and nuts. These foods contain over 20% of protein and soybean is the richest source containing over 40% of protein. Cereal and millets are moderate source of protein as they contain about 10% of protein.

FUNCTIONS OF DIETARY PROTEIN

- Proteins are necessary structural integrity of cells and growth of the body.
- They are required for the formation of enzymes, digestive juices, hemoglobin, and hormones.
- Required for the protection of the body against infection.
- Proteins help in the transport of oxygen and nutrients.
- Protein is required for tissue repair.
- They are needed for the production of milk proteins during lactation.
- To replace the daily loss of body proteins.

Proteins are also a source of energy. Each gram of protein provides 4 kcal. Therefore, when carbohydrates constitute to about 50% of the dietary intake it is referred to as protein sparing action wherein proteins are not utilized for giving energy to various cells of body and can fulfil its functions.

TYPES OF PROTEIN

Dietary protein can be classified in two forms (Table 1).

PROTEIN REQUIREMENTS

The current international Recommended Dietary Allowance (RDA) for protein is 0.8 g per kg of body weight, regardless of age (Table 2).[6] Individuals with

TABLE 1: Classification of dietary protein.[5]

Complete/class 1 protein	Incomplete/class 2 protein
• Provide all essential amino acids (EAAs) in adequate amounts and proportions needed by the body for growth and tissue maintenance	• These are deficient in one or more EAA
• Totally used by body and very little waste is left	• Not completely used by the body and produce more waste products
• Animal protein	• Plant protein
• Fish, chicken, eggs, meat, and dairy products	• Legumes, pulses, cereals, soybeans, and nuts

TABLE 2: Recommended dietary allowance (RDA) for protein (g/d) for Indians.

Group	Particulars	Body weight kg	Protein g/d
Man	Sedentary work	60	60
	Moderate work		
	Heavy work		
Woman	Sedentary work	55	55
	Moderate work		
	Heavy work		
	Pregnant woman		+23
	Lactation 0–6 months		+19
	6–12 months		+13
Infants	0–6 months	5.4	1.16 g/kg/d
	6–12 months	8.4	1.69 g/kg/d
Children	1–3 years	12.9	16.7
	4–6 years	18	20.1
	7–9 years	25.1	29.5
Boys	10–12 years	34.3	39.9
Girls	10–12 years	35.0	40.4
Boys	13–15 years	47.6	54.3
Girls	13–15 years	46.6	51.9
Boys	16–17 years	55.4	61.5
Girls	16–17 years	52.1	55.5

(*Source:* National Institute of Nutrition. Dietary guidelines for Indians—A manual, 2nd edition. Hyderabad: National Institute of Nutrition; 2011. Annexure 3: p. 89.)

low physical activity level (PAL) have decreased rates of nitrogen retention and therefore in order to maintain muscle tissue, they have increased protein requirements in comparison to those who are active. Physical activity decreases with age. This is an important factor when protein needs are evaluated.[2] Further, the daily protein requirement of healthy individuals over 65 years is 1.0–1.2 g protein/kg/bw. A further increase is recommended for individuals with acute or chronic illnesses (1.2–1.5 g protein/kg/bw) and severe illnesses, injuries, or malnutrition (2.0 protein g/kg/bw).[6]

PROTEIN INTAKES IN INDIA

In Indian diets, about 60% of protein is derived from cereals having relatively low quality and digestibility. In India, over the last 25 years, there have been many surveys of diets and protein intakes by the National Nutrition Monitoring Board (NNMB) conducted in rural and urban as well as in tribal populations and slum dwellers.

Therefore, while there is the burden of improving the quality of protein consumption in rural India, overall quality of diet is a challenge that needs to be met.[7]

PRODIGY Survey: 80% Indian diets are Protein deficient[8]
In India, we consume fat and starch but insufficient protein. Due to this, India is also known as a protein-deficient state. Unfortunately, IMRB conducted latest survey PRODIGY "Protein Consumption in the Diet of Adult Indians Survey" proves that 80% of Indians are protein-deficient. This survey was conducted in seven main cities of India amid 1,260 citizens in which about 91% of the vegetarians and 85% of the nonvegetarians Indians were found to be deficient in protein. In India, lack of adequate proteins in food can lead to undernourishment causing fatigue, decreased immunity, muscle mass failure, and a weakened cardiovascular system.[8]

Why Indian Cuisine Lacks Protein?

- *A vegetarian diet*: Majority of Indian population are vegetarians out of which statistics reveals that 91% vegetarians were found to have higher protein deficiency compared to 85% of nonvegetarians. Thirty-one percent of Indians are vegetarian, according to the 2006 The Hindu-CNN-IBN State of the Nation

Survey. Pulses are consumed by vegetarians as well as nonvegetarians in India. Indeed, despite the proportion of nonvegetarians, the quantity of consumed egg, fish, and meat is small. Thus, a large part of the protein requirement could be met by pulses.

- *Lack of knowledge:* Most Indians are unaware of the optimum protein intake needed in our daily diet. As a result of this lack of knowledge, working women and housewives are found to be 70–80% deficit in protein since they are the main food-masters of the household.[8]
- *Myth about protein sources:* India has been mapped as a protein deficient country. Seventy percent of women believe protein in fruits and vegetables are easily available and 73% urban Indian population think leafy vegetables contain more protein.
- *Lifestyle choices:* With a fast paced lifestyle, 70% of population relies on ready-to-eat and ready-to-cook foods which are usually loaded with either fat or sugar to make it palatable to our taste buds. These packed foods are often deficit in protein.
- *Over dependency on rice and wheat:* Indian diet is super dependent on rice and wheat products and our daily diet is majorly driven by it. But we should not forget that pulses are the powerhouse of nutrients. Many people do not know that combination of pulses not only gives a good calorie amount but also is low in glycemic index and are high in soluble fiber which is beneficial in controlling healthy blood sugar levels.
- *Fallacy about protein:* A mis-belief works among Indians that protein plays major role for athletes, weight lifters or sportsmen only. But the fact of the matter is that an optimum protein intake is needed for all.

Indians have higher insulin resistance and poor glucose utilization- Role of proteins in diabetes

- Type 2 diabetes have an altered adaptive mechanism for protein sparing, independent of protein quality
- It appears abnormalities of protein metabolism are present even with mild hyperglycemia
- The threshold for abnormal nitrogen synthesis and breakdown is reported to be at a fasting glycemia between 108 mg/dL and 125 mg/dL[9]
- Therefore, with moderate energy restriction there is need for a generous dietary protein intake (~1 g/kg body weight)

Clearly there is an increased requirement of protein in diabetes as:

- Plasma glucose does not increase after protein ingestion
- Substitution of dietary carbohydrate with protein improves glycemic control without increasing risk of atherosclerosis
- Plasma glucagon concentration is high with high protein diet
- Plasma triglyceride response is reduced
- High-protein diet (30%) results in 40% reduction in plasma glucose concentration.[9]

How to Optimize Protein in Indian Cuisine?

Good news for vegetarians. There is a dietary strategy called **mutual supplementation** in which you combine complementary partially complete protein food to supply adequate amounts of all the essential amino acids.[10] For example, though both beans and brown rice are quite rich in protein, each lacks one or more of the essential amino acids. However, when beans are combined with brown rice, the result is equivalent to a complete protein that can substitute chicken or meat. Unlike most beans, soybean products (such as tofu and soymilk) are complete proteins. They contain the essential amino acids. Tofu, soy flour, soy-based meat substitutes, soy cheese, and many other soy products are healthy ways to make a meatless diet "nutrient complete." Some more combinations that can be tried are soy curry and rice, milk and oats, etc.

Follow the plate method way of eating as every meal has to be balanced with protein (Fig. 1). Protein should be at least 25% of your plate and you should include it in major meals like breakfast, lunch, and dinner with judicious choice of protein snacks in between.[11] Apart from the total daily intake, per-meal protein quantity and daily frequency of protein ingestion have also been shown to play an important role in preserving muscle mass and function. It is estimated that consumption of two to three meals a day, each containing ~25–30 g of high-quality protein, is optimal for the stimulation of 24-hour muscle protein synthesis (MPS) in healthy adults.[10,11]

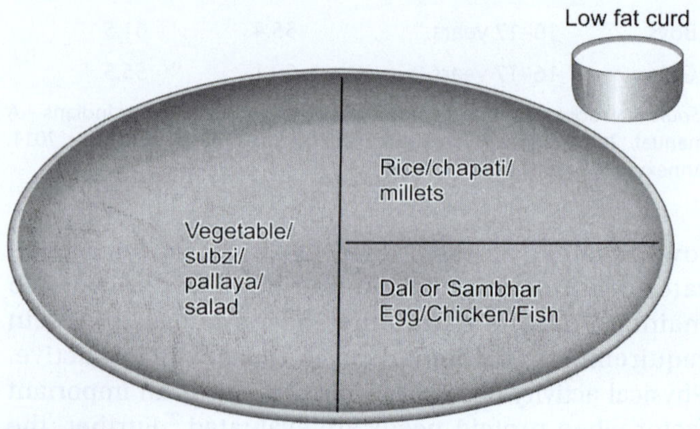

Figure 1 One portion/exchange of protein.

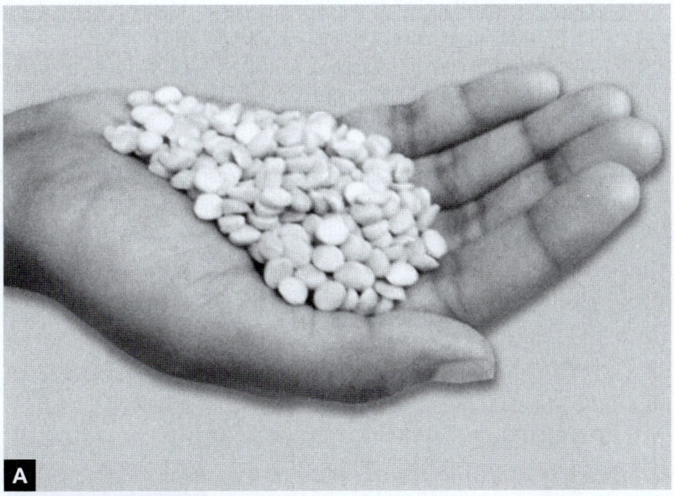

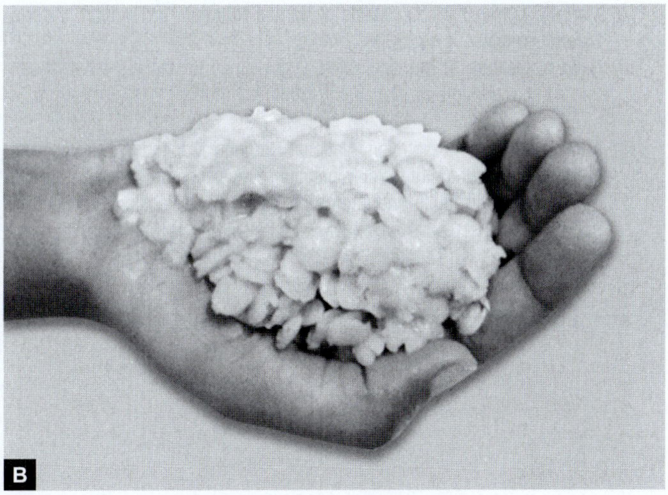

Figures 2A and B (A) Raw pulses/dals; (B) Cooked pulses/dals.

- Vegetarians can include combination of pulses along with cereals (to get all the essential amino acids) (Figs. 2A and B). Besides pulses, other sources are legumes (rajma/kidney beans, chaana/chickpeas, lobia/black eyed peas, cowpea), green peas, soybean, paneer, tofu, sprouts, amaranth seeds, etc.
- Among dairy sources milk, curd, yogurt, low fat cheese can also provide good amount of protein in diet.
- Rotation of whole grain cereal and millet are important for optimum protein intake.
- Include fistful of nuts, roasted peanuts or chana along with seeds cocktail as a protein snack.
- Nonvegetarians can include fish, eggs, and lean meat in their diet for high protein amount.
- Snack on protein rich foods like low fat yoghurt/sprouts/a cup of low-fat milk, etc.
- Keep consumption of lean cuts of chicken and fish to not more than 2–3 times/week. Avoid shell fish such as prawns, crabs, lobsters, and red meat.
- Besan and sattu have been an integral part of Indian cooking and perfect sources of protein.
- One part soy flour can be added to three parts of wheat flour or other cereals while making chapati dough to improve protein content of daily diet.
- Low fat skim milk powder is an excellent source to improve the protein quality and quantity of any Indian recipe.
- Newer versions of cereals like quinoa has also gained lot of popularity in recent years as it provides good amount of protein and fiber.
- In recent years, unconventional sources of protein like leaf proteins, single cell protein (SCP, viz. yeast) etc., have been proposed for human use, but they have not found wide acceptance or their safety for human consumption fully established.

CONCLUSION

The thin-fat India is protein deficient.[1] There is a need for improving the knowledge levels around protein sources and importance of physical activity, to improve daily protein intake and lean muscle mass. Which in turn will also help in tackling chronic diseases like diabetes, obesity, etc. Using plate method for each meal can be the fundamental approach in tackling the low dietary protein intake in India. Adding locally available pulses and legumes to each major meal and snacks should be reinforced. Animal based protein to be consumed in moderation. In addition novel proteins require the development of new value chains, and attention to issues, such as production costs, food safety, scalability, and consumer acceptance.[10]

REFERENCES

1. Lakshmi S, Metcalf B, Joglekar C, et al. Differences in body composition and metabolic status between white U.K. and Asian Indian children (EarlyBird 24 and the Pune Maternal Nutrition Study). Pediatr Obes. 2012;7: 347-54.
2. Lear SA, Kohli S, Bondy GP, et al. Ethnic variation in fat and lean body mass and the association with insulin resistance. J Clin Endocrinol Metab. 2009;94:4696-702.
3. Gluckman P, Hanson M. Echoes of the past: evolution, development, health and disease. Discov Med. 2004;4:401-7.
4. Rampal P. An analysis of protein consumption in India through plant and animal sources. Food Nutr Bull. 2018;39: 564-80.

5. Mann J, Truswell AS. Essentials of Human Nutrition, 3rd edition. Oxford: Oxford University Press; 2008.
6. National Institute of Nutrition. Dietary guidelines for Indians—A manual, 2nd edition. Hyderabad: National Institute of Nutrition; 2011. Annexure 3: p. 89.
7. National Institute of Nutrition. National Nutrition Monitoring Bureau: Diet and Nutritional Status of Rural Population, Prevalence of Hypertension and Diabetes among Adults and Infant and Young Child Feeding Practices—Report of Third Repeat Survey. NNMB Technical Report No. 26. Hyderabad: National Institute of Nutrition, ICMR; 2012.
8. Gopalan C, Rama Sastri BV, Balasubramanian SC. Nutritive value of Indian Foods. Hyderabad: National Institute of Nutrition, ICMR; 2007.
9. Manish M. "Protein consumption in diet of adult Indians: a general consumer survey (PRODIGY). Indian Medical Gazette. 2015;149-50.
10. Swaminathan S, Vaz M, Kurpad AV. Protein intakes in India. Br J Nutr. 2012;108:S50-8.
11. Comerford KB, Gonca Pasin G. Emerging evidence for the importance of dietary protein source on glucoregulatory markers and type 2 diabetes: Different effects of dairy, meat, fish, egg, and plant protein foods. Nutrients. 2016;8. pii: E446.

19 CHAPTER

Macronutrient Composition of Diet for Diabetes Mellitus Patients: Tips for Clinicians

Sanjeev Gulati, Sushil Jindal, Shalini Chutani

INTRODUCTION

Diabetes is a chronic illness, and management of diabetes requires a holistic approach. The most challenging and important part of diabetes management is determining and advising a meal plan to an individual. Nutritional science is constantly evolving, so what may be considered appropriate today might become outdated by tomorrow. Modern diet for an individual with diabetes is based on concepts from clinical researches; giving 1,800 calorie diet sheet, a "one size fits all" approach, might not work.[1] Every person with diabetes should be actively engaged in education, self-management, and treatment planning with his or her healthcare team, including development of an individualized eating pattern.[2]

GENERAL GOALS—GOALS OF MEDICAL NUTRITION THERAPY IN DIABETES

To promote and support healthy eating patterns, a variety of nutrient-dense foods in appropriate portion sizes has to be emphasized. This is done in order to improve overall health and specifically to:

- Achieve and maintain body weight goals
- Attain individualized glycemic, blood pressure, and lipid targets
- Delay or prevent the complications of diabetes
- Address individual nutritional needs based on personal and cultural preferences, access to healthy foods, willingness, and ability to make the behavioral changes
- Maintain pleasure of eating and limiting food choices, only if evidence based
- Provide the individual with diabetes with practical tools for meals planning
- Provide adequate nutrition to expectant mothers and growing children
- Energy balance—for overweight or obese adults with type 2 diabetes, reducing energy intake while maintaining a healthy eating pattern is recommended to promote weight loss.

MACRONUTRIENT COMPOSITION

There is no ideal ratio of carbohydrate, protein, and fat in the diet for people with diabetes. Macronutrient distribution should be individualized based on the assessment of current eating pattern, preferences, and metabolic goals.[1]

Carbohydrates

Carbohydrates are necessary for energy, some vitamins, fiber, and dietary palatability and as a major regulator of postprandial glucose levels.

There is no consistent definition of "low or (high) carbohydrate diets." The following definitions are used in different literature:[3]

- Very low carbohydrate diet: 21–70 g per day of carbohydrate
- Moderately low carbohydrate diet: 30–40% of total calories as carbohydrate
- Moderate carbohydrate diet: 40–65% of total calories as carbohydrate
- High carbohydrate diet: >65% of total calories as carbohydrate.

These definitions are not all inclusive, as 100 g/day carbohydrate may represent <30% of kcal, but all the published articles fit in one of these categories.[3]

In the Diabetes Remission Clinical Trial (DiRECT) study, the intervention group was given low-calorie diet with carbohydrate 59% initially and 50% in the maintenance phase. Fifteen percent of the low-calorie group lost 15 kg weight and 46% achieved remission in 1 year.[4]

In a study by Seidelmann et al.[5] on ARIC (atherosclerosis risk in communities) cohort to see the association of carbohydrate intake on mortality, the authors reported that there was a U-shaped association between percentage of energy consumed from carbohydrate (means 48%) and mortality; a percentage of 50–55% energy from carbohydrate was associated with the lowest risk of mortality. Both low-carbohydrate <40% (and hence, very high fat) consumption and high-carbohydrate consumption (>70%) conferred a greater mortality risk.[5]

Carbohydrate is the chief source of energy in many low- and middle-income countries, contributing to 70–80% of daily calories. Diets of Asian countries including India continue to derive two-thirds of carbohydrate calories from cereal staples. Excess carbohydrate in diet is linked to both increased susceptibilities to type 2 diabetes mellitus, proneness to poor glycemic control, and complications of diabetes. The take-home message for Asians would be to cut down the carbohydrate from present 65–80% to 50–55% and add enough proteins.[6]

Practical Tips for Carbohydrate Intake

- With evidence inconclusive about the ideal amount of carbohydrate for people with diabetes, it is the quality of carbohydrate which is more important. Carbohydrate intake from vegetables, legumes, whole grains, and fresh fruits should be advised over intake from other sources, especially those that contain added fat, sugars, and sodium.[7]
- Monitoring carbohydrate, whether by experience-based estimation or by carbohydrate counting, remains a key in achieving glycemic control.
- Start the day with whole grain, whole wheat porridge, oats, millets, quinoa, and sprouts without added sugars.
- Avoid white bread. Most of the commercially available breads are high in refined flour.
- Use whole grain bread (chapati) and brown rice for lunch or snacks.
- Beans and legumes are an excellent source of slowly digestible carbohydrate as well as a great source of proteins.
- Include a variety of fresh salad and vegetables in each meal.
- Mixing of wheat flour with gram flour or rice batter with lentils or peas batter adds to both proteins and fiber in the diet and provides healthier carbohydrates. (Prefer Missi roti over Naan in restaurants or parties.)
- Nuts such as walnut, peanut, and almonds are healthy carbohydrates.
- Seeds, such as chia seeds, pumpkin seeds, and tubers such as potatoes and sweet potatoes are good carbohydrate sources and contain proteins and fiber.
- Avoid consuming fruits with meals. This increases carbohydrate load and thus may increase postprandial blood sugar. Fruits consumed as mid-morning or evening snacks are better.
- Kneading chapati flour with leftover dals gives healthy carbohydrates and proteins as well.

Avoid carbohydrates from:
- Sugary drink and fruit juices
- White bread: These are refined carbohydrates that are low in essential nutrients and bad for metabolic health. This applies to most commercially available breads, pastries, cookies and cakes, ice-cream, candies, and chocolates.
- French fries and potato chips. Whole potatoes are healthy, but French fries and potato chips are not.

Proteins

The 2013 American Diabetes Association (ADA) nutrition recommendation for adults with diabetes position statement states the following.
- For individuals with diabetes and no evidence of diabetic kidney disease, evidence is inconclusive to recommend an ideal amount of protein intake for glycemic control or improving one or more cardiovascular disease (CVD) risk measures. Therefore, goals should be individualized.
- For individuals with diabetic kidney disease, reducing the amount of protein intake below the usual intake of 0.8 g/kg body weight/day is not recommended because it does not alter glycemic measures, cardiovascular risk measures, or the course of glomerular filtration rate (GFR) decline.
- In individuals with type 2 diabetes, ingested protein can increase insulin response without increase in plasma glucose concentrations. Therefore, carbohydrate sources high in protein should not be used to prevent or treat hypoglycemia.

Joslin Diabetes Center advocates a protein intake of 20–30% of total energy intake or not less than 1–2 g/kg ideal body weight for individuals with type 2 diabetes.[8]

On an average, in India the consumption of food per capita per day is 1.317 kg, which is 2,458 calories. Indians consume starchy diets which are rich in carbohydrates. This constitutes approximately 70–80% of their diet.

In an Indian diet, proteins are also sourced from carbohydrate-rich foods, because of their excess in regular diets. Actual protein sources such as dairy products, animal foods, and pulses are consumed in a comparatively limited quantity by Indians.

The Indian Market Research Bureau's 2017 report states that protein deficiency among Indians stands at more than 80%, measured against the recommended 60 g/day. The usual sources of proteins in a regular diet are a cup of lentil, a glass of milk, or a cup (200 g) of yoghurt that contains 7–8 g of protein.

To get the daily requirement of 60 g protein, it would be necessary to eat eight bowls of lentils or drink —seven to eight glasses of milk.

Protein from animal sources such as meat, poultry, fish, eggs, milk, cheese, and yogurt provide all nine essential amino acids and are considered "Complete Proteins," while proteins from vegan sources such as plants, nuts, seeds, legumes, and grains are deficient in one or more essential proteins, and are considered "Incomplete Proteins."

Practical Tips to Increase Protein Content in the Diet for Indian Patients

- Replace the cereals in breakfast with eggs: Most breakfasts are low in protein; eating three eggs for breakfast can provide 19 g of high-quality protein. Eating eggs for breakfast has a satiating effect for several hours.
- Including low-fat yogurt or curd in any one meal provides 10 g protein in each serving of 250 g.
- Breakfast options for vegetarians can be preparations made from legumes such as moong dal cheela, sprouts, and quinoa.
- Add high-protein sources to salad, such as chicken or turkey, and kidney beans, chickpeas, cottage cheese, or tofu for vegetarians.
- Commercially available meal replacement provides 10–15 g proteins per servings.
- Consume a high-protein dish with each meal such as chicken, fish, or legumes and cottage cheese for vegetarians
- Mixing wheat and gram flour or even soy flour can provide good protein.
- Studies have found cottage cheese to be as healthy as eggs.
- Peanut butter for breakfast or snacks, 2 tablespoons contains 8 g of proteins.
- Edamame, unripened soybeans, are an excellent protein source—100 g contains 11 g of proteins, used as a vegetable in many parts.
- Other vegetarian sources of proteins are—Seitan (wheat meat), a protein-rich food made from wheat gluten, chia seeds, pumpkin seeds, almonds, quinoa, spirulina, breads made from sprouted grains and legumes, soymilk, oats, and oatmeal.
- Protein-rich vegetables are broccoli, spinach, asparagus, potatoes, and sweet potatoes which contain 4–5 g protein per cooked cup.
- Fruits are generally low in proteins. Certain fruits such as guava, mulberries, and bananas contain 2–4 g proteins per cup.

Fat

An ideal amount of dietary fat for individual with diabetes is controversial. The quality of fat is more important than quantity. Lowering of fat intake infrequently improved glycemic control or CVD risk factors in clinical trials involving individuals with diabetes. Lowering fat intake in diabetes may improve total cholesterol and low-density lipoprotein (LDL) but may also lower high-density lipoprotein (HDL) cholesterol.[3] The National Institute of Medicine has defined AMDR for fat as 20–35% of the total daily calorie intake. AMDR is acceptable macronutrient distribution range, the range of intake for an energy source which is associated with a lower risk of chronic disease, while providing essential nutrient intake consumption. Exceeding this is associated with a risk of chronic disease. Below this leads to an insufficient intake of essential nutrients. Since diabetes is considered as a CVD risk factor, the amount and type of fat intake recommendation remain same as with an individual with CVD without diabetes.[7]

The 2013 standards of medical care from ADA recommend that:

- Saturated fat intake should be less than or equal to 10% of total calories and reducing the trans fat in the diet lowers LDL cholesterol and increases HDL cholesterol; therefore, intake of trans fat should be minimized.
- *Monounsaturated fatty acids (MUFA)*: Evidence from large prospective cohort studies, clinical trials, and

a systematic review of randomized controlled trials (RCTs) indicate that high MUFA diets are associated with improved glycemic control and improved CVD risk or risk factors.[9]

- *Polyunsaturated fatty acids*: The evidence of effects of omega-6 polyunsaturated fatty acids (PUFAs) on people with diabetes is limited. Controversy exists on the best ratio of omega-6 to omega-3 fatty acids.
- *Omega-3 fatty acids*
    - Evidence does not support recommending omega-3 [eicosapentaenoic acid (EPA) and docosahexaenoic acid (DHA)] supplements for people with diabetes for the prevention or treatment of cardiovascular events.[9]
    - As recommended for the general public, foods containing long-chain omega-3 fatty acids (EPA and DHA) and omega-3 linolenic acid (ALA) are recommended.[9]
- Mediterranean-style diet, which is rich in monounsaturated and polyunsaturated fat, improves glycemic control and reduces cardiovascular risk factors in people with diabetes, can be adapted and modified to suit Indian needs.

Practical Tips for Fat Intake

- Avoid saturated fat containing food such as red meat, poultry with skin, butter, cheese, full-fat milk products, palm oil, and coconut oil and completely avoid trans fats such as hydrogenated oils, deep fried food, and processed food containing trans fats.
- Use of items that are rich in MUFA and PUFA such as vegetable and nut oils including canola, corn, safflower, sunflower, peanut, sesame, soybean oil, mustard oil, vegetable oil spreads, whole nuts and nut butters, and avocado should be advised.
- Mustard oil is cheap and a good source of omega 3 fatty acids. Cooking one dry vegetable in mustard oil supplies good quantity of omega 3 fatty acid. Other good sources are fish, walnut, soybean oil, flax seeds, or flaxseed oil.

Fiber

The recommended intake for fiber is 25 g for adult women and 35 g for adult men. Fiber should be sourced from food. Since most of our patients are either overweight or obese and considering the very high ratio of carbohydrates in Indian diet, we should try to focus on correct balance of macronutrients in the diet. A diet having carbohydrates in the ratio of 50–55%, proteins 20–25%, and fats 25–30% is broadly recommended. More important is the quality of the macronutrients. Practitioners should advocate on a diet which suits the financial and cultural milieu of the patients. Repeated counseling and reinforcements are often needed.

CONCLUSION

All professional organizations have emphasized the role of MNT as an important part of diabetes management, with evidences inconclusive, focus should be on correct balance of macronutrients according to metabolic goals as BMI, blood sugar levels and lipid parameters. A diet having Carbohydrates in the ratio of 50–55%, Proteins 15–25% and fats 25–30% is broadly recommended. More important is the quality of the macronutrients, practitioners should advocate on a diet which suits the financial and cultural milieu of the patients. Repeated counselling and reinforcements are often needed

REFERENCES

1. American Diabetes Association. Lifestyle management: Standards of medical care in diabetes-2019. Diabetes Care. 2019;42(suppl 1):S46-60.
2. Franz MJ, MacLeod J, Evert A, et al. Academy of Nutrition and Diabetes Nutrition practice guidelines for Type 1 and Type 2 diabetes in adults: systematic review of evidence for medical nutrition therapy effectiveness and recommendations for integration into the nutrition care process. J Acad Nutr Diet. 2017;117:1659-75.
3. Wheeler ML, Dunbar SA, Jack LM, et al. Macronutrients, food groups, and eating patterns in the management of diabetes: A systematic review of literature, 2010. Diabetes Care. 2012;35:434-45.
4. Lean MEJ, Leslie WS, Barnes AC, et al. Primary care lead weight management for remission of type 2 diabetes (DiRECT). The Lantus. 2018;391(10120):P541-51.
5. Seidelmann SB, Clagget B, Cheng S, et al. Dietary carbohydrate intake and mortality: a prospective cohort study and meta-analysis. Lancet Public Health. 2018;3:e419-28.
6. Mohan V, Unnikrashnan R, Shobhana S, et al. Are excess carbohydrates the main link to diabetes and its complications in Asians. Indian J Med Res. 2018;148:531-8.
7. Evert AB, Boucher JL, Cypress M, et al. Nutrition therapy recommendations for the management of adults with diabetes. Diabetes Care. 2014;37(suppl 1): S120-43.
8. Campbell AP and Rains TM. Dietary protein is important in the practical management of prediabetes and type 2 diabetes. J Nutr. 2015;145(1):164S-9S.
9. Gray A. Nutritional recommendations for Individuals with diabetes (updated 2015 May 31). In: Feingold KR, Anawalt B, Boyce A, et al., (Eds). Endotext (Internet). South Dermoth (MA): MD Text.com, Inc; 2000. Available from https://www.ncbi.nlm.nih.gov/pubmed/24357208.

20

CHAPTER

What is more Important for Weight Loss: Carbohydrate Restriction or Fat Restriction?

Ramesh Kumar Goenka

INTRODUCTION

The incidence of obesity had almost doubled worldwide since 1980s as per World Health Organization (WHO). Worldwide, in 2008, 35% of people more than 20 years of age were characterized as overweight and 11% were obese. In adults, overweight and obesity are related with type 2 diabetes, cardiovascular disease (CVD), and particular types of carcinoma.[1,2] Diabetes is one of the largest public health problems in the world, which is associated with health, economic, and social costs. For slowing or even reversing this rising trend, urgent solutions are required, particularly from investment in modifiable factors comprising diet, weight, and physical activity.[3] As per global burden of disease study that was conducted in 188 countries, diet is a leading contributor to the mortality and morbidity globally.[4]

The importance of nutrition which is the most controversial and difficult part in the management and prevention of type 2 diabetes, is clearly established through its effect on weight and metabolic control. In a study published by Diabetes Care in 2009, it was shown that obesity promotes diabetes and weight loss (be it from diet or metabolic surgery) counteracts it (Fig. 1) by virtue of increased insulin sensitivity.[5]

Diabetic patients may have more difficulty in losing weight due to genetic differences, metabolic factors (inflammation, insulin resistance, adipokines), medications [insulin, thiazolidinediones (TZDs), sulfonylureas], increased food to avoid hypoglycemia, limited physical activity, and diet fatigue due to carbohydrate restrictions.[6] It is therefore necessary to further explore dietary measures that can most effectively make a contribution to reduce excess body weight and improve insulin sensitivity, as well as risk parameters for CVD.

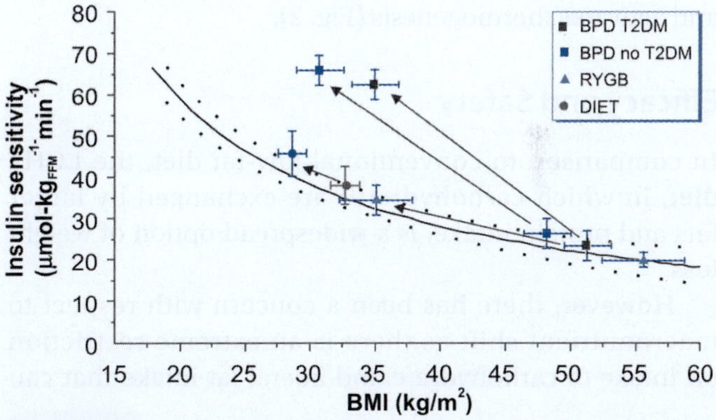

Figure 1 Correlation between insulin sensitivity and body mass index with respect to patients undergoing weight loss by diet.

Most of the guidelines recommend reducing energy intake to promote weight loss in obese and overweight people. Most evidence suggests that food intake high in fruits, vegetables, whole grains, nuts, dairy products, and legumes should be encouraged. Mostly two approaches are followed; a low-fat hypocaloric diet that reduces insulin resistance and prevent type 2 diabetes and a low-carbohydrate, high-fat (LCHF) diet which is proposed as a more effective alternative.

LOW-CARBOHYDRATE HIGH-FAT DIET

Limiting the daily consumption of carbohydrate, specifically that of rapidly digestible starches and sugars has recently been recommended by WHO and various national authorities. In the past there have been various popular diet plans which evolved around low-carbohydrate content like Atkins diet, the Zone diet, the South Beach diet, and the ketogenic diet. A significant reduction in carbohydrate content in these diets is accompanied by an increase in amount of fat and to a lesser extent, also protein. Hence these diets are more appropriately termed "LCHF" diet. The much described beneficial effect of such diet are due to the weight loss achieved, the safety concerns are still awaited in view of lack of long-term data. In these diet plans, carbohydrate intake is restricted to as low as 20 g per day which limits the food choices severely, resulting in monotony ending up in reduced caloric intake. The body depletes its glycogen stores and induces gluconeogenesis, using lean tissue for producing glucose as a source of energy for the brain. From adipose tissue, free fatty acids are also mobilized that result in the formation of ketone body. The appetite is diminished by mild ketosis and high intake of protein increases satiety and activates thermogenesis (Fig. 2).

Efficacy and Safety

In comparison to conventional low-fat diet, the LCHF diet, in which carbohydrates are exchanged by larger fats and protein intake, is a widespread option of weight loss.

However, there has been a concern with respect to macronutrient shift as there is an extreme restriction on intake of carbohydrate and liberal fat intake that can present detrimental impact on CVD risk factors.[7,8] Increase in intake of fat, specifically saturated fatty acid (SFA), has been related with increased low-density lipoprotein (LDL) cholesterol and therefore increase in risk of CVD.[7,9,10] WHO recommends limiting SFA intake to less than 10% of total energy intake whereas American Heart Association (AHA) recommends restricting it to less than 7%.[7] However, one of the meta-analyses challenged these recommendations, as it was concluded by the authors that there was no significant association between increase in risk of CVD and coronary heart disease (CHD) and intake of SFA.[11] In a review by American Diabetes Association (ADA), interventions of low-carbohydrate diet (less than 40% of calories) from 2001 to 2010 were analyzed and about half reported greater improvement in HbA1c on an LCHF diet versus a low-fat diet and a greater reduction in the use of medicine to lower blood glucose.[12]

As per a highly controlled study, which was an inpatient feeding study, a decrease in mean HbA1c levels from 7.3% to 6.8% (P = 0.006) was observed in just 14 days on an LCHF diet.[13] Those studies have supported LCHF diet plans where subjects on LCHF diets showed more weight loss, more reduction in both TG and total cholesterol, and increase in HDL cholesterol in comparison to their low-fat diet counterparts.[14,15] However, it is also reported by studies that there were significant increase or paucity of reduction in LDL cholesterol after consumption of an

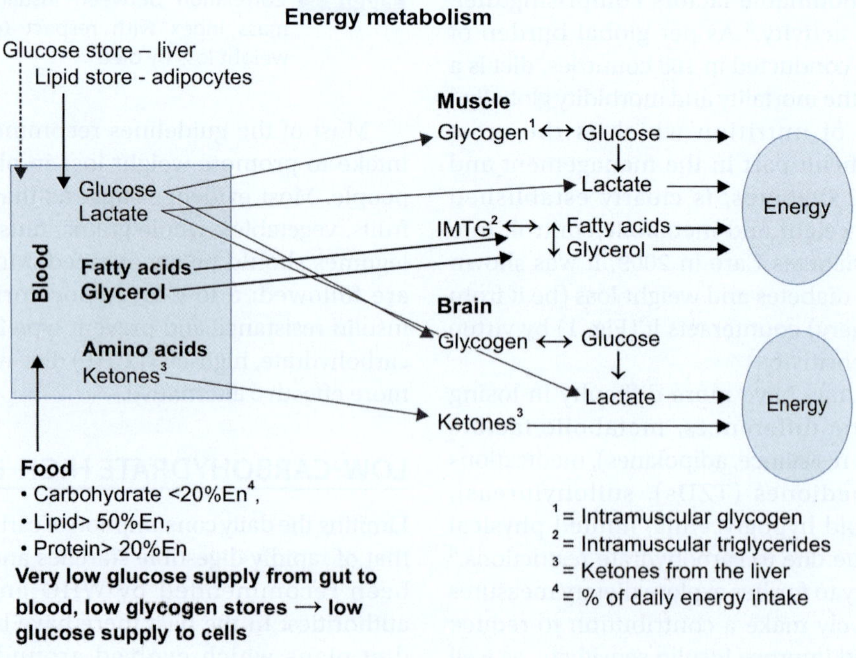

Figure 2 Energy metabolism during a high fat–low carbohydrate diet.

LCHF diet,[15-19] which potentially could be detrimental because LDL cholesterol is a significant risk factor in the CVD morbidity and mortality.[20-22] Therefore concerns have been raised with regards to the use of LCHF diet, especially by the patient with known CVD, type 2 diabetes mellitus (T2DM), dyslipidemia and/or hypertension.[23] Overall a LCHF diet are not recommended for weight loss and maintenance.

LOW-FAT DIET

A low-fat diet is one that restricts fat with often saturated fat and cholesterol as well. In general hypocaloric low-fat diets are high in carbohydrates (55–60% of total energy intake), low in fat (<30% of total energy intake) and reduced in energy (deficit of 500–1,000 calorie). Diets in this category have generally been supported by studies to have beneficial effect on CVD risk among high risk patients.[11,12] Diets in this category include National Cholesterol Education Program (NCEP) Step I Diet with energy intake restriction; the DASH diet, which is based on the US Department of Agriculture Food Guide Pyramid; and some commercial programs (e.g., Weight Watchers). Low-calorie diet should have high fiber content and a low-glycemic index. High-fiber and low-glycemic-index diets are related with enhanced satiety, reduced postprandial glycemic response, reduced levels of insulin, and thus are protective against diabetes and CVD. Studies have generally supported low-fat diet to have useful impact on CVD risk in high-risk patients (Fig. 3).[24,25]

Efficacy and Safety

The National Institute of Health reviewed 34 randomized controlled trials for evaluating the efficacy of low-calorie low-fat diets for weight loss, reducing abdominal fat and enhancing cardiorespiratory fitness; and reported that over a period of 3–12 months, total body weight was reduced by about 8%. In addition to reducing weight, such diets also reduced abdominal fat as shown by a 1.5–9.5 cm decrease in waist circumference and showed no improvement in cardiorespiratory fitness. Another meta-analysis of 16 trials, that were of 2–12 months duration, out of which 14 were randomized, reported that low-fat diets with no intentional limitation of energy intake lead to more weight loss (3.2 kg, 95% confidence interval (CI) 1.9–4.5 kg, $P < 0.001$) compared to the usual or medium-fat diets and weight loss was noted to be more substantial in heavier subjects. Another meta-analysis by Yu-Poth and colleagues of 37 studies using NCEP Step I and Step II diets reported that each 1% reduction in total fat energy was related with a 0.28 kg reduction in body weight and both the diets showed a 12% and 16% decline in circulating LDL cholesterol levels, respectively.

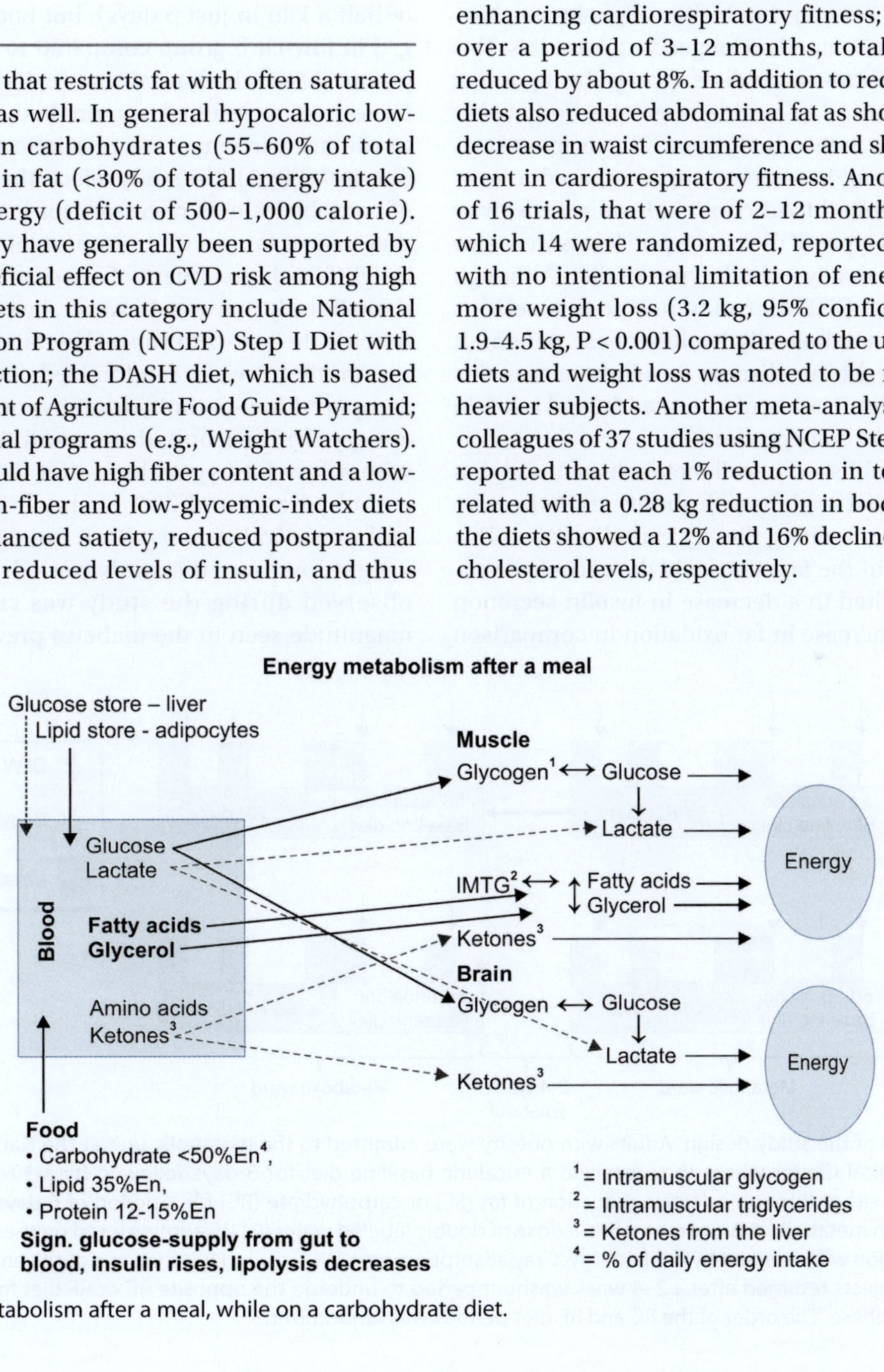

Figure 3 Energy metabolism after a meal, while on a carbohydrate diet.

COMPARING HYPOCALORIC LOW-FAT DIET VERSUS LOW-CARBOHYDRATE, HIGH-FAT DIET

Both low-fat and low-carb diet result in weight loss. Two studies, each 6 months in duration reported greater weight loss with low-carb diet than with low-fat diet and subsequently many more studies also showed more weight loss with low-carb diet than with low-fat diet. The greater weight loss with low-carb diet was concluded in short-term studies of less than 6 months but in this weight loss on low-carb diet was not maintained on longer duration trials. This excess weight loss in low-carb dieter group during initial few weeks was reported to be due to greater body water loss and greater loss in lean body mass. The dropout rates were very high among low-carb group compared to low-fat group due to limited food choices. Insulin sensitivity improved with both types of diet and leptin levels were also found to decrease equally in both types of diet. Although in the short term, LCHF diet may not pose a serious health threat to a metabolically healthy obese patient, it may pose a risk of chronic disease development, as this approach does not limit intake of saturated fat and is low in vegetables, fruits, and dairy products.

A latest study published in cell metabolism found that decreasing intake of fat in adults with obesity results in more loss of body fat than limiting dietary carbohydrates. This happened in spite of the fact that only the carbohydrate-restricted diet resulted in a decrease in insulin secretion and a substantial increase in fat oxidation in comparison with the baseline energy balanced diet. The study was conducted on 19 obese men and women who were rigorously enforced on either a 6 day low-fat or low-carb diet (Fig. 4). Low-fat group led to more fat loss but low-carb group lead to more weight loss. On the whole, both diets resulted in weight loss for 6 days, but people on low-carb lost significantly more weight.

After 6 days low-carb group lost about 1.85 kg compared to around 1.35 kg of low-fat group (difference of half a kilo in just 6 days), but body fat loss was 53 ± 6 g/d in low-carb group compared to 89 ± 6 g/d in low-fat group. Research showed that "calorie for calorie, dietary fat restriction resulted in more body fat loss as compared to dietary carbohydrate restriction among adults with obesity" (Fig. 5). The study rejects the claim that restriction of carbohydrate is necessary for loss of body fat, adding that loss of fat is a more important goal as compared to weight loss in treatment of obesity.[26] The findings of such a small study may not, however, be sufficiently convincing to settle the low-carb versus low-fat debate.

Another 8-week randomized controlled trial directly compared low-carbohydrate hypocaloric diet with 20% energy from carbohydrates and 60% energy from fat with a low-fat hypocaloric diet with 60% energy from carbohydrates and 20% energy from fat in overweight and obese individuals. Both the diets achieved similar weight loss over the study period. The 7% weight loss observed during the study was comparable with the magnitude seen in the diabetes prevention studies. Both

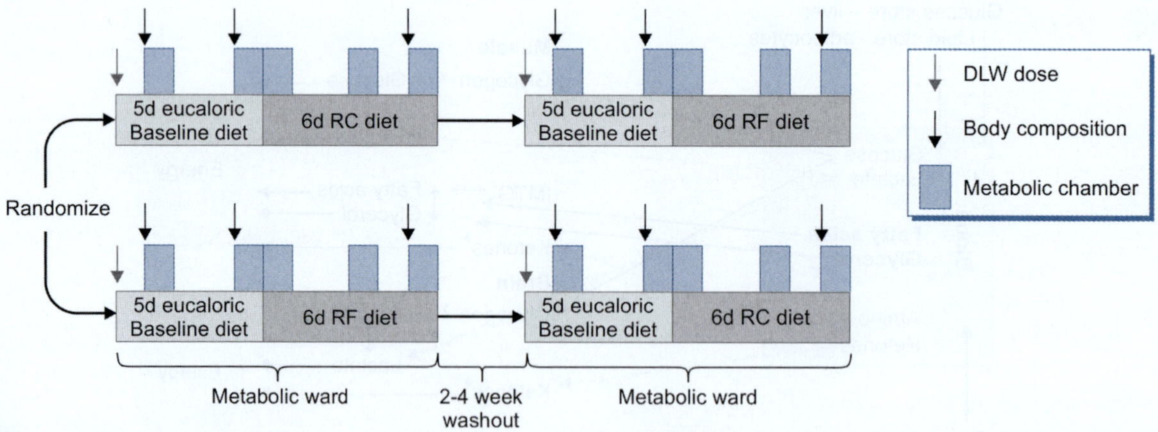

Figure 4 Overview of the study design. Adults with obesity were admitted to the metabolic unit at the National Institute of Health (NIH) Clinical Center where they received a eucaloric baseline diet for 5 days followed by a 30% energy restricted diet achieved either through selective reduction of fat (RF) or carbohydrate (RC) for a period of 6 days. Subjects spent 5 days residing in metabolic chambers and had a dose of doubly labeled water (DLW) administered on the first inpatient day. Body composition was assessed by dual-energy X-ray absorptiometry (DXA) during baseline and at the end of the reduced energy diets. Subjects returned after a 2–4 week washout period to undergo the opposite RC or RF diet following the same 5 day baseline phase. The order of the RC and RF diet periods was randomized.

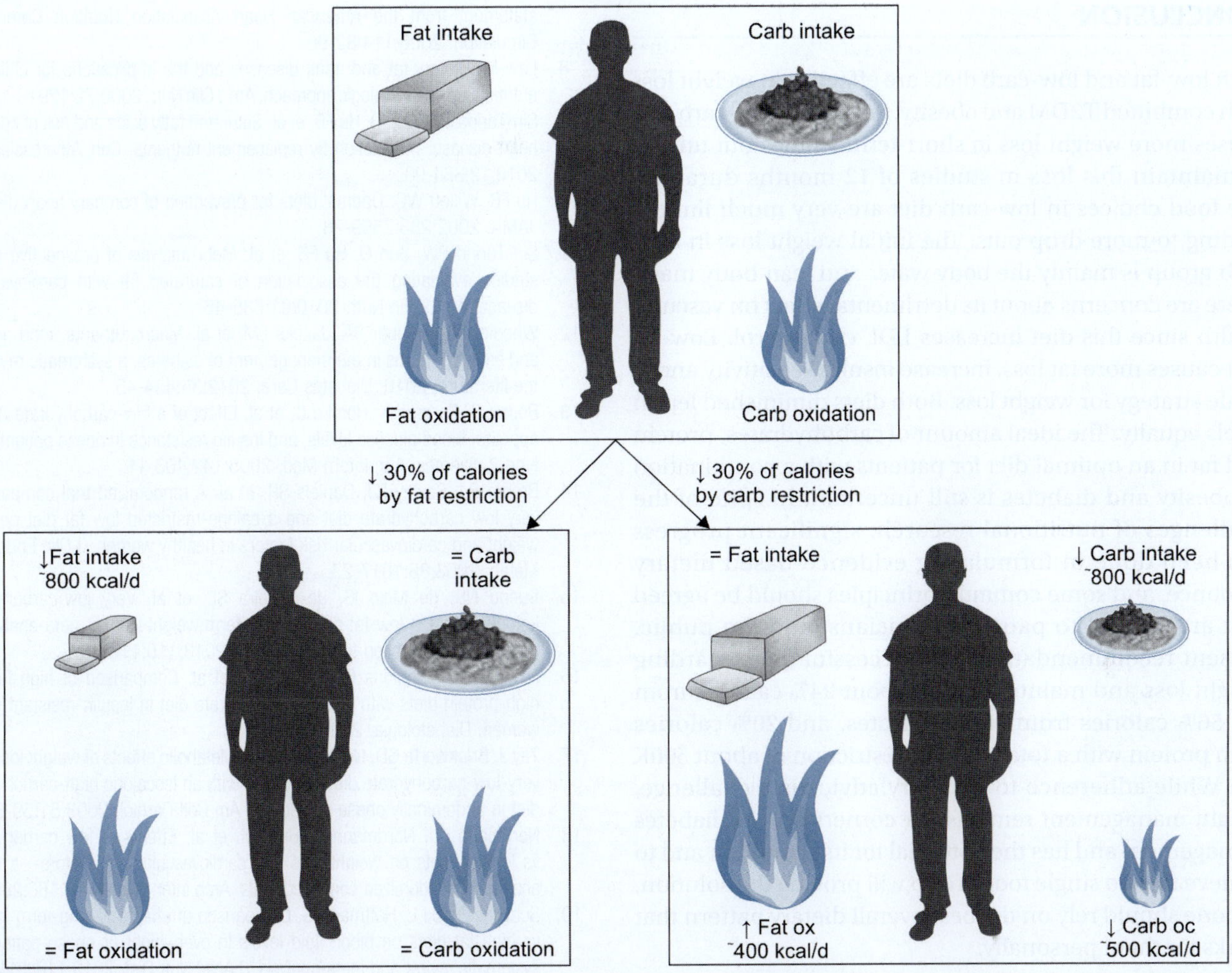

Figure 5 Human metabolism: process of release of energy by fat and carbohydrate oxidation.

the diet promoted weight loss from the central body region and were associated with comparable effect on insulin sensitivity. In this trial a significant difference was observed in augmentation index, a measure of vascular compliance that was not explained by changes in the conventional vascular risk factors and showed a negative impact of low-carb diet on vascular stiffening.[27]

Another study assessed the impact of low-fat versus low-carbohydrate diet on 12-month weight loss among overweight adults. This "Diet Intervention Examining the Factors Interacting with Treatment Success" (DIETFITS) randomized clinical trial enrolled total 609 adults in the age range of 18–50 years without diabetes and having a body mass index between 28 kg/m^2 and 40 kg/m^2. Randomization of the participants was done to either the 12-month healthy low-fat (HLF) diet or a healthy low-carbohydrate (HLC) diet.

Mean age of the participants was 40 (SD, 7) years; 57% were women. Mean body mass index of patients was 33 (SD, 3) kg/m^2; 40% (n = 244) had a low-fat genotype. 30% (n = 180) had a low-carbohydrate genotype; mean baseline INS-30 was 93 μIU/mL. Among 609 participants randomized, 79% (n = 481) completed the trial. In the HLF versus HLC diets, respectively, the mean 12-month macronutrient distributions were 48% versus 30% for carbohydrates; 29% versus 45% for fat; and 21% versus 23% for protein. Change in weight at 12 months was −5.3 kg for the HLF diet as compared to −6.0 kg for the HLC diet [mean between-group difference, 0.7 kg (95% CI, −0.2 to 1.6 kg)]. Therefore, it was concluded in the study that, in this 12-month weight loss diet study, no significant difference was noted in weight change between a HLF diet as compared to a healthy low-carbohydrate diet.[28]

CONCLUSION

Both low-fat and low-carb diets are effective in weight loss with combined T2DM and obesity. People on low-carb diet causes more weight loss in short-term studies but unable to maintain this loss in studies of 12 months duration. The food choices in low-carb diet are very much limited leading to more drop outs. The initial weight loss in low-carb group is mainly the body water and lean body mass. There are concerns about its detrimental effect on vascular health since this diet increases LDL cholesterol. Low-fat diet causes more fat loss, increase insulin sensitivity and is a safe strategy for weight loss. Both diets diminished leptin levels equally. The ideal amount of carbohydrates, protein and fat in an optimal diet for patients with a combination of obesity and diabetes is still uncertain. In spite of the challenges of nutritional research, significant progress has been done in formulating evidence-based dietary guidance, and some common principles should be agreed that are helpful to patients, clinicians, and the public. Present recommendations for successful diet regarding weight loss and maintenance is about 24% calories from fat, 56% calories from carbohydrates, and 20% calories from protein with a total calories restriction of about 500K cal. While adherence to a dietary advice is a challenge, weight management remains the cornerstone in diabetes management and has the potential for its remission and to achieve this no single food group will provide the solution, but one should rely on the best overall dietary pattern that works for them personally.

REFERENCES

1. World Health Organization (2014). Obesity and Overweight. [online] Available from https://www.who.int/mediacentre/factsheets/fs311/en/ (Last accessed September, 2019].
2. Basen-Engquist K, Chang M. Obesity and cancer risk: recent review and evidence. Curr Oncol Rep. 2011;13:71-6.
3. International Diabetes Federation. (2017). IDF Diabetes Atlas, 8th edition. [online] Available from https://www.diabetesatlas.org [Last accessed September, 2019].
4. GBD 2013 Risk Factors Collaborators, Forouzanfar MH, Alexander L, et al. Global, regional, and national comparative risk assessment of 79 behavioural, environmental and occupational, and metabolic risks or clusters of risks in 188 countries, 1990-2013: a systematic analysis for the Global Burden of Disease Study 2013. Lancet. 2015;386:2287-323.
5. Ferrannini E, Mingrone G. Impact of different bariatric surgical procedures on insulin action and beta-cell function in type 2 diabetes. Diabetes Care. 2009; 32:514-20.
6. Anderson JW, Kendall CW, Jenkins DJ. Importance of weight management in type 2 diabetes: review with meta-analysis of clinical studies. J Am Coll Nutr. 2003;22(5):331-9.
7. American Heart Association Nutrition Committee, Lichtenstein AH, Appel LJ, et al. Diet and lifestyle recommendations revision 2006: a scientific statement from the American Heart Association Nutrition Committee. Circulation. 2006;114:82-96.
8. Law M. Dietary fat and adult diseases and the implications for childhood nutrition: an epidemiologic approach. Am J Clin Nutr. 2000;72:1291S-1296S.
9. Siri-Tarino PW, Sun Q, Hu FB, et al. Saturated fatty acids and risk of coronary heart disease: modulation by replacement nutrients. Curr Atheroscler Rep. 2010;12:384-90.
10. Hu FB, Willett WC. Optimal diets for prevention of coronary heart disease. JAMA. 2002;288:2569-78.
11. Siri-Tarino PW, Sun Q, Hu FB, et al. Meta-analysis of prospective cohort studies evaluating the association of saturated fat with cardiovascular disease. Am J Clin Nutr. 2010;91:535-46.
12. Wheeler ML, Dunbar SA, Jaacks LM, et al. Macronutrients, food groups, and eating patterns in the management of diabetes: a systematic review of the literature, 2010. Diabetes Care. 2012;35:434-45.
13. Boden G, Sargrad K, Homko C, et al. Effect of a low-carbohydrate diet on appetite, blood glucose levels, and insulin resistance in obese patients with type 2 diabetes. Ann Intern Med. 2005;142:403-11.
14. Brehm BJ, Seeley RJ, Daniels SR, et al. A randomized trial comparing a very low carbohydrate diet and a calorie-restricted low fat diet on body weight and cardiovascular risk factors in healthy women. J Clin Endocrinol Metab. 2003;88:1617-23.
15. Bueno NB, de Melo IS, de Oliveira SL, et al. Very low-carbohydrate ketogenic diet v. low-fat diet for long-term weight loss: a meta-analysis of randomised controlled trials. Br J Nutr. 2013;110:1178-87.
16. McAuley KA, Hopkins CM, Smith KJ, et al. Comparison of high-fat and high-protein diets with a high-carbohydrate diet in insulin-resistant obese women. Diabetologia. 2005;48:8-16.
17. Tay J, Brinkworth GD, Noakes M, et al. Metabolic effects of weight loss on a very-low-carbohydrate diet compared with an isocaloric high-carbohydrate diet in abdominally obese subjects. J Am Coll Cardiol. 2008;51:59-67.
18. Nordmann AJ, Nordmann A, Briel M, et al. Effects of low carbohydrate vs low-fat diets on weight loss and cardiovascular risk factors—a meta-analysis of randomized controlled trials. Arch Inter Med. 2006;166:285-93.
19. Schwingshackl L, Hoffmann G. Comparison of effects of long-term low-fat vs high-fat diets on blood lipid levels in overweight or obese patients: a systematic review and meta-analysis. J Acad Nutr Diet. 2013;113:1640-61.
20. Dattilo AM, Kris-Etherton PM. Effects of weight reduction on blood-lipids and lipoproteins: a meta-analysis. Am J Clin Nutr.1992;56:320-8.
21. Berneis KK, Krauss RM. Metabolic origins and clinical significance of LDL heterogeneity. J Lipid Res. 2002;43:1363-79.
22. Krauss RM, Siri PW. Metabolic abnormalities: triglyceride and low-density lipoprotein. Endocrinol Metab Clin North Am. 2004;33:405-15.
23. Bravata DM, Sanders L, Huang J, et al. Efficacy and safety of low-carbohydrate diets: a systematic review. JAMA. 2003;289:1837-50.
24. Astrup A. The role of dietary fat in the prevention and treatment of obesity. Efficacy and safety of low-fat diets. Int J Obes Relat Metab Disord. 2001; 25:S46-50.
25. Ley SJ, Metcalf PA, Scragg RK, et al. Long-term effects of a reduced fat diet intervention on cardiovascular disease risk factors in individuals with glucose intolerance. Diabetes Res Clin Pract. 2004;63:103-12.
26. Hall KD, Bemis T, Brychta R, et al. Calorie for calorie, dietary fat restriction results in more body fat loss than carbohydrate restriction in people with obesity. Cell Metab. 2015;22:427-36.
27. Bradley U, Spence M, Courtney CH, et al. Low-fat versus low-carbohydrate weight reduction diets: effects on weight loss, insulin resistance, and cardiovascular risk: a randomized control trial. Diabetes. 2009;58:2741-8.
28. Gardner CD, Trepanowski JF, Del Gobbo LC, et al. Effect of low-fat vs low-carbohydrate diet on 12-month weight loss in overweight adults and the association with genotype pattern or insulin secretion: the DIETFITS randomized clinical trial. JAMA. 2018;319:667-79.

21 CHAPTER Artificial Sweeteners: Controversies and Consensus

Sandeep Rai, Dev Dutt Rai

INTRODUCTION

Sugar is a discovery from India in the pre-Alexander era (the word is derived from "*sharkara*", meaning "gravel" in Sanskrit). "Honey", "sweetheart", "candy" all conjure pleasant sensations (contrast to those that we associate "bitter" or "sour"). Sweet taste, therefore, is essential to our happiness. Artificial sweeteners have become the most commonly used food additives worldwide as they promise a guilt-free way to sweeten foods. By definition, artificial sweeteners (AS), otherwise are also referred to as very low-calorie sweeteners, non-nutrient sweeteners or intense sweeteners, which have a much greater intensity of sweetness than the caloric sweeteners such as sucrose, corn syrups, and concentrated fruit juice. As a sugar replacement, they are added in smaller quantities, hence, they provide no or only minimal calories. The Food and Drug Administration (FDA) has approved the use of six artificial sweeteners, which includes aspartame, sucralose, saccharin, advantame, neotame, and acesulfame potassium (Ace-K), in food and beverages (Table 1). Federal regulations require that any food that containing aspartame should bear this warning—"Phenylketonurics (PKU)—contains phenylalanine". This warning helps

TABLE 1: Artificial sweetener reference chart.

Artificial Sweeteners					
Generic name	Brand name	Sweetness factor/ Acceptable daily intake (ADI) (mg of sweetener/kg body weight/day)	Uses	Additional facts/ Metabolism	FDA approval
Saccharin	Sweet N Low Sweet Twin Necta Sweet Sweetex	200–700 times sweeter than sugar ADI—5 mg/kg	Tabletop sweetener, beverages, baked goods, jams, and gum	Heat stable/metabolism—nil, bitter, and metallic after taste	2001
Aspartame	NutraSweet/ Equal	200 times sweeter than sugar ADI—50 mg/kg	In processed foods and beverages	Not heat stable/metabolized to phenylalanine, aspartic acid, and methanol	1981
Acesulfame K	Sunett Sweet One	200 times sweeter than sugar ADI—15 mg/kg	General purpose	Heat stable to 392°F/ metabolism—nil	1998
Sucralose	Splenda/Sugar Free Natura	600 times sweeter than sugar ADI-5 mg/kg	General purpose	Can be used in home baking/metabolism—nil	1998
Neotame	Newtame	7,000–13,000 times sweeter than sugar ADI—18 mg/kg	General purpose/ metabolism by esterase	Similar to aspartame	2002

people with PKU avoid products that are a source of phenylalanine. Although artificial sweeteners are generally considered safe for human consumption, there is increasing controversy regarding their potential ability to promote metabolic derangements in humans.

ANY HEALTH RISKS OF USING ARTIFICIAL SWEETENERS?

This is still a highly controversial topic.[1] Artificial sweeteners have allegedly been linked to adverse effects such as cancer, weight gain, metabolic disorders, migraine, type 2 diabetes, vascular events, preterm delivery, hepatotoxicity, immune system disruptions, and alteration of gut microbiota activity.[2] Although these potential health problems have been studied for long, a firm conclusion has yet to be reached on these allegations due to a lack of credible and consistent evidence. We will discuss some of these controversial areas in the discussion below.

Artificial Sweeteners Fueling the Diabesity Epidemic?

A statement from the American Heart Association and the American Diabetes Association in 2011, pointed out that non-nutritive sweetener may be good for health by reducing or controlling weight and can have other beneficial metabolic effects too.[3] However, recent concerns regarding the safety of artificial sweeteners have arisen from few studies in humans. In a large meta-analysis of prospective studies[4,5] (17 cohorts with 38,253 cases), it has been shown that artificial sweeteners were associated with the risk of type 2 diabetes mellitus. Another similar study demonstrated that diets sweetened with either natural or artificial sugars are linked with an increase in type 2 diabetes.[6] In a recently published study, which collected 10-year-data from more than 10,000 women, who were consumers of artificial sweetener as packet and tablets,[7] showed an association between artificial sweetener usage and risk of diabetes. More importantly, they were also able to show a gradation of risk depending upon years of consumption and also the amount of artificial sweetener consumed per day.

The explanation given for a probable association between artificial sweeteners and type 2 diabetes (T2DM) in observation studies is the reverse causation bias because of increased intake of artificial sweeteners is otherwise also seen among obese people.[8] Another convincing explanation is that an orosensory stimulus is silently generated by sweet foods, telling the body about the likely inflow of calories that is going to follow. This is followed by several gastrointestinal reflexes that finally relay in brain and intimate the hypothalamus through negative feedback signals to decrease hunger sensation and increase satiety feeling as body has already received calories. When sweetness is sensed without inflow of calories (artificial sweetener ingestion), gastrointestinal reflexes do not send signals to hypothalamus to decrease hunger sensation (Fig. 1). The brain recalibrates and person's hunger sensation continues and this leads to increase in total calories consumed. This ultimately leads to weight gain and consequently increases the risk of diabetes.

A study was conducted in the University of San Diego, California on volunteers who were given sips of water mixed with either sugar or sucralose. Functional magnetic resonance imaging (fMRI) scans of the brain were then recorded. Images showed that sugar activated areas of the brain which were involved in food reward, whereas sucralose did not have the same effect. These results proved that artificial sweeteners may not be effective in managing cravings for sweets.[9]

Another study was carried out on more than 3,000 individuals, which saw the impact of artificially sweetened drinks on the body weight. Results showed that those who consumed these drinks had a 47% higher increase in body mass index (BMI) than those who did not.[10] Randomized controlled trials (RCTs) (1,003 participants; follow-up 6 months) and about 30 cohort studies (more than 400,000 participants; median follow-up 10 years) were critically analyzed. Evidence from RCTs does not support the benefits of artificial sweeteners for body weight management, and observational data suggest that routine intake of artificial sweeteners may be associated with increased BMI and cardiometabolic risk including coronary artery disease. In the cohort studies, it was found that consumption of artificial sweeteners was associated with increases in weight and waist circumference, and a higher incidence of obesity, metabolic syndrome, type 2 diabetes,[11] however publication bias was indicated for the studies with diabetes as an outcome.

Artificial Sweetener Safe in Pregnancy?

Although many artificial sweeteners are considered safe during pregnancy, women with any form of diabetes must limit their use of these substitutes. A study reported that saccharin causes effects such as depressed growth, iron and vitamin A deficiencies, anemia, and elevated levels of vitamin E in rats. They are also associated with premature deliveries, as reported by two observational studies published in 2010 and 2012. Therefore, at present

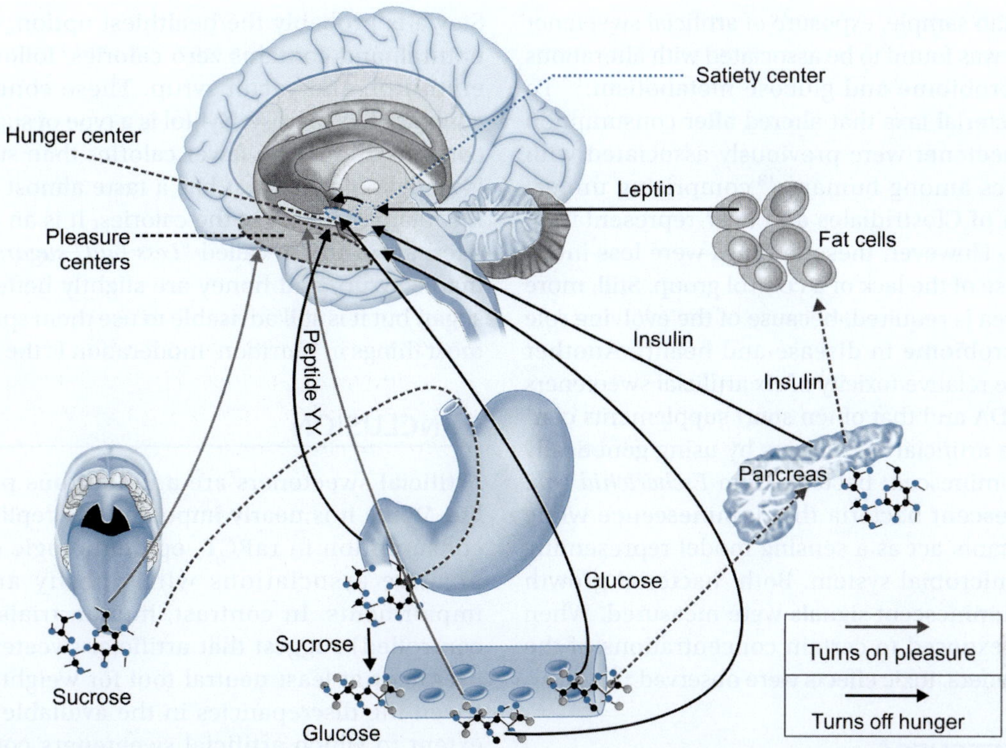

Figure 1 Sucrose ingestion leads to activation of pleasure centers in brain and the calorie inflow also activates multiple gastrointestinal (GI) negative feedback signals to hypothalamus to decrease hunger sensation, while artificial sweetener ingestion also results in activation of pleasure sensation but is followed by no calorie inflow and therefore, there is no feedback inhibition of hunger sensation from GI signals to hypothalamus, leading to increase in food intake and weight gain. ***(For color version see color plate No. 3)***

(*Source:* Gabymichel, Blaus B, Haggstrom M, et al. Medical gallery of Mikael Häggström. Wiki Journal of Medicine. 2014;1(2).)

time, till further large-scale studies are done, pregnant women must be advised to avoid these sweeteners.[12] It is also critical to investigate the effect of artificial sweetener in other populations, such as infants and young children, lactating women, and those with metabolic diseases.

Artificial Sweeteners and the Risk of Cancer?

In 1970, a research reported an association of saccharin with bladder carcinoma among laboratory rats. However, a different study raised suspicion when it reported that intake of aspartame is related with malignancies such as lymphoma, leukemia, and multiple myeloma (among men).[13] But this study had a limitation, that was its inability to quantify accurate intake of aspartame due to variable presence of aspartame in the dietary sources. One of the limitations of this study was that it was not able to describe the rationale behind preponderance of carcinoma risk in male. Similar to this, another study evaluated the possible impact of five non-nutritive sweeteners on cell proliferation, morphology, and DNA of cell. It was also observed that sucralose and sodium saccharin caused more DNA fragmentation in all the cell lines as compared to any other artificial sweetners.[14]

However, after careful review of the literature, Weihrauch and colleagues suggested that there was no significant evidence of consumption of artificial sweetener and cancer risk with presently accessible artificial sweeteners.[15] Another large study has also drawn similar conclusions. In this study, data was prospectively analyzed from more than 400,000 men and women over a 5-year period and found no association between aspartame consumption and risk of hematopoietic or brain tumors.[16]

Effect of Artificial Sweeteners on Gut Biome

Artificial sweeteners affect the oral mucosa's microbial composition, and the dental community views them positively. Therefore, it is not unusual that recently artificial sweeteners have been found to alter the gut microbiota, mainly in rodent models. There is limited experimental evidence of induced changes in gut microbiota of humans.

In a small human sample, exposure of artificial sweetener for only 1 week was found to be associated with alterations in the gut microbiome and glucose metabolism.[17] To note, many bacterial taxa that altered after consumption of artificial sweetener were previously associated with type 2 diabetes among humans,[18] comprising under-representation of Clostridiales and over-representation of Bacteroides. However, these findings were less interpretable because of the lack of a control group. Still, more study in this area is required, because of the evolving role of the gut microbiome in disease and health. Another study tested the relative toxicity of six artificial sweeteners approved by FDA and that of ten sport supplements consisting of these artificial sweeteners by using genetically modified bioluminescent bacteria from *Escherichia coli*. The bioluminescent bacteria that luminescence while detecting toxicants act as a sensing model representing the complex microbial system. Both bacterial growth and induced luminescent signals were measured. When bacteria were exposed to certain concentrations of the artificial sweeteners, toxic effects were observed.[19]

NOVEL SWEETENERS

It is difficult to fit novel sweeteners into a specific category due to what they are made from and how they are made. *Stevia* is obtained from the leaves of *Stevia rebaudiana*, which is a plant species native to Paraguay and Brazil. Stevia comprises steviol glycosides that are used as artificial sweeteners. The GRAS (Generally recognized as safe) status of specific high-purity steviol glycosides has not been questioned by FDA for their use in food. However, stevia leaf and crude stevia extracts are not known to be GRAS and are not approved for use in food by FDA. Tagatose is produced from lactose in dairy products and, due to its chemical structure, is also considered a sweetener. It is a naturally occurring low-carbohydrate sweetener similar to fructose. Tagatose is categorized by the FDA as a GRAS substance.

ALTERNATIVES TO ARTIFICIAL SWEETENERS

Instead of artificial sweeteners, several natural sweeteners, which are much safer, can be used. Most of these also provide added advantages of being rich in vitamins and minerals. These consist of coconut nectar, honey, fruits, molasses, maple syrup, sugar alcohols, agave nectar, stevia, apple sauce, and others. The key word here is alternatives—meaning they also contain sugar, but in less amount and should be used instead of refined sugar. Stevia is probably the healthiest option, which is 100% natural, and contains zero calories, followed by xylitol, erythritol, and yacon syrup. These contain less sugar compared to sucrose. Xylitol is a type of sugar alcohol that contains about 40% fewer calories than sugar. Erythritol is a sugar alcohol that has a taste almost like sugar, but it contains only 6% of the calories. It is an excellent sugar alternative. The so called *"Less bad" sugars* like molasses, maple syrup, and honey are slightly better than regular sugar, but it is still advisable to use them sparingly. As with most things in nutrition, moderation is the key.

CONCLUSION

Artificial sweeteners are a ubiquitous part of modern life. While it is nearly impossible to replicate "real-life" consumption in raRCT, epidemiologic studies report positive associations with obesity and metabolic impairments. In contrast, human trials (randomized controlled) suggest that artificial sweeteners may be a useful, or at least neutral tool for weight management. Given the discrepancies in the available literature, the extent to which artificial sweeteners could be helpful or harmful for weight management and chronic disease prevention needs further well-designed, large-scale studies. We conclude by saying that with all the evidence available till date, it is advisable that artificial sweeteners, if at all have to be used, should only be used in a very limited amount. If your sweet tooth keeps bothering you, it is safe to consume artificial sweeteners in small amounts. Physicians who advise these artificial sweeteners to their obese or diabetic patients need to take a step back and reevaluate their recommendations especially in light of the newer studies on various unfavorable metabolic effects that are emerging now. In fact, we may be dealing with a Wolf in a Sheep's clothing.

REFERENCES

1. Tandel KR. Sugar substitutes: Health controversy over perceived benefits. J. Pharmacol Pharmacother. 2011;2(4):236-43.
2. Marinovich M, Galli CL, Bosetti C, et al. Aspartame, low-calorie sweeteners and disease: regulatory safety and epidemiological issues. Food Chem Toxicol. 2013;60:109-15.
3. Gardner C, Wylie-Rosett J, Gidding SS, et al. Nonnutritive sweeteners: current use and health perspectives: A scientific statement from the American Heart Association and the American Diabetes Association. Circulation. 2012;126(4):509-19.
4. Imamura F, O'Connor L, Ye Z, et al. Consumption of sugar sweetened beverages, artificially sweetened beverages, and fruit juice and incidence of type 2 diabetes: systematic review, meta-analysis, and estimation of population attributable fraction. BMJ. 2015;351:h3576.

5. Fagherazzi G, Gusto G, Affret A, et al. Chronic consumption of artificial sweetener in packets or tablets and type 2 diabetes risk, evidence from the E3N-European Prospective Investigation into cancer and nutrition study. Ann Nutr Metab. 2017;70(1) 51-8.
6. Fagherazzi G, Vilier A, Saes Sartorelli D, et al. Consumption of artificially and sugar-sweetened beverages and incident type 2 diabetes. European Prospective Investigation into Cancer and Nutrition cohort. Am J Clin Nutr. 2013;97(3):517-23.
7. Anton SD, Martin CK, Han H, et al. Effects of stevia, aspartame, and sucrose on food intake, satiety, and postprandial glucose and insulin levels. Appetite. 2010;55(1):37-43.
8. Greenwood DC, Threapleton DE, Evans CE, et al. Association between sugar-sweetened and artificially sweetened soft drinks and type 2 diabetes: systematic review and dose-response meta-analysis of prospective studies. Br J Nutr. 2014;112(5):725-34.
9. Frank GK, Oberndorfer TA, Simmons AN, et al. Sucrose activates human taste pathways differently from artificial sweetener. Neuroimage. 2008;39(4):1559-69.
10. Fowler SP, Williams K, Resendez RG, et al. Fueling the obesity epidemic? Artificially sweetened beverage use and long-term weight gain. Obesity (Silver Spring). 2008;16(8):1894-1900.
11. Azad MB, Abou-Setta AM, Chauhan BF, et al. Nonnutritive sweeteners and cardiometabolic health: a systematic review and meta-analysis of randomized controlled trials and prospective cohort studies. CMAJ. 2017;189(28):E929-39.
12. Englund-Ögge L, Brantsæter AL, Haugen M, et al. Association between intake of artificially sweetened and sugar-sweetened beverages and preterm delivery, a large prospective cohort study. Am J Clin Nutr. 2012;96(3):552-9.
13. Schernhammer ES, Bertrand KA, Birmann BM, et al. Consumption of artificial sweetener and sugar-containing soda and risk of lymphoma and leukemia in men and women. Am J Clin Nutr. 2012;96(6):1419-28.
14. van Eyk AD. The effect of five artificial sweeteners on Caco-2, HT-219 and HEK-293 cells. Drug Chem Toxicol. 2015;38(3):318-27.
15. Weihrauch MK, Diehl V. Artificial sweeteners—do they bear a carcinogenic risk? Ann Oncol. 2004;15(10):1460-5.
16. Lim U, Subar AF, Mouw T, et al. Consumption of aspartame-containing beverages and incidence of hematopoietic and brain malignancies. Cancer Epidemiol Biomarkers Prev. 2006;15(9):1654-9.
17. Suez J, Korem T, Zeevi D, et al. Artificial sweeteners induce glucose intolerance by altering the gut microbiota. Nature. 2014;514:181-6.
18. Qin J, Li Y, Cai Z, et al. A metagenome-wide association study of gut microbiota in type 2 diabetes. Nature. 2012;490:55-60.
19. Harpaz D, Yeo LP, Cecchini F, et al. Measuring Artificial Sweeteners Toxicity Using a Bioluminescent Bacterial Panel. Molecules. 2018;23(10): piiE2454.

CHAPTER 22 How Exercise Helps in Management of Diabetes: Physiological Mechanism

Tvisha K Parikh

"Type 2 diabetes should be regarded as a deficiency state, with the deficiency being that of physical activity"
—*Exercise and Sport in Diabetes, 2005*[1]

INTRODUCTION

Exercise, along with diet and medications, is considered an important part of diabetes management.[2] Many studies worldwide have researched the effects of physical activity in diabetic patients and found beneficial effects. Whereas the terms "exercise" and "physical activity" (PA) are often used interchangeably in many of these research studies, they have distinct definitions. "Physical activity" is defined as bodily movement produced by the contraction of skeletal muscle that substantially increases energy expenditure.[3] "Exercise" is a planned, structured PA which is "a subset of PA done with the intention of developing physical fitness (i.e. cardiovascular, strength, and flexibility)".

The treatment goal in management of diabetes is to achieve and maintain optimal blood glucose levels, lipid levels, and blood pressure levels in order to prevent or delay the onset of diabetic complications.[3] At rest, blood glucose levels are optimally maintained by glucose production and clearance. Approximately 90% of this clearance occurs by uptake in the skeletal muscle, suggesting it is a potential site for interventions.[4] As part of management, an understanding of the mechanism of action of exercise in diabetes management can improve the exercise prescription by the physician, exercise compliance by the patient and hence ultimately achieve better patient health.

The physiological mechanism through which exercise aids diabetes management varies with the diabetes type and PA type. Whereas exercise is beneficial in all types of diabetes, exercise has more physiological effects on the blood glucose control in type 2 diabetes mellitus (T2DM). The beneficial effects exerted in type 1 patients differ to the type 2 patients. Physical activity is also of various types and intensities. The most common classification is low, moderate, and high-intensity activities, and aerobic and resistance exercises types. Glucose metabolism varies in the different forms of exercise.

NORMAL RESPONSE TO EXERCISE

Exercise and Glucose Kinetics in Healthy Nondiabetics

The onset of PA is accompanied by a number of metabolic changes in the blood, muscle, and liver.[5] There is an interaction of carbohydrates, fats, and to a small extent proteins to fuel the PA. The proportion of utilization of these three major fuels depends on the intensity and duration of activity.

During the transition from rest to exercise, glucose is an important fuel with increasing intensities of exercise. Muscle glycogen stores and blood glucose are an important source of glucose to fuel the exercising muscle. Glucose uptake is increased in the contracting muscles.[2,3] As these sources of glucose deplete, replacement of the blood glucose is achieved by glycogenolysis of liver glycogen stores. Insulin levels fall to facilitate liver glucose production.[6] The newly produced blood glucose can then be transported to the contracting muscle and used as fuel. Typically, exercise enhances this glucose uptake capacity of the muscle.[6] Glycogenolysis is dependent on enzyme phosphorylase which is activated at the onset of exercise through "calmodulin".[5] As the above sources deplete with progressing exercise, gluconeogenesis sets in. There is mobilization of free fatty acids to maintain blood glucose levels. The above glycogenolysis and gluconeogenesis is coordinated by increases in insulin, glucagon, catecholamines, and cortisol.[2,3,5,7]

As a result of the above metabolism trying to maintain the blood glucose, there is little change in blood glucose during mild to moderate exercise and euglycemia is usually preserved. However, strenuous short-term exercise may increase blood glucose levels due to higher epinephrine levels which promote glycogenolysis. During prolonged exercise lasting longer than 90 min, blood glucose may decrease. However, hypoglycemia rarely occurs in normal people.

Cellular Metabolism

At a cellular level, exercise training can enhance the responsiveness of skeletal muscles to insulin with increased expression and/or activity of proteins involved in glucose metabolism and insulin signaling. There is an upregulation of a protein adenosine monophosphate (AMP)-activated protein kinase (AMPK) with exercise training, which enhances glucose uptake by increasing both insulin-dependent as well as insulin-independent mechanisms.[8] The immediate effects of exercise on glucose are predominantly mediated through glucose transporter type 4 (GLUT4).[8] All forms of exercise increase the number of GLUT4 transporters increasing the velocity of blood glucose uptake into the muscles.[8,9] Muscle contractions also increase GLUT4 translocation. Contractions are an insulin-independent mechanism for glucose uptake. The contraction-mediated increased glucose uptake continues for hours postexercise. Exercise also increases the oxidative and nonoxidative enzyme concentrations in the muscles.[4]

Other Effects

Exercise is known to improve psychological well-being and improve quality of life.[2,3]

DIABETES AND EXERCISE

Type 2 Diabetes and Skeletal Muscle

Type 2 diabetes mellitus which accounts for nearly 90% of the cases is primarily a pathology of insulin resistance.[3] It begins as an inability of muscle cells to respond to insulin properly. The natural history of the disease suggests that increasing years of diabetes with prolonged hyperglycemia ultimately leads to β-cell dysfunction.[1] This leads to an inadequate insulin secretion ultimately.[3] Thus, T2DM is a combination of insulin resistance and inadequate compensatory insulin secretion producing a state of hyperglycemia. Since the skeletal muscle is an important site for insulin resistance, the normal insulin-mediated glucose uptake is affected.[3] Subsequently, in the insulin deficient or resistant states, storage of muscle glucose may be impaired because of incomplete transport and decreased glycogen synthase activity.[4]

At the cellular level, the insulin-mediated GLUT4 translocation is impaired in T2DM.[10] However, the contraction-mediated GLUT4 translocation appears to be intact in them.

Effect of Exercise on Type 2 Diabetes

Exercise and Glucose Kinetics

Exercise has an acute as well as long-term impact in diabetes. Most benefits of PA on diabetes management are realized through acute and chronic improvements in insulin action. Both aerobic and resistance training produce these changes.[3] Most simply, exercise benefits diabetics by utilizing the various glucose forms available in the body to fulfill the energy requirement of exercising muscles. Exercise is followed by a fall in the fasting as well as postprandial insulin levels suggesting an improvement in the insulin resistance.[1,11] However, in spite of circulating insulin levels falling, exercising muscle demonstrates a higher sensitivity to insulin. There is also a tendency toward an earlier insulin peak suggesting improvement in insulin secretion.[1] Some research also suggests that muscle contractions appear to directly stimulate glycogenolysis.[12]

Additionally, exercise has positive effects on risk factors and diseases, which often coexist with diabetes.[2,3] These include cardiovascular disease, obesity, hypertension, and dyslipidemia. These benefits of PA in T2DM were observed in a randomized controlled trial of 5,145 persons where the intensive lifestyle intervention arm markedly improved in risk factors and side effects in addition to some regression of diabetes.[13]

A common reason to exercise is fat loss. However, beneficial effects on blood glucose are observed even in the absence of weight loss.[1]

During moderate intensity aerobic exercise, normal to low blood glucose levels are seen in T2DM due to slightly higher glucose uptake than production.[1,3] The hepatic glucose production which maintains euglycemia in nondiabetics is not observed to a proportional extent. This is due to the impaired feedback between blood glucose and hepatic glucose production in T2DM.[1] Also, there are episodes when patients report a "higher blood glucose levels following a walk" and often an upward trend of glucose is noted on continuous glucose monitoring. Commonly, diabetics tend to have lower fitness levels especially when they begin an exercise routine. Hence, an activity which would otherwise be of moderate intensity may be of high intensity for the diabetic person. High intensity and short bout of exercise increases catecholamine levels which increases blood glucose levels.[3] Also in initial stages, patients might have a shorter duration of activity due to higher fatigue levels contributing to this hyperglycemia. These higher levels may continue for a short-period postexercise (unless external insulin is administered). However, there is a period of "insulin sensitization" noted postexercise which improves glucose utilization.[1] Thus, exercise has a heterogeneous impact on blood glucose postexercise in T2DM.

Cellular Metabolism

Exercise bypasses the impaired insulin-mediated GLUT4 translocation observed in T2DM and increases glucose uptake independently.[10] Aerobic and resistance exercises have the ability to increase GLUT4 abundance and blood glucose uptake even in the presence of T2DM. Exercise also improves insulin receptor numbers. Also, repeated contractions during exercise training in insulin-resistant muscles induce restoration of phosphatidylinositol 3-kinase activity enhancing the insulin signaling cascade.[8]

AMPK upregulation also increases lipid oxidation in the muscles.[8] This lipid oxidation is suggested to decrease the lipid species which accumulate in the muscle and inhibit insulin signal transduction.

Resistance Exercise

There is not enough research on physiological mechanism of glucose control by resistance exercises. However, the benefits that resistance training has in healthy population like increased muscle mass, strength, bone density, physical function, improved cardiovascular, and lipid profiles would be experienced in T2DM as well.[3] And most probably, the effect on enhanced glycemic control is exerted by increase in insulin sensitivity due to the increased/preserved muscle mass.[4] Also, diabetes is a risk factor for low muscular strength and hence resistance training is beneficial since it improves this.[2]

Tai chi, Yoga, Flexibility, and Balance Exercises

Scientific evidence that these exercises improve glycemic control is lacking. However, practically, an improvement in the range of motion around joints by doing flexibility-based exercises can improve the ability to perform aerobic and resistance exercises, ultimately improving glycemic control. Balance exercises would help improve mobility issues due to imbalance, and reduce falls ultimately ensuring continuous PA.

Diabetes, Inflammation, and Exercise

There is evidence that T2DM is associated with chronic inflammation. Interleukin 1b (IL-1b) is associated with β cell damage and tumor necrosis factor alpha (TNF-α) is associated with peripheral insulin resistance.[14] Mechanistic studies indicate that exercise has anti-inflammatory effects by inhibition of TNF-α and IL-1 receptor antagonist which inhibits IL-1b in turn.

Diabetes, Mental Health, and Exercise

There is no substantial research evidence reporting a psychological effect of exercise in diabetic patients. However, these effects are observed clinically and help in overall management of diabetes.[3]

Effect of Exercise on Type 1 Diabetes[2]

Response of blood glucose to PA is extremely variable in type 1 diabetes mellitus (T1DM). It depends on many factors like the meal timing, carbohydrate intake, exercise type, exercise duration, and timing of the insulin dose administered. Since the pathology is of insulin deficiency, the exercise benefits of improved insulin sensitivity are less marked. Nonetheless, there is overall glycemic improvement. All the cardiometabolic benefits of exercise observed in T2DM are experienced in T1DM and contribute to the overall diabetic management.

CONCLUSION

The role of exercise in the management of diabetes has been researched at both, the blood glucose kinematics level and cellular level. An increase in muscle glucose uptake by insulin-independent and dependent mechanisms is among the important physiological mechanisms by which exercise helps in diabetes. This benefit is predominantly observed in the insulin-resistant T2DM. T1DM also benefits from regular exercise but this benefit is more due to the accompanying cardiometabolic effects and other health improvements seen with exercise. Majority of the research has focused on aerobic type activities, but resistance training and other exercise forms like yoga, flexibility can also produce beneficial effects and a combination of aerobic and resistance exercises is recommended by the internationally published position statements.

REFERENCES

1. Nagi D. Exercise and Sport in Diabetes, 2nd edition. New Jersy: John Wiley and Sons, Ltd; 2005.
2. Colberg SR, Sigal RJ, Yardley JE, et al. Physical activity/exercise and diabetes: a position statement of the American Diabetes Association. Diabetes Care. 2016;39(11):2065-79.
3. Colberg SR, Albright AL, Blissmer BJ, et al. Exercise and type 2 diabetes: American College of Sports Medicine and the American Diabetes Association: joint position statement. Med Sci Sports Exerc. 2010;42(12):2282-303.
4. Peirce NS. Diabetes and exercise. Br J Sports Med. 1999;33(3):161-72.
5. Powers SK, Howley ET. Exercise Physiology, 7th edition. New York: McGraw-Hill; 2009.
6. Shugart C, Jackson J, Fields KB. Diabetes in Sports. Sports Health. 2010;2(1):29-38.
7. Chiang JL, Sue Kirkman M, Laffel LMB, et al. Type 1 diabetes through the life span: a position statement of the American Diabetes Association. Diabetes Care. 2014;37:2034-54.
8. Hawley JA, Lessard SJ. Exercise training-induced improvements in insulin action. Acta Physiol. 2008;192:127-35.
9. Goodyear LJ, Hirshman MF, Horton ES. Exercise-induced translocation of skeletal muscle glucose transporters. Am J Physiol. 1991;261:E795-E99.
10. Musi N, Fujii N, Hirshman MF, et al. AMP-activated protein kinase (AMPK) is activated in muscle of subjects with type 2 diabetes during exercise. Diabetes. 2001;50(5):921-7.
11. Wojtaszewski JF, Hansen BF, Gade J, et al. Insulin signaling and insulin sensitivity after exercise in human skeletal muscle. Diabetes. 2000;49:325-81.
12. Richter EA, Ruderman NB, Gavras H, et al Muscle glycogenolysis during exercise: Dual control by epinephrine and contractions. Am J Physiol. 1982;242:E25-E32.
13. Pi-Sunyer X. The look AHEAD trial: a review and discussion of its outcomes. Curr Nutr Rep. 2014; 3(4): 387-91.
14. Karstoft K, Pedersen BK. Exercise and type 2 diabetes: Focus on metabolism and inflammation. Immunol Cell Biol. 2015;94(2):146-50.

23 CHAPTER Exercise Prescription for Diabetes: Be SMART

Manoj Saluja

INTRODUCTION

The economic burden of diabetes requires sustainable, affordable and effective method of disease management. As the role of exercise is becoming better defined, its importance in the management of diabetes has increased many folds. Before making an exercise prescription for diabetes, it is very essential to learn standard recommendations for various subsets of diabetics. Besides discussing various types of physical activities and exercises as recommended by standard guidelines, this chapter also focuses on how a *SMART* prescription of exercise to a diabetic can help manage the disease more effectively on a long-term basis.

PHYSICAL ACTIVITY AS MEDICINE

Physical activity is any movement by skeletal muscle that requires energy; however, exercise is a planned, structured, and repetitive movement intended to improve or maintain physical fitness. Regular exercise has been shown to improve blood glucose control, reduce cardiovascular risk, contribute to weight loss, and improve well-being.[1]

Pre-exercise Testing

Risks associated with exercise program in diabetics include precipitation of myocardial ischemia, visual loss, damage to joints and ligaments, risk of hypoglycemia and even hyperglycemia. Patients in whom a new exercise program or even increasing usual patterns of physical activity is advised should undergo a detailed medical evaluation.[2]

Most people with diabetes can start a walking program without having any tests. Routine screening for coronary artery disease is not recommended. However, American Heart Association recommends having a stress (treadmill) test in patients with previous cardiovascular disease or in the presence of suggestive symptoms.[3]

TYPES OF EXERCISE

Aerobic Exercise

Activities involving continuous rhythmic movements of large muscle groups are known as aerobics or cardio. It improves glycemia, lipid profile and reduces blood pressure and insulin resistance in diabetics. People with diabetes should perform aerobic exercise regularly. Moderate (e.g. brisk walking, cycling, golf, etc.) to high intensity (e.g. running, hiking, swimming, etc.) aerobic exercise is associated with substantial reduction in HbA1c. Aerobic activity bouts should ideally last at least 10 minutes, with the goal of ~30 min/day or more, most days of the week for adults with type 2 diabetes. Not more than 2 days abstinence from exercise should be there. This should gradually increase in intensity, frequency, and/or duration to at least 150 min/week of moderate-intensity exercise.[4]

A newer form of exercise is high-intensity interval training (HIIT), or sprint interval training (SIT). This is a form of cardiovascular training in which alternating periods of high intensity exercise is combined with short lasting intervals of rest. Sessions are usually 30–40 minutes in duration. Such training has been demonstrated to result in greater insulin sensitivity and better overall blood glucose levels, at least in adults with type 2 diabetes.[4,5] This has also shown beneficial effects in patients with dyslipidemia and obesity.[6]

Resistance Exercise

This form of training includes exercises performed using weights, weight machines, resistance bands, or one's own body weight as resistance (e.g. pushups and squats). Resistance training can delay, prevent, and, in some cases, reverse the effects of sarcopenia.[7] Resistance exercise increase both muscle strength and endurance. Adults with diabetes should engage in 2–3 sessions per week of resistance exercise on nonconsecutive days.[8]

Resistance training exercise benefit in type 1 diabetes is unclear; however, it reduces risk of exercise induced hypoglycemia in such patients. When combining resistance training with aerobic exercise, risk of hypoglycemia is less when resistance training is done first as compared to the reverse.[9]

Flexibility and Balance Exercise

As a consequence of advanced glycation end (AGE) products in long-standing diabetes, joints become stiff with restricted mobility. Flexibility exercise increases range of motion; however, have little effect on HbA1c reduction. Balance training reduces the risk of fall and helps in improving gait in spite of established neuropathy.

Yoga and Tai chi exercise are mild exercises with mixed aerobic, flexibility, and balance exercise. They can be performed as additional training.

Daily Activity

Individual with diabetes are advised to remain physically active throughout the day to gain additional benefit. Being physically active in various forms of nonstructured physical activity helps reducing lean body mass. Remaining inactive for <30 minutes is advisable. This can be achieved through step counters with prefixed targets.[10] Average target of 10,000 steps is usually preferred.

Supervised versus Nonsupervised Exercise

Both supervised (structured) and non-supervised aerobic and resistance exercise helps in reducing HbA1c. However supervised training requires less dietary restrictions as compared to non-supervised training. American Diabetes Association (ADA) recommends supervised exercise training for individuals for type 2 diabetes.

EXERCISE GUIDELINES FOR PATIENTS WITH DIABETES

American Diabetes Association Recommendations for diabetics are as follows:[11]

- Pre-exercise medical clearance is generally unnecessary for asymptomatic individuals prior to beginning low- or moderate-intensity physical activity not exceeding the demands of brisk walking or everyday living (class B).
- Most adults with diabetes should engage in 150 minutes or more of moderate-to-vigorous intensity activity weekly, spread over at least 3 days/week, with no more than 2 consecutive days without activity. Shorter durations (minimum 75 minutes per week) of vigorous-intensity or interval training may be sufficient for younger and more physically fit individuals; class B (for type 2 diabetes), and class C (for type 1 diabetes).
- Children and adolescents with type 1 or type 2 diabetes should engage in 60 min/day or more of moderate or vigorous intensity aerobic activity, with vigorous, muscle-strengthening, and bone-strengthening activities included at least 3 days/week (class C).
- Adults with diabetes should engage in 2–3 sessions per week of resistance exercise on nonconsecutive days; class B (for type 2 diabetes), and class C (for type 1 diabetes).
- Flexibility training and balance training are recommended 2–3 times/week for older adults with diabetes. Yoga and tai chi may be included based on individual preferences to increase flexibility, muscular strength, and balance (class C).
- Individuals with diabetes or prediabetes are encouraged to increase their total daily incidental (nonexercise) physical activity to gain additional health benefits (class C).
- To gain more health benefits from physical activity programs, participation in supervised training is recommended over nonsupervised programs (class B).

EXERCISE IN SPECIAL POPULATION

Type 1 Diabetes

Type I diabetes is associated with variable glycemic control during exercise.[12] Individuals with type 1 are more likely to go into hypoglycemia. So, a decrease in pre-exercise insulin dose, short sessions of exercise training, frequent carbohydrate feeds, and glucose checks are recommended.

Pregnancy

Pregnant females with or at risk for gestational diabetes should engage in 20–30 minutes of moderate-intensity exercise on most of days of the week even before pregnancy.[13] Physical activity and exercise in gestational diabetes is associated with low risk of weight gain, reduced risk of preeclampsia and less chances of caesarian delivery.[14]

Elderly

Elderly patients experience important and specific issues; including the association of comorbidities, use of many medications, the presence of dependencies and frailty. Caution must be taken to prevent exercise related injuries, dehydration and hypoglycemia. Resistive activities are preferable for the frail and vulnerable diabetic elderly. Aerobic activities should be prescribed whenever possible, and the association of both modalities is the best choice.

MANAGEMENT OF EXERCISE RELATED MORBIDITY

Hypoglycemia

More common in patients with type 1 as compared to type 2 diabetes. Taking small amount of carbohydrate diet before or in between moderate intensity exercise sessions is helpful in preventing this. Exercise-induced nocturnal hypoglycemia occurs 6–15 hours post-exercise.[15] This can be prevented by reducing daily basal insulin dose by 20% and consuming low glycemic index carbohydrate feeds.[16] Supervised exercise with frequent blood glucose monitoring is recommended.

Hyperglycemia

Type 1 individuals may be prone to hyperglycemia if there is too much consumption of high glycemic foods between exercise sessions or pre-exercise insulin dose is reduced for the fear of hypoglycemia.[17] Type 2 individuals on insulin therapy may even develop hyperglycemia if post-exercise insulin is omitted.[18] Individuals with blood glucose ≥250 mg% should be tested for ketone bodies in urine. And exercise should be postponed if levels are ≥1.5 mmol/L.

Orthopedic Injuries

Glycemic variability results in changes in joint structure and increased fragility. Exercise training for each diabetic must be individualized and progressed gradually specially if patient is on statin therapy.[19]

Heat-related Effects

Autonomic dysfunction in diabetic individuals increases risk of raised body temperature during exercise.[20] Caution must be kept to avoid outdoor exercise during hot and humid weather conditions.

SMART GOAL

SMART is an acronym for **S**pecific, **M**easurable, **A**ttainable, **R**elevant, and Realistic and **T**ime-bound**.** Off late concept of *SMART* goals has emerged as a key for successful exercise prescription. World over this concept has been evaluated and found very effective in fetching long-term sustained benefits. Let us understand how *SMART* Goals can be applied to exercise training programs making it easier for individuals to train themselves.

- *Specific*: The clearer and more specific the goals are, greater are the chances to achieve them. Rather than just making goal to reduce weight, target to reduce weight of 15 kg is more specific and meaningful.
- *Measurable*: It means adding a number. Making a diary and keeping a record of your daily exercise will help to monitor progress. E.g. measurable targets like exercise for 4–5 times a week, running 5,000 steps a day.
- *Attainable*: Goals must be attainable otherwise failure to achieve daily targets will disappoint the patient and may result in drop-out from exercise schedule. In the starting of any exercise program doing 10 minutes exercise for 5 days in a week is attainable than making target for 40 minutes exercise in 5 days per week.
- ***Relevant or Realistic***: Set goals that are important for that individual patient and really achievable in the given time, according to his physical capacity. Consider all the obstacles that one would have to face, viz. family time, kids, self-study time, exercise associated weakness, leg pain, etc.
- *Time-bound*: Setting specific deadlines is essential for success of exercise program**.** Both the long-term and short-term goals should have deadlines. This helps in creating a future goal clearer and more focused so that it becomes achievable.

SMART goals are attainable and rewarding. Setting *SMART* goals helps keep big projects from being overwhelming. Steps for success are clearly spelled out so that one knows when he has made the goal. They help in reaching the long-term goal by use of small 1–2 week specific targets. At the bigger picture being small and of short duration these goals improve exercise capacity gradually and prepare oneself for greater achievable goals. The biggest payoff comes from terming short-term goals into long-lasting healthy habits.

CONCLUSION

The need of the hour is that the clinician should understand patient's profile and prepare a tailor-made recipe having a balanced and proportionate amalgamation of various types of exercises, with inbuilt checks and momentum to help a diabetic achieve favorable metabolic goals and overall a sound health. The bottom line is that an individualized approach, conformity to standard guidelines and setting *SMART* goals are the key elements of an exercise prescription for a diabetic patient which makes the whole exercise training program a success.

REFERENCES

1. Morrato EH, Hill JO, Wyatt HR, et al. Physical activity in U.S. adults with diabetes and at risk for developing diabetes, 2003. Diabetes Care. 2007;30(2):203-9.
2. American Diabetes Association. Physical activity/exercise and diabetes. Diabetes Care. 2004;27 (1):S58-S62.
3. Bax JJ, Young LH, Frye RL, et al. Screening for coronary artery disease in patients with diabetes. Diabetes Care. 2007;30(10):2729-36.
4. Little JP, Gillen JB, Percival ME, et al. Low-volume high-intensity interval training reduces hyperglycemia and increases muscle mitochondrial capacity in patients with type 2 diabetes. J Appl Physiol (1985). 2011;111(6):1554-60.
5. Jelleyman C, Yates T, O'Donovan G, et al. The effects of high-intensity interval training on glucose regulation and insulin resistance: a meta-analysis. Obes Rev. 2015;16(11):942-61.
6. Nybo L, Sundstrup E, Jakobsen MD, et al. High-intensity training versus traditional exercise interventions for promoting health. Med Sci Sports Exerc. 2010;42(10):1951-8.
7. Montero-Fernandez N, Serra-Rexach JA. Role of exercise on sarcopenia in the elderly. Eur J Phys Rehabil Med. 2013;49(1):131-43.
8. US Department of Health and Human Services. (2018). Physical Activity Guidelines Advisory Committee Report. [online]. Available from https://health.gov/paguidelines/2008/report/pdf/committeereport.pdf [Last accessed October, 2019].
9. Yardley JE, Kenny GP, Perkins BA, et al. Effects of performing resistance exercise before versus after aerobic exercise on glycemia in type 1 diabetes. Diabetes Care. 2012;35(4):669-75.
10. Bravata DM, Smith-Spangler C, Sundaram V, et al. Using pedometers to increase physical activity and improve health: a systematic review. JAMA. 2007;298(19):2296-304.
11. Colberg SR, Sigal RJ, Yardley JE, et al. Physical Activity/Exercise and Diabetes: A Position Statement of the American Diabetes Association. Diabetes Care. 2016;39(11):2065-79.
12. Biankin SA, Jenkins AB, Campbell LV, et al. Target-seeking behavior of plasma glucose with exercise in type 1 diabetes. Diabetes Care. 2003;26(2):297-301.
13. Sanabria-Martinez G, Garcia-Hermoso A, Poyatos-Leon R, et al. Effectiveness of physical activity interventions on preventing gestational diabetes mellitus and excessive maternal weight gain: a meta-analysis. BJOG. 2015;122(9):1167-74.
14. ACOG committee opinion no. 650: physical activity and exercise during pregnancy and the postpartum period. Obstet Gynecol. 2015;126(6):e135-42.
15. Tsalikian E, Mauras N, Beck RW, et al. Impact of exercise on overnight glycemic control in children with type 1 diabetes mellitus. J Pediatr. 2005;147(4):528-34.
16. Campbell MD, Walker M, Bracken RM, et al. Insulin therapy and dietary adjustments to normalize glycemia and prevent nocturnal hypoglycemia after evening exercise in type 1 diabetes: a randomized controlled trial. BMJ Open Diabetes Res Care. 2015;3(1):e000085.
17. Yardley JE, Zaharieva DP, Jarvis C, et al. The "ups" and "downs" of a bike race in people with type 1 diabetes: dramatic differences in strategies and blood glucose responses in the Paris-to-Ancaster Spring Classic. Can J Diabetes. 2015;39:105-10.
18. Gordon BA, Bird SR, MacIsaac RJ, et al. Does a single bout of resistance or aerobic exercise after insulin dose reduction modulate glycaemic control in type 2 diabetes? A randomised cross-over trial. J Sci Med Sport. 2016;19(10):795-9.
19. De Oliveira LP, Vieira CP, Guerra FD, et al. Structural and biomechanical changes in the Achilles tendon after chronic treatment with statins. Food Chem Toxicol. 2015;77:50-7.
20. Carter MR, McGinn R, Barrera-Ramirez J, et al. Impairments in local heat loss in type 1 diabetes during exercise in the heat. Med Sci Sports Exerc. 2014;46(12):2224-33.

24 CHAPTER Resistance Training Exercise: Impact on Glycemia and Cardiovascular Risk Factors

Suraj Prakash Sondhi, Amit Rastogi, Shafali Nandwani

INTRODUCTION

Diabetes mellitus is a very common disorder affecting more than 70 million people in India. Most of these belong to type 2 category, which is considered as a lifestyle disease. Sixty to seventy percent of these patients die of vascular complications (MI or stroke). Accordingly first and the foremost strategy in controlling this disease and its fall out, is lifestyle modifications, which includes diet and exercise. Together these two modalities could compete with most of the oral hypoglycemic agents in efficacy. A lot is known about the role of aerobic exercise in controlling glycemia and cardiovascular (CV) risk factors but there is not much clarity about resistance training (RT) exercise and its effect in diabetes mellitus. Skeletal muscle accounts for up to 40% of body weight and 75% of glucose uptake. Type 2 diabetic patients exhibit a decreased capacity to oxidize both glucose and fat in comparison to a healthy individual. Resistance training is known to increase both muscle mass and strength and thus justifiably stimulates interest in its use as an instrument to positively affect diabetes.

WHAT IS RESISTANCE TRAINING EXERCISE?

Exercises can broadly be divided into two kinds:

1. *Dynamic*: In which the muscle contraction produces a movement which could further be concentric (shortening of muscle) or eccentric (lengthening of muscle).
2. *Isometric or static* where there is no movement of limbs.

Exercises could further be *aerobic or anaerobic*. Whenever an exercise is done at moderate level for long period, e.g. long-distance running, the energy supplied is through increased amount of oxygen (higher heart rate and respiratory rate). Thus, exercise is called aerobic. While those exercises which are heavy and for very short duration require enormous energy, which cannot be supplied by oxygen and these are called anaerobic exercises, e.g. weight lifting.

Most exercises have both static or dynamic and aerobic and anaerobic components. But we basically classify the exercises on the basis of its major component.

Resistance training involves exercises that causes the muscles to contract against resistance with mainly a static or isometric component. Depending on whether lighter weights are repetitively done or heavier weights held for long, it has greater aerobic or anaerobic content.

The resistance could be external, e.g. weights, dumbbells, water bottles, bricks, any other object or rubber bands, exercise tubings or your own body weight. Resistance training works by causing microscopic damage or tears to the muscle cells, which in turn are quickly repaired by the body to help the muscles regenerate and grow stronger. Humans lose 5 pounds of muscle every 10 years after the age of 30 years. In the next 40 years (30–70) one can lose more than 25% of the type 2 muscle fibers, which are our strength fibers. Resistance training tries to overcome this loss and has many more advantages.

It could be of two types:

1. *Hypertrophy resistance training*: In which heavier weights are used for less numbers of repetitions. It increases both muscle mass and strength.
2. *Endurance training*: In which lighter weights are used for more repetitions.

PHYSIOLOGICAL RESPONSE

Depending upon the magnitude of resistance, duration of muscle contraction, and the intervening rest period, heart rate goes up and systolic blood pressure (SBP) and diastolic BP (DBP) goes up. Aerobic exercise will have similar effects except that DBP will not change or go down. Done under the instruction and only moderately, these responses may be very mild. Cardiac output goes up (mainly because of higher heart rate rather than stroke volume). The intramuscular pressure in the contracting muscle increases which gradually becomes more than the intravascular pressure causing muscular ischemia. The high cardiac output causes a reflex vasoconstriction in noncontracting muscles. Increased cardiac output against a backdrop of vasoconstriction ends up in high SBP, DBP, and mean BP. At the release of strain the venous return is increased but the vasoconstriction is still there, resulting in persistent high BP.

Jane E Yardley et al.[1] studied the acute effects of RT versus aerobic exercise in 12 patients of type 1 diabetes mellitus. The blood glucose levels came down significantly more in aerobic group (9.6–5.8 mmol/L) during the exercise than RT (8.4–6.8 mmol/L) but after the exercise it rebounded to the levels of the other group. There were more hypoglycemia in RT in the night after the exercise (nonsignificant). The conclusion was that aerobic exercise produces greater decline in blood glucose during activity but results in higher late postexercise levels.

FITNESS AND HEALTH BENEFITS

Potential benefits of resistance training:

- Improvement in muscular strength or mass or capacity to utilize glucose
- Improved lipid profile
- Lower blood glucose levels
- Decreased dosages of antidiabetic drugs, including insulin
- Improved muscle mitochondrial oxidative capacity
- Anti-inflammatory role.[2]

Randomized studies of more than 12 weeks consistently show an increase in muscle mass and quality. These are not age-dependent. In one study of elderly men and women (mean age 87 years) who lifted weights three times per week for 10 weeks, strength increased by a whopping 113%. The improvement in strength enabled them to walk faster (12%) climb 28% more stairs and the thigh muscle increased by more than 2.5%. With the increased muscle mass basal metabolic rate (BMR) goes up. BMD may also go up especially in the bones subjected to exercise. Intensive RT can result in a marginal increase in left ventricular mass, but is usually in the higher range of normal (physiological). Resting BP may come down and endothelial function may improve.

The effects of resistance training on glycemia in diabetics: There is enough evidence to indicate that aerobic exercise improves diabetic control and reduces harmful CV risk factors, but interest in RT is relatively new. Muscle contraction increases glucose uptake and increases insulin sensitivity. This provides a rationale to use this strategy in diabetic patients. The results of various studies on the effects of RT on HbA1c are variable depending upon the exercise regimen chosen and the duration of the study. Two RCT with 36 and 62 patients, respectively reported HbA1c reduction of 1.2 and 1.1. In the second study the diabetic medications were reduced for 72% in the RT group. Most of these studies also report an increase in skeletal muscle mass which supports the hypothesis that RT improves the glycemic control by pushing extra glucose into muscle as glycogen.

Some other studies have reported an improvement in insulin sensitivity even when there is no increase in the muscle mass suggesting a qualitative improvement in muscle function. Ibenza et al. reported decrease in visceral fat in patients put on RT which could also account for improved insulin sensitivity. Most of these studies are small and one has to be careful to draw definite conclusions.

Which Exercise is Better: Aerobic or RT or Both Combined?

Different studies have shown variable results. One small study which tried to look at A1c reduction randomized 43 patients into two groups for 4 months. RT group had a significant fall in HbA1c (1.2 vs 0.2%). Yavari et al. group[3] evaluated the effects of different exercises in 80 patients over 1 year of time. The maximum A1c reduction was observed in combined exercise group (1.74) followed by aerobic (1.33) and RT (0.55). Thus, to give optimal benefits to patients one may have to combine both the exercises. Maiorana et al. reported that combined exercise was better than no exercise with a difference of 0.6% in HbA1c. This study did not compare the two exercise regimen. One of the largest study (Baldacci et al.) in this field involved 120 patients followed up for 1 year. HbA1c was reduced by 1.2%. Low-density lipoprotein (LDL) and total cholesterol came down significantly and high-density lipoprotein (HDL) went up. Lukas Schwingshackl et al.[4] reported a meta-analysis in Diabetologia in 2014. They included 14 trials including 915 patients. Aerobic exercise was more effective than RT in improving A1c levels but the best reduction came when both the exercises were combined. ADA 2019 sums it up "clinical trials have provided strong evidence for the A1c lowering value of RT in older adults with type 2 diabetes and for an additive benefit of combined aerobic and resistance exercise in adults with type 2 diabetes". ADA recommends RT to be included in the exercise program of a diabetic unless there are contraindications. It further recommends that "people with diabetes should perform aerobic and resistance exercise regularly. Aerobic activity bouts ideally last at least 10 minutes, with the goal of ~ 30 min/day or more, most of the days (not allowing more than 2 days to lapse between sessions) to at least 150 min/week. *They should engage in 2–3 sessions/week of RT on nonconsecutive days (with each session consisting of at least one set of five or more different resistance exercises involving the large muscles group). Although heavier RT with free weights may improve glycemic control, RT of any intensity is recommended to improve strength, balance, and the ability to engage in activities of daily living"*.

American College of Sports Medicine and Sports Medicine, Australia, 2011 also recommends at least 2 sessions per week of 8–10 exercises repeated with 10–15 repetitions to fatigue.

INTERACTION BETWEEN METFORMIN AND RESISTANCE TRAINING

Metformin is the most widely prescribed first line oral antidiabetic drug recommended by ADA. The exact molecular mechanism of action remains unknown. One likely site of action is inhibition of respiratory system complex I within the mitochondria, increasing the AMP/ATP ratio and activating AMPK, resulting in improved insulin sensitivity.[5] Resistance training-induced increased insulin sensitivity also acts partly through AMPK activation, suggesting that it could have an additive effect with metformin. At least one trial (Boule NG Diabetologia, 2013) recently concluded that the effect of exercise (endurance) on A1c reduction was significantly more in patients on metformin (–0.57%) than in untreated ones (–0.17%). Conflicting findings were reported in another trial (Malin SK et al. in Diabetes care 2012) which revealed that metformin use blunted some of the beneficial effects of combined training. This controversy needs to be resolved to use exercise as a treatment option in type 2 diabetics, many of which are on metformin.

EFFECTS OF RESISTANCE TRAINING ON CARDIOVASCULAR RISK FACTORS

There is limited material available to conclude the effects of RT on CV risk factors. Study by Elizabeth C Shroeder et al. published in PLoS one December 2018 looked at these factors in an 8-week long exercise program on 69 hypertensive adults. It concluded that while both aerobic and RT exercises increased the lean body mass and body strength only combined exercise brought about a significant decrease in central diastolic BP (–4 mm Hg). Yavari et al. study[3] also looked at these parameters but found significant decrease in only triglyceride levels and that also only in aerobic group. A meta-analysis on role of RT in modifying the CV risk factors in syndrome X by Lemes et al. BMJ reported that SBP is reduced by 4.1 mm Hg. It is pertinent to mention here that even a small reduction of up to 2 mm Hg can reduce the stroke mortality by around 10% and mortality from heart disease by about 7%. Another systematic review published by Cybelle Nery et al. in Brazilian Journal of Physical Therapy July 2017 included 8 studies on 336 patients concluded that the quality of data was very poor. "Based on very low quality data the effectiveness of this (RT) exercise in glycemic control and lipid profile (HDL, LDL, TG, and total cholesterol) is still inconclusive". It concluded:

ACC/AHA 2019 Guidelines on The Primary Prevention of Cardiovascular Disease recommends that "Adults should engage in at least 150 min/week of accumulated moderate intensity or 75 min/week of vigorous intensity aerobic activity to reduce ASCVD risk (Class of Recommendation II A). Resistance exercise should also be encouraged because of its several health benefits, including improved physical functioning, improving glycemic control in individuals with diabetes and possible BP lowering. Whether resistance exercise lowers ASCVD risk is unclear."

CONCLUSION

Exercise as an option to control glycemia and decrease CV risk factors is an established method of treatment, but there is a lack of clarity about RT exercise which is different from aerobic exercises. There is not only a paucity of large randomized trials done in this field but also lack of uniformity among type of RT exercises used in different trials. Thus, results are not consistent. There is a reasonable agreement that RT is good for bringing down blood glucose levels, though the consensus is that combined exercise is better than alone. This has prompted most of the organizations including ADA to recommend both in diabetes. The effect of RT in improving CV risk factors is inconclusive and contradictory and there is a clear need to do more trials. Future research is likely to help in finding out which sets of exercises are better for which individual so that we can have an individualized prescription of exercise.

REFERENCES

1. Yardley JE, Kenny GP, Perkins BA, et al. Resistance versus aerobic exercise: acute effects on glycemia in type 1 diabetes. Diabetes Care. 2013:36:537-42.
2. Pedersen BK. The anti-inflammatory effect of exercise: its role in diabetes and cardiovascular disease control. Essays Biochem. 2006;42:105-17.
3. Yavari A, Najafipour F, Aliasgharzadeh A, et al. Effect of aerobic exercise, resistance training or combined training on glycaemic control and cardiovascular risk factors in patients with type 2 diabetes. Biol Sport. 2012;29:135-43.
4. Schwingshackl L, Missbach B, Dias S, et al. Impact of different training modalities on glycaemic control and blood lipids in patients with type 2 diabetes: a systematic review and network meta-analysis. Diabetologia. 2014;57:1789-97.
5. Pesta DH, Goncalves RLS, Madiraju AK, et al. Resistance training to improve type 2 diabetes: working toward a prescription for the future. Nutr Metab (Lond). 2017;14:24.

5 SECTION Therapeutics

25 CHAPTER Intensive Glycemic Control: Is it Achievable without Adverse Effects?

Arvind Gupta, Manoj Saluja

INTRODUCTION

Diabetes, a slowly growing epidemic, is becoming a growing burden to the nation's health and economy. Efforts to curb the complications as well as limit the disease by intense management was met with several challenges earlier, including metabolic side effects, fatal complications and sometimes raised overall mortality. In this chapter, we will discuss the studies done so far with the possible shortcomings and deliberate over newer possibilities which may aid in better management of the disease.

GLYCEMIC CONTROL

Diabetes and its complications are one of the leading causes of mortality and morbidity all over the world. As the disease and its complications are becoming rampant, a stringent management plan is essential. A 1% increase in the glycated hemoglobin (HbA1c) level is associated with an increase of 18% in the risk of cardiovascular (CV) events. Apart from that, an increase of 12–14% in the risk of death, and an increase of 37% in the risk of retinopathy or renal failure is also noted, implying a definite need to keep blood sugar in check.

Glycemic control has always been a delicately balanced act. The patient not only needs to maintain a euglycemic state but also should be educated enough to make or revise decision strategies, volitional control and the sense to avoid hypo- and hyperglycemia.[1] Strict glucose control, monitored via self-monitoring of blood glucose (SMBG) and glycated hemoglobin was strongly advocated keeping in mind the complications of uncontrolled blood sugar.

Trials involving patients with type 1 diabetes and patients with new-onset diabetes type 2 showed reduced microvascular complications with intensive glucose management. Significant reductions in incidence of CV incidents was not noted but follow-up observation studies indicated at a reduced risk of CV outcome and mortality.

Though DCCT-EDIC trial,[2] comparing intensive therapy to conventional therapy in type 1 diabetics, showed CV mortality benefit with lower incidence of retinopathy and nephropathy but with increased incidence of nonfatal hypoglycemia in the intensive control arm. The benefits of intensive glycemic control on microvascular and neuropathic complications are well established for both type 1 and type 2 diabetes. The ADVANCE[3] trial has added to that evidence by validating a significant reduction in the risk of new or worsening albuminuria when median A1c was lowered to 6.3% compared with standard glycemic control of 7.0%.

INTENSIVE SUGAR CONTROL: BOON OR BANE?

After a few years, intensive glucose control lost its charm owing to the increased risk of adverse effects like weight gain, incidents of hypoglycemia and sometimes raised risk of mortality whereas the benefits were almost similar to those attained with standard/recommended control, especially in patients with advanced type 2 diabetes.

Numerous trials involving patients with advanced type 2 diabetes like ACCORD (Action To Control Cardiovascular Risk In Diabetes) ADVANCE (Action In Diabetes And Vascular Disease: Preterax And Diamicron Modified Release Controlled Evaluation), VADT (Veterans Affairs Diabetes Trial) came to similar conclusions that improved glucose control over a median duration of 3–6 years provided a modest and nonsignificant reduction in CV events. The trials also showed that intensive control approach did not reduce CV-related mortality or total mortality.

One of the biggest studies, ACCORD study noted reduced microvascular complications but at a cost of more use of insulin, significantly more weight gain, and more episodes of severe hypoglycemia and increased mortality rates in the intensive arm (target A1c, 6.0%) than in standardized control arm (target A1c, 7.0–7.9%). In February 2008, the glycemic control study of ACCORD was stopped due to an increased rate of mortality in the intensive arm.[4]

The ADVANCE study noted that the overall or cardiovascular mortality in the intensive (target A1c, 6.5%) and the standard control arms (target according to 'local guidelines') were largely the same with no additional deaths noted in intensive arm. At the same time, intensive glycemic control significantly reduced the primary endpoint (nephropathy and retinopathy) and major adverse CV events.[4]

Type 2 diabetes patients with a median A1c of 9.4%, either on insulin or maximal dose oral agents were randomized in VADT where, in the 5.6-year follow-up period, the aggregate incidence of the primary outcome was not significantly lower in the intensive arm (HbA1c < 6.0%). A follow-up done after 10 years showed a benefit of 17% in intensive control arm but was negated by the study itself when the final data was compiled after 15 years.[4]

Most of these studies also observed that there was no 'legacy effect' of intense/standard control. VADT noted that the A1c levels of the last 3 years were significant higher values predisposing to worse clinical outcomes in both intensive and standard arms.

What caused the increased adverse effects with intensive control?

Though the increased adverse effects or at times the increased mortality raised concern regarding the safety of strict glycemic control, it is to be noted that they have been observational findings. Various post hoc analyses have failed to prove or find evidence regarding the cause.

The associated adverse effects in large trials by no means should be interpreted in a way that promotes poor glucose control. How meticulous should we be and where do we draw the line?

The downstream effects usually linked with the intensive arm are increased insulin use, drug combinations, weight gain, which may be associated with statistically significant mortality rate, but may or may not be causative. It is plausible that hypoglycemia or hypoglycemic unawareness could be increasing the risk of CV mortality in the high risk participant. Multiple oral agents along with or without multiple insulin doses, frequent therapy alteration to achieve the target A1c and low target self-monitored glucose may have led to drug interactions or effects that have not been accounted for.[4]

The difference in the outcomes of ACCORD and ADVANCE trials, despite a similar study design emphasized the differences between the two—the lower age of onset, less use of basal insulin and low A1c level at the time of entry into the trial. Both were carried out in participants with established diabetes (mean duration 8–11 years) who either had known cardiovascular disease (CVD) or several risk factors, signifying the presence of established atherosclerosis. Subset analyses suggested a significant benefit of intensive glycemic control on CVD in participants with shorter duration of diabetes, lower A1c at entry, and/or or absence of known CVD.[4]

The DCCT follow-up study (study on type 1 diabetes) found that strict glycemic control introduced in relatively young participants free of CVD risk factors a 57% reduction in major CVD outcomes was noted. This sufficiently favors the above hypothesis.[4] Almost 9 years were required for the benefit on CVD in the DCCT-EDIC[3] to be statistically significant and evident. This sheds light on another loophole that ACCORD and ADVANCE trials might have had, that is a short duration of study.

Various studies like J-DOIT3 also highlighted the importance of intensive glycemic control with the study reports showing significantly lower risks in CV mortality, even when compared to United Kingdom Prospective Diabetes Study (UKPDS) trial.

ADVENT OF NEW DRUGS AND NEW TRIALS

The third point in favor of intensive control is the arrival of newer and better oral antidiabetic drugs. The medications that were used in initial trials were either insulin or insulin secretagogues like sulfonylureas which accompanied a plethora of metabolic side effects. The newer agents such as DPP-4 inhibitors, GLP-1 agonists, alpha-glucosidase inhibitors, and SGLT-2 inhibitors not only have a safer drug profile, but some of them also provide CV benefit due to their pleiotropic effects.

Trials based on newer drugs like DPP-4 inhibitors, SGLT-2 inhibitors, and GLP-1 receptor agonists, originally done to prove noninferiority to placebo in CV mortality, brought out some interesting data. Noninferiority trials with DPP-4 inhibitors, viz. SAVOR-TIMI53 (saxagliptin), EXAMINE (Alogliptin), TECOS (Sitagliptin) showed no major event of hypoglycemia in latter two, while the increased incidence of hypoglycemia noted in saxagliptin arm was associated with the background drug given with it, usually sulfonylureas. All the three trials used participants with high-risk CV morbidity and yet were noninferior to placebos in terms of MACE.[5]

Absence of significant weight gain with DPP4 inhibitors was a highlight in the above trials. This may be attributed to its property of delayed gastric emptying, increased satiety and reduced events of hypoglycemia.

Two major trials CAROLINA and CARMELINA were based on linagliptin. CARMELINA[6] (The Cardiovascular and Renal Microvascular Outcome Study With Linagliptin) compared the effect of linagliptin in type 2 diabetic patients with high CV and renal risk factors. While, it did prove that it was noninferior to placebo when added to usual care in patients with high CV and renal risk; the trial failed to note any significant association between the drug and heart failure (as noted in SAVOR-TIMI53 and EXAMINE trials).[4]

Trials like EMPA-REG OUTCOME (empagliflozin), CANVAS-R (canagliflozin), CREDENCE (canagliflozin), DECLARE TIMI 58 (dapagliflozin) proved noninferiority of SGLT-2 inhibitors to placebo, showed definite benefit in CV mortality. Compared to placebo group, patients with type 2 diabetes at high risk for CV events who received empagliflozin had significantly lower rates of the primary composite CV outcome, death from any cause and lower rate of renal failure (EMPA-REG OUTCOME).[7] Dapagliflozin and canagliflozin showed similar results with low metabolic adverse effects but slightly increased risk of urinary tract infection (UTI).

The LEADER and SUSTAIN 6 trials, noninferiority trials for GLP-1a analogs, liraglutide and semaglutide, indicated lower rates of first occurrence of death from CV causes, nonfatal myocardial infarction, or nonfatal stroke among patients in type 2 diabetics with the drugs. Trials EXSCEL and REWIND (exenatide and dulaglutide respectively) merely proved noninferiority with no additional benefits unlike the previous two trials.[8]

ROLE OF LIFESTYLE MODIFICATION

The ACCORD and ADVANCE also vary in the strategies adopted to achieve the targets. The overall treatment approaches adopted to reach the A1c level might be the reason for increased mortality and not the reduced levels of A1c per se.[4] This emphasized the fact that lifestyle modification and other nonpharmacological approaches could be successfully used in keeping good blood sugar control with minimal side effects.

Look AHEAD[9] trial used intensive lifestyle modification in diabetes type 2 patients, especially obese. Though no CV benefits were noted, it was observed that significant weight loss along with improved biomarkers of glucose and lipid control, with better quality of life due to remarkably reduced complications and associated economic benefits.

The definite proven use of lifestyle changes could be used along with various drugs which would lead to lower requirement of pharmacotherapy and possibly lesser adverse effects. This may assist in achieving an intense control without fretting over the feared complications.

INDIVIDUALIZED MANAGEMENT

Subgroup analyses of clinical trials such as the DCCT and UKPDS suggest a small but incremental benefit in microvascular outcomes with A1c values closer to normal. Therefore, for selected individuals we may reasonably suggest lower A1c goals than the general goal of 7%. This set of patients includes those with short duration of diabetes, long life expectancy, and no significant CVD.

(ADA, B-level recommendation; ACC/AHA, class IIa recommendation)

Patients with a history of severe hypoglycemia, limited life expectancy, advanced micro- or macrovascular complications, or extensive comorbid conditions or those with longstanding diabetes, less stringent A1c goals may be appropriate for now. Meanwhile, to answer some of the pertaining questions, large and longer trials using newer drugs and clinical advances, randomized controlled trials with meaningful clinical outcomes are called for.

With the newer and less dangerous options available, it is highly likely that a better control would be attainable in this subset as well with comparable results if not equal to patients with less advanced comorbidities.

CONCLUSION

Keeping in mind the dire health and economic effects of diabetes and its complications as well as the substantial advantage glycemic control has shown, it is safe to say that intensive blood sugar control is not only desirable but also essential. Increase in awareness, intense lifestyle modification, use of newer drugs along with intelligent patient selection can definitely help us achieve near normal glycemic control with lesser adverse effects and much better clinical outcome.

REFERENCES

1. Perlmuter LC, Flanagan BP, Parinda H, et al. Glycemic control and hypoglycemia. Diabetes Care. 2008;31(10):2072-6.
2. Nathan DM, Cleary PA, Backlund JY, et al. Intensive diabetes treatment and cardiovascular disease in patients with type 1 diabetes. N Engl J Med. 2005;353:2643-53.
3. Patel A, MacMahon S, Chalmers J, et al. Intensive blood glucose control and vascular outcomes in patients with type 2 diabetes. N Engl J Med. 2008;358:2560-72.
4. Skyler JS, Bergenstal R, Bonow RO, et al. Intensive Glycemic Control and the Prevention of Cardiovascular Events: Implications of the ACCORD, ADVANCE, and VA Diabetes Trials. Diabetes Care. 2009;32(1):187-92.
5. Mannucci E, Mosenzon O, Avogaro A. Analyses of Results From Cardiovascular Safety Trials With DPP-4 Inhibitors: Cardiovascular Outcomes, Predefined Safety Outcomes, and Pooled Analysis and Meta-analysis. Diabetes Care. 2016;39(Suppl. 2):S196-204.
6. Rosenstock J, Perkovic V, Johansen OE, et al. Effect of Linagliptin vs Placebo on Major Cardiovascular Events in Adults With Type 2 Diabetes and High Cardiovascular and Renal Risk-The CARMELINA Randomized Clinical Trial. JAMA. 2019;321(1):69-79.
7. Zinman B, Wanner C, Lachin JM, et al. Empagliflozin, cardiovascular outcomes, and mortality in type 2 diabetes. N Engl J Med. 2015;373:2117-28.
8. Olmo-Garcia MI, Merino-Torres JF. GLP-1 receptor agonists and cardiovascular disease in patients with type 2 diabetes. J Diabetes Res. 2018;2018:4020492.
9. Look AHEAD Research Group, Wing RR, Bolin P, et al. Cardiovascular effects of intensive lifestyle intervention in type 2 diabetes. N Engl J Med. 2013;369(2):145-54.

CHAPTER 26 Continued Insulin Care: Monitoring Treatment to Suit Patient Needs

Ashutosh Chaturvedi, Divyansh Mathur, Girish Mathur

INTRODUCTION

Diabetes mellitus (DM) is now a rapidly growing global public health concern which imparts both social and economic burdens. Along with other pharmacologic and nonpharmacologic measures of treatment, insulin therapy is widely used in management of diabetes. Early insulin initiation not only significantly reduces the macro- and microvascular complications but can also lead to its reversal of diabetes.[1] To improve the care of patients, equitable and affordable access to insulin is necessary. Nowadays multiple formulations and regimens, and various delivery devices of insulin are available to individualize treatment for achieving the best possible glycemic control in diabetics. Various types of insulin ranging from ultrashort-acting to ultralong-acting differ in their onset, peak, and duration of action and also in safety profiles. With a surfeit of regimens and formulations of insulin, it is becoming increasingly challenging to initiate and intensify insulin therapy and also to match it with heterogenous patient profiles. Adult-onset diabetes has been stratified into subgroups to individualize treatment according to patient characteristics, disease progression, and risk of diabetic complications. There are barriers to insulin therapy, from both the patient and the physician's perspective, and the decision to initiate insulin therapy is influenced by cost, risk of hypoglycemia, convenience, and chances to gain weight. Patient characteristics such as age, body mass index, and bedtime or postbreakfast plasma glucose levels may change the efficacy of the regimen chosen, thus supporting the need to tailor treatment to meet an individual patient's requirements.

INSULIN TYPES AND FORMULATIONS

Table 1 lists the various types and formulations of insulin, along with information about their action profile and peak activity.

WHEN TO INITIATE INSULIN THERAPY?

When deciding that whether a patient should be put on insulin therapy or not, it is always useful to look at the guidelines for glycemic control. The patients who are unable to achieve their glycemic targets by using oral agents are usual candidates for insulin therapy. The most common indications of insulin use are summarized below.

Common indications for insulin initiation:

1. Type 1 DM—lifelong requirement
2. Type 2 DM
    a) At diagnosis when there is severe hyperglycemia with fasting plasma glucose (FPG) > 250 mg%, post prandial glucose (PPG) > 300 mg%, HbA1c > 9%.
    b) After failure of oral antidiabetic drugs that is a FPG > 150 mg%, PPG or random blood sugar (RBS) > 200 mg%, HBA1c > 8.5% despite after receiving optimal doses of 2 or 3 oral antidiabetic drugs.
    c) Special situations
        - Systemic infection
        - Acute myocardial infarction
        - Unstable angina
        - Sepsis
        - Diabetic ketoacidosis
        - Hyperosmolar non-ketotic coma

TABLE 1: Insulin and insulin analogs.

Type of insulin	Onset of action (min)	Time to peak concentration (min)	Maximum duration of action (hours)
Regular insulin	30–60	90–120	5–12
Insulin lispro (Humalog)	10–15	30–60	3–4
Insulin aspart	10–15	40–50	3–5
Insulin glulisine (Apidra)	10–15	55	3–5
Fiasp (faster insulin aspart)	16–20	91–133	5–7
NPH insulin	60–120	240–480	10–20
Premixed insulin (human) 70% NPH 30% regular 50% NPH 50% regular	30–60	Dual peak	16
Premixed insulin analogs 75% NPL 25% Lispro 50% NPL 50% Lispro 70% NPA 30% Aspart	5–15	Dual peak	10–16
Insulin glargine	60–120	None	24
Insulin detemir (Levemir)	60–120	None	20
Insulin Degludec (Tresiba) Available in 100 units/mL and 200 units/mL	30–90	No peak time	42–45
Insulin Glargine (Toujeo) 300 units/mL	60	Insulin delivered at a steady level	Up to 36

(NPA: neutral protamine aspart; NPH: neutral protamine Hagedorn; NPL: neutral protamine lispro)

- Pregnancy
- Diabetic kidney disease
- During major surgeries

MATCHING THE INSULIN REGIMEN TO THE PATIENT NEEDS

An ideal insulin regimen is that which mimics the physiological secretory pattern of insulin. Despite all advanced available formulations in the market, no single regimen can yet be considered ideal till date. It is important that insulin regimen is individualized and is based on various patient characteristics such as glycemic profile, dietary pattern, and personal lifestyle. The most commonly used regimens are basal, basal plus, basal bolus, and premixed regimens out of which the basal-bolus regimen comprising long-acting basal and rapid- or short-acting bolus insulin most closely mimics the physiological insulin secretion pattern.

A basal-bolus regimen—glargine at bedtime along with rapid- or short-acting insulin at each meal—is the ideal regimen in terms of physiological action and overall glycemic control but many patients are reluctant to start with a basal-bolus insulin regimen. The basal-bolus insulin regime management requires motivation of both patient and provider, and also a comprehensive training in carbohydrate counting (or some method of food or insulin matching) and adjustment of insulin doses. Therefore, the insulin regimen should be properly matched to the individual needs, concerns, and capabilities of each patient. Patients who resist basal-bolus therapy initially often shift to multiple daily injection (MDI) regimens after gaining self-confidence to safely and effectively use insulin through less intensive regimens. Table 2[2] presents commonly used insulin regimens based on a patient's clinical status and lifestyle attributes.

In patients whom postprandial blood sugar is not adequately controlled on combination therapy using basal insulin and oral agents, a twice-daily premixed-insulin regimen (prebreakfast and predinner) is preferred. Such patients can be initiated on once-daily injections at the evening meal and the second injection can be added then

TABLE 2: Insulin regimens based on different patient characteristics.

Regimen	HbA1c	Medication	Pattern	Diet history	Lifestyle	Monitoring
Basal insulin only	>7.5–10%	Oral anti diabetics (OAD) controlling PPG	High fasting plasma glucose (FPG)	Small, regular meals	Reluctance to do MDI	Fasting
Biphasic analog insulin	>7.5%	OAD Failure	Glucose rise during the day	Large dinner Small lunch	Consistent daily routine: reluctance to start MDI	Fasting and pre-dinner (if Insulin administered twice daily)
Biphasic human insulin	>7.5%	OAD Failure	Glucose rise during the day	Isocaloric meals or large lunches	Consistent daily routine: reluctance to start MDI	Fasting and pre-dinner (if Insulin administered twice daily)
Basal-bolus therapy	>7.5%		Can be matched to any pattern	Can be matched to any diet	Erratic schedule, motivated	Frequent (minimum before meals and bedtime)

as per the need. If the patient eats small lunches or misses lunch quite often, then rapid-acting analog premixed insulin is an option. For patients with glucose toxicity, i.e. fasting plasma glucose > 250 mg/dL, basal-bolus insulin therapy may be required.[3] Basal-bolus insulin therapy should also be the next option if premixed-insulin regimen fails in achieving the glycemic targets. After the glucose returns to near-normal levels, basal-bolus insulin therapy can be continued or modified accordingly.

INSULIN INITIATION AND INTENSIFICATION: START LOW AND TITRATE UNIFORMLY

A common initiating dose for insulin therapy in patients with type 2 diabetes is 0.15 units/kg body weight/day but because >90% of patients with type 2 diabetes are having insulin resistance,[4] usually significantly higher doses are often needed to attain the glycemic goals.[5]

In the Treat-to-Target study,[6] an initial dose of 10 units/day with glargine or Neutral Protamine Hagedorn (NPH) was used at bedtime with mean daily dosages being 0.48 units/kg for glargine and 0.42 units/kg for NPH at end point adjusted for body weight in patients who were maintained on one or two oral hypoglycemic agents throughout the study.

In a study of patients on oral agents, premixed insulin was initiated at a dose of 6 units/day; but surprisingly at 28 weeks, the average dosage was >75 units/day (0.85 units/kg/day), without any major episodes of hypoglycemia.[7] These studies have shown 10 units/injection to be a safe initiating dose for once-daily and twice-daily insulin regimens (Table 3).[2] It is important that glargine should be injected at the same time each day although it can be taken at any time during the day. Patients must record all their results from self-monitoring of blood glucose (SMBG) and insulin doses in their logbooks when initiating or adjusting insulin.

TABLE 3: Initiating dosages of various insulins.

Once-daily premix	10 units (pre-dinner)
Twice-daily premix	10 units (pre-breakfast), 10 units (pre-dinner)
Once daily basal	10 units (bedtime)
Multiple daily injections	Individualized doses as per blood sugar level (Basal plus or Basal bolus)

MONITORING AND ADJUSTING THE THERAPY TO ACHIEVE GLYCEMIC TARGETS

It is usually said that to be fruitful, insulin therapy needs timely and appropriate titration of dosages. A study showed that only half of patients with type 2 diabetes who are treated with insulin achieved hemoglobin A1c (HbA1c) < 7%.[8] Table 4[2] shows a titration schedule for once-daily and twice-daily regimens to do insulin adjustments safely and timely. Depending on their regimen, patients must

TABLE 4: Insulin dosage titration for once-daily or twice-daily insulin regimens based on pre-meal blood glucose values.

Blood glucose values	Dosage change
< 80 mg/dL	2 units
80–109 mg/dL	No change
110–139 mg/dL	2 units
140–179 mg/dL	4 units
≥ 180 mg/dL	6 units

Note: Do not increase dose if hypoglycemia (<70 mg/dL) or its symptoms are present.

BOX 1 Making a transition from one insulin regimen to another.

- **Current regimen basal → new regimen premix**
  - Divide total daily dose in half.
  - Initiate pre-breakfast and pre-dinner premix insulin.
  - Start new regimen 18–24 hours after last basal dose.
  - Based on SMBG data and diet history, titrate doses to achieve glycemic goals.
  - A larger proportion of insulin is usually required before the largest meal.
  - In case of recurrent hypoglycemia, reduce the total dose by 20%.
- **Current regimen premix → new regimen premix**
  - Divide total daily dose in half and initiate before breakfast and before dinner each.
  - Based on SMBG data and diet history, titrate doses to achieve glycemic goals.
  - A larger proportion of insulin is usually required before the largest meal.
  - In case of recurrent hypoglycemia, reduce the total dose by 20%.
- **Current regimen basal only → add rapid-acting insulin before the largest meal***
  - Initiate 10% of total daily dose as rapid-acting analog before the largest meal.
  - Decrease the basal insulin dose by 10%.
- **Current regimen premix → new regimen MDI**≠
  - Divide total daily dose in half.
  - Initial basal insulin dose = 0.8 × half of total daily dose.
  - Initial prandial insulin dose = Percentage of estimated calories for each meal ÷ 100 × half of total daily dose

* This regimen serves as a transition to MDI (Multi Daily Injections) therapy.

≠ *Example*: Patient is currently on 40 units total daily dose of premix insulin (20 units twice daily) and eats ~ 25% of total daily calories at breakfast, 25% at lunch, and 50% at dinner. The new regimen would be 16 units of basal insulin with 5 units of rapid-acting insulin at breakfast, 5 units at lunch, and 10 units at dinner.

(SMBG: self monitoring of blood glucose)

measure blood glucose once or twice daily (prebreakfast, predinner). The consulting physician can then make stepwise adjustments as per the average glucose values according to the blood glucose data recorded by the patient.

Prebreakfast dosage adjustments are made on the basis of predinner glucose values, whereas predinner dosage adjustments are based on prebreakfast glucose levels For example, in a patient who is on 10 units of premixed insulin twice daily and has a prebreakfast glucose level ranging from 147 mg/dL to 178 mg/dL over the last 4–7 days, the appropriate adjustment would be an addition of 4 units of insulin before dinner. To make timely adjustment is another key aspect of insulin titration. Similar to oral therapy, a delay in making adjustments in insulin dosages leads to excessive glycemic exposure to persist for months or years. Doctor–patient communication is of utmost importance to allow for timely insulin adjustments.

Diabetes education is an important aspect of patient care, especially for those who self-adjust their insulin dosages. If patients are unable to attain the glycemic goal even after 3–6 months of therapy or if there is recurrent hypoglycemia, thought must be given to change the regimen. Box 1[2] shows some strategical aspect for making this transition in insulin regimens. When assessing the need to change regimens, it is important to understand the main issue.

EDUCATING PATIENTS WITH TYPE 2 DIABETES MELLITUS TO MANAGE THEIR OWN INSULIN REGIMEN

Knowledge of glucose values with SMBG enables the patients to identify their blood glucose patterns and its relation to their medicines, exercise, and the quality and quantity of food chosen by them. Since basal insulin is generally started first, patients must check at least daily fasting sugar levels before they eat and when the target sugar levels are achieved, they can go for a twice-weekly testing. Patients need to be trained to identify which insulin, meal, or snack may be causing highs or lows during different times of the day. Use the patient's SMBG log to track glucose values, insulin dose as well as food and activity levels everyday. A minimum of 7 days of values should be used to help identify whether a blood glucose pattern can be established. Look for deviant values. The questions to be put up to the patient are as follows:

- How many doses of insulin have you missed in the last week?

- What particular food items, if any in your notice, make your glucose reading higher?
- Have you noticed any changes in your meals or activities in the last week?
    - If there are no significant changes present, then an insulin adjustment may be needed.
    - Restress the patient's target range, like morning glucose values of 80–130 mg/dL.
    - Ask the patient to identify the out-of-target blood sugar values during the last week.
    - Make one change at a time, even if blood sugar is elevated on several other times of the day. Adjustments are usually made in small (approximately 10%) increments.

KEY COUNSELING POINTS FOR PATIENTS USING INSULIN

The main message patients should understand is that insulin use does not have to be feared, and it can very quickly help control diabetes.

Benefits of insulin use:

- Very easy to use
- If injections are done with proper technique, they will not hurt
- Rapidly controls blood glucose values
- Patients gradually and consistently titrate upward on daily-insulin dosage to achieve glycemic targets, thus showing a direct objective impact on glucose levels.
- Usually, one injection per day of basal insulin along with a healthy diet and active lifestyle plan can control diabetes for a long time.

Key issues with insulin administration:

- Before using insulin, ensure that the correct type of insulin and dose are being administered.
- When used insulin can be stored at room temperature
- Insulin when not in use should be stored in a refrigerator.

Educate patient on how to prevent hypoglycemia and treat if it occurs:

- Advice not to skip meals.
- Test blood glucose regularly.
- Only take the prescribed insulin dose.
- Carry a source of glucose with yourself at all times.

Know how to prevent or minimize weight gain due to insulin therapy:

- Advice to eat healthy meals high in fiber and comprising fresh vegetables, whole grains, and lean meat.
- Teach about ways to become more physically active which are enjoyable as well.

ADDRESSING BARRIERS AND CHALLENGES TO INSULIN THERAPY

Type 2 diabetes is a progressive disease and many people with the condition inevitably require insulin therapy to achieve and maintain sufficient glycemic control. In clinical practice, initiation of insulin therapy is delayed in many patients who would benefit from such treatment. There are various patients' and physicians' beliefs and perceptions regarding insulin therapy that create barriers contributing to the delay in insulin initiation. Tables 5 and 6

TABLE 5: Addressing physician-related barriers to insulin initiation.

Barrier	Possible solution
Disbelief about effectiveness of insulin in real world setting	Available data shows that insulin is highly effective not only in controlled clinical trials, but also in routine clinical practice
Presumption that patients will be unwilling to initiate insulin	To establish a friendly repo with patients so that they can speak openly about their attitudes toward insulin and hence misconceptions can be dispelled
Belief that most patients will be unable to do self-management actively	Engage patients in shared decision making and problem solving
Concerns that patients will experience injection-related problems, dangerous episodes of hypoglycemia, and unacceptable weight gain with insulin	Inform patients about ways to minimize injection-related problems, avoid hypoglycemia, and limit weight gain

(*Source*: Peyrot M, Rubin RR, Lauritzen T, et al. Resistance to insulin therapy among patients and providers: results of the cross-national Diabetes Attitudes, Wishes, and Needs (DAWN) study. Diabetes Care. 2005;28(11):2673-9; Polonsky WH, Fisher L, Hessler D, et al. A survey of blood glucose monitoring in patients with type 2 diabetes: are recommendations from health care professionals being followed? Curr Med Res Opin. 2011;27(Suppl 3):31-7.)

TABLE 6 : Addressing patient-related barriers to insulin initiation.

Barrier	Clinician's explanation
Dubiousness about insulin's effectiveness	Insulin will improve glycemic control if used properly and will probably make the patient feel better and provide with more energy
Belief that disease has worsened	Insulin can improve glycemic control at any stage of diabetes and most patients will eventually need insulin therapy when their bodies would not produce sufficient insulin
Lack of confidence to self-manage insulin therapy	Explain personally the insulin injecting technique at least once to every patient. Most patients readily master the technique for taking basal insulin
Fear about injections	Injections are less painful than the lancets needed for SMBG, and prefilled pens readily facilitate insulin injection
Fear of hypoglycemia	Serious hypoglycemia is rare. Thorough training in preventing, recognizing, and treating hypoglycemia will be provided
Anxiety about weight gain	Some newer insulins cause little weight gain Daily exercise can minimize weight gain
Concerns about work and interpersonal relations	Insulin should not impair ability to work, but employer should be informed. Patients can ensure that others routinely surrounding them have necessary knowledge about insulin and its effects
Cultural barriers and health beliefs	Taking insulin is consistent with a variety of cultural values and health beliefs

(*Source*: Peragallo-Dittko V. Removing barriers to insulin therapy. Diabetes Educ. 2007;33(Suppl 3):60S-65S; Peyrot M, Rubin RR, Khunti K. Addressing barriers to initiation of insulin in patients with type 2 diabetes. Prim Care Diabetes. 2010;4(Suppl 1):S11-8; Petznick AM. Identifying and addressing barriers to insulin acceptance and adherence in patients with type 2 diabetes mellitus. J Am Osteopath Assoc. 2013;113(4 Suppl 2):S6-16; Campos C: Addressing cultural barriers to the successful use of insulin in Hispanics with type 2 diabetes. South Med J. 2007, 100: 812-820. ; Ho, E. Y., James, J. (2006). Cultural barriers to initiating insulin therapy in Chinese people with type 2 diabetes living in Canada. Canadian Journal of Diabetes. 30(4), 390–96.)

summarize the various important clinician and patient-related challenges to insulin therapy and their possible solutions.

CONCLUSION

Insulin is the most effective therapy available for treating hyperglycemia. There are evidences to state that early insulin initiation in T2DM may improve glycemic control leading to prevention or delay in the development of diabetes-related complications. Due to various physician-, patient-, and healthcare system-related barriers which can be easily avoided, insulin therapy is underutilized and mostly delayed. Patient education regarding the promising role of insulin therapy in diabetes treatment and destigmatizing its use helps in managing patient-related barriers and leads to increased patient adherence and self-management. Physicians should always actively listen to patients and proactively address their worries and concerns emphasizing the relative ease associated with today's insulin regimens and delivery systems. Individualization of insulin therapy with a regimen compatible with the patient's blood glucose profile and insulin secretion pattern also enables clinicians to overcome barriers and challenges to achieve the target glycemic control.

REFERENCES

1. Weng J, Li Y, Xu W, et al. Effect of intensive insulin therapy on b-cell function and glycaemic control in patients with newly diagnosed type 2 diabetes: a multicentre randomised parallel-group trial. Lancet. 2008;371(9626):1753-60.
2. Hirsch IB, Bergenstal RM, Parkin CG, et al. A real-world approach to insulin therapy in primary care practice. Clin Diabetes. 2005;23(2):78-86.
3. Mayfield JA, White RD. Insulin therapy for type 2 diabetes: rescue, augmentation, and replacement of beta-cell function. Am Fam Physician. 2004;70:489-500.
4. Haffner SM, D'Agostino R Jr, Mykkanen L, et al. Insulin sensitivity in subjects with type 2 diabetes: relationship to cardiovascular risk factors: the insulin resistance atherosclerosis study. Diabetes Care. 1999;22: 562-8.
5. Malone JK, Kerr LF, Campaigne BN, et al. Combined therapy with insulin lispro mix 75/25 plus metformin or insulin glargine plus metformin: a 16 week, randomized, open label, cross-over study in patients with type 2 diabetes beginning insulin therapy. Clin Ther. 2004;26:2034-44.
6. Riddle MC, Rosenstock J, Gerich J, the Insulin Glargine 4002 Study Investigators. The treat-to-target trial: randomized addition of glargine or human NPH insulin to oral therapy of type 2 diabetic patients. Diabetes Care. 2003;26:3080-6.
7. Raskin P, Rojas P, Allen E. Comparison of twice-daily biphasic insulin aspart 70/30 (BIAsp 70/30) with once-daily insulin glargine (GLA) in patients with type 2 DM on oral antidiabetic agents. Diabetes. 2004;53(Suppl 2): 602-P.
8. Koro CE, Bowlin SJ, Bourgeois N, et al. Glycemic control from 1988 to 2000 among U.S. adults diagnosed with type 2 diabetes: a preliminary report. Diabetes Care. 2004;27:17-20.

27 CHAPTER Insulin Initiation in Type 2 Diabetes: Why Basal Insulin should be Preferred?

Jay Chordia

INTRODUCTION

Type 2 diabetes mellitus (T2DM) is characterized by physiological insulin resistance and high blood glucose levels and can lead to microvascular and macrovascular complications, contributing to significant morbidity and mortality.[1] Insulin therapy is highly effective and could be considered a savior in the treatment of diabetes mellitus and its complications. Early insulin therapy allows the pancreas to rest by reducing β-cell stress thereby improving β-cell function, overcome the glucotoxic effects of hyperglycemia, preserve β-cell mass and improve insulin sensitivity. These will result in significant improvements in quality of life and treatment satisfaction. Current guidelines approved the initiation of insulin early in T2DM course, especially in patients with high glycated hemoglobin (HbA1c), as the use of oral agents alone in patients with uncontrolled diabetes is unlikely to attain glycemic targets. Once daily dosage of basal insulin such as insulin glargine with constant use of one or more oral antidiabetic drugs (OADs) in most insulin-naïve patients has confirmed to be an effective and safe glucose lowering treatment. It has numerous advantages—only one insulin injection can be needed every day; there is no need to mix distinct types of insulin, and titration can be done slowly and safely. Additionally, this combination therapy needs a lower total dose of insulin.[2]

WHEN TO INITIATE INSULIN THERAPY?

Translating the learning from the UK Prospective Diabetes Study (UKPDS) and the Kumamoto study, most of the clinical guidelines for diabetes advocate early glycemic target achievement to check the onset as well as progression of diabetes-related complications. It is accounted that roughly one-half of the patients with T2DM will achieve HbA1c target after 3 years with monotherapy while this is even worse after 9 years where only one-fourth of the patients achieve target. Early insulin initiation benefits T2DM patients in the recuperation and improvement of their β-cell function by providing "β-cell rest" and sustained glycemic control compared to treatment with OADs. This reinforces the rationale for the initiation of insulin therapy in people with T2DM whose glycemic targets are not achieved with lifestyle adjustments and OADs.[3]

Insulin should be initiated in a timely manner, preferably within 3–6 months of inadequate control, with the optimal use of OADs. Insulin may be initiated at the diagnosis also of diabetes, if severe hyperglycemic symptoms like polyuria, polydipsia, or catabolic symptoms like weight loss or ketosis are present and/or HbA1c is more than 9%. Insulin can also be initiated in patients on metformin or other first-line agents and HbA1c ≥7.5% or not achieving target HbA1c goal in 3 months of monotherapy. Insulin should be considered for glycemic control in patients with decompensated hepatic or renal insufficiency and when patients have suffered from myocardial infarction, stoke, or a major operation.[4]

HOW TO INITIATE INSULIN THERAPY?

Insulin therapy remains the most powerful agent for glycemic control than any antidiabetic medications available, but it may be associated with risks of hypoglycemia and weight gain. Since all insulins are not the same in this regard, the healthcare provider must choose the most appropriate insulin to start with. The best choice for a starter insulin in T2DM should be convenient

TABLE 1: Characteristics of available basal insulins.[6]

Basal insulin class	Insulin	Duration of action	CV safety	Risk of nocturnal hypoglycemia	Other considerations
Intermediate acting	NPH	16–18 hours	NA	+++	Needs resuspension. Administered twice daily
First-generation long-acting	Glargine-U100	Up to 24 hours	Neutral	++	Administered once daily, same time of day
	Detemir	20–24 hours	NA	++	Administered once or twice daily
Second generation long-acting	Glargine-U300	>24 hours	Neutral	+	Administered once daily with ± 3 hour flexibility
	Degludec	>24 hours	Neutral	+	Administered once daily with flexibility

for the patients and have proven efficacy with lower risk of hypoglycemia and weight gain. Basal insulin is the most convenient and effective option for insulin initiation in many patients with T2DM. Basal Supported Oral Therapy (BOT), i.e. basal insulin in combination with OADs is easy to administer and is the preferred starting insulin regime.[5]

Basal insulin includes both intermediate acting like neutral protamine Hagedorn (NPH), first-generation long-acting analogs like glargine-U100 and detemir and second-generation long-acting analogs like glargine-U300 and degludec. Table 1 summarizes some important characteristics of different types of available basal insulin. Long-acting basal analogs are preferred to NPH in T2DM due to their better convenience and safety profile.[6] The usual starting dose of basal insulin analogs is 10 U/day or 0.1–0.2 U/kg/day administered as once daily subcutaneous injection at the same time daily. Once initiated empower the patients for self-monitoring of blood glucose (SMBG) and titrate the insulin dose to achieve a fasting plasma glucose (FPG) target of 100–130 mg/dL. Titration of basal insulin is usually done once/twice a week based on three most recent FPG values. In case of hypoglycemia, reduce the basal insulin dose by 10–20% and determine the cause. BOT offers complementary mechanisms of action that can help maximize efficacy, reach target HbA1c goals, and minimize adverse events.[6]

WHY BASAL INSULIN IS PREFERRED?

Owing to its simplicity and lower risk of hypoglycemia, eminent experts in the field of diabetes care have agreed upon basal insulin as the usual starting point for insulin therapy in T2DM.[7] Studies have shown that premixed insulin regimen results in similar reductions in HbA1c compared with basal regimens, but is associated with more weight gain, an increased risk of hypoglycemia, and is more complex, which may affect adherence. It also has a higher dose requirement (Fig. 1). Basal insulin, on the other hand, is simple and has a lower risk of hypoglycemia. Thus, it is most convenient to start with a basal regimen, owing to its simplicity and favorable safety profile.[8,9]

In a 24-week, randomized, parallel-group trial that assessed the safety of twice daily premixed insulin (70:30 neutral protamine Hagedorn) with once daily glargine-U100 plus OADs in 371 T2DM patients inadequately controlled on OADs. The study showed significantly greater (~50%) confirmed hypoglycemic episodes with twice daily premixed insulin compared to once daily insulin glargine. Furthermore, severe hypoglycemia was noted only in the premixed insulin group (0.05/patient-year).[10] In another 24-week randomized comparative trial, patients with T2DM inadequately controlled with OADs were randomized to either glargine-U100 or human premixed insulin. To achieve the same efficacy, the risk of symptomatic hypoglycemia was significantly higher with human premix insulin versus insulin glargine (42 vs 12 hypoglycemic episodes). Additionally, weight gain with premix was found to be significantly higher versus glargine (1.4 kg vs 0.4 kg).[11] Similarly, a 28-week randomized controlled trial was done to assess the safety of twice daily biphasic insulin aspart 70/30 (BIAsp 70/30) with once daily insulin glargine-U100 in 233 insulin-naive patients with T2DM. The results reported a significantly greater incidence of minor hypoglycemic events in the biphasic insulin aspart (BIAsp) 70/30 group compared to the insulin glargine-U100 group. Similarly, minor hypoglycemia was reported by 43% patients in the BIAsp group as compared to only 16% in the insulin glargine-U100 group.[12] Due to these evident limitations with premixed insulin, it is considered as less adaptable method of glycemic control as compared to basal insulin and most guidelines do not endorse the use of premix insulin in the type 2 diabetes management algorithm. This suggests a conscious drift from the earlier approach to diabetes care to "basal first",

Basal

- Simple
- Lower risk of hypoglycemia

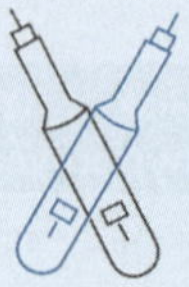

Premixed

- Associated with more weight gain
- Increased risk of hypoglycemia
- More complex' Less flexible, may affect adherence
- Higher insulin dose required

Figure 1 Advantages of basal insulin over premixed.[8,9]

considering the disadvantages associated with premixed-insulin regimen.[13]

The second-generation basal insulins like insulin glargine-U300 and insulin degludec had shown lesser risk of hypoglycemia than the first-generation basal insulins.[14] This is because the second-generation basal insulins offer lesser variability and prolonged duration of action compared to the first-generation. In a 24-week randomized controlled trial which compared the two second-generation basal insulins, it was shown that insulin glargine-U300 has lesser risk of anytime and nocturnal confirmed hypoglycemia than insulin degludec during the titration period (0–12 weeks).[15]

This "basal-first" approach has been unanimously recommended in all leading guidelines like American Diabetes Association (ADA), American Association of Clinical Endocrinologists (AACE), American College of Endocrinology (ACE), Canadian Diabetes Association (CDA), European Association for the Study of Diabetes (EASD), International Diabetes Federation (IDF), and National Institute for Health and Care Excellence (NICE).[7,13,16,17]

CONCLUSION

The decision of an insulin regimen, the timing of initiation, and optimization of insulin therapy is imperative in achieving optimal glycemic control. All leading international diabetes guidelines unanimously recommend the basal-first approach in T2DM patients with inadequate glycemic control. Basal insulin combined with oral agents is the most preferred and convenient initial insulin regimen owing to its simplicity and lower risk of hypoglycemia and weight gain compared to premixed insulins. Clinical evidence suggests that long-acting insulin analogs are preferred basal insulin due to their better safety profile.

REFERENCES

1. Zheng Y, Ley SH, Hu FB. Global aetiology and epidemiology of type 2 diabetes mellitus and its complications. Nat Rev Endocrinol. 2017;14(2): 88-98.
2. Lovre D, Fonseca V. Benefits of timely basal insulin control in patients with type 2 diabetes. J Diabetes Complications. 2015;29(2):295-301.
3. Owens D. Clinical evidence for the earlier initiation of insulin therapy in type 2 diabetes. Diabetes Technol Ther. 2013;15(9):776-85.
4. Garber AJ, Abrahamson MJ, Barzilay JI, et al. Consensus statement by American association of clinical Endocrinologists and American college of Endocrinology on the comprehensive type 2 diabetes management algorithm–2019 Executive Summary. Endocr Prac. 2019; 25(1): 69-100.
5. Kuritzky L. Addition of basal insulin to oral antidiabetic agents: a goal-directed approach to type 2 diabetes therapy. Med Gen Med. 2006;8(4):34.
6. Thomas N, Kapoor N, Velavan J, et al. A practice guide to diabetes mellitus, 6th edition. New Delhi: Jaypee Brothers Medical Publishers Ltd.; 2012.
7. LaSalle JR, Berria R. Insulin therapy in type 2 diabetes mellitus: a practical approach for primary care physicians and other health care professionals. J Am Osteopath Assoc. 2013;113(2):152-62.
8. Lau AN, Tang T, Halapy H, et al. Initiating insulin in patients with type 2 diabetes. CMAJ. 2012;84(7):767-76.
9. Berard L, Antonishyn N, Arcudi K, et al. Insulin matters: A practical approach to basal insulin management in type 2 diabetes. Diabetes Ther. 2018;9(2): 501-19.
10. Janka HU, Plewe G, Riddle MC, et al. Comparison of basal insulin added to oral agents versus twice-daily premixed insulin as initial insulin therapy for type 2 diabetes. Diabetes Care. 2005;28:254-9.
11. Singhai A, Banzal S, Joseph D, et al. Comparison of insulin glargine with human premix insulin in patients with type 2 diabetes inadequately controlled on oral hypoglycemic drugs in a 24-week randomized study among central Indian population. Indian J Clin Prac. 2013;23(10): 619-23.
12. Raskin P, Allen E, Hollander P, et al. Initiating insulin therapy in type 2 Diabetes: a comparison of biphasic and basal insulin analogs. Diabetes Care. 2005;28(2):260-5.
13. Bajaj S, Das AK, Kalra S, et.al. BE-SMART (Basal Early Strategies to Maximize HbA1c Reduction with Oral Therapy): Expert opinion. Diabetes Ther. 2019;10(4):1-16.
14. Roussel R, Ritzel R, Boëlle-Le Corfec E, et al. Clinical perspectives from the BEGIN and EDITION programmes: Trial-level meta-analyses outcomes with either degludec or glargine 300 U/mL vs glargine 100 U/mL in T2DM. Diabetes Metab. 2018;44(5):402-9.
15. Rosenstock J, Cheng A, Ritzel R, et al. More similarities than differences testing insulin glargine 300 Units/mL versus insulin degludec 100 units/mL in insulin-naive type 2 diabetes: The randomized head-to-head Bright TRIAL. Diabetes Care. 2018;41:2147-54.
16. CDA (2018). Clinical Practice Guidelines Committees [online] Available from: http://guidelines.diabetes.ca/docs/CPG-2018-full-EN.pdf [Last accessed September, 2019].
17. NICE (2002). Final Appraisal Determination Long-acting insulin analogues for the treatment of diabetes–insulin glargine. [online] Available from https://www.nice.org.uk/guidance/ta53/documents/final-appraisal-determination-longacting-insulin-analogues-for-the-treatment-of-diabetes-insulin-glargine-2 [Last accessed September, 2019].

28 CHAPTER Intensification of Insulin Therapy in Patients Started on Basal Insulin

Ajay Shah

INTRODUCTION

In patients with uncontrolled type 2 diabetes (T2D), timely treatment intensification and blood glucose control are critical for reducing the risks of long-term complications related to diabetes.[1] As there is a progressive loss of beta-cell function inT2D, majority of the patients may finally need insulin therapy for achieving and maintaining glycemic targets.[2] It is unfortunate that delays in initiation of insulin and intensification of treatment among patients having uncontrolled T2D are persistent challenges in management of diabetes.[3] Such challenges are due to several factors, such as reluctance of patient to intensify, non-adherence of medication, and nonpersistence; all of these can play a role of barriers in timely control of diabetes. Other factors include increasing of the age, the duration of diabetes, the presence of multiple diabetes chronic complications, and the use of multiple oral antihyperglycemic agents. Clinical inertia to intensify also contributed toward this problem with both specialists and nonspecialists (primary care physicians) being equally guilty, and only about one-third of eligible patients for insulin treatment intensification had it done.

PREVALENCE AND TIMING

Treat-to-target titration preliminaries have characterized the initiation and titration of basal insulin analogs, dependent upon accomplishing fasting plasma glucose (FPG) targets.[4] However, albeit basal insulin gives a consistent level of insulin for the duration of the day and controls FPG levels by bringing down baseline plasma glucose, as it has no immediate impact on postprandial plasma glucose (PPG).[5] As per estimates by researches, minimum 60% of patients with T2D treated with basal insulin alone are uncontrolled being dependent on their hemoglobin A1c (HbA1c) values (HbA1c >7%).[6] A latest trial[7] advised that the increase in PPG and nighttime glucose change measurements were more valuable predictors than HbA1c for recognizing individuals with T2D on basal insulin treatment, with or without oral anti-diabetic drugs, who can get most benefit by intensification with bolus insulin. In addition, the nighttime glucose change may for sure perform just as well as PPG increase, while being simpler to measure. Another retrospectively analyzed data[8] suggests that in the patients where the difference between a patient's blood glucose level at bedtime and the following morning before breakfast is negative, there is no benefit from supplementation of basal-supported oral therapy with prandial insulin.

In routine clinical practice, it is hard to recognize, in a timely manner, the patients having T2D who would most possibly get advantage from intensification with use of bolus insulin. Further increase in dosages of basal insulin in certain patients has limitedly affected PPG, and higher doses may lead to "over-basalization" which additionally results in building the risk of hypoglycemia and weight gain.[9] At present, the recommendations advise intensification of treatment when the dose surpasses 0.5 IU/kg/d of the basal insulin and HbA1c stays above target levels. A basal insulin dose of more than 0.4 IU/kg/d ought to be a sign for clinicians to begin considering anti-diabetic agents that address PPG excursions in a better way, comprising prandial insulin, or oral or injectable incretin therapies, with the goal that treatment intensification can be started before basal insulin doses surpasses 0.5 IU/kg/d (although ADA/EASD algorithm propose up to 0.7U/kg/d).[9]

OPTIONS

Latest updates to treatment guidelines support adding sodium-glucose co-transporter-2 (SGLT2) inhibitors or dipeptidyl peptidase-4 (DPP-4) inhibitors among patients having existing cardiovascular disease or in whom weight reduction is needed and glycemic targets are not being accomplished.[10]

The other traditionally followed options available for patients who need further intensification of their insulin regimen are—the addition of rapid-acting insulin with one of the daily meals (basal plus regimen), the addition of rapid insulin with two to three daily meals (basal bolus), or a switch to premix insulin before two to three daily meals.[11-13]

It is recommended by the ADA/EASD consensus statement[10] that intensification of treatment should be done by combining basal insulin and mealtime bolus insulin, when glycemia is not controlled on basal insulin only. Rapid-acting analogs (such as Glulisine, Aspart, or Lispro) are preferable over regular insulin due to a faster onset and offset of action and are related with less hypoglycemia. The simplest approach is covering the largest meal with a prandial injection of rapid-acting insulin analog (start with 10% of basal dose or 5U) prior to the largest meal (i.e. Basal Plus 1). In case of not achieving glycemic goal, progressive intensification of treatment should be done by addition of bolus injections prior to two (i.e. Basal Plus 2) or three meals (Basal Plus 3). Alternative way of intensifying insulin treatment is switching to a full basal-bolus program, which gives more flexibility in patients having varying mealtimes and carbohydrate content (Flowchart 1).

In this program, the total daily dose (TDD) of insulin (0.3–0.5 U/kg) is divided as 50% prandial insulin and 50% basal insulin. The 50% prandial insulin dose is then distributed into three doses, given prior to each major meal. For reaching the desired glycemic goal, titration of insulin dose can be performed every 2–3 days. If 2-hour postprandial or next premeal glucose is steadily more than 140 mg/dL, prandial dose can be increased by 10% or 1–2 U. In hypoglycemia, TDD basal and/or prandial insulin can be decreased by 10–20% or 20–40%, in case blood glucose level is steadily less than 70 mg/dL and less than 40 mg/dL, respectively. It is also recommended by IDF 2012 that insulin therapy intensification should be done with basal and meal-time prandial insulins (Flowchart 2).

Premixed (biphasic) insulins (70/30 aspartmix; 75/25 or 50/50 lispro mix; NPH/regular 70/30) give less flexibility of dosing but do provide the benefit of simplified dosing

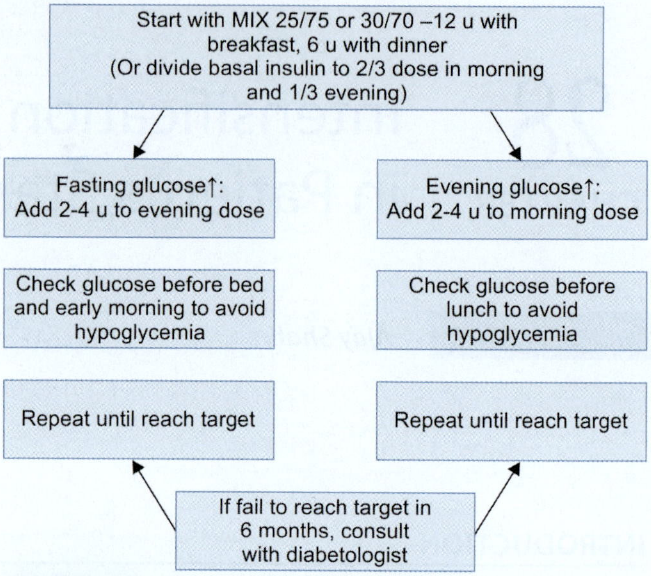

Flowchart 1 Initiation and intensification of premix insulin analogs.[13]

TABLE 1: Which patient should be offered a premix versus basal-bolus/basal plus regimen?[13]

Premix insulin analogs	Basal plus/basal bolus
Patient preference	Type 1 diabetes (any age)
Older age	Younger age
Need assistance with injections	Highly motivated and compliant
Organized lifestyle	Active lifestyle
Two meals a day or evening main meal	High variability in eating habits

regimen in comparison to basal-bolus, which can make them specifically appropriate for selected patients, namely those who struggle for managing multiple daily injections. However, in all, premixed insulins are less effective as compared to basal bolus regimens for attaining the target HbA1c and their usage has been related to a higher rate of hypoglycemia and with more weight gain. The initial premix dose ought to be on the basis of the current basal insulin dose, distributed into two-thirds AM and one-third PM, with once or twice weekly titration (1–2 units or 10–15 %) to target. Patients who take premixed insulins are required to obey a regular schedule of meal and exercise for reducing the risk of hypoglycemia (Table 1).

The key patient barriers to intensification to basal-bolus are the complexity of the basal-bolus regimen, along with additional injections, and negative side effects like weight gain and hypoglycemia.

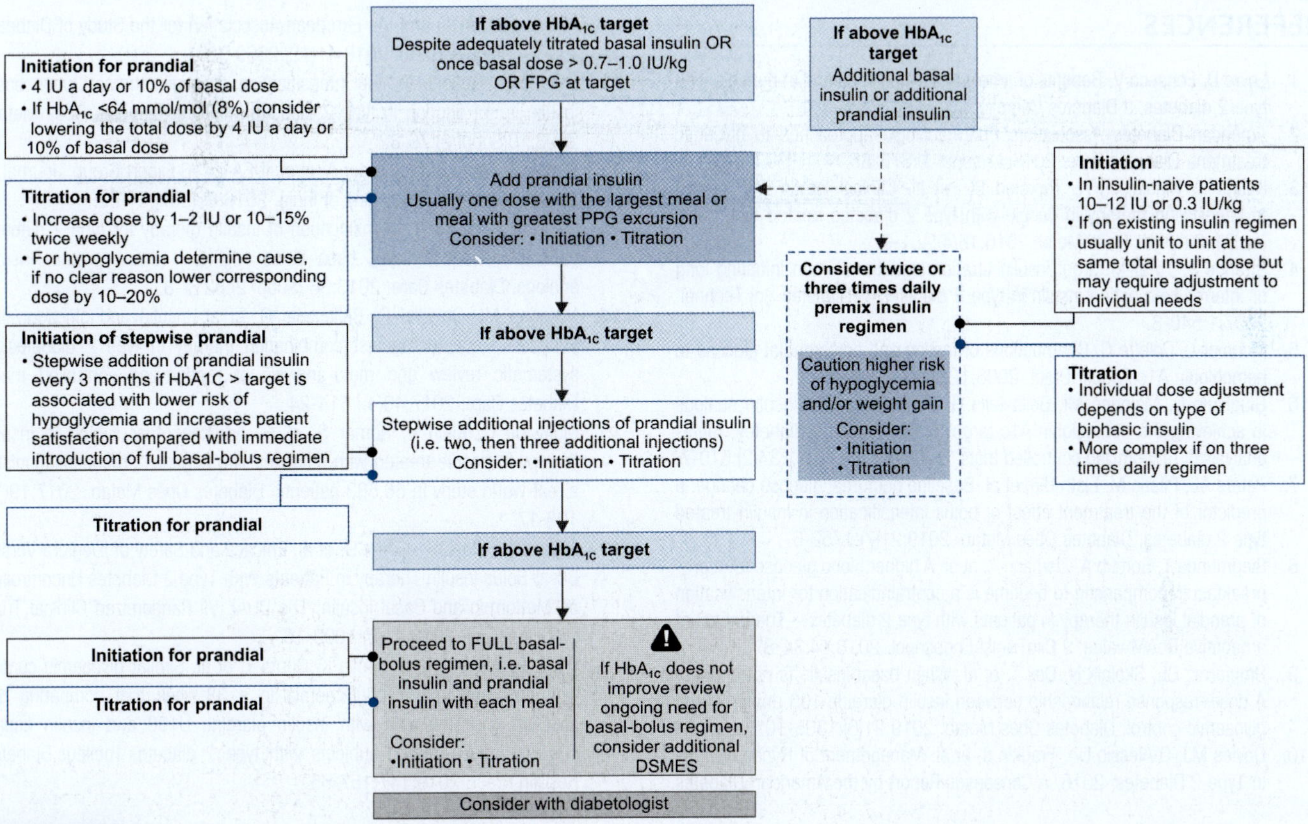

Flowchart 2 Timely tradition to insulin intensification.[4,10]

These regimes, hence, are considered inconvenient by many patients, who look forward to more simple, and patient-friendly pathways for glycemic control.

The American Diabetes Association (ADA) Standards of Medical Care recommends intensification of injectable therapy among patients having type 2 diabetes, who are failing on basal insulin therapy by addition of a glucagon-like peptide-1 receptor agonist (GLP-1RA).[10] Previous meta-analyses of randomized controlled trials (RCTs)[14] have reported a mean reduction of HbA1c of about 0.45% in favor of the GLP-1RA/insulin combination (combo) in comparison to other injectable treatment strategies, with no increase in hypoglycemia and decreased body weight. Additionally, the findings of the expanding real-world use of the combo strategies are likely to verify the results of RCTs.[15] The successful utilization of a single daily dose of fixed ratio combination injectable anti-diabetic therapy (liraglutide/degludec), shows that it is presently possible to co-formulate two different drugs and give them in a single patient-friendly device.[16] Dose titration can be performed by utilization of simple schemes that are easily understood by the patient or his/her caregiver. Efficacious glycemic control can be achieved with much low-insulin doses, therefore minimizing hypoglycemia and facilitating weight loss. Less number of injections that can be flexibly administered, irrespective of injection-meal gaps or meal times, increase the attraction of this drug regimen.[17] However, recurrently reported causes of patient refusal to intensify with GLP-1RA were insurance coverage/costs and negative side effects of GLP-1 RA.

CONCLUSION

Much obliged to these medicines and regimens, people having type 2 diabetes presently have a much broader, people-friendly, and convenient choice of therapeutic options. These therapies enable safer and convenient control with a reduced intrusion index. Choosing a suitable option that is most commensurate with patient characteristics, will determine the success for glycemic control.

ACKNOWLEDGMENT

Dr Nimisha Jain, for providing the references and proof reading of the manuscript.

REFERENCES

1. Lovre D, Fonseca V. Benefits of timely basal insulin control in patients with type 2 diabetes. J Diabetes Complic. 2015;29(2):295-301.
2. American Diabetes Association. Pharmacologic approaches to glycemic treatment. Diabetes Care. 2018;41(suppl 1):S73-85.
3. Khunti K, Nikolajsen A, Thorsted BL, et al. Clinical inertia with regard to intensifying therapy in people with type 2 diabetes treated with basal insulin. Diabetes Obes Metab.2016;18(4):401-9.
4. Strange P. Treat-to-target insulin titration algorithms when initiating long or intermediate acting insulin in type 2 diabetes. J Diabetes Sci Technol. 2007;1:540-8.
5. Monnier L, Colette C. Contributions of fasting and postprandial glucose to hemoglobin A1c.Endocr Pract. 2006;12(suppl 1):42-6.
6. Giugliano D, Maiorino MI, Bellastella G, et al. Efficacy of insulin analogs in achieving the hemoglobin A1c target of 7% in type 2 diabetes: meta-analysis of randomized controlled trials. Diabetes Care. 2011;34(2):510-7.
7. Peters AL, Piletic M, Ejstrud J, et al. Baseline nocturnal glucose change: a predictor of the treatment effect of bolus intensification in insulin-treated type 2 diabetes. Diabetes Obes Metab. 2019;21(7):1752-6.
8. Siegmunda T, Borckb A, Zismanc A, et al. A higher blood glucose level pre-breakfast in comparison to bedtime is a contraindication for intensification of prandial insulin therapy in patients with type 2 diabetes – The impact of a negative BeAM value. J ClinTransl Endocrinol. 2018;14:34-8.
9. Umpierrez GE, Skolnik N, Dex T, et al. When basal insulin is not enough: A dose–response relationship between insulin glargine 100 units/mL and glycaemic control. Diabetes Obes Metab. 2019;21(6):1305-10.
10. Davies MJ, D'Alessio DA, Fradkin J, et al. Management of Hyperglycemia in Type 2 Diabetes, 2018. A Consensus Report by the American Diabetes Association (ADA) and the European Association for the Study of Diabetes (EASD). Diabetes Care. 2018;41(12):2669-70.
11. Raccah D. Options for the intensification of insulin therapy when basal insulin is not enough in type 2 diabetes mellitus. Diabetes Obes Metab. 2008;10(Suppl 2):76-82.
12. Ghosal S, Sinha B, Majumder A, et al. IDEA-2016 Expert Group. Journal of the Association of Physicians of India. 2016;65(207):51-62.
13. Mosenzon O, Raz I. Intensification of insulin therapy for type 2 diabetic patients in primarycare: basal-bolus regimen versus premix insulin analogs. Diabetes Care. 2013:36 (Suppl 2):S212-8.
14. Maiorino MI, Chiodini P, Bellastella G, et al. Insulin and glucagon-like peptide 1 receptor agonist combination therapy in type 2 diabetes: a systematic review and meta-analysis of randomized controlled trials. Diabetes Care. 2017;40(4): 614-24.
15. Montvida O, Klein K, Kumar S, et al. Addition of or switch to insulin therapy in people treated with glucagon-like peptide-1 receptor agonists: a real-world study in 66,583 patients. Diabetes Obes Metab. 2017;19(1): 108-17.
16. Billings LK, Doshi A, Gouet D, et al. Efficacy and Safety of IDegLira Versus Basal-Bolus Insulin Therapy in Patients With Type 2 Diabetes Uncontrolled on Metformin and Basal Insulin: The DUAL VII Randomized Clinical Trial. Diabetes Care. 2018;41(5):1009-16.
17. Philis-Tsimikas A, Astamirova K, Gupta Y, et al. Similar glycaemic control with less nocturnal hypoglycaemia in a 38-week trial comparing the IDegAsp co-formulation with insulin glargine U100 and insulin aspart in basal insulin-treated subjects with type 2 diabetes mellitus.Diabetes ResClin Pract. 2019;147:157-65.

29 CHAPTER

Premixed Insulin Therapy versus Basal-Bolus Insulin Therapy: Comparative Analysis

Girish Mathur, Ashutosh Chaturvedi, Divyansh Mathur, Rahul Ramchandani

INTRODUCTION

Diabetes mellitus has now become one of the most common and dreadful public health concerns of this century. The United Kingdom Prospective Diabetes Study (UKPDS) showed that half of the beta cell functions are lost at the time of diagnosis itself in the type 2 diabetes mellitus (T2DM) patients with a progressive reduction by 5% annually.[1] It is also well known that over the time oral antidiabetic agents usually become ineffective and patients require exogenous insulin therapy. Numerous guidelines exist for the insulin selection, initiation, optimization, and intensification but still there is no universal consensus regarding the selection of an optimal regimen for insulin therapy. Various factors influencing the decision to begin insulin therapy are related to the cost, convenience, and safety profile of the insulin regime. Basal-bolus insulin regime and twice-daily premix insulin are commonly used for insulin initiation and intensification but there are few studies comparing these two treatment regimens. The key point to follow always is the individualization of diabetes care and treatment as per each patient's needs. Various types and preparations of insulin are summarized in Table 1.[2]

PREMIXED INSULIN THERAPY

Premixed insulins comprises fixed proportion combination of rapid or short-acting and intermediate- or long-acting insulins and are meant for both fasting and postprandial control of blood sugar. These combinations include the traditional premixed formulations with human insulin, premixed analogs, and a premixed combination of rapid-acting and ultra-long-acting basal insulin analogs (Table 1). Depending upon patient needs premixed insulins can be given once, twice, or thrice daily.

Premixed insulin therapy is suitable for patients who have uniform eating patterns and steady lifestyle. NICE guidelines[3] recommends starting premixed insulin, if hemoglobin A1c (HbA1c) is more than 9.0%. For initiation of premix insulin a twice daily dose has been recommended but a once daily dose has been found to be

TABLE 1: Various insulin types and preparations available in market.

Description	Insulin and insulin analog preparation
Ultra-fast acting insulin	Aspart (Fiasp)
Short acting insulin	Regular/soluble insulin
Rapid-acting insulin	Lispro Aspart Glulisine
Intermediate-acting insulin	NPH or Isophane insulin
Long-acting insulin	Glargine Detemir Degludec (Ultra-long acting) Toujeo (High strength Glargine insulin U-300)
Premixed insulin (Human)	30% Regular 70% NPH 50% Regular 50% NPH
Premixed insulin (Analogues)	25% Lispro 75% NPL 50% Lispro 50% NPL 30% Aspart 70% Protamine aspart
Biosimilar insulin	Basaglar (Glargine)

(NPL: neutral protamine lispro; NPH: neutral protamine Hagedorn)

good for patients who are unwilling to initiate insulin and require less than 20 units per day.[4] The common standards to initiate premixed insulin are as follows:[5]

- 10 U/day once daily either in the morning or evening or 0.3–0.5 U/kg/day, as per blood glucose level.
- For patients with HbA1c < 9%–0.2 U/kg/day and 0.4 U/kg/day for those with HbA1c > 9%.
- Twice a day premixed insulin is recommended, if total daily dose of insulin (TDD) is more than 20 U, dosed along with breakfast and evening meal as per the carbohydrate content in meal and daily activity.
- The 50:50 ratio can be considered for premix analogs, if a single dose exceeds 30 U.

The conventional premixed biphasic human insulin comprises regular human insulin and neutral protamine Hagedorn (NPH) in ratio of 30/70 or 50/50. Their pharmacokinetics permits a 24-hour effective action and patient convenience both which leads to high adherence rates and better glycemic control with premixed insulins.[6] Conventional premixed insulins are given 30 minutes before meals, and their action lasts for about 10–16 hours while the analog premixed formulations (Lispro 25/75, Lispro 50/50, BIAsp 30/70, and BIAsp 50/50) can be administered up to 15 minutes before meals because of a quicker onset of action. They also have a longer duration of action ranging from 12 hours to 24 hours as compared to the conventional premixed formulations. IDegAsp (70/30) is a combination of the ultra-long-acting insulin degludec (IDeg) and rapid-acting analog insulin aspart (IAsp) that is safe, well-tolerated, and offers good control of both fasting and prandial hyperglycemia. IDegAsp 70/30 has a quicker onset (10–20 minutes) and longer duration of action (24 hours) and also provides the mealtime flexibility.[6] Titration of premixed insulins can be done once or twice weekly for 12 weeks and thereafter every 2 weeks, according to the fasting plasma glucose (FPG) targets as per algorithm below[5] (Table 2).

Tanaka and Ishii[7] in their study found that the lispro mix 50/50 insulin was better in controlling the postprandial glucose (PPG) and also stabilized the diurnal blood glucose variations in patients who were poorly controlled on insulin 70/30 or 75/25.

TABLE 2: Dose titration for premixed insulin.

Premeal plasma glucose level	Dose titration units (U)
≤80 mg/dL (≤4.4 mmol/L)	–2U
80–110 mg/dL (4.4–6.1 mmol/L)	0 (No change)
111–140 mg/dL (6.2–7.8 mmol/L)	+2U
141–180 mg/dL (7.9–10 mmol/L)	+4U
≥180 mg/dL (≥10 mmol/L)	+6U

BASAL-BOLUS INSULIN THERAPY

When target glycemic control is not achieved with basal insulin alone an intensified insulin therapy in the form of basal-bolus regimen is used. This regimen mimics the physiological secretion of insulin by the pancreas. The rapid- or short-acting insulin is prescribed as bolus insulin before meal and the intermediate- or long-acting insulin is given as basal insulin. Frequent and active self-monitoring along with titration of insulin doses is required to achieve target glycemic control with this regimen. The basal or basal plus regimen can be intensified to initiate the basal-bolus insulin regimen. The TDD is first calculated as 0.6–1.0 units/kg. Fifty percent of TDD is given as basal insulin which is administered at bedtime while the remaining 50% is divided between bolus doses for breakfast, lunch, and dinner.[8] Dose titration can be done by adjusting 2–3 units as required every 3–7 days till the target is achieved. FPG is used to titrate the basal insulin whereas titration of bolus insulin is based on pre prandial or PPG levels at mentioned in Table 3.[8]

Insulin dose is increased or decreased by 10% depending on blood glucose reading shown in Table 3. To titrate the basal dose, sometimes Treat-to-Target Trial's titration schedule is also used as per Table 4.

TABLE 3: Titration of basal-bolus insulin dose as per blood glucose level.

Basal/bolus insulin	Time of self-monitoring blood glucose
Basal insulin	Fasting (pre-breakfast) blood glucose
Pre-breakfast bolus insulin	2-hours post-breakfast or pre-lunch blood glucose
Pre-lunch bolus insulin	2-hours post-lunch or pre-dinner blood glucose
Pre-dinner bolus insulin	Post-dinner or bedtime blood glucose

TABLE 4: Titration of basal insulin as per blood glucose levels.

Pre-meal plasma glucose level	Dose titration units (U)
≤100 mg/dL (≤5.5 mmol/L)	-2U
100–120 mg/dL (5.5–6.7 mmol/L)	No change
121–140 mg/dL (6.8–7.8 mmol/L)	+2U
141–160 mg/dL (7.9–8.9 mmol/L)	+4U
161–180 mg/dL (9.0–10.0 mmol/L)	+6U
≥180 mg/dL (≥10 mmol/L)	+8U

EVIDENCE-BASED USE OF PREMIXED AND BASAL-BOLUS INSULIN REGIMENS

When initiating insulin, the healthcare providers can initiate with premixed or basal insulin, depending on clinical situation. Various studies have been performed to compare the efficacy and safety of these two types of insulin regimens.

Ligthelm et al.[9] in their multicentric trial in 2006 involving 394 patients compared Human isophane insulin (NPH) and insulin aspart (IAsp) thrice daily with biphasic IAsp (BIAsp) thrice daily meal-BIAsp 70 (BMI 30) or BIAsp 50 (BMI > 30) with breakfast and lunch and BIAsp 30 with dinner. They found that mean HbAlc (±SD) reduced from 9.1 ± 0.7% to 7.8 ± 1.0% with both regimens. Glycemic control provided by BIAsp was noninferior to that obtained by the IAsp + NPH patient group. The incidence of hypoglycemic episodes and adverse events was also similar in the two study groups.

Rosenstock et al.[10] in 2008, (Fig. 1) in a 24-week, multicenter, open-label trial assigned patients randomly to premixed-insulin regime (lispro mix 50/50: 50% insulin lispro protamine suspension, and 50% lispro; n = 187) thrice daily with meals or basal-bolus regime (glargine at bedtime plus mealtime lispro; n = 187). It was found that at 24 weeks A1c was lower with basal-bolus therapy (BBT) (6.78 vs 6.95%) while the rates of hypoglycemia were similar for both groups.

Fritsche, Larbig, Owens, and Haring in 2010[11] in their 52-week, open-label, randomized, multinational, multicenter GINGER study (Fig. 2) involved 310 patients with type 2 diabetes (T2D) on premix regime, with or without metformin, and were randomized to a basal-bolus regimen with glargine and glulisine or twice-daily premix. The main

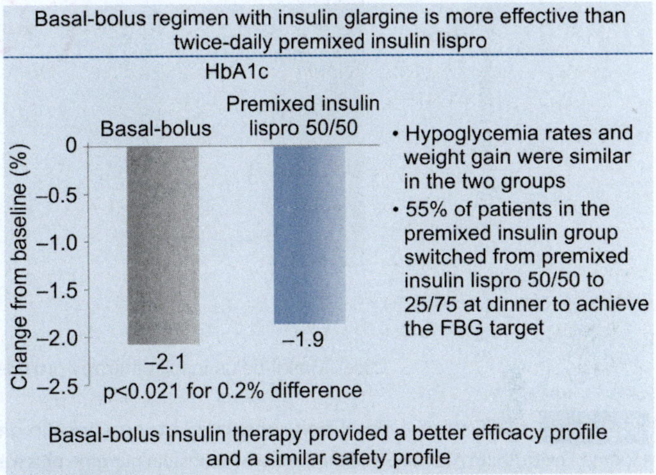

Figure 1 Basal-bolus regimen with insulin glargine is more effective than twice daily premixed insulin lispro.

(*Source:* Rosenstock J, Ahmann AJ, Colon G, et al. Advancing insulin therapy in type 2 diabetes previously treated with glargine plus oral agents prandial premixed (insulin lispro protamine suspension/lispro) versus basal/bolus (glargine/lispro) therapy. Diabetes Care. 2008;31(1): 20-5.)

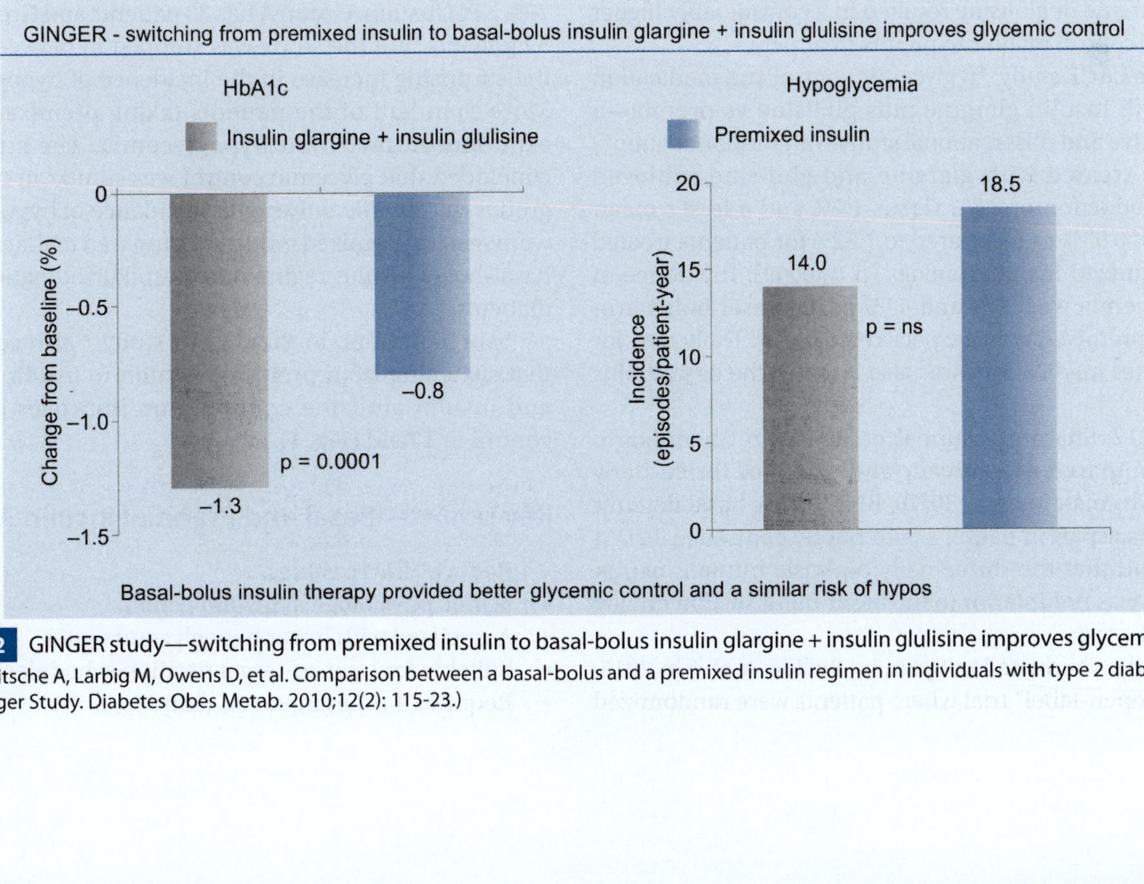

Figure 2 GINGER study—switching from premixed insulin to basal-bolus insulin glargine + insulin glulisine improves glycemic control.

(*Source:* Fritsche A, Larbig M, Owens D, et al. Comparison between a basal-bolus and a premixed insulin regimen in individuals with type 2 diabetes results of the Ginger Study. Diabetes Obes Metab. 2010;12(2): 115-23.)

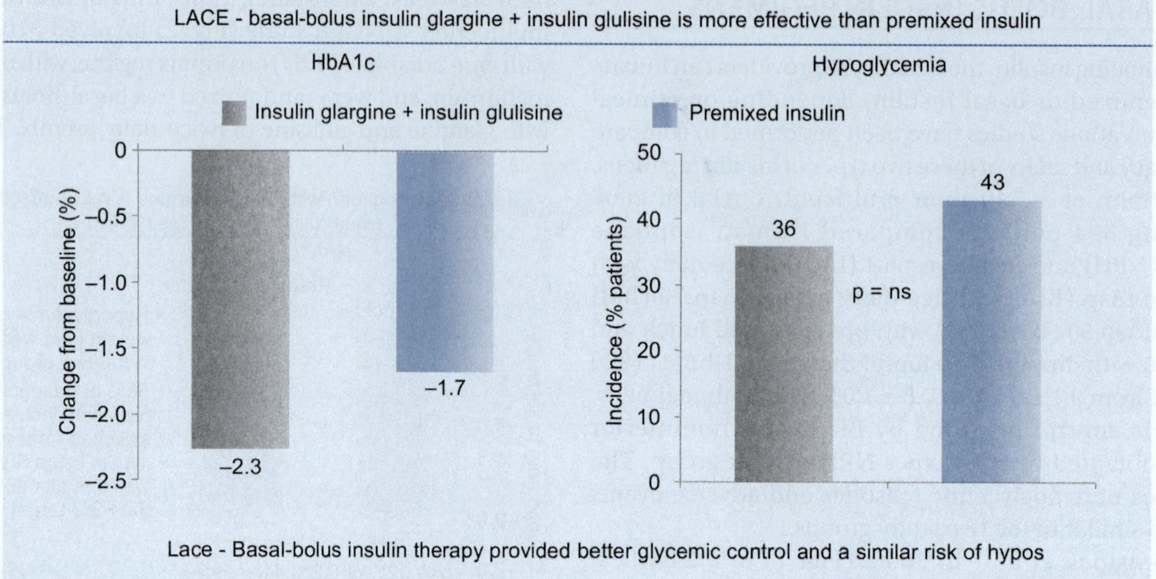

Figure 3 LACE study—basal-bolus insulin glargine + insulin glulisine is more effective than premixed insulin.
(*Source:* Levin, Philip A. et al. Glycemic control with insulin glargine plus insulin glulisine versus premixed insulin analogues in real-world practices: A cost-effectiveness study with a randomized pragmatic trial design. Clinical Therapeutics, Volume 33, Issue 7, 841-50.)

endpoint was change in HbA1c from baseline to endpoint. The study concluded that in a population with long-standing insulin-treated diabetes, with no increase in the rates of hypoglycemia, an intensified basal-bolus regimen using glargine or glulisine resulted in a considerably higher glycemic control relative to premix treatment.

In the LACE study[12] ("glycemic control and medication costs with insulin glargine plus glulisine vs premix—a prospective and observational study with randomization") patients treated with glargine and glulisine achieved HbA1c reduction of 2.3% versus 1.7% and a lesser mean HbA1c of 6.93% as compared to 7.52% for patients treated with premixed insulin analogs ($p = 0.009$). Incidence of hypoglycemia was 36% and 42% in the basal-bolus arm and the premixed arm, respectively (Fig. 3). Daily cost for all diabetes medications was also lower in the basal-bolus group.

In 2012, Shanmugasundar et al.[13] from Chandigarh, India compared the efficacy and safety of thrice-daily biphasic human insulin (30/70, BHI) versus basal detemir and bolus aspart in patients with poorly controlled T2DM and found that the thrice daily biphasic human insulin regimen was noninferior to the basal-bolus insulin analog regimen.

A study, conducted in Spain by Bellido et al.[14] in 2015, was an "open-label" trial where patients were randomized to either Group A to receive a basal-bolus regimen with glargine as the long-acting insulin and glulisine as the rapid-acting premeal insulin, or in Group B on twice-daily premixed human insulin having 30% regular insulin and 70% NPH insulin. Group A has 33 patients and Group B had 39 patients. But the study was stopped in between due to the surprising increase in the incidence of hypoglycemia. More than half of the patients taking premixed insulin experienced recurrent hypoglycemia. The study thus concluded that glycemic control was similar in two study groups but significantly higher incidence of hypoglycemia were seen in premixed group as compared to that receiving basal-bolus insulin regimen in hospitalized patients with diabetes.

Schreiber et al. in their LADI study[15] also concluded that switching from premixed insulin to insulin glargine and insulin glulisine combination improves glycemic control in T2DM (Fig. 4).

Key points—Basal and Prandial Insulin Analogs

- Reduce HbA1c values.
- Mimic physiological insulin action.
- Associated with lower hypoglycemia rates.
- Suitable for treat-to-target titration schedules.
- Requires 4 times injection daily.

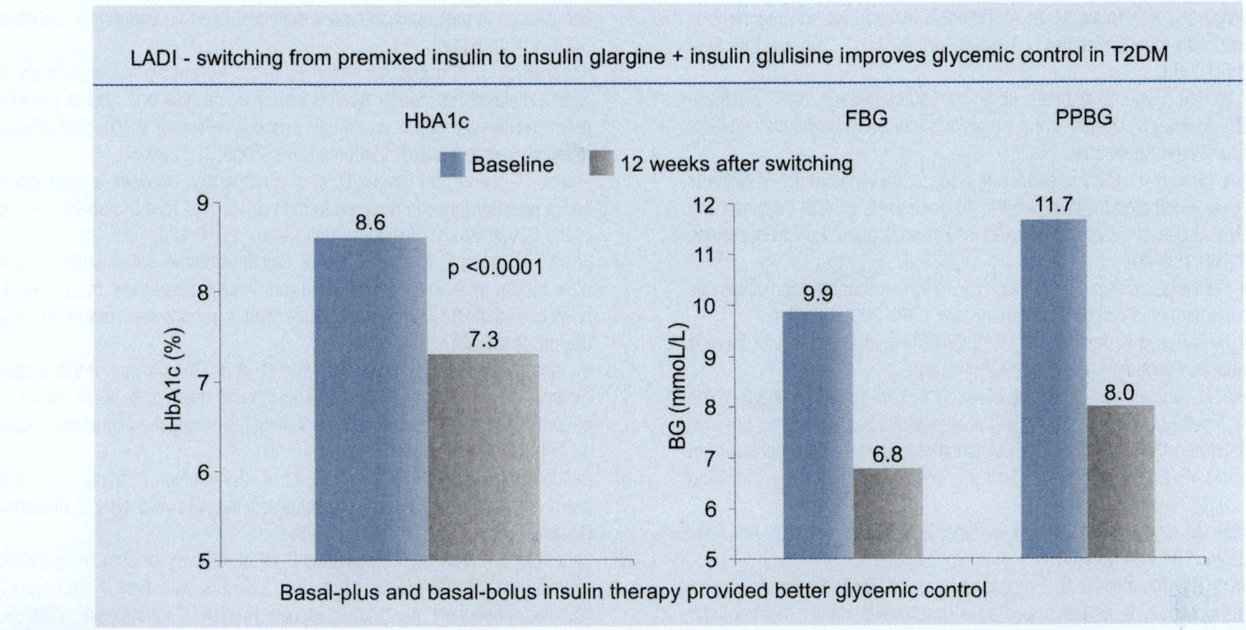

Figure 4 LADI study—switching from premixed insulin to insulin glargine + insulin glulisine improves glycemic control in T2DM. (*Source:* Schreiber S, Ferlinz K, Donaubauer B, et al. Efficacy of combining insulin glulisine with basal insulin glargine in patients with type 1 and type 2 diabetes previously on premix insulin therapy. Diabetologia. 2007;50 (suppl 1): S410-11.)

- Provide meal plan and schedule flexibility.
- Can be individualized to suit a patient's lifestyle.

Key points—Premixed Insulin Analogs

- Reduce HbA1c values.
- Do not mimic physiological insulin action.
- Associated with higher hypoglycemia chances.
- Fixed ratio of the basal and prandial insulin components.
- Difficult to monitor and titrate.
- Not suitable for treat-to-target titration schedules.
- Usually required 2–3 times daily.
- Require structured meal plans and schedules.
- Cannot be easily individualized.

CONCLUSION

Clinicians should individualize the diabetes treatment and various available options should be discussed with patients along with educating them regarding insulin therapy. There are a number of important factors that affect insulin therapy and need to be considered. These are number of daily injections, total daily dose of insulin, difficulties in monitoring blood glucose, weight gain, chances of hypoglycemia, and cost of therapy, adherence and quality of life.

If we consider that initiating insulin-naive patients on premix versus basal-bolus regimens has the similar effect in terms of blood glucose control, then hypoglycemia and weight gain are the other two key factors to consider. It is an established fact that the basal-bolus insulin regimen is associated with lesser weight gain and fewer chances of hypoglycemia than the premix insulins. On the other hand whereas basal-bolus insulin regimen requires four injections per day, premix insulins are administered twice or thrice daily. The basal-bolus regimen also resembles the physiological insulin secretion.

Therefore, it can be concluded that although similarities in glycemic control, fewer incidences of hypoglycemia, less weight gain, and convenience with basal-bolus regime promotes its use, premixed analogs are also a good option with their lesser demand for glucose monitoring and convenient injection schedule. As titration of insulin over time is critical for glycemic control and to prevent the occurrence of diabetes-related complications,[8] so an individually centered regimen that minimally disrupts the patient lifestyle will surely be the key factor for the successful management.

REFERENCES

1. Harris MI, Klein R, Welborn TA, et al. Onset of NIDDM occurs at least 4e7 yr before clinical diagnosis. Diabetes Care. 1992;15(7):815-9.

2. Ali MM, Aung KT, Young M, et al. Different insulin initiation regimens in patients with type 2 diabetes - A review article. Int J Diabetes Clin Res. 2018;5(1):083.
3. NICE (2015). Type 2 diabetes in adults: Management. NICE guideline [NG28] [online] Available from https://www.nice.org.uk/guidance/NG28 [Last accessed September, 2019].
4. Vaag A, Lund S. Therapy of endocrine disease: Insulin initiation in patients with type 2 diabetes mellitus: Treatment guidelines, clinical evidence and patterns of use of basal vs premixed insulin analogues. Eur J Endocrinol. 2011;166:159-70.
5. Indian Consensus Group. Premix insulin: Initiation and continuation guidelines for management of diabetes in primary care. JAPI. 2009;57:42-6.
6. Silver B, Ramaiya K, Andrew SB, et al. EADSG guidelines: insulin therapy in diabetes. Diabetes Ther. 2018;9(2):449-92.
7. Tanaka M, Ishii H. Pre-mixed rapid-acting insulin 50/50 analogue twice daily is useful not only for controlling post-prandial blood glucose, but also for stabilizing the diurnal variation of blood glucose levels: switching from premixed insulin 70/30 or 75/25 to pre-mixed insulin 50/50. J Int Med Res. 2010;38:674-80.
8. Petznick A. Insulin management of type 2 diabetes mellitus. Am Fam Physician. 2011;84:183-90.
9. Ligthelm RJ, Mouritzenz U, Lynggaard H, et al. Biphasic insulin aspart given thrice daily is as efficacious as a basal-bolus insulin regimen with four daily injections: a randomised open label parallel group four months comparison in patients with type 2 diabetes. Exp Clin Endocrinol Diabetes. 2006;114(9):511-9.
10. Rosenstock J, Ahmann AJ, Colon G, et al. Advancing insulin therapy in type 2 diabetes previously treated with glargine plus oral agents prandial premixed (insulin lispro protamine suspension/lispro) versus basal/bolus (glargine/lispro) therapy. Diabetes Care. 2008;31(1):20-5.
11. Fritsche A, Larbig M, Owens D, et al. Comparison between a basal-bolus and a premixed insulin regimen in individuals with type 2 diabetes results of the Ginger Study. Diabetes Obes Metab. 2010;12(2):115-23.
12. Levin PA, Zhang Q, Mersey JH, et al. Glycemic control with insulin glargine plus insulin glulisine versus premixed insulin analogues in real-world practices: a cost-effectiveness study with a randomized pragmatic trial design. 2011;33(7):841-50.
13. Shanmugasundar G, Bhansali A, Walia R, et al. Comparison of thrice daily biphasic human insulin (30/70) versus basal detemir & bolus aspart in patients with poorly controlled type 2 diabetes mellitusea pilot study. Indian J Med Res. 2012;135(1):78-83.
14. Belido V, Suarez L, Rodriguez MG, et al. Comparison of basal-bolus and premixed insulin regimens in hospitalized patients with type 2 diabetes. Diabetes Care. 2015;38(12):2211-6.
15. Schreiber S, Ferlinz K, Donaubauer B, et al. Efficacy of combining insulin glulisine with basal insulin glargine in patients with type 1 and type 2 diabetes previously on premix insulin therapy. Diabetologia. 2007;50 (suppl 1):S410-11.

CHAPTER 30 Beta Cell Preservation

Sanjeeb Kakati, Arpita Ray

INTRODUCTION

The global prevalence of diabetes has rapidly risen over the last two decades with more than 425 million people (20–79 years) living with diabetes worldwide. It is estimated that around 629 million people will be affected by diabetes and its complications by 2045.[1]

Type 2 diabetes mellitus (DM) is characterized by hyperglycemia, insulin resistance, and relative impairment in insulin secretion. The pathogenesis of type 2 DM is multifactorial such as genetic, environmental, and lifestyle influences making it difficult to determine the exact cause in an individual patient. Type 2 diabetes occurs when the insulin producing beta- (β) cells of pancreatic islets are unable to produce or release sufficient insulin to overcome peripheral insulin resistance, resulting in hyperglycemia. Hyperglycemia itself causes a state of glucotoxicity which causes irreversible damage to the β-cell thereby causing a vicious cycle leading to progressive β-cell decline. Obesity, visceral adiposity, results in increased free fatty acid (FFA) levels that lead to a state of lipotoxicity which has been shown to correlate with decreased insulin gene expression and β-cell death. Several metabolic and inflammatory cellular stresses such as oxidative and endoplasmic reticulum (ER) stress, proinflammatory responses, and islet amyloid deposition have been found to impair insulin synthesis and release from the β-cells and eventually lead to β-cell failure.

Islet amyloid is formed by the abnormal aggregation of islet amyloid polypeptide, i.e. cosecreted with insulin. Almost 90% patients of type 2 DM were found to have islet amyloid as a pathological lesion in the pancreas.[2] This pathological deposition of extracellular islet amyloid polypeptide (IAPP) within the pancreatic islets have been found to be a major cause of increased β-cell apoptosis. The aggregations of these proteins lead to formation of amyloid fibrils which further worsen the glucotoxicity.[3]

Various studies have demonstrated a reduction in the total β-cell mass in patients with type 2 DM.[4] The presence of decreased β-cell volume in individuals with impaired fasting glucose suggests that this process occurs early on in the process of developing diabetes.[4]

Initially, the insulin resistance is marked by a compensatory increase in the β-cell secretion of insulin however with persisting glucotoxicity, lipotoxicity, proinflammatory markers, and IAPP deposition, there is a progressive decline in the β-cell function and mass leading to decreased glycemic control. This remains a major challenge in the management of type 2 DM.

STRATEGIES TO PRESERVE BETA CELL FUNCTION

The aim of management of type 2 diabetes is to reduce the plasma glucose levels and thereby the long-term micro and macrovascular complications. Various therapeutic options have been studied that have different mechanism of action and some may even exhaust the remaining β-cells.

Interventions that reduce the load on β-cells by decreasing the demand for insulin have better durability on glycemic control and have been found to decrease the development of diabetes in high-risk population.

Lifestyle Modification and Intensive Glycemic Control

Weight gain increases insulin resistance and thereby increased secretory demand for insulin on the β-cells. Exercise and weight loss on the contrary enhances insulin sensitivity, reducing the workload on the β-cells.

Physical exercises have been shown to increase circulating levels of growth hormone (GH), insulin-like growth factor 1 (IGF-1), glucagon-like peptide 1 (GLP-1), interleukin (IL-6), and IL-1 receptor agonist (IL-1ra), which have a positive effect on beta cell mass.[5]

The XENical in the Prevention of Diabetes in Obese Subjects (XENDOS) study reported that orlistat, a gastrointestinal lipase inhibitor resulted in greater weight loss and a 37% reduced relative risk for diabetes compared with lifestyle intervention alone in obese adults with normal and impaired glucose tolerance.[6]

However, lifestyle modifications with weight control alone have not been sustainable in prevention of diabetes.

Intensive Glycemic Control

The United Kingdom Prospective Diabetes Study (UKPDS), Diabetes Control and Complications Trial (DCCT), and Epidemiology of Diabetes Interventions and Complications (EDIC) study have demonstrated that intensive glycemic control is foremost in preventing progressive β-cell loss.

Early Insulin Intensification and Early Glycemic Control

Early initiation and intensification of insulin have been found to be effective in delaying the progression of β-cell decline by having a detrimental effect on the glucotoxicity and lipotoxicity. Its role however in already established diabetes is uncertain.

In a study conducted by Lindsay B Harrison et al.[7] to establish the β-cell function preservation after 3.5 years of intensive diabetes therapy, they found that β-cell function can be preserved for at least 3.5 years after diagnosis of type 2 diabetes when intensive therapy is initiated early in the disease process. This was true regardless of the method used to attain intensive control (insulin-based regimen or a triple combination of oral agents, both after an initial 3-month insulin treatment period).

The Kumamoto trial showed maintenance of HbA1c of approximately 7.2% for 8 years and prevention of progression of microvascular complications with an early treatment with multiple insulin injections.

Therapeutic Strategies

Metformin

Metformin reduces hyperglycemia by reducing the hepatic glucose production and increasing the insulin sensitivity in the peripheral tissues. In certain, in vitro studies, metformin has been found to have beneficial effects on the human islet cell by reducing glucotoxicity and lipotoxicity.

Diabetes Prevention Program research Group USA, and Indian DPP study showed that metformin reduced the conversion from IGT to type 2 DM by 31%.[8] However, the UKPDS and ADOPT study showed that though the initial durability of metformin was promising yet it resulted in 21% failure rate at 5 years in patients recently diagnosed with type 2 diabetes.[9]

Thiazolidinediones

Thiazolidinediones (TZD) are potent insulin sensitizers that act via the peroxisome proliferator activator receptor (PPAR). TZD also exert a potent effect to preserve β-cell function.[10] They improve the muscle insulin sensitivity by reducing the plasma FFA and intramyocellular lipid content, alteration of the fat topography,[11,12] and direct insulin-sensitizing effect mediated via PPAR receptor.[12]

Thiazolidinediones have been found to augment the β-cell function by various mechanisms: (1) improving the insulin sensitivity by unloading the β-cells, (2) decreasing the plasma levels of FFA, (3) reverting lipotoxicity (toxic lipid metabolites are mobilized out of the β-cells), (4) increase serum adiponectin, (5) decreases β-cell apoptosis.

Several clinical trials have shown these beneficial effects such as Troglitazone in Prevention of Diabetes (TRIPOD), Pioglitazone in Prevention of Diabetes (PIPOD), Diabetes Reduction Assessment with Ramipril and Rosiglitazone Medication (DREAM), and Actos now (ACT-NOW). In DPP, troglitazone reduced IGT conversion to diabetes by 23% after 3 years.[13,14]

In DREAM, rosiglitazone reduced the IGT to type 2 diabetes conversion by 62%. In females with history of gestational diabetes, both troglitazone (TRIPOD) and pioglitazone (PIPOD) markedly reduced IGT progression to type 2 diabetes.

In summary, the TZD besides having an insulin sensitizing effect also thus improve and preserve the β-cell function, cause a durable HbA1c reduction and prevent conversion of IGT to type 2 DM.

Glucagon-like Peptide-1 Analogs

The rise in insulin in response to glucose ingestion is two- to threefold more than its response to the same level of hyperglycemia produced by intravenous (IV) glucose. This is called as the incretin effect.

Glucagon-like peptide-1, released by L cells in response to meal ingestion, and glucose-dependent insulinotropic polypeptide (GIP), released by K cells, account for 90% of the incretin effect. GLP-1 and GIP both act as potent insulin secretagogues. They also inhibit the secretion of glucagon promote weight loss by delaying the gastric emptying and its additional appetite suppressant effect. GLP-1 however is degraded rapidly by dipeptidyl peptidase-IV, i.e. present on the cell membranes.

Liraglutide, exenatide are close to ideal antidiabetic agents as they are potent insulin secretagogues, they reduce the postprandial glucose levels without a risk of hypoglycemia, promote weight loss and are resistant to dipeptidyl peptidase-IV degradation. They have been found to have a durable HbA1c reduction, improved β-cell function.[15] They have also been found to have effect on the *PDX1* gene expression thereby stimulating insulin gene transcription.

Glucagon-like peptide-1 analogs have thus found to have the potential of preventing β-cell exhaustion, replenish the insulin stores, and preserve β-cell function.

Dipeptidyl Peptidase IV Inhibitors

Dipeptidyl peptidase IV inhibitors inhibit the enzyme dipeptidyl peptidase-IV thereby slowing down the inactivation of the incretin hormones GLP-1 and GIP.

Dipeptidyl peptidase IV inhibitors have been found to stimulate β-cell survival, facilitate islet neogenesis and enhance insulin biosynthesis thereby preserving β-cell mass and function, in diabetic animal models.[16] They have been found to have an additional anti-inflammatory effect which alleviates the loss of β-cell function.

Treatment of patients with type 2 diabetes with DPP-IV inhibitors have shown to have beneficial effects on the HbA1c increased postprandial insulin secretion, and C-peptide, and β-cell responsiveness.

In conclusion, DPP-IV inhibitors when used as a monotherapy or as an add-on therapy in type 2 DM have been found to improve β-cell function but have doubtful effect on insulin resistance.

Alpha Glucosidase Inhibitors

Acarbose is an α-glucosidase inhibitor that inhibits the activity of small intestinal enzymes thereby reducing the glucose absorption. This reduces the postprandial glucose surge and has also been found to augment the incretin effect. Acarbose alters the gut microbiota which in turn has been found to have a beneficial effect on the glucose homeostasis. The study to prevent NIDDM (STOP-NIDDM) found a 25% relative risk reduction in the development of type 2 DM over 3.3 years in patients with impaired glucose levels treated with acarbose compared with placebo.[17]

Angiotensin-converting Enzyme Inhibitors

Angiotensin-converting enzyme (ACE) inhibitors or angiotensin receptor blockers (ARBs) found to improve the glucose tolerance and insulin sensitivity through inhibition of the renin-angiotension system (RAS) complex. This may be due to improvement of the microcirculation in the skeletal muscles, enhancing the delivery of insulin and glucose to the insulin sensitive tissues thereby improving the insulin signaling mechanism at the cellular level and hence better insulin secretion by the β-cells. ACE inhibitors and ARBs reduce the harmful effect of angiotensin II on vasoconstriction, inflammation, fibrosis, apoptosis, and β-cell death, thus preserving β-cell mass.

Cytokine Suppressors

It is found that the expression of IL-1 receptor antagonist is reduced in the pancreatic islets in patients with type 2 DM. High glucose concentrations have been found to induce production of IL-1 beta in human pancreatic islet β-cells thereby impairing insulin secretion and β-cell loss by apoptosis. It was found in a study conducted by Larsen CM et al. that blockade of IL-1 with anakinra improved the glycemia and β-cell secretory function and reduced markers of inflammation preventing β-cell loss.[18]

K^+ Channel Activators

K-ATP channel openers, such as diazoxide counteract the chronic over stimulation of β-cells and protect against toxic conditions such as relative hypoxia. The mechanism may include indirect (counteracting over-stimulation) and direct mitochondrial effects. A 6-month intervention with diazoxide failed to result in better preservation of β-cell function in newly diagnosed type 1 diabetics. K-ATP channel openers may improve β-cell function in some type 2 diabetes patients who are simultaneously treated with bedtime insulin.[19]

Bariatric Surgery

Bariatric surgery, which conventionally encompasses four surgical procedures, including, (1) Roux-en-Y gastric bypass (RYGB), (2) laparoscopic adjustable gastric banding (LAGB), (3) biliopancreatic diversion (BPD), and (4) laparoscopic sleeve gastrectomy (LSG), provides substantial improvement in the glycemic control in obese type 2 diabetic patients.

Weight loss occurs with gastric volume reduction, intestinal malabsorption or a combination of the two. Bariatric surgery has been shown to prevent onset of type 2 diabetes in almost 99–100% of patients with IGT and reduce the symptoms of diabetes in 64–93% of the patients with diabetes. The benefits of β-cell function appear to be greatest when weight loss is achieved before β-cell function is completely impaired.

BETA CELL PRESERVATION IN PATIENTS WITH TYPE 1 DIABETES

Type 1 DM is a chronic autoimmune disease that leads to destruction of pancreatic β-cells, with early development of complications and a lifelong dependence on insulin. Preservation of residual β-cells in type 1 diabetes has to be initiated at a very early stage owing to the disease pathology. A variety of immune interventions have been studied based on the various stages of the disease pathology including nonspecific immunosuppression, pathway-specific immune modulation, antigen specific therapies, and cellular therapies.

TARGETS FOR IMMUNE INTERVENTION

As the pathogenesis of type 1 diabetes was established to be autoimmune[20] attempts were made to induce remission with nonspecific immunosuppressive agents such as cyclosporine, azathioprine, and prednisolone. These agents however lacked long-term benefits and had the prospect of lifelong immunosuppression and concomitant toxicity, for which they were withdrawn.

Interleukin-1 has been known to be directly toxic to the pancreatic β-cells and hence randomized trials of anti-IL-1 agents, anti-IL-1β mAb, canakinumab, and the IL-1 receptor antagonist anakinra were established. However, they failed to show significant benefit in new onset type 1 diabetic patients.

Recently, clinical trials of two other anti-cytokine agents, tocilizumab (anti IL-6 receptor mAb) and Ustekinumab (anti-IL-12/23 mAb), that block the key inflammatory mediators in the immune pathway have been studied.

A combination therapy targeting innate, adaptive pathway, co-stimulatory blockade, and antigen-specific blockade may be theoretically possible however clinical trials for its feasibility are required, for example, combination might include an induction agent that can deplete key subsets of effector T cells (such as alefacept or teplizumab), followed by a pro-tolerogenic agent (such as tocilizumab or IL-2) combined with autoantigens (such as proinsulin peptides or DNA) that facilitate expansion of antigen-specific Tregs.

CONCLUSION

Type 2 DM involves a progressive failure of β-cell function and its associated complications. Various recent trials have highlighted the importance of early initiation of therapy and a tight glycemic control to prevent progressive β-cell loss.

Glucagon-like peptide 1 analogs and DPP-IV inhibitors, via the incretin effect and various other beneficial metabolic effects have shown to improve the glucose metabolism, preserve the β-cell function and also prevent the development of new onset type 2 diabetes in patients with IGT.

Interventions that reduce body fat (such as diet and exercise, GLP-1 receptor agonists, or bariatric surgery) or that change fat biology (TZDs) provide the best evidence for slowing or arresting the deterioration of β-cell function that causes type 2 DM. These agents hence should be initiated early in the course of the disease.

Preservation of residual β-cells after restoration by transplantation, differentiation from stem cells, or neogenesis (drug-induced) are potential immune interventions in type 1 DM.

REFERENCES

1. International Diabetes Federation (IDF). Facts and Figures, 8th edition. 2017.
2. Jurgens CA, Toukatly MN, Fligner CL, et al. β-cell loss and β-cell apoptosis in human type 2 diabetes are related to islet amyloid deposition. Am J Pathol. 2011;178:2632-40.
3. Park YJ, Woo M, Kieffer TJ, et al. The role of caspase-8 in amyloid-induced beta cell death in human and mouse islets. Diabetologia. 2014;57:765-75.
4. Butler AE, Janson J, Bonner-Weir S, et al. Beta-cell deficit and increased beta-cell apoptosis in humans with type 2 diabetes. Diabetes. 2003;52:102-10.
5. Jensen J, Galsgaard ED, Karlsen AE, et al. STAT5 activation by human GH protects insulin-producing cells against interleukin-1β, interferon-γ and tumour necrosis factor-α-induced apoptosis independent of nitric oxide production. J Endocrinol. 2005;187:25-36.
6. Torgerson JS, Hauptman J, Boldrin MN, et al. XENical in the prevention of diabetes in obese subjects (XENDOS) study: a randomized study of orlistat as an adjunct to lifestyle changes for the prevention of type 2 diabetes in obese patients. Diabetes Care. 2004;27:155-61.

7. Harrison LB, Raskin P, Adams-Huet B, et al. β- cell function preservation after 3.5 years of intensive diabetes therapy, Diabetes Care. 2012;35:1406-12.
8. Knowler WC, Barrett-Connor E, Fowler SE, et al. Reduction in the incidence of type 2 diabetes with lifestyle intervention or metformin. N Engl J Med. 2002;346:393-403.
9. UK Prospective Diabetes Study (UKPDS) Group. Intensive blood-glucose control with sulphonylureas or insulin compared with conventional treatment and risk of complications in patients with type 2 diabetes (UKPDS 33). Lancet. 1998;352(9131):837-53.
10. Gastaldelli A, Ferrannini E, Miyazaki Y, et al. Thiazolidinediones improve β–cell function in type 2 diabetic patients. Am J Physiol Endocrinol Metab. 2007;292:E871-83
11. Bays H, Mandarino L, DeFronzo RA. Role of the adipocytes, free fatty acids, and ectopic fat in pathogenesis of type 2 diabetes mellitus: peroxisomal proliferator-activated receptor agonists provide a rational therapeutic approach. J Clin Endocrinol Metab. 2004;89:463-78.
12. Yki-Järvinen H. Thiazolidinediones. New Engl J Med. 2004;351:1106-18.
13. Xiang AH, Peters RK, Kjos SL, et al. Effect of pioglitazone on pancreatic beta-cell function and diabetes risk in Hispanic women with prior gestational diabetes. Diabetes. 2006;55:517-22
14. Hanley AJ, Zinman B, Sheridan P, et al. Effect of Rosiglitazone and Ramipril on {beta}-cell function in people with impaired glucose tolerance or impaired fasting glucose: the DREAM trial. Diabetes Care. 2010;33:608-13.
15. DeFronzo RA, Ratner RE, Han J, et al. Effects of exenatide (synthetic exendin-4) on glycemic control and weight over 30 weeks in metformin-treated patients with type 2 diabetes mellitus. Diabetes Care. 2005;28: 1092-100
16. Pospisilik JA, Martin J, Doty T, et al. Dipeptidyl peptidase IV inhibitor treatment stimulates beta-cell survival and islet neogenesis in streptozotocin induced diabetic rats. Diabetes. 2003;52:741-50.
17. Chiasson JL, Josse RG, Gomis R, et al. Acarbose for prevention of type 2 diabetes mellitus: the STOP-NIDDM randomised trial. Lancet. 2002;359:2072-7.
18. Larsen CM, Faulenbach M, Vaag A, et al. Interleukin-1 receptor antagonist in type 2 diabetes mellitus. N Engl J Med. 2007;356(15):1517-26.
19. Grill V, Radtke M, Qvigstad E, et al. Beneficial effects of K-ATP channel openers in diabetes: an update on mechanisms and clinical experiences. Diabetes Obes Metab. 2009;11(Suppl 4):143-8.
20. Eisenbarth GS. Type I diabtes mellitus: a chronic autoimmune disease. N Engl J Med. 1986;314(21):1360-8.

31 CHAPTER Comparing Cardiovascular Outcome Data of All Antidiabetic Drugs

Sailesh Lodha

INTRODUCTION

The management of type 2 diabetes mellitus (T2DM) mainly involves maintaining quality of life and preventing or delaying complications, which is possible with glycemic control and cardiovascular risk prevention.[1] However, almost half of the T2DM patients achieve less than 7% hemoglobin (Hb) A1C target.[2] Patients who have controlled glycemia, blood pressure, or cholesterol levels and without smoking are only 14%.[3]

Administration of either oral or injectable drugs is often needed to control glycemic levels in T2DM patients.

Compared to conventional glycemic control, an intensive glycemic control as demonstrated by randomized controlled trials (RCTs) in T2DM is associated with an absolute difference of 0.90% in mean HbA1C at completion of follow-up. Nevertheless, inconsistency has been noted with tight glycemic control to reduce the cardiovascular (CV) complications in T2DM patients. Residual vascular risk refers to intensive and successful glycemic control followed by high, very high or unchanged risk of macrovascular (major cardiovascular events) and microvascular (retinopathy, nephropathy and neuropathy) complications.[4] Long-term macrovascular risk may be reduced by early intervention.[5] With microvascular complications, the onset is delayed and severity is reduced with management of chronic hyperglycemia. Apart from its glucose-lowering action, reduced cardiovascular risk makes metformin the preferred first-line therapy to manage hyperglycemia of T2DM.[6] The cardiovascular benefits offered by the glucose-lowering drugs seem largely independent of their glucose-lowering efficacy.

CARDIOVASCULAR OUTCOME TRIALS OF AVAILABLE ANTIDIABETIC DRUGS

The completed and ongoing postmarketing cardiovascular outcome trials (CVOTs) of antidiabetic drugs that are designed to fulfil the Food and Drug Administration (FDA) criteria have been discussed as follows (Table 1). A 3-point MACE (Major adverse cardiovascular events) including CV death, nonfatal myocardial infarction (MI) and nonfatal stroke are the primary end points. Some trials like TECOS and ELIXA have a 4-point MACE (the 3-point MACE mentioned above along with hospitalization for unstable angina).

TABLE 1: Completed large post-marketing prospective CV outcome studies with glucose-lowering agents in type 2 diabetes. Most of these trials were designed to fulfil FDA criteria to confirm CV safety versus placebo.

Trial	Test agent	Start	End	Years	n =	1˙ endpoint
SAVOR-TIMI 53	Saxagliptin	2010	2013	2.1	16492	3Pt MACE
EXAMINE	Alogliptin	2009	2013	1.5	5380	3Pt MACE
TECOS	Sitagliptin	2008	2015	2.8	14671	4Pt MACE
CARMELINA	Linagliptin	2013	2018	~4	7003	3Pt MACE

Contd...

Contd...

Trial	Test agent	Start	End	Years	n =	1° endpoint
CAROLINA	Linagliptin vs SU	2010	2019	~4	6103	3Pt MACE
ELIXA	Lixisenatide	2010	2015	2.1	6068	4Pt MACE
LEADER	Liraglutide	2010	2016	3.8	9340	3Pt MACE
SUSTAIN-6	Semaglutide sc	2012	2016	2.1	3297	3Pt MACE
EXSCEL	Exenatide QW	2010	2017	3.2	14752	3Pt MACE
FREEDOM ICTA 650	Exenatide implant	2013	2016	1.2	4156	4Pt MACE
HARMONY	Albiglutide	2015	2018	~2	9574	3Pt MACE
REWIND	Dulaglutide	2011	2018	~5	9622	3Pt MACE
PIONEER-6	Semaglutide oral	2016	2018	~1.6	3176	3Pt MACE
EMPA-REG OUTCOME	Empagliflozin	2010	2015	3.1	7020	3Pt MACE
CANVAS (& CANVAS-R)	Canagliflozin	2009	2017	2.4	10142	3Pt MACE (& albuminuria)
DECLARE TIMI 58	Dapagliflozin	2013	2018	~4	17276	3Pt MACE
DEVOTE	Degludec vs glargine	2013	2017	1.8	7637	3Pt MACE
TOSCA.IT	Pioglitazonevs SU	2008	2017	4.7	3028	3Pt + coronary revasc
ACE (in IGT)	Acarbose	2009	2017	5	6522	5Pt MACE(3pt + angina + hHF)

The design of these studies showed non-inferiority for the primary CV composite outcome. Experimental therapy and placebo have been compared with sequential hierarchical testing for superiority in the background of glucose-lowering treatment. A large number of patients who have already encountered an adverse CV event (secondary prevention) have been selected for these trials. In contrast, most of the diabetic patients are treated with glucose-lowering drugs even before a CV event occurs (primary prevention) in routine clinical practice.

Dipeptidyl Peptidase-4 Inhibitors

Dipeptidyl peptidase-4 (DPP4) inhibitors enhance incretin effect by decreasing the degradation of glucagon-like peptide-1 (GLP-1), thus lowering blood glucose. The CV safety of drugs like saxagliptin, alogliptin, and sitagliptin have been proved with the results of the postmarketing CV outcome trials that indicate no change in MACE in T2DM treated with these drugs.[7-9] EXAMINE (Examination of Cardiovascular Outcomes with Alogliptin versus Standard of Care) trial showed nonsignificant increase in CV risk with alogliptin. TECOS (Trial Evaluating Cardiovascular Outcomes with Sitagliptin) showed no heart failure signal with sitagliptin.[8]

The CV status of patients randomized into these trials was somewhat different—SAVOR included a mix of patients with either prior CV disease or high CV risk, whereas EXAMINE restricted inclusion to patients 15–90 days after an acute MI or hospitalization for unstable angina. More than 50 years old CV patients were only studied in TECOS.

The CAROLINA (Cardiovascular Outcome Study of Linagliptin Versus Glimepiride) study evaluated the CV safety of 6,033 T2DM patients with increased CV risk or established cardiovascular disease (CVD), who were administered linagliptin, 5 mg once daily.[10] The results showed that linagliptin, a DPP-IV inhibitor that met primary end points was non-inferior when compared to glimepiride till the initial adverse cardiovascular event (CV death, nonfatal MI or nonfatal stroke) occurred in T2DM patients with high CV risk. This was the first and only active-comparator CV outcome trial for a DPP-IV inhibitor that compared linagliptin (Tradjenta) and glimepiride during a median follow-up of 6 years.

The safety of linagliptin (Tradjenta, Boehringer Ingelheim/Eli Lilly) was also demonstrated in CARMELINA (CArdiovascular and Renal Microvascular OutcomE Study with LINAgliptin in Patients with Type 2 Diabetes Mellitus) subanalyses done in a large set of high-risk patients with type 2 diabetes. The study suggested linagliptin to be the choice for patients who are at high risk for hypoglycemia in particular.

The potential to reduce degradation of many hormones remain the same for all DPP4 inhibitors; though their metabolism and elimination characteristic subtly vary for each drug. Further, the potential cardioprotective effects of DPP4 inhibitors may include improving the blood lipid profile and lowering blood pressure, slightly.[11]

Glucagon-like Peptide-1 Receptor Agonists

Glucagon-like peptide-1 receptor agonists (GLP-1RAs) exert various effects on the CV system besides the following:

- Lowering of glucose and weight
- Enhancing insulin secretion induced by glucose
- Reduce glucagon secretion,
- Delay gastric emptying and induce satiety.

The action of GLP-1RAs in T2DM patients vary from reducing blood pressure, though heart rate is increased, reducing inflammation and plasminogen activator inhibitor-1 to improving the lipid profile.[12] They have favorable CV outcomes according to evidences from many studies.[13]

Of the four major studies, Liraglutide in LEADER and semaglutide in SUSTAIN-6 are CV studies that reveal a significant reduction in a 3-point MACE. Study on exenatide in EXSCEL and lixisenatide in ELIXA showed no change.[14-17] The LEADER trial studied 9,340 T2DM patients with high CV risk and randomized them to placebo or liraglutide at a dosage of 0.6–1.8 mg/day for 3.1 years. The 3-point MACE result revealed 13% reduction in the liraglutide group, 22% reduction in CV death and 15% reduction in total mortality.

FREEDOM is a completed CV outcome trial with a depot formulation of exenatide but the results are not yet fully reported. Other ongoing CV outcome trials include REWIND with dulaglutide, PIONEER-6 with oral semaglutide and HARMONY with albiglutide.

Sodium/Glucose Cotransporter-2 Inhibitors

Sodium/glucose cotransporter-2 (SGLT2) inhibitors act by reducing renal glucose reabsorption and lowering blood glucose through glucosuria. EMPA-REG OUTCOME and CANVAS programs are two post-marketing CV outcome studies with the SGLT2 inhibitors empagliflozin and canagliflozin, respectively which showed significant improvements in the 3-point MACE with these agents.[18,19]

The effect of empagliflozin was found with the EMPA-REG OUTCOME study which randomized 7,020 T2DM patients with CV disease. A dose of 10 or 25 mg/day empagliflozin or placebo was administered and the patients were followed for 3.1 years. More than 75% treatment of the CV risk of patients in EMPAREG OUTCOME trial included the following—received statin, more than 95% received antihypertensive therapy and about 90% received anticoagulant/antiplatelet drugs. Though empagliflozin did not affect the onset of nonfatal MI and stroke, it seemed to significantly reduce hospitalization for heart failure.[20] Rapid divergent rates of the MACE, mortality, and heart failure hospitalization between the empagliflozin and placebo groups was a notable feature of this CV trial, recorded within the first 6 months after randomization.

CANVAS (Canagliflozin Cardiovascular Assessment Study) and CANVAS-R are two trials, which altogether randomized 10,142 T2DM patients at high CV risk to placebo or canagliflozin at a dosage of 100–300 mg/day. The two trials were integrated to form the CANVAS program.[19] A follow-up of 3.1 years revealed that canagliflozin significantly reduced the 3-point MACE by 14%. On the contrary, CV death or overall mortality did not alter with canagliflozin in contrast to empagliflozin. However, it was found that canaglifozin significantly reduced hospitalization for heart failure, as seen with empagliflozin in the EMPA REG OUTCOME trial. Gradual divergent rates of MACE between canagliflozin and placebo patients were reported in contrast to the rapid divergence rates in EMPA-REG OUTCOME trial.

CONCLUSION

Lessons from CVOTs

- The safety of glucose-lowering agents, such as DPP4 inhibitors, GLP-1RAs and SGLT2 inhibitors usage in T2DM have been confirmed by many placebo controlled trials which demonstrate no increase in adverse CV events such as CV death, non-fatal MI and stroke.
- Favorable CV outcomes with significant reduction in 3-point MACE have been shown with SGLT2 inhibitors empaglifozin and canagliflozin, as well as the GLP-1RAs liraglutide and semaglutide.
- It is not simple and easy to compare the results of the trials discussed because of differences in trial population, patient CV risk status, trial design, and data collection and analysis strategies.
- The lowering of glucose in microvascular diseases has not been focused as much as that in macrovascular diseases in the CV outcome trials. This should not be neglected as the microvascular diseases may impact the severity of some macrovascular diseases.

- The results of the latest CV outcome trials have reassured the use of newer glucose-lowering agents to manage hyperglycemia in T2DM with no adverse CV risks including CV death, non-fatal MI or stroke, and some agents may offer cardioprotective benefits as well.

REFERENCES

1. Giugliano D, Meier JJ, Esposito K. Heart failure and type 2 diabetes: From cardiovascular outcome trials, with hope. Diabetes, Obes Metab. 2019;21(5): 1081-7.
2. Lipska KJ, Yao X, Herrin J, et al. Trends in drug utilization, glycemic control, and rates of severe hypoglycemia, 2006–2013. Diabetes Care. 2017;40(4):468-75.
3. Ali MK, Bullard KM, Saaddine JB, et al. Achievement of goals in U.S. diabetes care, 1999-2010. N Engl J Med. 2013;368(17):1613-24.
4. Giugliano D, Maiorino MI, Bellastella G, et al. Glycemic control in type 2 diabetes: from medication nonadherence to residual vascular risk. Endocrine. 2018;61(1):23-7.
5. Stratton IM, Adler AI, Neil HA, et al. Association of glycaemia with macrovascular and microvascular complications of type 2 diabetes (UKPDS 35): prospective observational study. BMJ. 2000;321(7258):405-12.
6. Control G, Turnbull FM, Abraira C, et al. Intensive glucose control and macrovascular outcomes in type 2 diabetes. Diabetologia. 2009;52(11): 2288-98.
7. Scirica BM, Bhatt DL, Braunwald E, et al. Saxagliptin and cardiovascular outcomes in patients with type 2 diabetes mellitus. N Engl J Med. 2013;369(14):1317-26.
8. White WB, Cannon CP, Heller SR, et al. Alogliptin after acute coronary syndrome in patients with type 2 diabetes. N Engl J Med. 2013;369(14): 1327-35.
9. Green JB, Bethel MA, Armstrong PW, et al. Effect of Sitagliptin on Cardiovascular Outcomes in Type 2 Diabetes. N Engl J Med. 2015;373(3):232-42.
10. Rosenstock J, Perkovic V, Alexander JH, et al. Rationale, design, and baseline characteristics of the CArdiovascular safety and Renal microvascular outcomE study with LINAgliptin (CARMELINA®): a randomized, double-blind, placebo-controlled clinical trial in patients with type 2 diabetes and high cardio-renal risk. Cardiovasc Diabetol. 2018;17(1):39.
11. Avogaro A, Fadini GP. The pleiotropic Cardiovascular Effects of Dipeptidyl peptidase-4 Inhibitors. Br J Clin Pharmacol. 2018;84(8): 1686-95.
12. Nauck MA, Meier JJ, Cavender MA, et al. Cardiovascular Actions and Clinical Outcomes With Glucagon-Like Peptide-1 Receptor Agonists and Dipeptidyl Peptidase-4 Inhibitors. Circulation. 2017;136(9):849-70.
13. Bethel MA, Patel RA, Merrill P, et al. Cardiovascular outcomes with glucagon-like peptide-1 receptor agonists in patients with type 2 diabetes: a meta-analysis. Lancet Diabetes Endocrinol. 2018;6(2):105-13.
14. Pfeffer MA, Claggett B, Diaz R, et al. Lixisenatide in Patients with Type 2 Diabetes and Acute Coronary Syndrome. N Engl J Med. 2015;373(23): 2247-57.
15. Marso SP, Daniels GH, Brown-Frandsen K, et al. Liraglutide and Cardiovascular Outcomes in Type 2 Diabetes. N Engl J Med. 2016;375(4):311-22.
16. Marso SP, Bain SC, Consoli A, et al. Semaglutide and Cardiovascular Outcomes in Patients with Type 2 Diabetes. N Engl J Med. 2016; 375(19): 1834-44.
17. Holman RR, Bethel MA, Mentz RJ, et al. Effects of Once-Weekly Exenatide on Cardiovascular Outcomes in Type 2 Diabetes. N Engl J Med. 2017; 377(13):1228-39.
18. Zinman B, Wanner C, Lachin JM, et al. Empagliflozin, Cardiovascular Outcomes, and Mortality in Type 2 Diabetes. N Engl J Med. 2015;373(22): 3117-28.
19. Neal B, Perkovic V, Mahaffey KW, et al. Canagliflozin and Cardiovascular and Renal Events in Type 2 Diabetes. N Engl J Med. 2017; 377(7): 644-57.
20. Zinman B, Inzucchi SE, Lachin JM, et al. Empagliflozin and Cerebrovascular Events in Patients With Type 2 Diabetes Mellitus at High Cardiovascular Risk. Stroke. 2017;48(5):1218-25.

32 CHAPTER Newer Therapies in Heart Failure with Preserved Ejection Fraction

Jotideb Mukhopadhyay, Soumyadip Kar

INTRODUCTION

Heart failure with preserved ejection fraction is a complex clinical syndrome. This condition is characterized by the presence of signs and symptoms of heart failure, including reduced exercise capacity and/or retention of fluid in the setting of normal or near normal left ventricular ejection fraction (LVEF) and impaired diastolic function (relaxation is *impaired*).[1]

It has now been well established that around half of those patients who are hospitalized present with the clinical symptoms of heart failure with preserved ejection fraction (HFpEF),[2] So far there have been no established therapies that have shown to improve the morbidity and mortality in patients with HFpEF, unlike for patients with heart failure with reduced ejection fraction (HFrEF).

PATHOPHYSIOLOGY OF HFPEF

Heart failure with preserved ejection fraction has a quite complex pathophysiology and, thus by far, it is not completely understood. It is associated with the alterations in the cardiac structure and functions, which together with systemic and pulmonary vascular abnormalities leads to left ventricular (LV) abnormalities. Along with these LV abnormalities, coronary disease, chronotropic incompetence, poor vasodilator reserve, and microvascular changes can also be seen.[3] Most patients with HFpEF present a normal size of left ventricle and ejection fraction but due to enlarged LV mass or relative wall thickness with concentric remodelling, the systolic function is frequently compromised.[4] Studies have demonstrated that in HFpEF longitudinal strain is usually decreased and radial strain is preserved, thus leading to the appearance of a preserved EF. Diastolic dysfunction, the hallmark of HFpEF leads to futile left atrium (LA) emptying and LV filling, along with decreased capacity to enhance cardiac output (Flowchart 1).

On exertion, and thus results in an elevated pulmonary artery pressure and ensuing clinical sequelae of fluid retention.[5,6]

Increased LV stiffness due to hypertrophy and interstitial fibrosis or abnormal LV relaxation secondary to abnormal calcium cycling can cause diastolic dysfunction. Studies in animals have shown that cytoskeletal titin which functions as a bidirectional spring, accountable for early diastolic and late diastolic distensibility, are impaired in subjects with HFpEF.[7,8] A recent study has demonstrated that LV relaxation is virtually impaired in every patient with HFpEF, independent of the presence of LVH or increased stiffness.[9] It is more likely to be responsible to pharmacological interventions considering that LV relaxation is an active physiological relaxation process, rather than just being a structural change.

THERAPEUTIC TARGETS FOR HFPEF

There has been no therapy to date that has shown to improve the mortality in patients with HFpEF. Any significant reduction in morbidity and mortality in patient with HFpEF has not even been shown by the clinical trials including several pharmacological interventions. However, as we continue to boost our knowledge and understanding regarding the pathophysiology of HFpEF, we can start exploring potential targets for this increasingly prevalent condition (Flowchart 2).

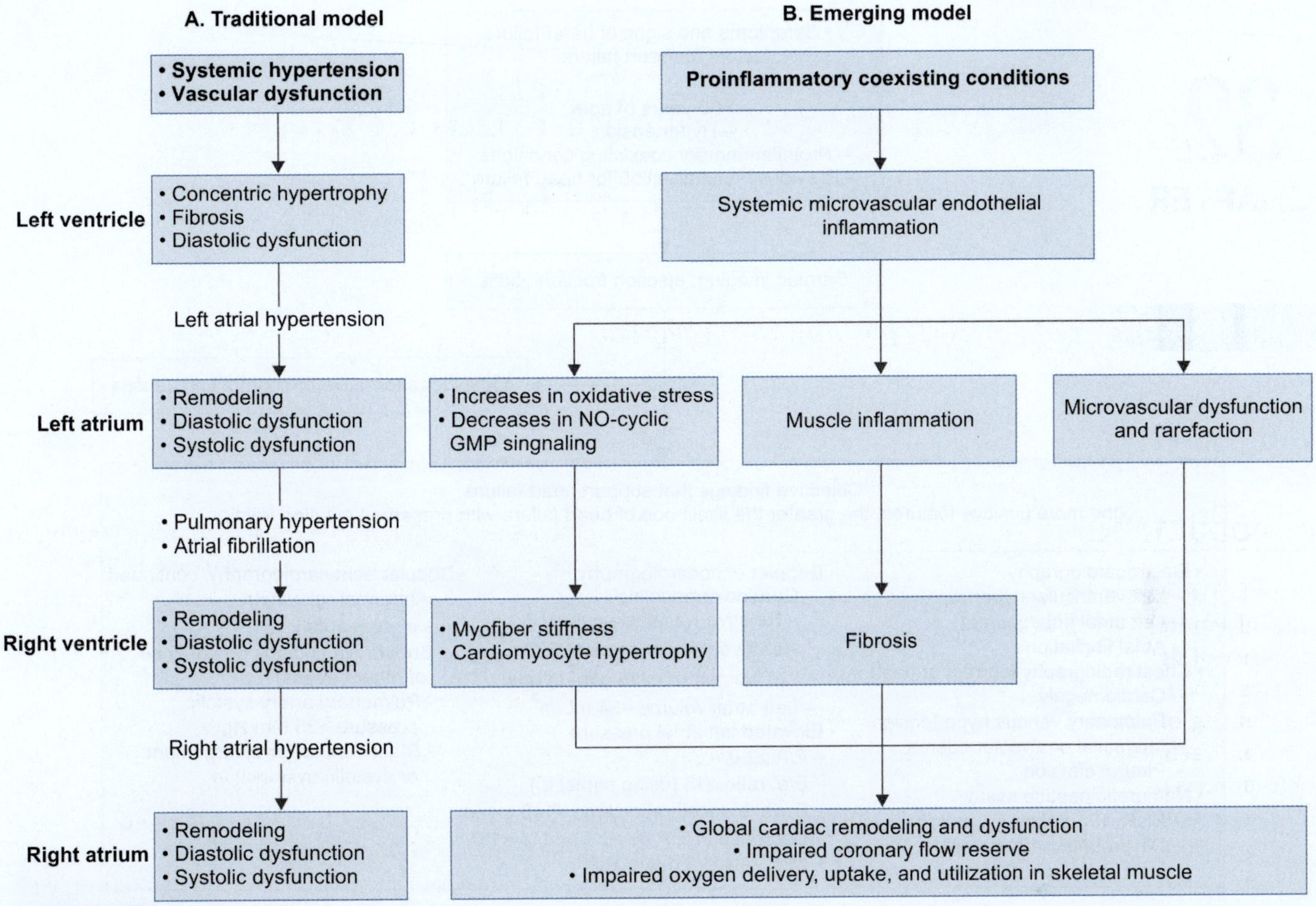

Flowchart 1 Traditional and emerging pathophysiological models of heart failure with preserved ejection fraction.

(*Source*: Margret M. Heart Failure with Preserved Ejection Fraction. N Engl J Med. 2016;375:1868-77.)

Therapies Targeting Diastolic Dysfunction

Diastolic dysfunction leads to an increased LV mass, mass/volume ratio, left atrial (LA) area and stress in the diastolic wall in patients with HFpEF.[6] Titin, a giant cytoskeletal structural protein, is expressed in sarcomeres which functions as molecular spring.[7,8] Diastolic monocyte stiffness is increased by a stiffer titin. Studies have demonstrated that therapies that increase cyclic guanosine monophosphate (cGMP) can reduce myocardial diastolic stiffness in HFpEF by activating protein kinase G, which then phosphorylates the stiff titin isoform and thus improves the LV diastolic dysfunction (Flowchart 3).[10]

Therapies Targeting Late Sodium Current Inhibition

Another proposed potential mechanism of HFpEF pathophysiology is increased cytosolic calcium during diastole. When ischemia or HF sets in, there is an increase in the number of late sodium currents that occur during the process of myocyte depolarization.[11] This process results in an excess calcium accumulations during diastole via the sodium/calcium exchange pump, which leads to impaired relaxation.[12] In studies using nonischemic cardiac myocytes, ranolazine was found to decrease late sodium current and there by decrease calcium overload and diastolic dysfunction. Studies shows decrease in LV end-diastolic pressure (LVEDP) and pulmonary capillary wedge pressure (PCWP) in the ranolazine group than in placebo group.

Therapies Targeting LV Fibrosis and RAAS Inhibition

Aldosterone mediates vascular and cardiac remodelling. It also gets bound to the mineralocorticoid receptor

- Symptoms and signs of heart failure
- Risk factors for heart failure:
  - >60 years of age
  - Hypertension
  - Proinflammatory coexisting conditions
  - Previous hospitalization for heart failure

↓

Cardiac imaging: ejection fraction ≥50%

↓ → Consider alternative or contributing causes

Objective findings that support heart failure
(the more positive features, the greater the likelihood of heart failure with preserved ejection fraction)

- Electrocardiography
  - Left ventricular hypertrophy
  - Left atrial enlargement
  - Atrial fibrillation
- Chest radiography (current or past)
  - Cardiomegaly
  - Pulmonary venous hypertension
  - Interstitial or alveolar edema
  - Pleural effusion
- Natriuretic peptide assay
  - BNP>100 pg/mL
  - NT-proBNP >400 pg/mL
- Doppler echocardiography
  - Cardiac remodeling
    - Relative wall thickness >0.42
    - Left ventricular mass >95 g/m^2 in women or >115 g/m^2 in men
  - Left atrial volume >34 mL/m^2
- Elevated left atrial pressure
  - E/A ≥2.0
  - E/e′ ratio ≥15 (using septal e′)
  - E-wave deceleration time ≤140 msec
  - Decrease in E/A by ≥0.5 and to <1.0 with Valsalva maneuver
- Doppler echocardiography, continued
  - Abnormal relaxation
    - e′ <8 (septal)
  - Supportive findings (in absence of other causes)
    - Pulmonary artery systolic pressure >35 mm Hg
    - Right ventricular enlargement or systolic dysfunction

↓

Consider specialized testing in selected patients

- Stress imaging or coronary angiography
  - Angina or cardiovascular risk factors
- Right heart catheterization
  - Diagnosis in indeterminate cases
  - Define severity and mechanism of pulmonary hypertension
  - Exercise hemodynamic testing: to detect abnormal exercise but normal resting hemodynamic status
- Cardiopulmonary exercise testing
  - Quantify severity of functional limitation
  - Exclude pulmonary limitation
  - Detect chronotropic incompetence
  - Detect exaggerated hypertensive response
- Technetium-99m pyrophosphate or technetium-99m 3, 3-diphosphono-1, 2-propanedicarboxylic acid scintigraphy
  - Exclude suspected transthyretin cardiac amyloidosis

Flowchart 2 Systematic approach to the diagnosis of heart failure with preserved ejection fraction.

(*Source*: Margret M. Heart Failure with Preserved Ejection Fraction. N Engl J Med. 2016;375:1868-77.)

stimulating cardiac fibroblasts and cause an increase in the collagen synthesis and deposition. These events will eventually result in myocardial fibrosis and increased stiffness of left ventricle. Use of angiotensin-converting enzyme (ACE) inhibitors and angiotensin II receptor blockers (ARBs) to block the renin–angiotensin–aldosterone system (RAAS) aims at improving the outcomes in patients with HFpEF. However, the major outcome trials, namely CHARM-preserved (Candesartan), PEP-CHF (Perindopril), I-preserve (Irbesartan), RAAM-PEF (Eplerenone), TOPCAT, and Aldo-DHF (Spironolactone), were unsuccessful to show any mortality benefit in patients with HFpEF. However, such a therapeutic strategy does not emerge as a harmful one and should be considered for the treatment of appropriate concomitant frequent comorbidities in HFpEF.

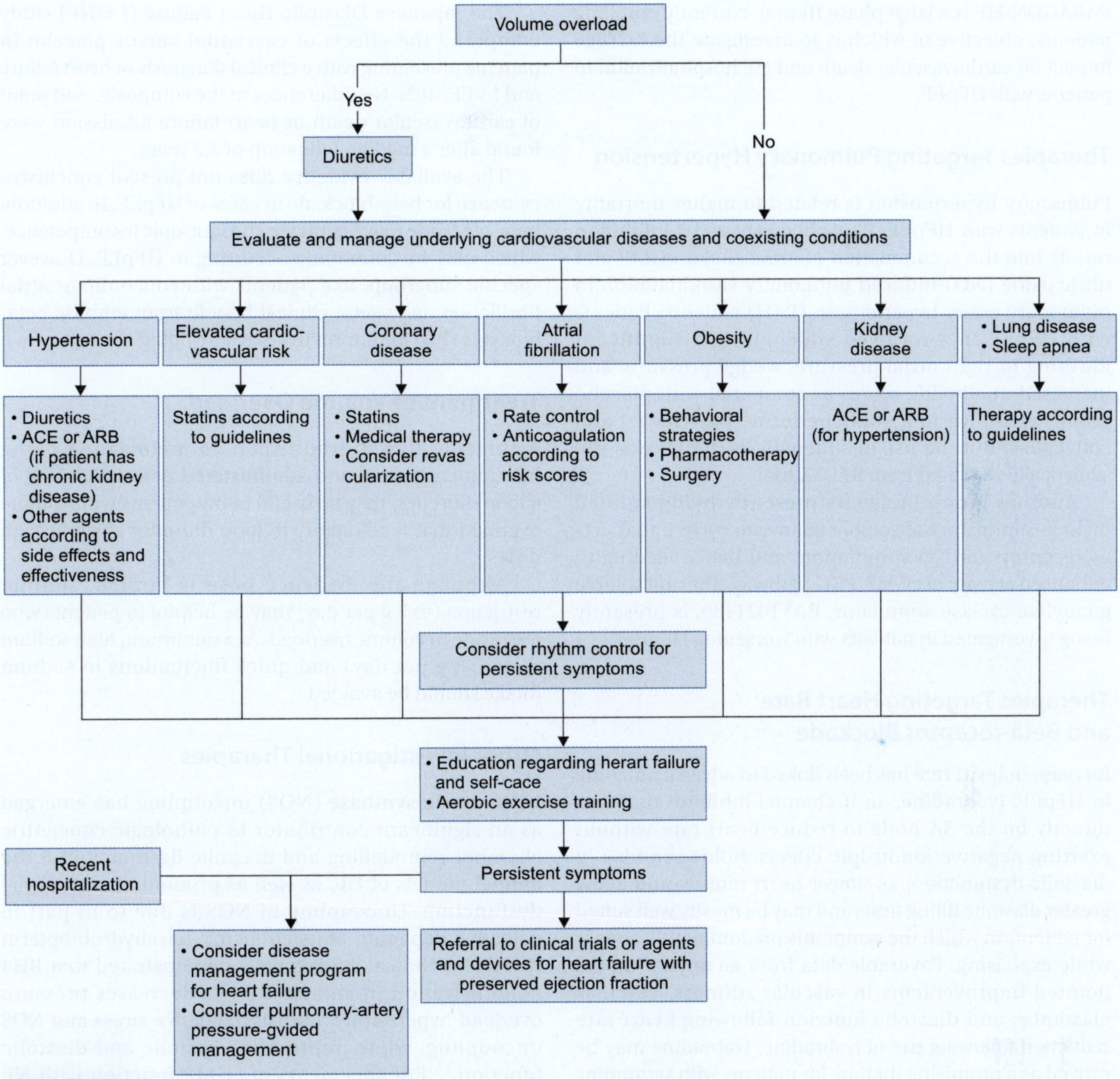

Flowchart 3 Treatment algorithm for heart failure with preserved ejection fraction.

(*Source*: Margret M. Heart Failure with Preserved Ejection Fraction. N Engl J Med. 2016;375:1868-77.)

Therapies Targeting Natriuretic Peptide

Natriuretic peptides (NP), including brain NP (BNP) and atrial NP (ANP) exhibits both antiproliferative and natriuretic properties and play a vital role in fluid homeostasis. Neprilysin is a protease enzyme that degrades NPs, thus enzyme inhibition could be of potential help in decreasing fluid overload. The new drug LCZ696, contains both angiotensin receptor inhibitor (Valsartan) and neprilysin inhibitors, has demonstrated promising results in HFpEF.[13] The PARAMOUNT 31 trial in phase II compared LCZ696 with valsartan in 308 patients. Patients in the LCZ696 arm showed more improvement in left atrial size, along with improvement in the symptom severity.

PARAGON-HF is a large phase III trial, currently enrolling patients, objective of which is to investigate the LCZ696 impact on cardiovascular death and HF hospitalization in patients with HFpEF.

Therapies Targeting Pulmonary Hypertension

Pulmonary hypertension is related to higher mortality in patients with HFpEF. Phosphodiesterase-5 inhibition results into the accumulation of intracellular cGMP and nitric oxide (NO)-induced pulmonary vasodilatation in pulmonary artery hypertension (PAH) patients. Patients with HFpEF that received sildenafil had significant lowering of right atrial pressure, wedge pressure, and increased quality life scores as compared with placebo group, as shown in a study performed by Guazzi and colleagues. But the use of sildenafil in HFpEF was not statistically validated from RELAX trial.

Another group of agents presently being studied include stimulators of soluble guanylate cyclase that acts as receptors for NO stimulation, and hence leading to enhanced activity of cGMP-PKG pathway. The oral soluble guanylate cyclase stimulator, BAY1021189, is presently being investigated in patients with worsening HFpEF.[14]

Therapies Targeting Heart Rate and Beta-receptor Blockade

Increase in heart rate has been linked to adverse outcome in HFpEF. Ivabradine, an If-channel inhibitor that acts directly on the SA node to reduce heart rate without exerting negative ionotropic effects, holds promise in diastolic dysfunction; as slower heart rates would allow greater diastolic filling time, and may be mostly well suited for patients in which the symptoms predominantly appear while exercising. Favorable data from an animal model pointed improvements in vascular stiffness, vascular elastance, and diastolic function following heart rate reduction following use of ivabradine. Ivabradine may be proved as a promising therapy for patients with symptoms that only appear while exercising.

Patients with HFpEF have increased serum levels of norepinephrine similar to patients with HFrEF, which suggests a potential target for therapy. The Effect of Long-term Administration of Nebivolol on clinical symptoms (ELANDD) trial demonstrates that there was no alteration in 6-minute walk test distance and peak oxygen uptake. The investigators suggested that the negative chronotropic effects of nebivolol could be drawn in the lack of response to exercise capacity.

The Japanese Diastolic Heart Failure (J-DHF) study compared the effects of carvedilol versus placebo in patients presenting with a clinical diagnosis of heart failure and LVEF>40%. No differences in the composite end point of cardiovascular death or heart failure admission were found after a median follow-up of 3.2 years.

The available evidence does not present conclusive evidence for beta-blockade in cases of HFpEF. In addition, beta-blockade may aggravate chronotropic incompetence, which may be commonly occurring in HFpEF. However specific subgroup, like patients with concomitant atrial fibrillation, may get a clinical benefit from empiric beta-blockers (BB) for improving diastolic filling.

Treatment of Volume Overload

A thiazide-like diuretic such as metolazone being intermittently used and administered before the dose of a loop diuretics, may be useful in outpatients with volume overload that is refractory to loop diuretics given in high doses.

Although the evidence base is limited, sodium restriction (to 2 g per day) may be helpful in patients who are prone to volume overload. At a minimum, high sodium diets (>6 g per day) and quick fluctuations in sodium intake should be avoided.

Other Investigational Therapies

Nitric oxide synthase (NOS) uncoupling has emerged as an significant contributor to pathologic concentric chamber remodelling and diastolic dysfunction in the animal models of HF, as well as promoting endothelial dysfunction. Uncoupling of NOS is due to in part to oxidative depletion of its co-factor, tetrahydrobiopterin (BH4). Preclinical studies have demonstrated that BH4 administration in animal models decreases pressure overload hypertrophy, fibrosis, oxidative stress and NOS uncoupling, while improvising systolic and diastolic function.[15] Enhancements of cGMP function with NP or also may moderate pathologic increases in LV filling pressures during exercise.

Rho-kinase inhibitors, like fasudil and Y-27632, have vasodilatation properties and have demonstrated the ability to blunt hypertrophic remodelling progression in animal models of HF.[16] Intriguingly, 3-HMG CoA reductase inhibitors (statins) also hold back rho-kinase signaling; and a case series reported that statin use was linked with the improved outcome in HFpEF, whereas other conventional HF therapies such as ACE Inhibitors or BB were not.

Autonomic dysfunction has prevalence in HFpEF, and improvement in parasympathetic tone via carotid sinus stimulation has been proposed as a treatment but data are not existing. Dyssynchrony is common in HFpEF, but in contrast to HFrEF, delay in electrical conduction is not, and it remains unidentified whether resynchronization therapy may play a role in HFpEF.

Alagebrium chloride (ALT-711) is a new compound that break glucose cross links and improvises ventricular and arterial compliance in animals and decreases blood pressure and vascular stiffness in human hypertension.[17]

Transforming growth factor-beta (TGF-β) is a profibrotic cytokine and infusion of TGF-β neutralizing antibody in a rat model of pressure overload was found to reduce fibrosis and diastolic dysfunction.

FUNCTIONAL IRON DEFICIENCY AND ANEMIA

In a small study, functional iron deficiency was there in almost 50% of HFpEF. FAIR-HFpEF trial is in progress to observe the effect of intravenous (IV) iron (ferric carboxymaltose) on exercise tolerance, symptoms, and quality of life in patients with HFpEF and also iron deficiency with or without anemia.

Bendavia

Bendavia (mitochondrial enhancer) is being evaluated in Mito-HFpEF trial, an ongoing study.

TREATMENT OF COEXISTING CONDITIONS

Treatment of hypertension, dyslipidemia, coronary artery disease, and atrial fibrillation to be done according to the current guidelines.

OTHER THERAPIES TO REDUCE SYMPTOMS OR INCREASE EXERCISE TOLERANCE

Nitrates are very frequently prescribed for patients who have HFpEF. However, a randomized, placebo-controlled trial of isosorbide mononitrate did not demonstrate increases in submaximal exercise capacity or quality-of-life sores in these patients.

In small studies, exercise training has constantly been shown to generate clinically meaningful increase in exercise capacity and a lessening of symptoms. Clinicians should advise a daily target of 30 minutes of aerobic exercise tailored to the abilities and resources in particular to every patient.

NONPHARMACOLOGICAL TREATMENT

Autonomic Modulation and Chronotropic Incompetence

One of the factors implicated in the pathophysiology of HFpEF is autonomic dysfunction.. Modulation of autonomic function, e.g. by baroreceptors activation, vagal nerve stimulation, and renal artery denervation, is under investigation for treating patients with HFpEF.

Controlled Left-to-right Interatrial Shunt

In patients with HF and EF more than or equal to 40%, creation of an interatrial shunt with the interatrial shunt device (IASD) leads to unloading of left atrium and reduction of PCWP during exercise (REDUCE LAP-HF I trial).

Implantable Hemodynamic Monitoring

The wireless CardioMEMS pulmonary artery monitoring device has been approved by the USFDA for monitoring pulmonary artery pressure and heart rate in patients with New York Heart Association (NYHA) class III HF, who have been hospitalized during the previous year (Fig. 1).

The CHAMPION randomized, single-blind trial found that transmission of pulmonary artery pressure data from device reduced HF-related hospitalization at 6 months. An exploratory subgroup analysis found that device-guided management reduce HF-related hospitalization in patients with HFpEF as well as in patients with HFrEF. However, the efficacy of the CardioMEMS device in this population has not been established.

CONCLUSION

The ideal treatment modality of HFpEF should be one that is capable enough to alleviate symptom but also provide benefit in mortality or morbidity. Regrettably, to date, there has been no treatment that has confirmed to achieve both arms. Studies of neurohumoral blocking agents in patients with HFpEF have been unsuccessful in showing a mortality benefit, although one should continue using inhibitors of RAAS and sympathetic nervous system in the population of patients with HFpEF who present with other comorbidities. While the usage of drugs like LCZ696 seems promising, research is still ongoing with respect to whether this would actually help the patients with multiple comorbidities such as atrial

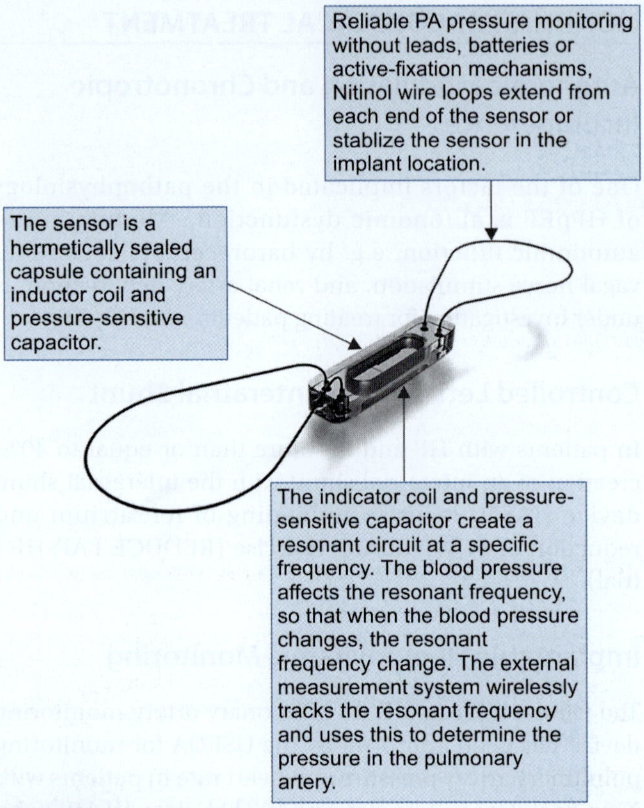

Figure 1 Wireless CardioMEMS pulmonary artery pressure monitoring system.

fibrillation, which renders the myocardium less receptive to intervention. Research are still ongoing for suitable combination of medications to decrease the mortality and morbidity in these patients.

REFERENCES

1. Paulus WJ, Tschöpe C, Sanderson JE, et al. How to diagnose diastolic heart failure: a consensus statement on the diagnosis of heart failure with normal left ventricular ejection fraction by heart failure and echocardiography Associations of the European Society of Cardiology. Eur Heart J. 2007;28(20):2539-50.
2. Steinberg BA, Zhao X, Heidenreich PA, et al. Trends in patients hospitalized with HFpEF: prevalence, therapies, and outcomes. Circulation. 2012;126(1):65-75.
3. Lam CS, Roger VL, Rodeheffer RJ, et al. Cardiac structure and ventricular-vascular function in person with HFpEF from Olmsted county, Minnesota. Circulation. 2007;115(15):1982-90.
4. Kötter S, Gout L, Von frieling-Salewsky M, Müller AE, et al. Differential changes in titin domain phosphorylation increase myofilament stiffness in failing human hearts. Cardiovasc Res. 2013;99(4):648-56.
5. Grewal J, McKelvie RS, Persson H, et al. Usefulness of N-terminal pro-brain natriuretic peptide and brain natriuretic peptide to predict cardiovascular outcomes in patients with heart failure and preserved left ventricular ejection fraction. Am J Cardiol. 2008;102:733(6)-7.
6. Rossi A, Cicoira M, Florea VG, et al. Chronic heart failure with preserved left ventricular ejection fraction: diagnostic and prognostic value of left atrial size. Int J Cadiol. 2006;110(3):386-92.
7. Chung CS, Hutchinson KR, Methawsin M, et al. Shortening of the elastic tandem of the immunoglobulin segment of titin leads to diastolic dysfunction. Circulation. 2013;128(1):19-28.
8. Baurlag BA, Nishimura RA, Sorajja P, et al. Exercise hemodynamics enhance diagnosis of early heart failure with preserved ejection fraction. Circ Heart Fail. 2010;3(5):588-95.
9. Asp MI, Martindale JJ, Heinis FI, et al. Calcium mishandling in diastolic dysfunction: mechanisms and potential therapies. Biochim Biophys Acta. 2013;1833(4):895-900.
10. Borbély A, van Heerebeek L, Paulus WJ. Transcriptional and posttranscriptional modifications of titin: implications for diastole. Circ Res. 2009;104(1):12-14.
11. Jacobshagen C, Bellardineli L, Hasenfuss G, et al. Ranolazine for the treatment of heart failure with preserved ejection fraction: background, aims and design of the RALI-DHF study. Clin cardiol. 2011;34(7):426-32.
12. Maier LS, Layug B, Karwatoska-Prokopczuk E, et al. Ranolazine for the treatment of diastolic heart failure in patients with preserved ejection fraction: the RALI-DHF: proof-of-concept study. JACC Heart Fail. 2013;1(2):115-22.
13. Solomon SD, Zile M, Pieske B, et al. The angiotensin inhibitor neprilysin inhibitor LCZ696 in heart failure with preserved ejection fraction: a phase 2 doubled blind randomized controlled trial. Lancet. 2012;380(9851):1387-95.
14. National Institute of Health. (2013). Phase IIb safety and efficacy study of four dose regimens BAY1021189 in patients with heart failure with preserved ejection fraction suffering from worsening chronic heart failure. (SOCRATES-PRESERVED). [Online]. Available from https://clinicaltrials.gov/ct2/show/NCT01951638. [Last accessed September, 2019].
15. Moens AL, Takimoto E, Tocchetti CG, et al. Reversal of cardiac hypertrophy and fibrosis from pressure overload by tetrahydrobiopterin: efficacy of recoupling nitric oxide synthase as a therapeutic strategy. Circulation. 2008;117(20):2626-36.
16. Lai A, Frishman WH. Rho-kinase inhibition in the therapy of cardiovascular disease. Cardiol Rev. 2005;13(6):285-92.
17. Kass DA, Shapiro EP, Kawaguchi M, et al. Improved arterial compliance by a novel advanced glycation end-product crosslink breaker. Circulation. 2001;104(13):1464-0.

33 CHAPTER Antidiabetic Agents and Gut Microbiome

Ranjit Unnikrishnan

INTRODUCTION

The human body is home to more than 100 trillion microorganisms, which exceed the number of human cells by 2–3 folds. The majority of these microorganisms reside in the gut, primarily the large intestine. The microbial flora of the gut is termed the gut microbiota.

The human gut is sterile at birth but becomes colonized during passage through the maternal birth canal. Further changes in the microbiome occur upon introduction of solid food, but once the adult microbiome is established, it remains remarkably consistent unless disturbed by disease or medication. While there exists diversity of bacterial species in the gut, most of the human gut microbiome can be considered to belong to three major phyla—*Actinobacteriaceae*, *Firmicutes*, and *Bacteroidetes*.

Gut microbiota have been postulated to play a major role in several forms of human disease, including obesity and type 1 and type 2 diabetes. They are also influenced by various medications, including antibiotics. Various studies have assessed the changes in gut microbiota occurring in type 2 diabetes (T2D). In general, these studies have shown that there is moderate to severe gut microbial dysbiosis in T2D, characterized by a reversal of the normal *Bacteroidetes: Firmicutes* ratio as well as a decline in the abundance of butyrate-producing bacteria that are otherwise numerous in a healthy gut.[1] These changes might lead to a proinflammatory state whereby products of bacterial metabolism or components of the cell wall (such as lipopolysaccharides) are able to access the systemic circulation and promote release of inflammatory cytokines. It has been shown that a diet rich in calories and refined sugars can promote these changes in the gut microbiota.[2] Alterations of gut microbiota have also been postulated to increase propensity to type 1 diabetes by increasing the leakiness of the intestinal tight junctions and allowing absorption of immunogenic elements into the bloodstream.[3]

Conversely, a diet rich in whole grains and fiber has been shown to reverse these changes to a great extent. Use of probiotics and prebiotics has also been shown to favorably modulate the gut microbial profile, and has also been associated with metabolic benefits in T2D.[4]

There are several classes of antidiabetic medications available at present. Several of them have effects on the gastrointestinal tract and can be expected to affect the gut microbiota also. Indeed, the gut, as a member of the "ominous octet", might play a more important role in the pathogenesis of T2D than has been assumed previously. The relationship between antidiabetic medications and gut microbiome may take one of three forms.

1. The medication may favorably alter the gut microbiome, helping in metabolic control of diabetes.
2. The metabolism and efficacy of the drug may be dictated in part by the nature of the gut microbiome; and
3. The gut microbiome may influence the gastrointestinal tolerability of the drug.

In this chapter, we will discuss the current evidence linking antidiabetic medications to changes in the gut microbiota.

METFORMIN

Metformin is a biguanide drug, currently recommended as the first line of therapy in most patients with T2D. Its advantages include low risk of hypoglycemia, modest weight loss, and low cost. The exact mechanism of action remains unclear even after 60 years of clinical use.

There is, however, some evidence to suggest that at least part of the antidiabetic effect of metformin is mediated through the gut. For instance, metformin is effective orally but not intravenously. Metformin has also been shown to alter the enterohepatic circulation of bile acids. In another recent study, extended release metformin (which is not absorbed systemically but releases active drug in the large intestine) was found to lower HbA1c to a greater extent than conventional sustained release metformin.[5]

In rodents, metformin has been shown to favorably alter gut microbiota, but only under conditions of a high-fat diet (HFD). Metformin has been shown to alter the relative abundances of *Firmicutes* and *Bacteroidetes*, and reduce bacterial diversity, in mice on HFD. Metformin also increases the abundance of butyrate producers such as *Blautia*, *Bacteroides*, *Butyricicoccus*, and *Phascolarctobacterium*.[6]

In humans, metformin increase the abundance of *Akkermansia* and *Lactobacillus*, as also of the butyrate producers such as *Bifidobacterium*, *Prevotella*, *Megasphaera*, and *Butyrivibrio*. *Akkermansia* is a mucin-degrading bacterium while *Bifidobacterium* has been shown to negatively correlate with HbA1c. Restoration of abundance of these genera could play a role in the antidiabetic efficacy of metformin. However, there is some evidence to show that the GI side effects of metformin may also be mediated by its effects on the gut microbiota.[7]

ALPHA-GLUCOSIDASE INHIBITORS

Alpha-glucosidase inhibitors (AGIs) reduce postprandial glucose spikes by inhibiting the digestion and absorption of dietary poly- and di-saccharides. They perform this action by inhibiting the alpha glucosidase enzymes found in the small intestinal brush border.

The AGIs have potent direct and indirect effects of bacterial metabolism and thereby influence the structure and function of the gut microbiome. In mice, use of the AGI miglitol has been shown to reverse the increase in abundance of *Erysipelotrichaceae* and *Coriobacteriaceae* induced by a HFD, and thereby reduce inflammation. Use of acarbose has been shown to increase short chain fatty acid-producing bacteria such as *Lactobacillus*, *Bifidobacterium*, *Faecalibacterium*, and *Prevotella*, and also to reduce the utilization of starch by propionate-producing bacteria. Voglibose has been shown to restore the *Bacteroidetes* to *Firmicutes* ratio that is deranged in T2D.[8]

GLUCAGON LIKE PEPTIDE-1 RECEPTOR AGONISTS

Glucagon like peptide-1 (GLP-1) is an incretin hormone secreted from the gut in response to a carbohydrate load. This hormone acts on the beta cells of the pancreatic islets of Langerhans to promote glucose-dependent insulin release. It also inhibits release of glucagon from the alpha cells. It reduces gut motility and induces satiety. Native GLP-1 has a short half-life because it is rapidly inactivated by the enzyme dipeptidyl peptidase-4 (DPP-4). Numerous synthetic analogs of GLP-1 have been developed, that are resistant to inactivation by DPP-4 and these are now important agents in the treatment of T2D.

The GLP-1 receptor agonist (GLP-1 RA) liraglutide has been shown to reduce bacterial diversity in HFD-fed mice, by enriching *Firmicutes* and depleting *Bacteroidetes*, *Proteobacteria*, and *Actinobacteria*. Interestingly, liraglutide enhances the abundance of several genera of bacteria associated with weight loss, such as *Lactobacillus*, *Turicibacter*, *Blautia*, and *Coprococcus*, while it depletes obesity-related bacteria such as *Erysipelotrichaceae incertae sedis*, *Marvinbryantia*, *Roseburia*, *Candidatus Arthromitus*, and *Parabacteroides*.[8]

DIPEPTIDYL PEPTIDASE-4 INHIBITORS

Another approach to enhancing the incretin effect is to minimize the degradation of native GLP-1 by inhibiting DPP-4. The DPP-4 inhibitors are potent oral antidiabetic agents that prolong the half-life of GLP-1.

The effects of DPP-4 inhibitors on the gut microbiome are milder than those of GLP-1 RA. In mice, treatment with saxagliptin increased the abundance of *Firmicutes* (particularly *Lactobacillus*, *Allobaculum*, and *Turicibacter*) at the expense of *Bacteroidetes* (particularly *Bacteroides* and *Prevotella*). In contrast to liraglutide, saxagliptin reduced the abundance of only one genus of obesity-related phylotype viz. *Candidatus Arthromitus*.[8]

SODIUM GLUCOSE COTRANSPORTER-2 INHIBITORS

The sodium glucose cotransporter-2 (SGLT-2) inhibitors reduce hyperglycemia by inhibiting the SGLT2 transporter found on the proximal convoluted tubule of the nephron. This leads to loss of a significant proportion of the filtered glucose by means of glycosuria. Recently, dual inhibitors have been developed, that inhibit not only SGLT-2, but also SGLT-1, which is responsible for glucose absorption from the gut as well as the distal (S3) segment of the proximal convoluted tubule of the nephron.

There is little data on the effect of SGLT2 inhibitors on gut microbiota. Use of dapagliflozin has been shown to decrease the gut microbial diversity in mice, as well as the *Firmicutes*: *Bacteroidetes* ratio. Dapagliflozin administration has also been shown to increase the abundance of *A. muciniphila*, which is associated with favorable metabolic outcomes.[8] Use of dual SGLT inhibitors can be expected to induce greater changes in the gut microbiome, but data, thus far, is lacking.

ORLISTAT

Orlistat is an inhibitor of pancreatic lipase enzyme, which has been used as an agent for weight loss due to its effect in reducing fat absorption. There is also evidence that this agent can delay or prevent the progression of prediabetes to diabetes. By increasing the availability of fat to the colon, orlistat may cause alterations in the gut microbiome. However, there have been no large studies assessing this effect of orlistat thus far, with the only (small) study showing no effect from the increased fat delivery to the colon.[9].

OTHER AGENTS

There are several other agents used for the treatment of T2D, such as sulfonylureas, meglitinides. thiazolidinediones, bromocriptine, and hydroxychloroquine. There is as yet little evidence for any effect of these agents on the gut microbiome.

EFFECTS OF GUT MICROBIOTA ON DRUG METABOLISM

All orally administered drugs have to pass through the gut and its epithelium in order to reach the systemic circulation. During this course, they may be acted upon by various microbial as well as host enzymes, with significant consequences for their efficacy. Gut microbes elaborate several enzymes such as beta-glucuronidase, azo-reductase, nitroreductase, N-acetyltransferase, and proteases which can either act on a prodrug or drug conjugate and activate it, or degrade an active drug and inactivate it.[9] The effect of gut microbiota on drug kinetics has been best studied for acarbose, which is activated to form more potent inhibitors by means of bacterial enzymes in the intestinal wall. The effect on other antidiabetic agents remains to be studied.

CONCLUSION

The role of gut microbiota in metabolic disease is an emerging topic of research. The gut microbiome influences susceptibility to disease and can be successfully manipulated in order to better manage disease. There is now considerable evidence to show that antidiabetic agents exert their effects, at least in part, through modulation of the gut microbiome. This is particularly so for agents such as metformin, alpha glucosidase inhibitors, and GLP-1 receptor agonists, which have a GI-based mechanism of action. The efficacy of drugs as well as the propensity to side effects may also be mediated through the gut microbiome. Further studies are needed to elucidate how best this knowledge can be utilized for the better management of T2D.

REFERENCES

1. QinJ, Li Y, Cai Z. A metagenome-wide association study of gut microbiota in type 2 diabetes. Nature. 2012;490:55-60.
2. Cani PD, Neyrinck AM, Fava F, et al. Selective increases of bifidobacteria in gut microbiota improve high-fat-diet-induced diabetes in mice through a mechanism associated with endotoxemia. Diabetologia. 2007;50: 2374-83.
3. Sanz Y, Olivares M, Moya-Perez A, et al. Understanding the role of gut microbiota in metabolic disease risk. Pediatr Res. 2015;77(1-2):236-44.
4. Houghton D, Hardy T, Stewart C et al. Systematic review assessing the effectiveness of dietary intervention on gut microbiota in adults with type 2 diabetes. Diabetologia. 2018;61(8):1700-11.
5. Buse JB, DeFronzo RA, Rosenstock J, et al. The primary glucose-lowering effect of metformin resides in the gut, not the circulation: results from short-term pharmacokinetic and 12-week dose-ranging studies. Diabetes Care. 2016;39(2):198-205.
6. Montandon SA, Jornayvaz FR. Effects of antidiabetic drugs on gut microbiota composition. Genes (Basel). 2017;8(10):E250.
7. Lv Y, Zhao X, Guo W, et al. The relationship between frequently used glucose-lowering agents and gut microbiota in type 2 diabetes mellitus. J Diabetes Res. 2018;2018:1890978.
8. Whang A, Nagpal R, Yadav H. Bi-directional drug-microbiome interactions of anti-diabetics. EBioMed. 2019;39:591-602.
9. Morales P, Fujio S, Navarrete P, et al. Impact of dietary lipids on colonic function and microbiota: An experimental approach involving orlistat-induced fat malabsorption in human volunteers. Clin Transl Gastroenterol. 2016;7:e161

CHAPTER 34 Metformin: Simple Drug with Mysterious Benefits

Puneet Rijhwani, Aviral Gupta, Shilpi Rijhwani

INTRODUCTION

Synthesized nearly 100 years ago, metformin has been gaining recognition in the past few decades for its role in diabetes and its multitude of benefits in preventing the associated complications. Despite an abundance of research and technological advances, the exact mechanisms of action of this simple drug still elude us, but the mysterious benefits it provides are a subject of great interest to both researchers and clinicians. Regarded as one of the first-line drugs in management of type 2 diabetes, could this drug have the potential to stop the diabetes juggernaut?

HISTORY OF METFORMIN

Dimethylbiguanide or metformin, the only biguanide currently approved for use in treatment of type 2 diabetes, is the most commonly prescribed oral antidiabetic drug in the world. A herbal medicine derived from *Galega officinalis* (also known as French lilac, goat's rue), described for use in symptoms of what is now known to be diabetes, has been dated back to the 17th century.[1] Later, in 1918, it was identified that guanidine was the active substance with blood glucose lowering properties, which led to the synthesis and discovery of guanidine derivatives and biguanides. These compounds, with the exception of metformin, were used to treat diabetes throughout the 1920s and 1930s, but needed to be discontinued in view of their toxicity and the increasing availability of insulin.

Metformin (which was then forgotten) was rediscovered in the 1940s, when guanidine-based derivative proguanil was undergoing research for the treatment of malaria and influenza, and it was noted that its modified form metformin (called flumamine) could lower blood glucose.[1] Jean Sterne, in 1957, then published the landmark paper which led to the reemergence of metformin as an antidiabetic drug. Between 1977 and 1980, phenformin and buformin (the other biguanides) were withdrawn in most countries due to their risk of lactic acidosis, but metformin survived this biguanide cull.[1] Throughout the 1980s and the early 1990s, clinical and scientific data continued to accumulate on the safety profile of metformin and in 1994, the Food and Drug Administration (FDA) approved the use of metformin as an antidiabetic agent.

Metformin is now recommended as the first-line oral agent for type 2 diabetes by the European Association for the Study of Diabetes (EASD) and American Diabetes Association (ADA) since 2009.[2]

MECHANISM OF ACTION OF METFORMIN

The exact mechanism of action of metformin remains unclear. Metformin concentrates in the jejunal mucosa and hepatic circulation, which might be responsible for its gastrointestinal side effects and indicate its therapeutic efficacy. It causes reduced intestinal glucose uptake and alters the intestinal microbiome, which might contribute to its weight-lowering effect.[3] Increased levels of postprandial glucagon-like peptide-1 (GLP-1) and its receptor, along with a mild decrease in dipeptidyl peptidase 4 (DPP-4) activity, has been noted.[4] In the liver, metformin inhibits complex 1 of the mitochondrial respiratory chain, leading to activation of adenosine monophosphate (AMP)-activated protein kinase (AMPK). AMPK-independent effects are also responsible for some of the actions of metformin. The net result is a lowering of blood glucose due to decreased hepatic glucose output and gluconeogenesis. Metformin also increased the sensitivity of peripheral tissues to insulin, resulting in decreased circulating glucose and insulin levels.

Metformin has many nonglycemic effects, with some mechanisms being common with its glycemic actions.

PHARMACODYNAMIC EFFECTS OF METFORMIN

Cardiovascular Effects

In 1998, the United Kingdom Prospective Diabetes Study (UKPDS)[5] and its 10-year follow-up[6] showed that in addition to glycemic control, low hypoglycemia risk, and weight neutrality, long-term metformin therapy had potentially advantageous effects on micro- and macrovasculature endothelium, reducing cardiovascular events and improving survival.[5,6] It demonstrated a 39% lower risk of myocardial infarction in patients on metformin. This improvement in cardiovascular outcomes is independent of its glycemic control as indicated by multivariate analysis in the Prevention of Restenosis with Tranilast and its Outcomes (PRESTO) trial.[7] The proposed mechanisms of vascular protection are improvements in endothelial function (by AMPK-dependent eNOS stimulation), coagulation and inflammatory pathway, and antithrombotic activity (by reducing insulin resistance).

The UKPDS trial showed that metformin significantly reduced diabetes-related mortality by 42% and the all-cause mortality by 36%.[5] Metformin promotes myocardial preconditioning, improves ischemic adaptation of cardiomyocyte metabolism, has a protective effect against development of heart failure, and reduces cardiomyocyte programmed cell death during ischemia.

Metformin and Atherosclerosis

Insulin resistance lies at the core of type 2 diabetes. This leads to high circulating levels of insulin, high serum triglycerides, high levels of low-density lipoprotein (LDL) cholesterol, low levels of high-density lipoprotein (HDL) cholesterol, and high concentrations of C-reactive protein and plasminogen activator inhibitor-1 (PAI-1). Metformin, by causing activation of AMP-dependent protein kinase, increases glucose consumption in muscles while decreasing hepatic glucose output. AMPK-independent mechanisms are also noted which decrease hepatic gluconeogenesis. AMPK activation has several other benefits, such as antiatherogenic activity, increased cell antioxidant defense, decreased inflammatory cell adhesion to endothelium, and increased nitric oxide synthesis.

Metformin has a direct atheroprotective effect, which is unrelated to plasma lipid levels, by preventing plaque formation in atherosclerosis. There is an inhibition of inflammatory cell adhesion to endothelium, foam cell proliferation, platelet aggregation, and smooth muscle cell proliferation. AMPK-dependent improvements in vascular endothelial cell function, prevent micro- and macrovascular complications of diabetes. Machado et al. concluded that metformin use was protective against macrovascular complications of diabetes and was associated with increased systolic carotid artery diameter and total systolic blood flow.[8] The undiscovered potential of metformin in treatment of complications associated with cerebral blood flow is interesting to say the least.

Effects on Lipid Metabolism

Metformin increases insulin sensitivity by increased insulin receptor tyrosine kinase activity, increased glycogen synthesis, higher translocation, and activity of GLUT-4 transporters. Metformin also increases plasma GLP-1 levels and its receptor expression via peroxisome proliferator activated receptor-α (PPAR-α). In adipose tissue, it inhibits lipolysis and promotes reesterification of fatty acids.

Metformin's favorable effect on lipid profile was noted in a review of several clinical studies, where it leads to reduced plasma triglyceride and LDL cholesterol levels. Animal studies indicated that metformin therapy in type 2 diabetes leads to decreased plasma LDL cholesterol and total cholesterol. In a cohort study in type 2 diabetes patients with metabolic syndrome, metformin significantly reduced body mass index (BMI), waist circumference, and total cholesterol, while simultaneously improving glycemic control.[9]

Effects on Coagulation

Diabetic patients are at an increased risk of thrombosis and have impaired fibrinolysis, which can often result in life-threatening consequences. The Diabetes Prevention Program Research Group revealed that increased levels of fibrinogen are found in diabetic patients, which did not correlate with demographic variables, improvement in blood glucose, or insulin resistance index; and metformin therapy resulted in a modest, yet significant reduction in fibrinogen levels.[10] Numerous studies on metformin's fibrinolytic potential show that there is a reduction in the concentration of PAI-1, which net results in increased fibrinolysis. Machado et al. also indicated that metformin increased plasminogen levels, thus increasing fibrinolytic activity.[8]

Effects on Glycemic Control and Diabetes Progression

The efficacy of metformin in lowering blood sugar was supported in a meta-analysis of randomized controlled trials, which revealed that metformin monotherapy contributed to a 0.9% reduction in HbA1c and a 36 mg/dL reduction in fasting blood glucose.[11] The benefits on reduced proinflammatory and procoagulant state coupled with its antiatherogenic activity might contribute to the reduced risk of cardiovascular events in type 2 diabetes.[12]

Some preclinical studies have shown the potential of metformin to decrease advanced glycation end-products (responsible for complications of diabetes), improve diabetic nephropathy, and decrease endothelial oxidative stress while improving outcomes in heart failure patients (irrespective of the improvement in glycemic control).[13]

It was hypothesized that since insulin resistance lies at the core of diabetes progression, metformin by improving insulin resistance could prevent diabetes. This was supported by the Diabetes Prevention Program (DPP) trial, which showed a significant 31% reduction in the incidence of diabetes with metformin, as compared to placebo.[14] Hostalek et al. also reported that metformin prevents progression of impaired glucose tolerance to type 2 diabetes, reduces hyperinsulinemia, and can even facilitate weight reduction in obese patients, while improving dyslipidemia in some individuals.[15]

Metformin and Weight Loss

Metformin can facilitate weight loss by increasing insulin sensitivity, decreasing appetite and changing the way the body metabolizes and stores fat.[15] Meta-analysis indicates that metformin leads to weight loss and combination of metformin and lifestyle changes can reduce BMI by 1.42.[16] The benefit of weight reduction has also been noted when used with medications that cause weight gain (such as antipsychotics).

Anti-inflammatory Actions

The anti-inflammatory properties of metformin were studied *in vivo* by Chakraborty et al. who evaluated stress and inflammatory parameters in patients with diabetes. They found reduced generation of reactive oxygen species and advanced oxidation protein products in patients on treatment with metformin, as compared to placebo.[17]

All these effects help ameliorate risk factors for coronary heart disease and a lower atherogenic blood profile.

Antineoplastic Properties of Metformin

Diabetics are at an increased risk of cancer such as those of the liver, pancreas, breast, and colon and metformin has been proposed to reduce that risk. Metformin has been used in chemotherapy in various malignancies (e.g., prostate, breast, colorectal, pancreas, and lung), both as monotherapy and as an adjuvant, based on its broad anticancer activity. The inhibition of mitochondrial complex I in cancer cells reduces tumorigenesis and the reduced levels of insulin and insulin-like growth factor 1 (IGF-1), which are tumorigenic, might explain this effect. Metformin also modifies inflammatory pathways, reduces secretion of proinflammatory cytokines by blocking transcription factor—nuclear factor κB (NF-κB), and enhances immune response to cancer cells. Both AMPK-dependent and AMPK-independent inhibition of the mammalian target of rapamycin (mTOR) pathway (which reduces cell proliferation), apoptosis and induction of cell cycle arrest are the mechanisms of its antineoplastic activity. Numerous observational studies have suggested a protective effect of metformin against cancer. However, recent studies provide conflicting data, with a meta-analysis of the available randomized controlled trials not supporting this hypothesis.[18] More investigation and data are required and are underway on this effect.

Molecular mechanism involved in antineoplastic properties of Metformin are not clear. The wound healing assays and transwell chamber were used to see the effects of this drug on the movement and invasion of women cancer cells of cervix and to study the novel antineoplastic mechanisms. This study demonstrated that it can prevent the MALAT1/ miR-142-3p sponge from emerging antineoplastic properties in cervical cancer cells of women and these cells xenografts in nude mice.[19]

Antiaging Properties

Aging is primarily caused by two mechanisms—reactive oxygen species and the TOR signaling theory. Reduced caloric intake has long been associated with increased life span, by suppressing the mTOR signaling pathway. Metformin mimics the benefits of calorie restriction without an actual reduction in caloric intake by indirectly inhibiting mTOR signaling via AMPK-dependent pathway.[20]

Nutrient deficiency mimicked by metformin also activates apoptosis (via suppressed signaling along the mTOR and IGF pathways), which is critical for extending the life span. The antiaging effect of metformin has thus been attributed to increased insulin sensitivity, reduced cholesterol and LDL levels, increased AMPK activity, antioxidant and alteration in folate and methionine metabolism. The UKPDS showed these long-term benefits of metformin, including reduced cardiovascular and all-cause mortality.[5,6]

Prospective Future in Fatty Liver

Insulin resistance and inflammation in prediabetes and diabetes lead to nonalcoholic fatty liver disease (NAFLD). Beneficial alterations in lipid metabolism have also been noted with metformin. By increasing fatty acid esterification and inhibiting lipogenesis (probably via AMPK-dependent mechanisms), metformin might be beneficial in fatty liver. Meta-analysis shows that metformin can improve insulin resistance and could potentially offer benefit in NAFLD.[21] However, this improvement in insulin resistance has not been demonstrated with a simultaneous improvement in liver histology, and currently there is insufficient evidence for its use in NAFLD.

ADVERSE EFFECTS OF METFORMIN

The most serious and life-threatening adverse event is lactic acidosis, at a rate of <10 per 100,000 patient years. Transient gastrointestinal intolerance such as abdominal pain, diarrhea, and flatulence occur frequently. Malabsorption of vitamin B_{12} can lead to vitamin B_{12} deficiency, predisposing patients to anemia, which is dose and duration related. Elevation of liver transaminases may require monitoring and withdrawal of the drug. Contraindications of therapy are metabolic acidosis, renal impairment, liver dysfunction, and dehydration.

CONCLUSION

The role of metformin in the treatment of type 2 diabetes is already well established. Its multitude of actions and good safety profile have made it the most prescribed oral antidiabetic drug. Recent literature and ongoing studies of its benefits on a wide variety of risk factors and complications of diabetes (such as lipid profile, body weight, cardiovascular risk, antiaging, and antineoplastic) are providing promising results. The potential of this safe and simple drug to shape the future of diabetes should not be underestimated.

REFERENCES

1. Bailey CJ. Metformin: historical overview. Diabetologia. 2017;60:1566.
2. Nathan DM, Buse JB, Davidson MB, et al. Medical management of hyperglycemia in type 2 diabetes: a consensus algorithm for the initiation and adjustment of therapy: a consensus statement of the American Diabetes Association and the European Association for the Study of Diabetes. Diabetes Care. 2009;32(1):193-203.
3. Forslund K, Hildebrand F, Nielsen T, et al. Disentangling type 2 diabetes and metformin treatment signatures in the human gut microbiota. Nature. 2015;528(7581):262-6.
4. Maida A, Lamont BJ, Cao X, et al. Metformin regulates the incretin receptor axis via a pathway dependent on peroxisome proliferator-activated receptor-alpha in mice. Diabetologia. 2011;54(2):339-49.
5. King P, Peacock I, Donnelly R. The UK prospective diabetes study (UKPDS): clinical and therapeutic implications for type 2 diabetes. Br J Clin Pharmacol. 1999;48(5):643-8.
6. Holman RR, Paul SK, Bethel MA, et al. 10-year follow-up of intensive glucose control in type 2 diabetes. N Engl J Med. 2008;359:1577-89.
7. Kao J, Tobis J, Mc Clelland RL, et al. Relation of metformin treatment to clinical events in diabetic patients undergoing percutaneous intervention. Am J Cardiol. 2004;93:1347-50.
8. Machado H, Vieira M, Cunha MR, et al. Metformin, but not glimepiride, improves carotid artery diameter and blood flow in patients with type 2 diabetes mellitus. Clinics. 2012;67:711-7.
9. Mourão-Júnior CA, Sá JR, Guedes OMS, et al. Effects of metformin on the glycemic control, lipid profile, and arterial blood pressure of type 2 diabetic patients with metabolic syndrome already on insulin. Braz J Biol Res. 2006;39:489-94.
10. Haffner S, Temprosa M, Crandall J, et al. Intensive lifestyle intervention or metformin on inflammation and coagulation in participants with impaired glucose tolerance. The Diabetes Prevention Program Research Group. Diabetes. 2005;54:1566-72.
11. Johansen K. Efficacy of metformin in the treatment of NIDDM. Meta-analysis. Diabetes Care. 1999;22:33-7.
12. Bailey CJ. Metformin: effects on micro and macrovascular complications in type 2 diabetes. Cardiovasc Drug Ther. 2008;22:215-24.
13. Evans JM, Doney AS, AlZadjali MA, et al. Effect of metformin on mortality in patients with heart failure and type 2 diabetes mellitus. Am J Cardiol. 2010;106(7):1006-10.
14. Diabetes Prevention Program Research Group. Ten-year followup of diabetes incidence and weight loss in the Diabetes Prevention Program Outcomes Study. Lancet. 2009;374:1677-86.
15. Hostalek U, Gwilt M, Hildemann S. Therapeutic use of metformin in prediabetes and diabetes prevention. Drugs. 2017;75:1071-94.
16. Bouza C, Lopez-Cuadrado T, Gutierrez-Torres LF, et al. Efficacy and safety of metformin for treatment of overweight and obesity in adolescents: an updated systematic review and meta-analysis. Obes Facts. 2012;5(5):753-65.
17. Chakraborty A, Chowdhury S, Bhattacharyya M. Effect of metformin on oxidative stress, nitrosative stress and inflammatory biomarkers in type 2 diabetes patients. Diabetes Res Clin Pract. 2011;93:56-62.
18. Stevens RJ, Ali R, Bankhead CR, et al. Cancer outcomes and all-cause mortality in adults allocated to metformin: systematic review and collaborative meta-analysis of randomised clinical trials. Diabetologia. 2012;55:2593-603.
19. Xia C, Liang S, He Z, et al. Metformin, a first-line drug for type 2 diabetes mellitus, disrupts the MALAT1/miR-142-3p sponge to decrease invasion and migration in cervical cancer cells. Eur J Pharmacol. 2018;830:59-67
20. Anisimov VN. Metformin: do we finally have an anti-aging drug? Cell Cycle. 2013;12:3483-9.
21. Mazza A, Fruci B, Garinis GA, et al. The role of metformin in the management of NAFLD. Exp Diabetes Res. 2012;2012:716404.

35 CHAPTER Sulfonylurea Saga after CAROLINA (Recent Trial)

Yashasvi Gautam, Akanksha Gautam

INTRODUCTION

Sulfonylurea (SU) saga started in 1942 with the discovery of this class of drug by Marcel Janbon and coworkers who were conducting a study on sulfonamide antibiotics and revealed that the compound sulfonylurea induced hypoglycemia in animals.

The first SU, tolbutamide, was marketed in the 1950s in Germany. This was followed by introducing the other first-generation agents—chlorpropamide, acetohexamide, and tolazamide. The next advancement in SU therapy in the United States did not happen until the release of the more potent second-generation agents that include glipizide and glyburide in 1984. These agents had been used in Europe for many years before this. Glimepiride, the next SU agent, sometimes referred to as a third-generation agent, was released in 1995.

Over last 70 years, SUs have chequered history but still they are extensively used, usually safe, low-cost, and relatively predictable. Their prime use-limiting side effect is hypoglycemia, though they are also related to weight gain. Usually, a reduction in glycated hemoglobin (HbA1c) of 1–2% can be expected in a responsive patient with type 2 diabetes. Despite the large number of anti-diabetic agents existing, sulfonylureas stay the most extensively used drugs for treating patients with type 2 diabetes.

SULFONYLUREA

Sulfonylureas are the oldest class of Orally administered antihyperglycemic agents (OHAs) as recommended by current guidelines for type 2 diabetes mellitus (T2DM) treatment.[1-4] The American Diabetes Association/European Association for the Study of Diabetes (ADA/EASD) position statement recommends use of sulfonylurea as first line if metformin intolerant, after metformin as second-line, or when glycemic goals are not achieved as third-line.[5] The Scottish Intercollegiate Guidelines Network (SIGN), the International Diabetes Federation (IDF), and National Institute for Health and Clinical Excellence (NICE) guidelines also recommend SUs as first- or second-line agents in patients who are not obese, with intolerance or contraindications to metformin therapy, and those needing a rapid response due to hyperglycemic symptoms.[1,2,4]

In addition, the use of SUs as first- or second-line agents for the management of T2DM has been recommended by the national guidelines from South Africa, China, Japan, and Korea.[6-9] As per Japan Diabetes Society, SUs are to be considered early on in the course of diabetes where patients present with considerable number and function of β-cells. The Indian Council of Medical Research (ICMR) guidelines for T2DM management advocate SU use, either alone, or in combination with metformin, and suggests not combining an SU with other SUs or meglitinide, as both have comparable mechanism of action.

If available, SU-containing dual or triple fixed dose combinations, (with drugs that have complementary modes of action) decrease cost, offer convenience, and improvise patient adherence.

Differences in the pharmacodynamic/pharmacokinetic (PK/PD) profiles (Table 1) of individual SUs also elucidate the variations in anti-diabetic activity, specificities to different tissue-specific SURs, hypoglycemic risk, impact on myocardial ischemic preconditioning, and insulin secretory effects.[9] In light of this, it may be astute to opt for modern SUs that pose lesser risk of hypoglycemia and are cardiac friendly. However, lack of comparable data from

TABLE 1: PK/PD profile of frequently prescribed SUs.

PK/PD properties	Glibenclamide	Gliclazide	Glipizide	Glimepiride	Glipizide XL	Gliclazide MR
Duration of action	16–24 h	10–24 h	12–24 h	24 h	>24 h	>24 h
Volume of distribution	9–10 L	13–24 L	10 –11 L	19.8–37.1 L	10 L	19 L
Protein binding (%)	99	85–99	98–99	99	98–99	>90
Metabolism	Hepatic	Hepatic (no active metabolites)	Hepatic (no active metabolites)	Hepatic (active metabolites)	Hepatic (no active metabolites)	Hepatic, (no active metabolites)
Bioavailability (%)	99	80	100	100	100	97
Half-life	10 h	8–12 h	2–5 h	5±4.1 h	2–5 h	16 h
Time to peak	2–4 h	2–4 h	1–3 h	2–3 h	6–12 h	<60–70% renal
Excretion	50% renal	80% renal	80% renal	60% renal	80% renal, 10% feces	10–20% in feces
Drug-drug interaction	May interact with CYP2C9 inducers or inhibitors	Likely increase half-life and slower elimination	No significant differences in PK properties			
PK changes in elderly	Slow elimination; higher volume of distribution					
PK changes in renal and hepatic impairment	May be altered increasing the risk of toxic reactions to drug	May affect the distribution and may also reduce the capacity for neoglucogenesis	Metabolism and excretion may be slowed	No significant differences in PK properties in renal impairment while it is not evaluted in hepatic impairment	May affect the disposition of drug and also diminish gluconeogenic capacity	May affect the distribution and may also reduce the capacity for neoglucogenesis increasing the risk of hypoglycemia

(MR: modified release; XL: extended release; PK/PD: pharmacodynamic/pharmacokinetic; SUs: sulfonylureas)

clinical trials needs careful evaluation of SUs with respect to patient-relevant endpoints.[10]

Sulfonylureas in Comorbid Conditions

Shorter-acting drugs, particularly those metabolized in the liver (glipizide), should be the favored SU in patients with moderate/severe impairment of renal functions. Gliclazide and glimepiride may also be used in mild/moderate renal impairment, preferably at lower doses.

Decline in dose and longer intervals between dose adjustments for SUs are recommended in patients with mild/moderate impairment of hepatic functions.

Sulfonylureas with a reduced risk of hypoglycemia such as gliclazide MR and glimepiride are recommended in the elderly patients. Alternatively, short-acting SUs, or SUs in low dose can be employed.

SUs are not indicated to be used in children and adolescents, and should be avoided during pregnancy and lactation (If the patient absolutely refuses for insulin, and if metformin is not tolerated/contraindicated, glibenclamide may be prescribed in pregnancy and lactation).

SULFONYLUREA: LANDMARK TRIALS

Sulfonylureas have a strong evidence base for lowering glycemia, both as monotherapy and in combination with other OHAs. In a recent systemic review and meta-analysis, monotherapy of SU was found to reduce HbA1c by 1.51% more than placebo (95% CI, 1.25, 1.78). Overall, in placebo comparator studies, SUs therapy was found to decrease the fasting plasma glucose by 20–40 mg/dL and HbA1c by 1.0%–2.0%.[5,10] Several landmark trials that include UKPDS, ADVANCE, ADOPT, and VADT-FS demonstrated that intensive glycemic control with SU-based therapy (chlorpropamide, glibenclamide, glipizide in UKPDS, gliclazide MR in ADVANCE, glibenclamide in ADOPT, and glimepiride in VADT-FS) was linked to decrease in HbA1c reduction and improvement in the long-term outcomes (Table 2).[11,12] A meta-analysis of randomized clinical trials (RCTs) that compared the metformin and glimepiride monotherapy efficacy, reported that glimepiride was as effectual as metformin in achieving glycemic control.[13]

In combination therapy with metformin,[14] rosiglitazone,[15] insulins[16] or DPP-4 inhibitor,[17] SUs yielded better glycemic control with comparatively favorable safety profiles. A systemic review reported decline in HbA1c of 1.62% (95% CI: 1.0, 2.24) with SU + OHAs, and 0.46% (95% CI: 0.24, 0.69) with SU + insulin (with reduced dose of insulin). The DiaRegis registry that examined the impact of various treatment intensification options in T2DM patients following failure of metformin, suggested that adding SU to metformin resulted into greater HbA1c reduction than incretin therapy (–0.6% vs –0.5%, $P = 0.039$) with no difference in the hypoglycemic event rates.[18]

CAROLINA Trial

CAROLINA® (Cardiovascular Outcome study of linagliptin vs glimepiride in patients with type 2 diabetes) is a multinational, randomized, double-blind, active-controlled clinical trial that involved 6,033 adults with type 2 diabetes from 43 countries at more than 600 sites observed for a median duration of more than 6 years.[19] Adults with early type 2 diabetes—adults with a median disease duration of 6.2 years, who either received no

TABLE 2: Outcomes of treatment with SUs in landmark trials.

Study	Interventions	Glycemic efficacy		Safety (rate of major hypos episode/year)	Weight gain (kg)	Outcomes
		6 months	Long-term			
UKPDS33	Intensive (chlorpropamide/ glibenclamide or insulin) versus conventional (diet alone)	HbA1c reduced to 7.0% HbA1c reduced to 7.9%		Chlorpropamide 1.0% Glibenclamide 1.2% Diet 0.7%	Chlorpropamide +2.6 Glibenclamide +1.7	12% lower risk of any diabetes-related endpoint
ADVANCE	Intensive (gliclazide MR + combination) versus standard-control therapy	6.5% 7.3%		Gliclazide MR 2.7% Control 1.5%	Gliclazide MR +0.0	Incidence of complications decreased (18% vs. 20%, HR: 0.9, $P = 0.01$)
ADOPT	Glyburide versus metformin versus rosiglitazone	Reduction in FPG and HbA1c, greatest with glyburide	Increase in FPG and HbA1c, greatest with glyburide	Serious hypos, percentage of patients Glyburide 0.6% Metformin 0.1% Resiglitazone 0.1%	Glyburide +1.6 Metformin –2.9 Rosiglitazone +4.8	Treatment failure (FPG > 180 mg/dL) at 5 years Glyburide 34% Metformin 21% Rosiglitazone 15%
ADVANCE ON	Post-observational follow-up study from ADVANCE Intensive (gliclazide MR + combination) versus standard-control therapy	HbA1c levels maintained over 10 years		Overall low	The mean body weight was similar in the intensive and standard glucose control groups	Persistent benefit of intensive glucose control with respect to end-stage renal disease (HR: 0.54; 95% CI: 0.34–0.85; $P = 0.007$) observed
VADT/ VADT-FS	Intensive versus standard care (SU used was glimepiride)	6.9% versus 8.4% (different 1.5%)	0.2–0.3% different at end of follow-up	Higher in the intensive-therapy group than standard-therapy ($P<0.001$)	4 kg gain in intensive group	At 10 years, significantly lower risk of major CV events with intensive therapy (HR, 0.083; 95% CI: 0.70–0.99; $P = 0.04$)

(FPG: fasting plasma glucose; HbA1c: glycated hemoglobin; MR: modified release; CI: confidence interval; OR: odds ratio; SUs: sulfonylureas; HR: hazard ratio)

treatment at all, or received 1–2 glucose-lowering agents (e.g. metformin) were included in the trial.[19] It was designed to evaluate the Tradjenta® (linagliptin) effect (in the doses of 5 mg once daily) compared to the sulfonylurea glimepiride (both added to stable background glucose-lowering medication and cardiovascular standard of care) on cardiovascular safety in adults with type 2 diabetes and elevated cardiovascular risk or well-known cardiovascular disease.[19] These people mirror patients that doctors typically deal with in their daily clinical practice.[5]

It is critical that we view sulfonylurea-related cardiovascular outcome data objectively, keeping in mind the nature of the sulfonylurea studied, and the limitations of the trial design used. The CAROLINA study, which compares cardiovascular outcomes with linagliptin versus glimepiride, is a welcome attempt to settle the cardiovascular safety controversy of sulfonylureas.

The CAROLINA study assessed dipeptidyl peptidase-4 (DPP-4) Inhibitor safety over the glimepiride. This study conducted longest period ever in a DPP-4 inhibitor Cardiovascular outcome trial, with a median follow-up of more than 6 years. Linagliptin was alike glimepiride in the secondary endpoint.

The CAROLINA study demonstrates similar overall effects on HbA1c, but decreased the relative risk for hypoglycemia (low blood sugar) by 77%. This reduction in the risk was consistent across all hypoglycemia categories, including severe hypoglycemia needing hospitalization. There were no differences in the overall composite endpoint of cardiovascular death (fatal stroke and fatal myocardial infarction [MI]), nonfatal MI (excluding silent MI), or nonfatal stroke. On the whole, the 3-point MACE (major adverse cardiovascular events) occurred in 11.8% of the 3,023 participants who receive linagliptin compared with 12.0% of the 3,010 participants receiving glimepiride (hazard ratio [HR], 0.98; P = .7625).

Likewise, insignificant differences were seen between linagliptin and glimepiride for each individual component of cardiovascular (CV) death (HR 1.00; 5.6% vs 5.6%; P = .9863), nonfatal MI (HR, 1.01; 4.8% vs 4.7%; P = .9060), and nonfatal stroke (HR, 0.87; 3.0% vs 3.5%; P = .3352).

The same holds relevance for secondary endpoints that includes hospitalization for heart failure (HR, 1.21; 3.7% vs 3.1%; P = .1761), CV death (HR, 1.00), non-CV death (HR, 0.82), and all-cause mortality (HR, 0.91).

No variations were seen in glycemic control. HbA1c levels dropped more hastily with glimepiride, but by the end of the trial both groups had returned to a baseline of around 7.0%. There were no differences in the proportion of patients for whom new glucose-lowering therapies, including insulin, were needed (about 40% in both groups).

Those in the glimepiride group at first gained about 0.6 kg in weight while the linagliptin group lost about 1.0 kg. The glimepiride group weighed about 1.5 kg more than the linagliptin participants, by the end of the trial.

No variations were seen between the groups in systolic or diastolic blood pressure, or in LDL cholesterol, HDL cholesterol, or triglycerides.

Hypoglycemia occurred considerably more often in the glimepiride group, including hypoglycemia overall (37.7% vs 10.6%; P< .0001), moderate to severe hypoglycemia (30.9% vs 6.5%; P < .0001), severe hypoglycemia (2.2% vs 0.3%; P < .0001), and hospitalization due to hypoglycemia (0.9% vs 0.1%; P = .0004).

CONCLUSION

The infamous 1970 publication by the University Group Diabetes Program (UGDP) study with tolbutamide, which has been discontinued since long had evoked the concerns about the cardiovascular safety of sulfonylureas. Subsequent studies with newer-generation of sulfonylureas, have not demonstrated increase in cardiovascular risk in comparison to placebo, but each of those were not capable in answering the cardiovascular safety question. The CAROLINA study resolves the decades-long highly debated cardiovascular safety of sulfonylureas, especially glimepiride.

The CAROLINA trial has done great service to diabetes care. It has provided robust proof that two commonly prescribed drugs, linagliptin and glimepiride, can continue to be used for the benefit of persons with diabetes.

It can be concluded that sulfonylureas are an effective, safe, well-tolerated, affordable, and convenient therapeutic option in the management of T2DM.

REFERENCES

1. Inzucchi SE, Bergenstal RM, Buse JB, et al. Management of hyperglycemia in type 2 diabetes, 2015: a patient-centered approach: Update to a position statement of the American Diabetes Association and the European Association for the Study of Diabetes. Diabetes Care. 2015;38(1):140-9.
2. Garber AJ, Abrahamson MJ, Barzilay JI, et al. American Association of Clinical Endocrinologists' comprehensive diabetes management algorithm 2013 statement-Executive summary. Endocr Pract. 2013;19(3):536-57.
3. National Institute for Health and care excellence (NICE) Clinical Guideline [CG87]. (2009). Type 2 Diabetes: The Management of Type 2 Diabetes. [Online]. Available from https://www.nice.org.uk/guidance/cg87. [Last accessed September, 2019].
4. Scottish Intercollegiate Guidelines Network (SIGN). (2010). Management of Diabetes. A National Clinical Guideline. [Online]. Available from https://

services.nhslothian.scot/DiabetesService/InformationHealthProfessionals/Documents/sign116.pdf. [Last accessed September, 2019].
5. Japan Diabetes Society. Treatment Guideline for Diabetes; 2012-2013. Available from: http://www.jds.or.jp/modules/en/index.php?content_id=44
6. Chinese Diabetes Society. China Guideline for type 2 Diabetes. Chin J Diabetes. 2010;2(Suppl2):1-56.
7. Ko SH, Kim SR, Kim DJ, et al.Clinical practice guidelines for type 2 diabetes in Korea.Diabetes Metab J.2011;35:431-6.
8. ICMR 2005. Available from: http://www.icmr.nic.in/guidelines_diabetes/section7.pdf. [Last accessed on 2015 Apr 03].
9. Proks P, Reimann F, Green N, et al. Sulfonylurea stimulation of insulin secretion. Diabetes. 2002;51(Suppl 3):S368–76.
10. Pfeiffer AF, Klein HH. The treatment of type 2 diabetes. DtschArztebl Int. 2014;111:69-81.
11. ADVANCE Collaborative Group, Patel A, MacMahon S, et al. Intensive blood glucose control and vascular outcomes in patients with type 2 diabetes.N Engl J Med. 2008;358:2560-72.
12. Kahn SE, Haffner SM, Heise MA, et al. Glycemic durability of rosiglitazone, metformin, or glyburide monotherapy.N Engl J Med. 2006;355:2427-43.
13. Zhu H, Zhu S, Zhang X, et al. Comparative efficacy of glimepiride and metformin in monotherapy of type 2 diabetes mellitus: meta-analysis of randomized controlled trials. Diabetol Metab Syndr. 2013;5(1):70.
14. Charpentier G, Fleury F, KabirM, et al. Improved glycaemic control by addition of glimepiride to metformin monotherapy in type 2 diabetic patients. Diabet Med. 2001;18(10):828-34.
15. McCluskey D, Touger MS, Melis R, et al. Results of a randomized, double-blind, placebo-controlled study administering glimepiride to patients with type 2 diabetes mellitus inadequately controlled with rosiglitazone monotherapy. ClinTher. 2004;26(11):1783-90.
16. Fritsche A, Schweitzer MA, Häring HU. Glimepiride combined with morning insulin glargine, bedtime neutral protamine hagedorn insulin, or bedtime insulin glargine in patients with type 2 diabetes. A randomized, controlled trial. Ann Intern Med. 2003;138:952-9.
17. Hermansen K, Kipnes M, Luo E, et al. Efficacy and safety of the dipeptidyl peptidase-4 inhibitor, sitagliptin, in patients with type 2 diabetes mellitus inadequately controlled on glimepiride alone or on glimepiride and metformin. Diabetes Obes Metab. 2007;9:733-45.
18. Gitt AK, Bramlage P, Binz C, et al. Outcome of sulfonylurea and insulin versus incretin-based treatment in type 2 diabetes patients uncontrolled on prior metformin monotherapy: Results of Dia Regis. J Am Coll Cardiol. 2014;63(12 Suppl):A1336.
19. Boehringer Ingelheim and Eli Lilly and Company. Patients and clinical practice. Data on file. Available from: https://clinicaltrials.gov/ct2/show/NCT01243424.

36 CHAPTER Glitazones: When and Why?

Amit Gupta, Jugal Kishor Sharma

INTRODUCTION

Glitazone belongs to the thiazolidinediones group of drugs.[1] At present two molecules pioglitazone and rosiglitazone are available for clinical use. The key pathophysiological defect in type 2 diabetes mellitus (T2DM) is insulin resistance and there exists an unmet need of addressing insulin resistance by means of pharmacotherapy. Two classes of drugs biguanides (i.e. metformin) and glitazones (pioglitazone and rosiglitazone) improve glycemia by acting as insulin sensitizers.[2] The clinical journey of glitazones is fascinating and marked with several ups and downs. Recent cardiovascular (CV) outcome trials has shown improved cardiovascular outcomes with two classes of drugs namely SGLT-2 inhibitors (empagliflozin in EMPA REG and canagliflozin in CANVAS Trial)[3,4] and GLP1 (glucagon-like peptide 1) analogs (liraglutide in LEADER and semaglutide in SUSTAIN-6 Trial).[5,6] In the light of these recent developments, established CV benefits of thiazolidinedione in particular pioglitazone has taken a backseat. The current review aims to address when to use glitazones and why?

HISTORICAL BACKGROUND

The first drug in this class, troglitazone was banned in the United States and the United Kingdom as it caused severe hepatic dysfunction and liver failure. The medical fraternity ever since looked at glitazones with some degree of suspicion as use of glitazones has been associated with safety issues. In 2010, sales of rosiglitazone were suspended by European medical agencies and US Food and Drug Administration (FDA) imposed restrictions on the use of rosiglitazone due to concerns regarding CV safety [increased risk of myocardial infarction (MI) and CV death] after considering the findings of the RECORD (Rosiglitazone Evaluated for Cardiac Outcomes and Regulation of Glycaemia in Diabetes) study.[7] However FDA removed its restrictions on rosiglitazone after reevaluation of RECORD study in 2013. The US FDA has also discontinued Risk Evaluation and Mitigation Strategy for rosiglitazone in 2015. In 2011, French and German medical agencies suspended the use of pioglitazone sighting safety reasons and increased risk of bladder carcinoma.

MECHANISM OF ACTION

The glitazones act by improving insulin sensitivity and reducing insulin resistance by increasing peripheral utilization of glucose by increasing the uptake of glucose in adipose tissue, muscles and liver. The exact mechanism of action of thiazolidinediones remains elusive till date however they act by binding on a nuclear receptor—peroxisome proliferator-activated receptors (PPAR).[1,2] There are two types of PPAR alpha and gamma. PPAR-alpha receptors are principally expressed in hepatic cells, cardiac muscles, skeletal muscles, and vascular walls. PPAR-gamma is expressed predominantly in adipose tissues, beta cells of the pancreas, vascular endothelium, macrophages, and central nervous system (CNS). Thiazolidinediones differ in their actions by having variable effects on PPAR alpha and gamma. Rosiglitazone is an exclusive agonist of PPAR-gamma while pioglitazone has agonist effects on PPAR-alpha also. In patients with diabetes and obesity concentration of PPAR-gamma is increased in skeletal muscles. Glitazones improve insulin responsiveness of muscles by promoting glucose uptake in skeletal muscles, increasing muscle glycogen synthesis and glucose oxidation. Thiazolidinediones promotes lipid storage by regulating production of adipokines from adipose tissue by activation of PPAR-gamma. Activation of PPAR-gamma in CNS contributes to weight gain associated with thiazolidinediones use; however, this may also be one of the possible mechanisms of improving hepatic insulin sensitivity. Pioglitazone also reverses hepatic steatosis [Nonalcoholic fatty liver disease and NASH (nonalcoholic steatohepatitis)].

GLITAZONES AND CLINICAL EFFECTS (THE GOOD AND THE BAD)

Glycemic Efficacy

Thiazolidinediones decrease A1c by 0.5–1.4% and fasting glucose by 29.6–55 mg% when used as monotherapy. Pioglitazone has glycemic efficacy as good as or even better than many other oral antidiabetic drugs including DPP4 inhibitors. Not only this durability is also better then sulfonylureas. They can be combined with metformin and other oral drugs. However, combination of insulin and glitazones in patients with heart failure resulted in an increased incidence of heart failure hence should be avoided in patients with heart failure.

Cardiovascular Effects

Rosiglitazone increases low-density lipoprotein (LDL) cholesterol levels, while LDL levels remain unaffected or rises to a less extent with pioglitazone. High-density lipoprotein (HDL) levels increase by up to 10% with both the glitazones. Pioglitazone decreases triglyceride levels to a greater extent than rosiglitazone. Both the glitazones are associated with an increase in risk of heart failure; however, the risk is higher with rosiglitazone than pioglitazone. Meta-analysis of trials studying rosiglitazone in diabetes suggests an increase in relative risk of MI with rosiglitazone. The results of an interim analysis of the RECORD data were inconclusive on MI (small number of events, higher use of statins) however it suggested an increase in risk of heart failure with rosiglitazone.[7] The data from meta-analysis of 19 trials on pioglitazone for management of diabetes and largest trial like PROactive (Prospective Pioglitazone Clinical Trial in Macrovascular events) has shown favorable CV effects. PROactive trial evaluated the effect of pioglitazone in 5,238 patients with a previous history of MI, stroke, coronary artery bypass graft surgery, acute coronary syndrome and symptomatic peripheral vascular disease. PROactive trial was terminated prematurely because of a significant decrease in the "main" secondary composite endpoint of all-cause mortality, MI (excluding silent MI), or stroke in the pioglitazone group.[8] However, there are concerns over terminating the trial prematurely, before achieving the primary outcome, late definition of a "main" secondary endpoint after the trial was underway, the analytic strategy and doubt over results if trial was to be completed.

Bladder Cancer

There is no data to suggest that rosiglitazone causes bladder and data with pioglitazone is conflicting. In PROactive trial there were more cases of bladder cancer in pioglitazone group than placebo (14 with pioglitazone and 5 with placebo).[8] However in an ongoing observational study no significant association was found between pioglitazone and bladder cancer. The risk of bladder cancer was highest with the longest duration of exposure and highest cumulative doses. A large population studies has reported that incidence of bladder carcinoma is five times less in general population with diabetes when compared to incidence of liver, colon and lung cancer. Use of pioglitazone has shown decreased incidence of liver cancer, colorectal cancer, and lung cancer, and the effect is related to duration and cumulative dose of pioglitazone.

Skeletal Fractures

Thiazolidinediones decrease bone density and increases the risk of fractures, especially in women. The absolute risk of fractures is small; however, it is advisable that thiazolidinediones be avoided in women with reduced bone density or increased fracture risk. The same cannot be said convincingly in men as results from observational studies are conflicting. Glitazones activate PPAR gamma-2 isoform of PPAR-gamma in bones, leading to decreased bone formation and increased adipogenesis in bone. The health ABC (Health Ageing and Body Composition study) has shown greater bone loss, while ADOPT (A Diabetes Outcome Progression Trial)[9] and RECORD trial has shown a higher rate of fracture in women than men with diabetes on rosiglitazone therapy. The RECORD study also highlighted that fractures occurred more frequently in upper and distal lower limbs.[7] The pioglitazone also increases the risk of bone fracture. Both pioglitazone and rosiglitazone increase the risk of low-trauma fractures in both men and women.

Hypoglycemia

Glitazone monotherapy is unlikely to cause hypoglycemia as it acts by improving insulin sensitivity; however, hypoglycemia can occur when used in combination with insulin or sulfonylureas.

Weight Gain

Both rosiglitazone and pioglitazone can cause weight gain, which are dose as well as time-dependent. In one study, rosiglitazone resulted in weight gain of up to 4.5 kg over a period of 26 weeks, while in another cohort use of pioglitazone for 30 months lead to a weight gain of up to 5.3 kg. The weight gain results from fluid retention, activation of PPAR-gamma in CNS and proliferation of new adipocytes.

Fluid Retention

Peripheral edema results from fluid retention (4–6% of cases) and is seen more often in patients with heart failure. The fluid retention may result in worsening or precipitation of heart failure. The PPAR-gamma is found in abundance along the collecting tubules of nephron. The PPAR-gamma activation in nephrons leads to reabsorption of sodium in collecting tubules in the same way as caused by aldosterone.

Hepatotoxicity

Troglitazone was associated with severe hepatotoxicity and even hepatic failure, hence the drug was withdrawn. Rosiglitazone and pioglitazone may cause mild elevation of aminotransferases. There are occasional case reports of severe hepatotoxicity and fulminant hepatic failure with pioglitazone and rosiglitazone. FDA recommends assessment of liver functions at baseline and periodically thereafter guided by clinical judgment.

Macular Edema

Glitazone can cause macular edema in patients with diabetes and the risk is highest in those who also have peripheral edema.

WHEN NOT TO USE GLITAZONES?

Glitazones are contraindicated in patients with symptomatic heart failure, New York Heart Association (NYHA) class III or IV heart failure, in patients with active bladder cancer or a history of bladder cancer. They are also contraindicated in patients with high risk of fracture like postmenopausal women with osteoporosis. They are also contraindicated in patients with type 1 diabetes, pregnancy and active liver disease.

WHY WE STILL NEED GLITAZONES?

Rosiglitazone has gone into disrepute and because of its tainted history and bad press there are few takers if any to revive interest in rosiglitazone. But Pioglitazone is still attractive as it is an inexpensive drug. It has good glycemic efficacy as well durability of effect. It addresses the basic pathophysiological defect of T2DM which is insulin resistance and also improves beta-cell function. It has a low risk of hypoglycemia when used as monotherapy. It has once a day dosing, can be combined with other antidiabetic drugs. It increases HDL, decreases triglycerides and has little or no effect on LDL. It has shown improvement in carotid intima media thickness (CIMT)—CHICAGO Trial[10] and IVUS (PERISCOPE STUDY).[11] PROactive and IRIS trial suggest positive CV benefits.[12] Weight gain can be managed by using doses of 15 mg or 30 mg and by avoiding use with insulin and combining with GLP1 agonist or SGLT 2 inhibitors. Fat deposition is more in subcutaneous stores than in viscera. In ACT NOW study pioglitazone reduced the risk of developing T2DM by 70%.[13] The QUARTET studies, has shown that pioglitazone has a consistent lowering effect on microalbuminuria. Pioglitazone also addresses the multiple pathophysiological pathways of metabolic syndrome and has a great potential as drug for NASH and fatty liver.

CONCLUSION

Diabetes care has entered a new era where the focus is on individualization of pharmacotherapy of diabetes based on the available evidence. The guidelines by all the societies are now emphasizing on choosing a therapy that not only improves glycemia and reduces the risk of CV complications but also improves CV outcomes. Myocardial infarction and stroke are the greatest cause of mortality in patients with diabetes. Pioglitazone has shown to reduce MI, stroke and CV mortality in various studies (PROactive, IRIS and Meta-analysis of several prospective studies). Most of the guidelines do not place pioglitazone higher up in hierarchy when it comes to recommendations; however, pioglitazone has a favorable

risk benefit profile if selected carefully for an appropriate patient. Thus, pioglitazone is an effective and useful drug in the management of diabetes.[14]

REFERENCES

1. Yki-Järvinen H. Thiazolidinediones. N Engl J Med. 2004;351(11):1106-18.
2. Park KS, Ciaraldi TP, Abrams-Carter L, et al. PPAR-γ gene expression is elevated in skeletal muscle of obese and type II diabetic subjects. Diabetes. 1997;46(7):1230-4.
3. Zinman B, Wanner C, Lachin JM, et al. Empagliflozin, cardiovascular outcomes, and mortality in type 2 diabetes. N Engl J Med. 2015;373(22): 2117-28.
4. Neal B, Perkovic V, Mahaffey KW, et al. Canagliflozin and cardiovascular and renal events in type 2 diabetes. N Engl J Med. 2017;377(7):644-57.
5. Marso SP, Daniels GH, Brown-Frandsen K, et al. Liraglutide and cardiovascular outcomes in type 2 diabetes. N Engl J Med. 2016;375(4): 311-22.
6. Marso SP, Bain SC, Consoli A, et al. Semaglutide and cardiovascular outcomes in patients with type 2 diabetes. N Engl J Med. 2016;375(19):1834-44.
7. Home PD, Pocock SJ, Beck-Nielsen H, et al. Rosiglitazone evaluated for cardiovascular outcomes in oral agent combination therapy for type 2 diabetes (RECORD): a multicentre, randomised, open-label trial. Lancet. 2009;373(9681):2125-35.
8. Asanuma H, Kitakaze M. Prospective pioglitazone clinical trial in macrovascular events. Nihon rinsho. Japanese J Clin Med. 2012;70:301.
9. Viberti G, Kahn SE, Greene DA, et al. A diabetes outcome progression trial (ADOPT): an international multicenter study of the comparative efficacy of rosiglitazone, glyburide, and metformin in recently diagnosed type 2 diabetes. Diabetes Care. 2002;25(10):1737-43.
10. Mazzone T, Meyer PM, Feinstein SB, et al. Effect of pioglitazone compared with glimepiride on carotid intima-media thickness in type 2 diabetes: a randomized trial. JAMA. 2006;296(21):2572-81.
11. Nissen SE, Nicholls SJ, Wolski K, et al. Comparison of pioglitazone vs glimepiride on progression of coronary atherosclerosis in patients with type 2 diabetes: the PERISCOPE randomized controlled trial. JAMA. 2008;299(13):1561-73.
12. Bath PM, Appleton JP, Sprigg N. The Insulin Resistance Intervention after Stroke trial: A perspective on future practice and research. Int J Stroke. 2016;11(7):741-3.
13. DeFronzo RA, Tripathy D, Schwenke DC, et al. Prevention of diabetes with pioglitazone in ACT NOW: physiologic correlates. Diabetes. 2013;62(11):3920-6.
14. Davidson MA, Mattison DR, Azoulay L, et al. Thiazolidinedione drugs in the treatment of type 2 diabetes mellitus: past, present and future. Crit Rev Toxicol. 2018;48(1):52-108.

37

CHAPTER

Tackling the Cardiovascular Burden of Type 2 Diabetes in Greater Manchester: The Manchester Cardiometabolic Pathway

Naresh Kanumilli, Nicola Milne

INTRODUCTION

Diabetes affects 9% of the United Kingdom adult population with type 2 diabetes (T2D) accounting for approximately 90% of all cases of diabetes.[1] T2D is associated with increased risks of a range of complications which affect a person's quality of life, care needs, and survival. Inevitably this leads to additional demands on the National Health Service (NHS) budget for more complex care and subsequent burden on social care budgets.

An estimated £10 billion, which is approximately 10% of the NHS budget, is spent on diabetes annually and a staggering 80% of this cost is for the treatment of diabetes complications such as heart disease, lower limb amputation, and renal failure.

The failure to manage T2D effectively at an early stage is resulting in a current NHS cost for diabetes of £315 per second.[2]

The most prevalent cause of mortality and morbidity in T2D is from the macrovascular complications of heart disease. Statistics show that 1 in 4 persons in hospital having had a stroke or heart attack have diabetes[2] and nationally each week there are:

- 500 premature deaths from diabetes complications,
- 2,000 new cases of heart failure,
- 680 strokes, and
- 530 heart attacks.

In Greater Manchester, 7.2% of the population are living with T2D with 8.6% thought to have T2D but are undiagnosed and 10.9% have prediabetes thus at high-risk of developing T2D.[3] Increasing obesity rates are fueling this explosion in numbers and there is much to be done in the areas of diabetes prevention and diabetes remission. Innovations such as the National Diabetes Prevention Plan,[4] digital diabetes support/well-being apps, DiRECT[5] like dietary plans and Cities Changing Diabetes[6] within Greater Manchester are gaining momentum and outcomes are keenly anticipated in terms of impact on halting the tide of numbers with T2D.

In terms of reducing the risk of onset and progression of T2D-related microvascular and macrovascular complications, studies such as STENO-2[7] show the benefits of ensuring optimal blood pressure, lipids, and glycemic control early and ongoing in a person's journey with diabetes. A potential 60% reduction in microvascular complications and a 50% reduction in macrovascular complications can be achieved with just under an estimated 8 year increased life span by treating blood pressure, lipids, and hemoglobin A1c (HbA1c) (the three treatment targets), effectively. Greater Manchester has among its diabetes priorities outlined in its Diabetes Strategy: Tackling Diabetes Together,[8] the achievement of these three treatment targets.

In February 2019, the Nuffield Health Economics Research Centre published a paper, which examined the impact of achieving these targets for T2D on health outcomes and costs and showed that achieving all three targets led to a lower incidence of diabetes-related complications and reductions in healthcare costs.[9]

Figure 1 shows the improvement gained by achieving one, two, and three of the treatment targets for each diabetes-related complication with the biggest impact made on the reduction of strokes, heart attacks [myocardial infarction (MI)], and cardiovascular disease (CVD) deaths with a relative-risk reduction of nearly a third when all three targets are achieved.

Greater Manchester has the poorest outcomes in terms of cardiovascular (CV) mortality in those aged under

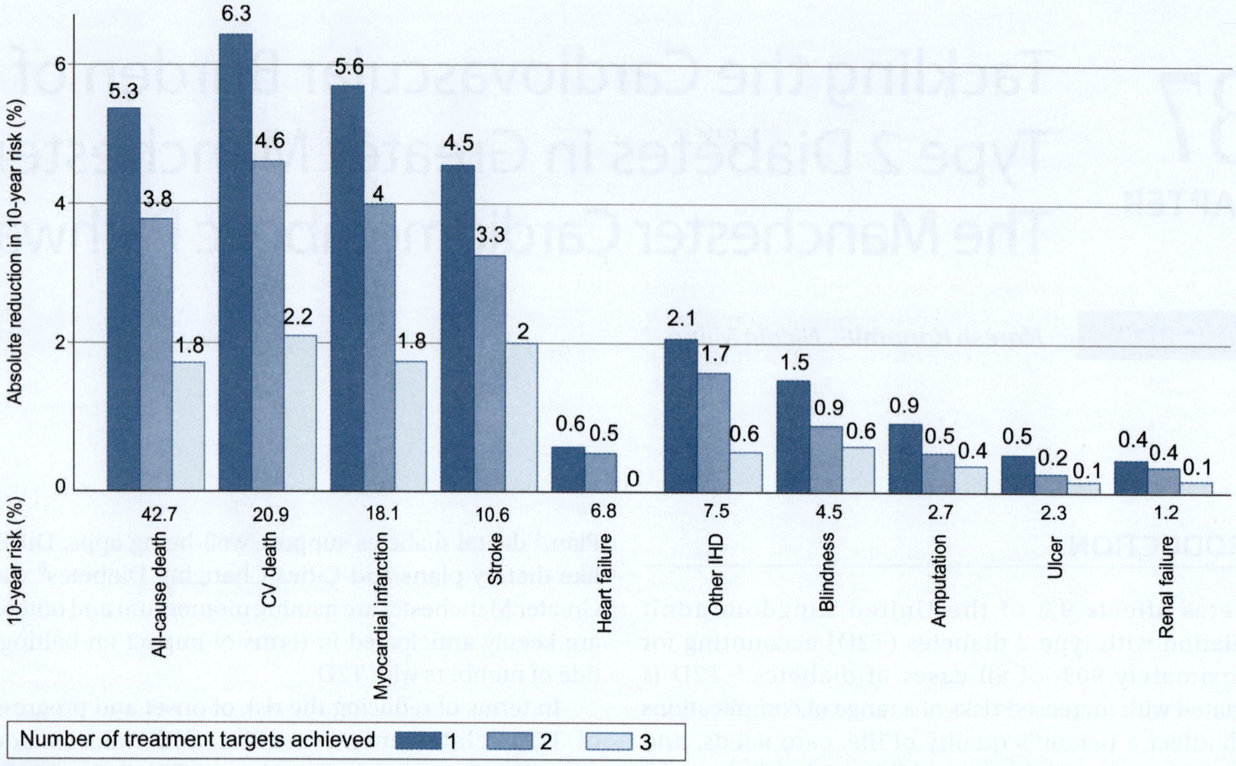

Figure 1 The improvement gained by achieving the treatment targets for each diabetes-related complication.

75 years in the UK and in the last year alone over £10 million extra has been spent on admissions for CV events in those with T2D.[10] This is unsustainable.

Within Greater Manchester against this backdrop of poor CV outcomes there has been an impetus to go even further in achieving improved outcomes. In addition to achieving the three treatment targets as above, contemplation was given to the growing evidence base of improved CV outcomes with certain anti-glycemic therapies used in T2D.[11] It has been clearly established that certain sodium-glucose cotransporter 2 (SGLT2) is and glucagon-like peptide 1 receptor agonist (GLP1-RA) therapies show a clear benefit in terms of reducing further CV events in those who have already experienced a CV event[12-16] and more recently we have seen benefit in those with heart failure and reduced ejection fraction and having no diabetes taking Dapagliflozin.[17]

Current English guidelines[18] in terms of a pathway for escalating medications when individualized HbA1c targets are unmet were developed ahead of many of the CVOT outcomes data. There is a lack of clear guidance in terms of direction of escalation of specific, more suitable medications when a person has T2D and a comorbidity to include CVD. As most T2D diabetes care in England is undertaken by generalist doctors and nurses as only a part of their overall role in terms of holistic care this lack of direction can often lead to confusion and clinical inertia.[19]

Two healthcare professionals (HCPs) within a primary care setting devised an informal, simplified pathway, based on CVOT data for those persons with T2D, and established CVD. Sharing good practice, it was soon established that there was a need to promote and disseminate this pathway across the whole of Greater Manchester (486 practices) to enhance T2D care, reduce variability in care and ultimately improve outcomes.

It was important to have a consensus of expert opinion and thus a group of local experts were brought together to devise the Greater Manchester cardiometabolic pathway.

AIMS

To develop a fit for purpose, easy to use, evidence-based guideline for use across Greater Manchester hosted on Greater Manchester Medicines Management Group (GMMMG) website. This was to be based on previously published and emerging evidence from CVOTs.

This aim aligned with and further enhanced the importance of the Greater Manchester Diabetes Strategy-Tackling Diabetes together,[8] laying out the principles of best diabetes care for the population of Greater Manchester.

METHODS

The local experts comprised a general practitioner (GP) with a special interest in diabetes, three diabetologists (one a professor in cardiometabolic medicine), a cardiologist, and a community diabetes specialist nurse. The group scanned and reviewed research papers and other guidelines. There was a paucity of guidelines, which considered the evidence from the CVOTs.

Four face-to-face meetings were held over a period of a year to discuss the research and develop the guideline. Agreement was reached such that it was to be a one-page guidance with clear and concise advice.

Once the guideline was developed, it was shared with the local medicines management team, GMMMG, through their pathways group. Commissioning managers and pharmacists were actively encouraged to input into the pathway.

A consultation period of 6–8 weeks was allocated—during which period 90 comments were received from across Greater Manchester. One meeting was set aside to review and consider each of the comments and this was achieved during this meeting with no further comments received prior to the submission to the Directors of Commissioning.

Meetings were supported by pharmaceutical companies who had a hands-off approach to the process. No honorariums were paid to any of the participants.

RESULTS

The guidelines were launched on the 8th of May 2019, at a meeting where all stakeholders from across the region were invited. This included commissioners, pharmacists, HCPs, voluntary sector organizations, such as Diabetes UK and medicines management teams. The pathway was endorsed by NHS England by the presence of their Associate Director for Diabetes.

This "Manchester" pathway has now also been adapted and adopted in other regions and has been successfully applied and "live" in those areas.

In the Central Manchester region, the CoDES (Community Diabetes Education and Support) team has been one of the pioneers in initiating therapy based on the pathway and positively identifying suitable persons which has accounted for approximately 7% of the work they have undertaken in consultations.

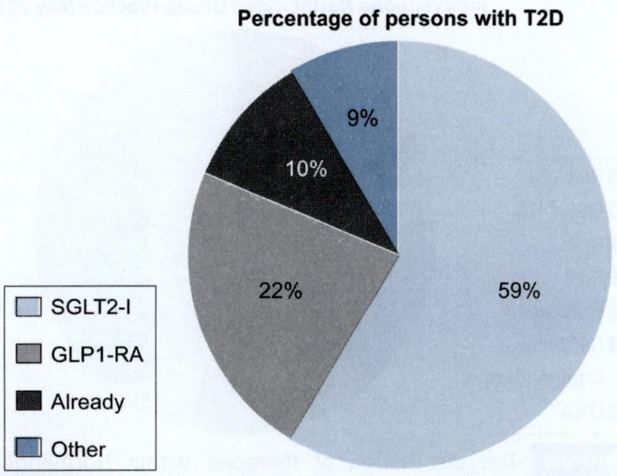

Figure 2 Percentage of persons with type 2 diabetes (T2D).

The CoDES Team actively identified 25% of their cohort as having T2D and established CVD. Ten percent of persons were already on an anti-hyperglycemic agent with cardio-protective benefits, 56% were initiated onto an SGLT2-I, 23% a GLP1-RA, and 9% either had contraindications to initiation or refused treatment (Fig. 2).

In the GP practice where the initial philosophy around the cardiometabolic pathway was developed: 23% of the practice population were identified as having coexisting T2D and CVD, very similar to the CoDES cohort. The Figure 3 shows again the distribution of therapies used within this group of persons. The practice is continuing to actively run searches and audit those suitable for consideration of the pathway as the cohort is ever changing as persons experience a CV event, are newly diagnosed with T2D or who go from being well-controlled to poorly controlled in terms of HbA1c.

In addition, the CoDES Team has been providing for education and the dissemination of resources so that all HCP within primary care feel supported and confident in being able to initiate and use SGLT2-is and GLP1-RAs. For example, a baseline review of confidence levels in using these therapies scored only 5/10 for each one and only 7% of HCPs felt confident to give sick day guidance. It is vital that education is in place so that the pathway can be used safely. There have been educational meetings, study days, and dissemination of resources packs and newsletters which include "traffic light" benefit/risk tools[20,21] for using these newer therapies. Confidence level among HCPs has increased significantly.

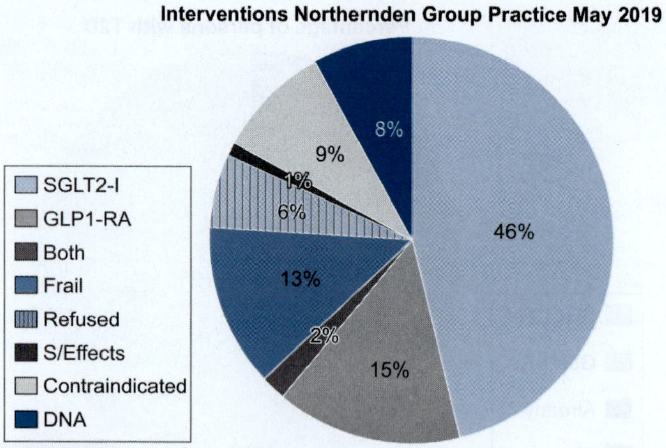

Figure 3 The distribution of therapies within Northenden group of persons.

CONCLUSION

A simplified and directive pathway has been welcomed by HCP. It is clear that such a pathway cannot only improve outcomes by enhancing knowledge and confidence in the newer therapies and their benefits, but it also helps overcome clinical inertia among HCPs which in itself is a huge contributor to the increase of the disease burden in terms of progression to the complications of diabetes.

In a climate of limited economic resources and financial scrutiny however, there has been a huge focus of ensuring that the pathway makes a sound financial argument for usage of these therapies, in the long term.

Although there is robust evidence and economic modeling available via the Nuffield Foundation and other modeling based on the cardiovascular outcome trials (CVOTs), there has been a request for validation of any financial modeling.

This has led to the delay of the publication in Greater Manchester onto the GMMMG website, but ironically as previously mentioned, the pathway has been established in other areas with little resistance from management teams.

NEXT STEPS

We continue to collaborate with health innovation Manchester and GMMMG to get some robust economic modeling. However, while awaiting this modeling, we continue to disseminate the pathway via educational workshops and there is a move to embed the pathway within the Manchester Standard (a document which establishes standards of care for the population of Manchester) so that we can make a difference across the whole population rather than targeting certain areas and clinics.

Continued education and refresher courses is the key area that we intend to focus on with ongoing development of resources and using technology to enable better usage of the pathway.

With emerging evidence and advances in therapy in this field, continued updates to pathway are an essential component to further improve outcomes for the citizens of Greater Manchester.

A current project is to develop a Diabetes Kidney Disease Pathway. We also hope to develop heart failure and Post-MI pathways all of which will complement the Greater Manchester Cardiometabolic Pathway.

REFERENCES

1. Diabetes UK. (2019). Facts and Figures. [online] Available from https://www.diabetes.org.uk/professionals/position-statements-reports/statistics [Last accessed September, 2019].
2. Diabetes UK. (2019). US, diabetes and a lot of facts and stats. [online] Available from https://www.diabetes.org.uk/resources-s3/2019-02/1362B_Facts%20and%20stats%20Update%20Jan%202019_LOW%20RES_EXTERNAL.pdf [Last accessed September, 2019].
3. Public Health England. (2019). Local Health Authority Profiles. [online] Available from https://fingertips.phe.org.uk/profile/health-profiles [Last accessed September, 2019].
4. NHS England. (2019). NHS Diabetes Prevention Programme. [online] Available from https://www.england.nhs.uk/diabetes/diabetes-prevention/ [Last accessed September, 2019].
5. Lean MEJ, Leslie WS, Barnes AC, et al. (2019). Two-year results of the randomised Diabetes Remission Clinical Trial (DiRECT). [online] Available from https://www.directclinicaltrial.org.uk/Pubfiles/Final%20accepted%20draft,%20prior%20to%20editing%20and%20corrections.pdf [Last accessed September, 2019].
6. Cities Changing Diabetes. (2014). Bending the Curve Together. [online] Available from http://www.citieschangingdiabetes.com/home.html [Last accessed September, 2019].
7. Gaede P, Oellgaard J, Carstensen B, et al. Years of life gained by multifactorial intervention in patients with type 2 diabetes mellitus and microalbuminuria: 21 years' follow-up on the Steno-2 randomised trial. Diabetologia. 2016;59(11): 2298-307.
8. The Greater Manchester Health and Social Care Partnership. (2018). Tackling diabetes together: Diabetes clinical best practice strategy 2018–2023. [online] Available from https://www.gmhsc.org.uk/wp-content/uploads/2018/05/Diabetes-Clinical-Strategy-2018-2023-11.05.18.pdf [Last accessed September, 2019].
9. Keng MJ, Tsiachristas A, Leal J, et al. (2019). Impact of achieving primary care targets in type 2 diabetes on health outcomes and healthcare costs. J Diabetes Obes Metab. [online] Available from https://onlinelibrary.wiley.com/doi/abs/10.1111/dom.13821 [Last accessed September, 2019].
10. NHS Digital. (2019). Hospital Episodes Statistics. [online] Available from https://digital.nhs.uk/data-and-information/publications/statistical/hospital-admitted-patient-care-activity/2017-18 [Last accessed September 2019].
11. Wilding J, Fernando K, Milne N, et al. SGLT2 inhibitors in type 2 diabetes management: Key evidence and implications for clinical practice. Diabetes Ther. 2018;9(5):1757-73.

12. Zinman B, Wanner C, Lachin JM, et al. Empagliflozin, cardiovascular outcomes, and mortality in type 2 diabetes. N Eng J Med. 2015;373:2117-28.
13. Wiviott SD, Raz I, Bonaca MP, et al. Dapagliflozin and cardiovascular outcomes in type 2 diabetes. N Eng J Med. 2019;380:347-57.
14. Neal B, Perkovic V, Mahaffey KW, et al. Canagliflozin and cardiovascular and renal events in type 2 diabetes. N Eng J Med. 2019;377:644-57.
15. Marso SP, Daniels GH, Brown-Frandsen K, et al. Liraglutide and cardiovascular outcomes in type 2 diabetes. N End J Med. 2016;375:311-22.
16. Marso SP, Bain SC, Consoli A, et al. Semaglutide and cardiovascular outcomes in patients with type 2 diabetes. N Eng J Med. 2016;375:1834-44.
17. European Society for Cardiology. (2019). Dapagliflozin reduces death and hospitalisation in patients with heart failure. [online] Available from https://www.escardio.org/The-ESC/Press-Office/Press-releases/dapagliflozin-reduces-death-and-hospitalisation-in-patients-with-heart-failure [Last accessed September, 2019].
18. National Institute for Clinical Excellence. (2015). NG28 Type 2 Diabetes in Adults: Management. [online] Available from https://www.nice.org.uk/guidance/NG28. [Last accessed September, 2019].
19. Khunti S, Davies MJ, Khunti K, et al. Clinical Inertia in the Management of Type 2 Diabetes Mellitus: A focused literature review. Br J Diabetes Vasc Dis. 2015;15:65-9.
20. Brown P. How to use SGLT2 inhibitors safely. J Diabetes Prim Care. 2018;20(5):173-4.
21. Milne N. How to use GLP-1 receptor agonist therapy safely and effectively. Diabetes Prim Care. 2019;21(2):45-6.

38 CHAPTER Resurgence of Sulfonylurea Wave: Lessons We could Learn!

AG Unnikrishnan, Suganthi Kumaran

INTRODUCTION

Sulfonylureas have been used as oral antidiabetic drugs since 1954, either alone or in combination with other antidiabetic medications. Modern sulfonylureas such as Glimepiride and Gliclazide modified release (MR) are both economical and associated with a better safety profile. They are recommended as second-line agents in type 2 diabetic patients who do not have atherosclerotic cardiovascular disease (ASCVD) or chronic kidney disease (CKD) and in whom cost is a major issue.[1] With the CAROLINA trial, cardiovascular safety of sulfonylureas has been proved to be as good as DPP4 inhibitor. Hence, sulfonylureas can be considered as second-line agents after metformin, in uncontrolled type 2 diabetes patients with no established cardiovascular disease, in whom cost is a major issue and who are not willing to take injections.

BACKGROUND/HISTORY

Sulfonylureas are derivatives of sulfonamides which stimulate pancreatic beta cells to produce insulin. Their hypoglycemic effect was serendipitously discovered during the typhoid epidemic in France in 1942, by Marcel Jabon while investigating the cause of hypoglycemia in the patients treated with sulfonamide derivative. Further studies led to the development of prototype sulfonylurea.[2]

MECHANISM OF ACTION

Sulfonylureas are insulin secretagogues, causing insulin release from the beta cells of pancreas. Beta cells in the pancreas produce insulin in response to high levels of plasma glucose. Glucose enters the beta cells via glucose transporter, type 2 (GLUT2) receptor, which is insulin independent. The glucose sensor of the beta cells, glucokinase enzyme, phosphorylates glucose to glucose-6-phosphate once the glucose enters the cell. This glucose-6-phosphate participates in the metabolic process of the cell, leading to production of adenosine triphosphate (ATP), which is the main source of energy. High levels of ATP in the cell lead to the closure of ATP-sensitive potassium channel (KIR), which results in increase in the potassium concentration of the cell, causing depolarization. Depolarization causes the entry of calcium ions into the cytoplasm from the extracellular fluid and endoplasmic reticulum. High calcium levels in the beta cells cause insulin release from the cell.

Sulfonylureas bind to the sulfonylurea receptors (SUR) which are closely associated with the KIR channels, causing them to close, resulting in high potassium in the cell leading to depolarization, calcium entry, and insulin release. This insulin release action of sulfonylureas is independent of plasma glucose levels, which explains the common side effect of hypoglycemia.

CLASSIFICATION

There are first and second generation of sulfonylurea agents. First-generation sulfonylureas include tolbutamide (short-acting) and chlorpropamide (long-acting). Second-generation sulfonylureas include Glibenclamide, Glipizide, Gliclazide, and Glimepiride. First-generation sulfonylureas are not in use these days due to severe side effects such as prolonged hypoglycemia. Second-generation sulfonylureas are commonly used because of high potency and less serious side effects.

Glibenclamide (Glyburide)

The usual dose varies from 2.5 mg to 20 mg per day with a duration of action about 16–24 hours. It is the most potent sulfonylurea. It also releases duodenal insulin-releasing agent (DIRA) which is probably responsible for its sustained effect.

Glipizide

The usual dose varies from 2.5 mg to 20 mg per day with a duration of action about 8–12 hours. As it is short- acting, it is useful for better control of postprandial hyperglycemia. Since it is metabolized in the liver, it can be used in patients with renal impairment.

Gliclazide

Dosage of Gliclazide varies from 40 mg to 320 mg per day with a duration of action about 8–12 hours. In addition to the pancreatic effects, it also has beneficial effects on platelet aggregation and fibrinolysis.

Gliclazide Modified-Release/Gliclazide Extended-Release

Dosage of Gliclazide MR and Gliclazide extended release (XR) varies from 30 mg to 120 mg per day with a duration of action about 24 hours. It selectively acts on pancreatic beta cell SUR1 rather than myocardial-SUR2 thus preserving protective ischemic preconditioning of myocardium, thereby rendering it cardiosafe.[3]

Glimepiride

Dosage of Glimepiride varies from 1 mg to 8 mg per day with a duration of action about 16–24 hours. It binds to a different receptor than Glibenclamide and has a faster rate of association and dissociation with the receptor. Hence, it has both rapid onset and longer duration of action. It is excreted by both liver and kidney. It can be used in mild renal insufficiency. The risk of hypoglycemia is less. It also has peripheral action by enhancing GLUT-4 translocation. It has high glucose-lowering action with low insulin-releasing action. It also has inhibitory effects on platelet aggregation.

PHARMACOKINETICS

Sulfonylureas are well absorbed after oral administration, metabolized in the liver, and excreted in the urine and bile. They have to be administered 30 minutes before meals.

SIDE EFFECTS

The main side effect of sulfonylureas is hypoglycemia. This can be quite severe and prolonged, especially with long-acting sulfonylureas such as Glibenclamide. Also, patients with hepatic and renal impairment are at high risk for sulfonylureas-induced hypoglycemia. Any patient with severe hypoglycemia should be admitted for at least 36 hours for recurrence of late hypoglycemia.

Weight gain is another known side effect. Usually, gastrointestinal side effects are not severe. Even though sulfonylureas are sulfa derivatives, patients who are allergic to sulfa do not exhibit cross-reactivity to sulfonylureas. Severe allergic reactions such as Stevens-Johnson syndrome are rare.

Increased Cardiovascular Risk: Older Sulfonylureas

The University Group Diabetes Program (UGDP) launched in 1960s was a placebo-controlled, multicentered randomized efficacy trial which showed an increased cardiovascular death risk with the first-generation sulfonylurea and tolbutamide.[4] With the advent of new antiglycemic agents which show good cardiovascular benefits besides being a good antidiabetic drug, it has become mandatory to check for the cardiovascular outcomes for all the antidiabetic drugs. Hence, after lifestyle intensification and first line of drug management with metformin, the American Diabetes Association (ADA) recommends addition of either sodium glucose co-transporter 2 (SGLT 2) inhibitor or glucagon-like peptide 1 receptor agonist (GLP-1 RA) in type 2 diabetes individuals with ASCVD. However, these agents are expensive and GLP-1 RA are taken as injections which make it cumbersome for patients. An end to this controversy of using sulfonylureas as second-line agents dawned with CAROLINA trial.[5]

CAROLINA (Cardiovascular Outcome Study of Linagliptin versus Glimepiride in Type 2 Diabetes Patients) Trial

CAROLINA trial is the first cardiovascular outcome trial to use an active comparator drug as opposed to others which used a placebo. The results of cardiovascular outcome trial of Linagliptin versus Glimepiride in type 2 diabetes (CAROLINA) were presented on June 10, 2019, at the American Diabetes Association 2019 Scientific Session and it showed that the cardiovascular safety with Glimepiride is similar to that with Linagliptin.[6] This study involved about 6,033 subjects from 607 sites in 43 countries. It was conducted on type 2 diabetes patients with relatively new-onset diabetes of about 6.3 years. There were no differences in the cardiovascular endpoint including the fatal and nonfatal myocardial infarction (MI) (excluding silent MI), fatal, and nonfatal stroke. The three-point MACE occurred in 11.8% of 3,023 patients taking Linagliptin when compared to 12% of 3,010 patients taking Glimepiride. Similarly, nonsignificant differences were noted in the secondary end points such as hospitalization due to heart failure, cardiovascular death, noncardiovascular death, and all-cause mortality between the two groups. Thus, there was no superior cardiovascular safety profile with Linagliptin when compared with Glimepiride. The glycemic control with glycated-hemoglobin reduction was about the same in both groups. However, hypoglycemia and weight gain were higher in the Glimepiride group compared to the Linagliptin group.

RECOMMENDATION

Modern sulfonylureas like Gliclazide MR/XR and Glimepiride can be considered as second-line antidiabetic agents after metformin in type 2 diabetes subjects who have not achieved the target glycemic goals. Besides being cardio safe (STENO-2 study), Gliclazide XR has better glucose-lowering efficacy when compared to other oral antihyperglycemic agents and a longer time to insulin initiation (14.5 years vs. 8 years) when compared to other sulfonylureas.[7,8] Also, intensive glycemic control with Gliclazide XR-based regimen reduces the risk of end-stage renal disease (ESRD), new micro- and macro-albuminuria as evidenced by ADVANCE study (which involved 11,140 patients with a 5-year period of follow-up).[9,10] In fact as per clinical practice recommendations during Ramadan 2017, Gliclazide can be effectively and safely recommended in Indian patients with type 2 diabetes because of advantages of fewer hypoglycemia and cardiovascular safety with low cost.

CONCLUSION

Modern sulfonylureas like Glimepiride and Gliclazide MR or XR are a safe addition to metformin in type 2 diabetes subjects when glycemic targets are not at goal. They are the second-line agents in type 2 diabetic patients who do not have established ASCVD or chronic kidney disease (CKD) and whom cost is a major issue.[11] Nowadays, new antidiabetic drugs are being tested for their cardiovascular safety before they are introduced in the market. As per ADA, antidiabetic drugs such as SGLT 2 inhibitors and GLP-1 RA are recommended as the next line of drugs after metformin in type 2 diabetic patients with ASCVD and/or cardiovascular risk factors. Modern sulfonylureas now have made a major comeback, especially with CAROLINA trial. It has been shown in this trial that there are no major cardiovascular outcome differences between dipeptidyl peptidase inhibitor like Linagliptin and sulfonylurea like Glimepiride in recently diagnosed type 2 diabetes subjects (about 6.3 years duration) at increased risk for cardiovascular events. Modern sulfonylureas also have the added advantage of being low cost, high efficacy, taken orally with fewer hypoglycemic episodes, compared to older generation sulfonylureas.

REFERENCES

1. American Diabetes Association. Standards of Medical Care in Diabetes—2019 Abridged for Primary Care Providers. Clin Diabetes. 2019;37(1):11–34.
2. Mohan V, Unnikrishnan R, Anjana RM. Management of diabetes mellitus – oral antidiabetic agents and non-insulin therapies. Dr. Mohan's Handbook of Diabetes Mellitus, 5th edition. New Delhi: Elsevier. pp. 49-51.
3. Colagiuri S, Matthews D, Leiter LA, et al. The place of gliclazide MR in the evolving type 2 diabetes landscape: A comparison with other sulfonylureas and newer oral antihyperglycemic agents. Diabetes Res Clin Pract. 2018;143:1-14.
4. Azoulay L, Suissa S. Sulfonylureas and the risks of cardiovascular events and death: A methodological meta-regression analysis of the observational studies. Diabetes Care. 2017;40(5):706-14.
5. CAROLINA shows neutral cardiovascular profile for modern sulfonylurea. [online] Available from: https://diabetes.medicinematters.com/linagliptin/glimepiride/carolina-neutral-cardiovascular-profile-for-modern-sulfonylurea/16790758 [Last accessed on September, 2019]
6. Tuker ME. CAROLINA reassures on CV safety for linagliptin, Glimepiride in Type 2 Diabetes. Medscape. 2019.
7. Jia Y, Lao Y, Zhu H, et al. Is metformin still the most efficacious first-line oral hypoglycaemic drug in treating type 2 diabetes? A network meta-analysis of randomized controlled trials. Obesity Rev. 2019;20(1): 1-12.
8. Satoh J, Takahashi K, Takizawa Y, et al. Secondary sulfonylurea failure: comparison of period until insulin treatment between diabetic patients treated with gliclazide and glibenclamide. Diabetes Res Clin Pract. 2005;70(3):291–7.
9. Heller SR. Diabetes and cardiovascular disease: A summary of the ADVANCE Trial. Diabetes Care. 2009;32(suppl 2):S357–61.
10. The ADVANCE Collaborative Group. Intensive blood glucose control and vascular outcomes in patients with type 2 diabetes. N Engl J Med. 2008;358:2560–72.
11. Varvaki Rados D, Catani Pinto L, Reck Remonti L, et al. The association between sulfonylurea use and all-cause and cardiovascular mortality: A meta-analysis with trial sequential analysis of randomized clinical trials. PLoS Med. 2016;13(4):e1001992. Epub 2016 Apr 12.

39 CHAPTER Lorcaserin: A Novel Anti-obesity Agent

Awadhesh Kumar Singh

INTRODUCTION

Obesity was known since ancient times. There is documentation in writings of ancient Greece, Egypt and India mentioning obesity as an obstacle to good health and long life. Sushruta, an ancient Indian physician considered obesity to be a "disease" in circa 600 BC.[1] In June 2014, American Medical Association declared obesity [Body Mass Index (BMI) ≥ 30] as a "disease" in its "Resolution 420" and recommended interventions for obesity treatment and prevention. Because obesity is closely linked with the development and progression of other coexisting complication that includes type 2 diabetes, hypertension, dyslipidemia, coronary artery disease, stroke, heart failure, osteoarthritis, obstructive sleep apnea, malignancy and an increase in all-cause death.

Emerging data clearly indicates that obesity is burgeoning problem and it has already reached an epidemic proportion worldwide with nearly 1.9 billion overweight and 650 million obese adults according to World Health Organization (WHO).[2] Noncommunicable disease (NCD) risk factors collaborators reported a staggered rise in obesity even in developing countries. China currently (in 2014) ranked at the top representing 16.3% of global obesity in men, replacing US. India also jumped to third (obesity in women, representing 5.3% of global obesity) and fifth rank (men, representing 3.7% of global obesity in men) in 2014, from rank 19, in year 1975. Interestingly, increase in obesity prevalence were even higher (>4-fold) in women.[3] One survey in 2016 also suggests that as high as ≈40% of people in the USA and 26% adult in England has obesity like many other countries, indicating at least a threefold increase in obesity in last 40 years.[4,5] Additionally, 40% people are overweight (BMI 25–29 kg/m^2) worldwide. By the current estimates, the prevalence of obesity and overweight in India is ≈23%.[6]

Fortunately, weight loss of 5–10% has been associated with significant improvement in glycemic control, hypertension, dyslipidemia and thus overall improvement in the cardiovascular (CV) risk beside improvement of joint pains, obstructive sleep apnea and overall quality of life.[7] Development of new type 2 diabetes has also been significantly reduced (5-year risk by 58%) by a modest 5% weight loss as observed in DPP (Diabetes Prevention Program) study.

In 2007, Food and Drug Administration (FDA) laid down certain criteria to qualify an agent to be an effective anti-obesity drug. Criteria set forth required at least one of the following criteria to be met after 1 year of treatment—(a) 'Mean' efficacy criterion: the difference in mean weight loss between the active product and placebo-treated groups is ≥5% and the difference are statistically significant or, (b) "Categorical" efficacy criterion: the proportion of subjects losing ≥5% of baseline body weight in the active-product group is ≥35%, is approximately double the proportion in the placebo-treated group, and the difference between groups is statistically significant.[8]

While lifestyle modification (LSM) is the gold standard method to tackle this menace, sustainability to maintain it does remain to be the biggest challenge. To mitigate this problem at least to some extent, drug therapy has been considered as a second tool. Pharmacotherapy has been considered for people who have not had satisfactory benefit with LSM or, having difficulty to maintain initial weight loss accrued through LSM or, where LSM is difficult due to chronic medical diseases. Recommendation-wise, drug is indicated along with LSM, in people with BMI

≥ 30 kg/m^2 or ≥ 27 kg/m^2 with at least one weight-related comorbidity, such as type 2 diabetes, hypertension or dyslipidemia.[9]

A wide range of anti-obesity drugs have been developed in the past few decades, for long-term use targeting different mechanisms that includes: (i) sympathomimetic adrenergic drugs—fenfluramine (only short-term use) and dexfenfluramine, (ii) selective cannabinoid 1 receptor blocker—rimonabant, (iii) serotonin (5-HT) reuptake inhibitor—sibutramine. Unfortunately, all these drugs were withdrawn, owing to some severe adverse side effects. While both fenfluramine and dexfenfluramine were associated with significant increase in pulmonary hypertension and valvular heart disease, rimonabant had increased suicidal risk and sibutramine had significantly higher increase in CV risks. Table 1 summarizes evolution of all anti-obesity drugs and their current status.

LORCASERIN

Lorcaserin is a selective agonist of the 5-hydroxytryptamine 2C serotonin receptor (5-HT$_{2C}$) which was approved for long-term use by FDA in 2012, as an adjunct to LSM, after an initial rejection in 2010. Unlike fenfluramine and dexfenfluramine which has nonselective serotonergic agonistic activity on all 5-HT receptors (5-HT$_{2A, 2B, 2C}$), lorcaserin has 8–15-fold greater potency for 5-HT$_{2C}$ compared to 5-HT$_{2A}$, and 45–90-fold greater potency for 5-HT$_{2C}$ compared to 5-HT$_{2B}$.[10] Therefore, off-target activation of 5-HT$_{2A}$ and 5-HT$_{2B}$ appears highly unlikely although theoretically still plausible, depending upon the plasma drug level.

Mechanism of Action

The mechanism by which lorcaserin reduces body weight is akin to decrease in energy intake though promotion of satiety.[11] This is mediated through the 5-HT$_C$ receptor on POMC/CART (pro-opiomelanocortin/cocaine and amphetamine-regulated transcript) neuron in the arcuate nucleus of hypothalamus. Stimulation of POMC/CART causes release in α-MSH (alpha-melanocyte-stimulating hormone) which acts on MC4Rs (melanocortin-4 receptors) on the neurons of PVN (paraventricular nucleus) which

TABLE 1: Evolution of anti-obesity drugs and their current status.

Drugs	Year approved	Year withdrawn	Reason for withdrawal or other special notes
For short-term use (≈12 weeks)			
Phentermine	1959	2000 (Eu)	Most prescribed drug in US but withdrawn in Europe due to higher risk-to-benefit ratio
Diethylpropion	1959	–	Abuse potential
Phendimetrazine	1959	–	Abuse potential
Benzphetamine	1960	–	Abuse potential
Mazindol	1973	1999	Discontinued by manufacturer
Fenfluramine	1973	1997	Increased risk of valvular heart disease
For long-term use (>12 weeks)			
Dexfenfluramine	1996	1997	Increased risk of valvular heart disease
Sibutramine	1997	2010	Increased risk of MACE (HR = 1.16; 95% CI = 1.03–1.31; P = 0.02)
Orlistat	1999	–	Also approved for pediatric obesity in 2003 at lower dosage. Lower dose (60 mg) approved in 2007 even without prescription
Rimonabant	2006 (Eu)	2008 (Eu)	NDA withdrawn from FDA. Withdrawn in Europe due to serious psychiatric adverse events
Phentermine + Topiramate	2012	–	Marketed under REMS to reduce risks of teratogenicity
Lorcaserin	2012	–	Marketing delayed due to Drug Enforcement Administration
Naltrexone + Bupropion	2014	–	Unfavorable effect on blood pressure
Liraglutide 3.0 mg	2014	–	Lower dose (0.6–1.8 mg) approved for diabetes

(CI: confidence interval; Eu: Europe; FDA: Food and Drug Administration; HR: hazard ratio; MACE: major adverse cardiac events; NDA: new drug application; REMS: risk evaluation mitigation strategy; US: United States)

promotes satiety.[10-12] An additional action on mesolimbic reward circuit has also been suggested through 5-HT_{2C} that might be helpful in obesity.[13] The majority of weight loss is ascribed to decrease in fat mass and only little due to decrease in lean mass as measured by DEXA-scan.[14]

Efficacy

There are several clinical studies that investigated lorcaserin versus placebo in the clinical setting, results of which have been summarized in Table 2. The first phase 3 study of lorcaserin demonstrated a mean Δ –2.9 kg weight reduction versus placebo and 31.2% of completers population showed ≥5% weight loss compared to 2.3% in placebo arm at 12-weeks.[15] All other phase 3 randomized controlled trials (RCTs) conducted with lorcaserin such as BLOOM (Behavioral Modification and Lorcaserin for Overweight and Obesity Management), BLOSSOM (Behavioral Modification and Lorcaserin Second Study for Obesity Management) and BLOOM-DM (Behavioral Modification and Lorcaserin for Obesity and Overweight Management in Diabetes Mellitus) study showed significant weight reduction versus placebo and fulfilled the *categorical efficacy* criterion (≥35% patients with ≥5% weight loss in active arm); however, they failed to achieve *mean efficacy* criterion (placebo subtracted ≥ 5% weight loss, at 1 year) of anti-obesity drug (Table 2).[16-18]

The reason for initial rejection of lorcaserin by FDA in 2010 was based on—(a) the difference in mean weight loss versus placebo was about 3% and thus did not satisfy the first "mean" efficacy criteria, although lorcaserin did fulfill 'categorical' efficacy criteria by a slim margin; (b) concerns related with increase in mammary and brain tumors in preclinical studies. However, FDA re-review in 2012, approved lorcaserin, with a requirement of cardiovascular outcome trial (CVOT).[19]

TABLE 2: Results from Phase 3 trials of lorcaserin (10 mg BID): MITT-LOCF data.

First author/Trial Eponyms, year	N	Study criteria	Active arm (max. dose/day)	Studies duration (Weeks)	Δ PBO-subtracted weight loss (kg)	% weight loss (Drug vs PBO)	Δ PBO-subtracted weight loss (%)	% of patients with ≥ 5% weight loss (Drug vs PBO)	% of patients with ≥ 10% weight loss (Drug vs PBO)
Smith et al., 2009	234	BMI 30–45 kg/m^2	10 mg BID	12	2.9	NR	NR	31.2 vs 2.3†	0
TULIP, 2011	57	BMI 27–45 kg/m^2	10 mg BID	8	1.6	NR	NR	NR	NR
BLOOM*, 2010	3,182	BMI 30–45 kg/m^2 or BMI 27–45 kg/m^2 if at least one comorbidity	10 mg BID	104	3.6	5.8 vs 2.2	3.6	47.5 vs 20.3	22.6 vs 7.7
BLOSSOM*, 2011	4,008	BMI 30–45 kg/m^2 or BMI 27–29.9 kg/m^2 if comorbidity	10 mg BID	52	2.9	5.8 vs 2.8	3.0	47.2 vs 25	22.6 vs 9.7
BLOOM-DM*, 2012	604	DM with BMI 27–45 kg/m^2	10 mg BID	52	3.1	4.5 vs 1.5	3.0	37.5 vs 16.1	16.3 vs 4.4
CAMELLIA*, 2018	12,000	BMI ≥ 27 kg/m^2 with or without established CVD	10 mg BID	Median (3.3 Year)	2.8	4.2 vs 1.4	2.8	38.7 vs 17.4	14.6 vs 4.8

*Data at 1 year.

†Completers analysis.

(MITT-LOCF: modified intention-to-treat analysis- last observation carried forward; BID: twice daily; BMI: body mass index; CVD: cardiovascular disease; DM: diabetes mellitus; max.: maximum; PBO: placebo)

Metabolic and Cardiovascular Effect

CAMELLIA-TIMI 61 (Cardiovascular and Metabolic Effects of Lorcaserin in Overweight and Obese Patients-Thrombolysis in Myocardial Infarction 61) was a large (N = 12,000) CVOT that has demonstrated a CV neutrality [hazard ratio (HR) = 0.99; 95% confidence interval (CI) = 0.85–1.14; $P < 0.001$ for non-inferiority] of lorcaserin, on the composite of MACE (major adverse cardiovascular events—CV death, myocardial infarction, or stroke) compared to placebo, in patients with high CV risk (≈75% had established CV disease) after a median follow-up of 3.3 years.[20] Moreover, lorcaserin significantly decreased the developmental rate of incident diabetes from no diabetes (HR = 0.77; 95% CI = 0.63–0.94; $P = 0.012$) and prediabetes (HR = 0.81; 95% CI = 0.66–0.99, $P = 0.038$).[21] Furthermore, lorcaserin significantly reduced the microvascular complication (HR = 0.79; 95% CI = 0.69–0.92; $P = 0.001$) primarily by reducing microalbuminuria (HR = 0.77; 95% CI = 0.66–0.90; $P = 0.001$).[20] Further analysis of CAMELLIA showed a significant reduction (HR = 0.87; 95% CI = 0.79–0.96; $P = 0.006$) in composite of renal outcome (new or worsening persistent micro- or macroalbuminuria, new or worsening chronic kidney disease, doubling of serum creatinine, end-stage renal disease, renal transplant or renal death).[22]

Safety

Nausea, headache and dizziness were common and consistent side effects observed with lorcaserin in all the phase 3 RCTs; however, no significant increase in FDA-defined valvulopathy [defined as mild or greater aortic regurgitation (AR) and/or moderate or greater mitral regurgitation (MR)], depression and suicidal risk were observed with lorcaserin in any studies.[16-18] FDA review also found an increase in nausea, dizziness and transient headache; however, no significant increase in FDA-defined valvulopathy or neuropsychiatric symptoms (depression or suicidal risk) were observed with lorcaserin.[19] Likewise, in the large and long CVOT CAMELLIA TIMI 61, there was no significant increase in FDA-defined valvulopathy, depression and suicidal risk with lorcaserin compared to placebo.[20]

CONCLUSION

Collectively, available data points toward a significant role of lorcaserin in improving body weight and other clusters of metabolic syndromes, with no obvious serious adverse side effects. However, the weight loss seems to be modest at its best. Another issues that have commonly lingered with all anti-obesity drug including non-responders and loss of maintenance of weight after a certain time-point, have also been observed with lorcaserin. A 12-week pilot study suggested only 28% of patients showing ≥5% weight loss to lorcaserin.[23] Likewise, BLOOM showed modest regain in weight at 2 year, despite significant weight loss at 1 year.[16] Another study suggested that lorcaserin failed to maintain weight loss at 1 year, despite achieving significantly weight loss initially.[24] FDA also recommended to withdraw the drug if weight loss of 5% is not achieved during first 12-weeks.

Finally, caution must be exercised while using lorcaserin with other drugs that also act through the serotonergic pathway, such as selective-serotonin reuptake inhibitors and serotonin-norepinephrine reuptake inhibitors, considering the increased chance of developing hyperserotonergic syndrome. Also, lorcaserin is currently not indicated in obese less than 18-year-old. Future trials (NCT 03338296) which are currently underway and are expected to be completed in 2021 will further explore the safety and efficacy of lorcaserin in the obese adolescent (12–17 years).[25]

REFERENCES

1. Tipton CM. Susruta of India, an unrecognized contributor to the history of exercise physiology. J Appl Physiol. 2008;104(6):1553-6.
2. World Health Organization (WHO). Obesity and Overweight. Geneva: WHO; 2017.
3. NCD Risk Factor Collaboration (NCD-RisC). Trends in adult body-mass index in 200 countries from 1975 to 2014: a pooled analysis of 1698 population-based measurement studies with 19·2 million participants. Lancet. 2016;387(10026):1377-96.
4. Hales CM, Fryar CD, Carroll MD, et al. Trends in obesity and severe obesity prevalence in US youth and adults by sex and age, 2007-2008 to 2015-2016. JAMA. 2018;319:1723-5.
5. NHS Digital. Statistics on obesity, physical activity and diet - England, 2018. England: NHS Digital; 2018.
6. Prabhakaran D, Singh K, Roth GA, et al. Cardiovascular Diseases in India Compared With the United States. J Am Coll Cardiol. 2018;72(1):79-95.
7. Després JP, Lemieux I, Prud'homme D. Treatment of obesity: need to focus on high risk abdominally obese patients. BMJ. 2001;322(7288):716-20.
8. U.S. Department of Health and Human Services Food and Drug Administration Center for Drug Evaluation and Research (CDER). (2007). Guidance for Industry Developing Products for Weight Management. [online] Available from www.fda.gov/media/71252/download. [Last accessed September, 2019].
9. Jensen MD, Ryan DH, Apovian CM, et al. 2013 AHA/ACC/TOS guideline for the management of overweight and obesity in adults: a report of the American College of Cardiology/American Heart Association Task Force on Practice Guidelines and The Obesity Society. J Am Coll Cardiol. 2014;63:2895-3023.

10. Food and Drug Administration. (2010). FDA briefing document, NDA 22529. Advisory committee meeting for lorcaserin. Endocrinologic and Metabolic Drugs Advisory Committee. [online] Available from www.sefap.it/farmacovigilanza_news_201011/UCM225631.PDF [Last accessed September, 2019].
11. Burke LK, Heisler LK. 5-hydroxytryptamine medications for the treatment of obesity. J Neuroendocrinol. 2015;27:389-98.
12. Martin CK, Redman LM, Zhang J, et al. Lorcaserin, a 5-HT(2C) receptor agonist, reduces body weight by decreasing energy intake without influencing energy expenditure. J Clin Endocrinol Metab. 2011;96(3): 837-45.
13. Valencia-Torres L, Olarte-Sanchez CM, Lyons DJ, et al. Activation of ventral tegmental area 5-HT2c receptors reduces incentive motivation. Neuropsychopharmacology. 2017;42(7):1511-21.
14. Apovian C, Palmer K, Fain R, et al. Effects of lorcaserin on fat and lean mass loss in obese and overweight patients without and with type 2 diabetes mellitus: the BLOSSOM and BLOOM-DM studies. Diabetes Obes Metab. 2016;18(9):945-8.
15. Smith SR, Prosser WA, Donahue DJ, et al. Lorcaserin (APD356), a selective 5-HT(2C) agonist, reduces body weight in obese men and women. Obesity. 2009;17(3):494-503.
16. Smith SR, Weissman NJ, Anderson CM, et al. Multicenter, Placebo-Controlled Trial of Lorcaserin for Weight Management. N Engl J Med. 2010;363(3):245-56.
17. Fidler MC, Sanchez M, Raether B, et al. A one-year randomized trial of lorcaserin for weight loss in obese and overweight adults: the BLOSSOM trial. J Clin Endocrinol Metab. 2011;96(10):3067-77.
18. O'Neil PM, Smith SR, Weissman NJ, et al. Randomized placebo-controlled clinical trial of lorcaserin for weight loss in type 2 diabetes mellitus: the BLOOM-DM study. Obesity. 2012;20(7):1426-36.
19. Food and Drug Administration. (2012). FDA news release. FDA approves Belviq to treat some overweight or obese adults. [online] Available from www.fda.gov/NewsEvents/Newsroom/PressAnnouncements/ucm309993.htm. [Last accessed September, 2019].
20. Bohula EA, Wiviott SD, McGuire DK, et al. Cardiovascular Safety of Lorcaserin in Overweight or Obese Patients. N Engl J Med. 2018;379(12):1107-17.
21. Bohula EA, Scirica BM, Inzucchi SE, et al. Effect of lorcaserin on prevention and remission of type 2 diabetes in overweight and obese patients (CAMELLIA-TIMI 61): a randomised, placebo-controlled trial. Lancet. 2018;392(10161):2269-79.
22. Scirica BM, Bohula EA, Dwyer JP, et al. Lorcaserin and Renal Outcomes in Obese and Overweight Patients in the CAMELLIA-TIMI 61 Trial. Circulation. 2019;139(3):366-75.
23. Smith SR, Garvey WT, Greenway FL, et al. Coadministration of lorcaserin and phentermine for weight management: a 12-week, randomized, pilot safety study. Obesity (Silver Spring). 2017;25(5):857-65.
24. Shaw Tronieri J, Wadden TA, Berkowitz RI, et al. A randomized trial of lorcaserin and lifestyle counseling for maintaining weight loss achieved with a low-calorie diet. Obesity (Silver Spring). 2018;26(2):299-309.
25. Clinicaltrials.gov. (2017). Study to evaluate the efficacy and safety of belviq XR® in conjunction with lifestyle modification for weight loss in obese adolescents, age 12 to 17 years. [online] Available from clinicaltrials.gov/ct2/show/NCT03338296. [Last accessed September, 2019].

40 CHAPTER

Teneligliptin: An Emerging Evidence on Safety and Efficacy—TREAT INDIA-2 Update

Sambit Das, Mahesh Rath

INTRODUCTION

Diabetes is a health emergency of this century. India has witnessed a rapid rise of type 2 diabetes mellitus (T2DM), affecting more than 74 million Indians, according to International Diabetes Federation (IDF) data from 2017.[1] Moreover India has the highest number of people with diabetes still undiagnosed and by 2045 number of diabetics are expected to cross 134.3 million (103.4–165.2).[1] The steady migration of people from rural to urban areas, the economic boom, and corresponding change in lifestyle are all affecting the level of diabetes.[2] While managing Indian patients with diabetes it is imperative to recognize that due to associated obesity and inadequate lifestyle modifications, only metformin along with lifestyle management may not just be enough in initial management of patients at least in some of them. While choosing oral antidiabetic agents (ADAs), apart from risk of hypoglycemia, it is important to also look into impact on weight, renal safety, cardiac safety and possible beta-cell preservation. Awareness of the disease and its aggressive management is considered as a cornerstone to control the disease in India.

Dipeptidyl peptidase-4 (DPP-4) inhibitors are the novel class of hypoglycemic agents widely used in the management of T2DM.[3] Though the mechanism of action of all DPP-4 inhibitors is same, there lies an important difference in the pharmacokinetics, pharmacodynamics and potency among all gliptins.[4] Gliptins usage has recently increased considerably in India after introduction of teneligliptin in the year 2015 (by Glenmark Pharmaceuticals). One of the most important factors while choosing any ADAs, is cost of therapy, keeping in mind that majority of patients in India are not covered by insurance and also due to other comorbidities could be on other therapies too.

Teneligliptin is a class 3 DPP-4 inhibitor with unique structural ability which enhances its potency and selectivity.[5] It has fivefold higher activity than other gliptins and produces more extensive inhibition of DPP-4.[6] Apart from its high potency and selectivity, the economic advantage of teneligliptin, that, it is available at one-fourths to one-fifths cost of other gliptins has made teneligliptin as the most commonly prescribed gliptin in India. Given the widespread use of teneligliptin, there was need for large-scale data on teneligliptin in real world setting of India, which will help patient populations with this challenging disease, where personalized therapeutic approaches are commonly considered taking into consideration the patients' age and associated comorbidities, among other factors. In India, previous studies, which have reported the real world evidence of teneligliptin, has been small in number as compared to RUBY Surveillance conducted by Kadowaki T et al. in T2DM patients in Japanese population.[7]

There are no large-scale data published from India on T2DM patients' population, which is needed to understand factors important in control of diabetes in real-world setting.

The TREAT INDIA-2 Study was thus designed to evaluate effectiveness of teneligliptin in large population of T2DM in India.

METHODOLOGY

This was retrospective cohort analysis, where a predesigned structured case record form (CRF) was used to collate patient's profile information from hospital records of 18 centers across India after obtaining approval from ethics committee *(Suraksha Ethics Committee, Registration No: ECR/644/Inst/MH/2014/RR-17)*. Patients who were prescribed teneligliptin as a monotherapy or part of combination therapy and continued for a minimum period of 3 months without any addition of other ADA, were considered for the retrospective analysis. Patient's record details were collected either from hard copy or digital medical records of hospital or collated on the TREAT INDIA-2 CRF forms and it was further analyzed. Out of total 18 centers from where the data was collected and analyzed, seven centers were from south, followed by four centers in north and west each, and three centers were from east.

RESULTS

Total 10,623 patients' data was available for analysis as per eligibility criteria. The average age of enrolled patients was 51.9 year with male-to-female ratio of 1.1:1. There was statistically significant improvement in mean glycated hemoglobin (HbA1c), fasting plasma glucose (FPG) and postprandial plasma glucose (PPG) with 3 month teneligliptin therapy. Means changes in HbA1c, FPG and PPG were –0.99% (95% confidence interval of this difference was from 0.9572 to 1.0228; $P < 0.0001$), –43.11 mg/dL (95% confidence interval of this difference was from 42.5025 to 43.7175; $P < 0.0001$), and –87.76 mg/dL (95% confidence interval of this difference was from 86.5329 to 88.9871; $P < 0.0001$), respectively (Table 1). This data was further analyzed for teneligliptin as monotherapy and add-on therapy [added to metformin; added to metformin plus sulfonylureas (SUs); added to metformin plus SUs plus alpha-glucosidase inhibitors (AGIs); and added to metformin plus SGLT-2 inhibitors]. There was significant reduction in FPG, PPG and HbA1c in all the sub-groups of monotherapy and as an add-on therapy compared to baseline. Additionally further sub-analysis of this data

TABLE 1: Mean change in the glycemic parameters among study population.

Overall patients	FPG	PPG	HbA1c
Baseline	160.14 ± 23.05	257.06 ± 47.39	8.66 ± 1.15
12 week	117.03 ± 22.01	169.3 ± 43.57	7.67 ± 1.28
Difference	43.11	87.76	0.99
P value	$P < 0.0001$	$P < 0.0001$	$P < 0.0001$

(FPG: fasting plasma glucose; HbA1c: glycated hemoglobin; PPG: postprandial plasma glucose)

was carried out in special population such as the effect of teneligliptin across the all age groups (below 60 years, between 60 years and 75 years, and above 75 years). Patients with renal impairment (patients with mild, moderate and severe CKD patients), teneligliptin added in patients uncontrolled on insulin therapy with or without other ADAs. In patients where teneligliptin was switched over to from other gliptins and also in gliptins naïve patients. Significant improvement in glycemic parameters was observed in all these patient profiles after addition of teneligliptin.

DISCUSSION

This real-world evidence study is the largest nationally representative data of teneligliptin in Indian patients and to our knowledge probably this is also the largest available real world data worldwide on teneligliptin. In this study, data of 10,623 patients was collected to analyze the effectiveness of teneligliptin on various blood sugar parameters. The previously available large-scale data was in Japanese study from 10,532 patients.[7] The average age of patients in TREAT INDIA-2 study was 51.9 years with higher male-to-female ratio. The age and gender-wise association of diabetes in India was highlighted in the ICMR-INDIAB population-based study,[8] where the prevalence was higher in the age group of 35–65 years and was higher in males than females in this age group and beyond which it is higher in females. The management of diabetes in patients above 65 years of age is difficult because of the associated comorbid conditions and increased risk of weight gain as the age progress, which itself is an independent risk factor for diabetes.

The DPP-4 inhibitors are usually prescribed in patients who have not responded well to drugs such as metformin and SUs. In TREAT INDIA-2 study, teneligliptin was preferred as an add-on therapy (96%) in T2DM patients who have not responded to primary therapy of metformin and/or SUs. This prescription pattern of teneligliptin was also highlighted in study conducted by Kumar PKM et al.,[9] where teneligliptin was preferred as an add-on therapy to metformin and sulfonylurea. As a part of add-on therapy, teneligliptin was added to first-line metformin in 40% cases and to combination of metformin and SU in 34% cases in TREAT INDIA-2 study. Metformin and SU still remain the mainstay of first-line therapy in India, probably because of its direct action on pathogenic mechanism of diabetes. But chronic use of SUs has shown to decrease the beta-cell function with worsening of hyperglycemia and thus there exists the need of additional pharmacological agent.[10,11] Teneligliptin, a novel class of DPP-4 inhibitor, offer convenience of single dosing without affecting the survival of beta-cell and is weight neutral with lower risk of hypoglycemia, hence commonly used as a combination agent to metformin and/or SUs.[12]

Effectiveness of teneligliptin in India was first highlighted in real-world evidence study (TREAT INDIA, *n* = 4,305, conducted by Ghosh S et al.,[13] where teneligliptin, as a monotherapy and as an add-on therapy showed significant reduction in HbA1c, FPG and PPG. In the present (TREAT INDIA-2) study, conducted over large pool of patient population (n = 10,623) having representatives from different regions of country, 12-week teneligliptin therapy still significantly ($p < 0.001$) decrease the FFG (–43.11), PPG (–87.76) and HbA1c (–0.99%). The finding of above two large-scale RWE studies in Indian population reflects the effectiveness of teneligliptin, without any concerns of safety. Similar findings were reported in another real-world efficacy study conducted in India by Nashikkar N et al.[14] The effectiveness was also highlighted in a systematic meta-analysis by Xiaoxuan Li[15] of 10 randomized controlled trials (RCTs) where teneligliptin was shown to significantly ($p < 0.00001$) decrease HbA1c (0.82%), FFG (–18.32 mg/dL%) and PPG (–46.94%). Thus teneligliptin effectively improves glycemic control and thus suggests its useful role in treatment of patients who are uncontrolled with other ADA.

Subgroup analysis of TREAT INDIA-2 study population highlights the difference in the reduction of glycemic parameters with teneligliptin as a monotherapy and add-on therapy. Teneligliptin monotherapy was also effective in subset of population (n = 390) in our study, with significant ($p < 0.001$) reduction in glycemic parameter. Kutoha E et al.[16] evaluated the first-line use of teneligliptin in newly diagnosed T2DM patients. The result showed significant reduction in HbA1c ($p < 0.0001$) and fasting blood glucose ($p < 0.0002$). Raghavan V[17] compared the effectiveness of teneligliptin with metformin in newly diagnosed T2DM, this 12 week randomized trial showed similar efficacy of teneligliptin and metformin in reducing mean HbA1c, FBG and PPG. Suryawanshi et al.[18] reported, in an Indian study, a significant decrease in mean HbA1c (P = 0.0043) and PPG (P = 0.0070) in phase 3, 16-week, multicentric, double-blind, placebo-controlled trial with higher percentage (43.6%) of patient achieved target HbA1c of <7% with teneligliptin.

When used as an add-on therapy, teneligliptin was added to almost all classes of antidiabetic medications prescribed currently except GLP1 receptor agonists. In TREAT INDIA-2, teneligliptin was added to insulin with or without other ADAs. Insulin therapy, are considered as the most potent antihyperglycemic therapy for patients with uncontrolled T2DM; however, increasing insulin dosage is associated with increased risk of hypoglycemia and weight gain.[19] Teneligliptin when added to insulin therapy had shown to decrease the fluctuation of oral glucose level, increase proportion of time in the normal glucose range than in hyperglycemia over 24-hour period.[20] Such fluctuations are important triggering factor for oxidative stress and cardiovascular diseases.[21] Kadowaki T et al. in their 16-week RCT reported significant decrease in blood glucose parameter when teneligliptin was added to insulin therapy.[22]

Alpha-glucosidase inhibitors by its complementary and different mechanism of action to teneligliptin, increases GLP-1 action may provide valuable option to patients.[23]

CONCLUSION

In TREAT INDIA-2 study, AGIs and teneligliptin was used along with other ADAs and showed significant decrease in glycemic parameters. Several trials have evaluated efficacy and safety of gliptins with SUs and have reported a significant improvement in glycemic control.[24] In TREAT INDIA-2, almost 11% of patients (n = 1118) were given combination of teneligliptin and SGLT2 inhibitors like empagliflozin, canagliflozin, and dapagliflozin with other ADAs. Study conducted by Kadowaki T[25] showed significant improvement in long-term safety and efficacy of canagliflozin as add-on therapy to teneligliptin in Japanese patients and suggested effectiveness of combination in improving HbA1c, FPG and body weight.

Thus in TREAT INDIA-2 study, the largest retrospective study till date, showed regardless of other type of ADA, teneligliptin as an add-on therapy showed significant glucose lowering effect and can be considered as an ideal add-on ADA.

REFERENCES

1. International Diabetes Federation. (2017). IDF Diabetes Atlas, Eighth edition. [online] Available from https://diabetesasia.org/content/diabetes_guidelines/IDF_guidelines.pdf. [Last accessed on September, 2019].
2. Kaveeshwar SA, Cornwall J. The current state of diabetes mellitus in India. Australas Med J. 2014;7(1):45-48.
3. Gupta V, Kalra S. Choosing a Gliptin. Indian J Endocrinol Metab. 2011;15(4):298-308.
4. Chen XW, He ZX, Zhou ZW. Clinical pharmacology of dipeptidyl peptidase 4 inhibitors indicated for the treatment of type 2 diabetes mellitus. Clin Exp Pharmacol Physiol. 2015;42(10):999-1024.
5. Kishimoto M. Teneligliptin: a DPP-4 inhibitor for the treatment of type diabetes. Diabetes Metab Syndr Obes. 2013;6:187-95.

6. Nabeno M, Akahoshi F, Kishida H. A comparative study of the binding modes of recently launched dipeptidyl peptidase IV inhibitors in the active site. Biochem Biophys Res Commun. 2013;434(2):191-6.
7. Kadowaki T, Haneda M, Ito H, et al. Safety and efficacy of long-term treatment with teneligliptin: Interim analysis of a post-marketing surveillance of more than 10,000 Japanese patients with type 2 diabetes mellitus. Expert Opin Pharmacother. 2018;19(2):83-91.
8. Anjana RM. Prevalence of diabetes and prediabetes in 15 states of India: results from the ICMR-INDIAB population-based cross-sectional study. Lancet Diabetes Endocrinol. 2017;5(8):585-96.
9. Kumar PKM, Ingole S, Tamboli T, et al. Management of type 2 diabetes mellitus: insights into prescribing trends. Int J Res Med Sci. 2017;5:1306-11.
10. Defronzo RA. From the triumvirate to the ominous octet: A new paradigm for the treatment of type 2 diabetes mellitus. Diabetes. 2009;58:773-95.
11. Sawada F, Inoguchi T, Tsubouchi H, et al. Differential effect of sulfonylureas on production of reactive oxygen species and apoptosis in cultured pancreatic beta-cell line, MIN6. Metabolism. 2008;57:1038-45.
12. Maladkar M, Sankar S, Kamat K. Teneligliptin: Heralding change in type 2 diabetes. J Diab Mel. 2016;6:113-31.
13. Ghosh S, Trivedi S, Sanyal D, et al. Teneligliptin real-world efficacy assessment of type 2 diabetes mellitus patients in India (TREAT INDIA study). Diabetes Metab Syndr Obes. 2016;9:347-53.
14. Nashikkar N, Panikar V, Joshi S, et al. Retrospective real-life efficacy assessment of teneligliptin in Indian T2DM patients. Int J Res Med Sci. 2018;6:3571-5.
15. Li X, Huang X, Bai C, et al. Efficacy and safety of teneligliptin in patients with type 2 diabetes mellitus: A systematic review and meta-analysis of randomized controlled trials. Front Pharmacol. 2018;9:449.
16. Kutoha E, Hiratea M, Ikenoa Y. Teneligliptin as an initial therapy for newly diagnosed, drug naive subjects with type 2 diabetes. J Clin Med Res. 2014;6(4):287-94.
17. Raghavan V, Lahiri A, Akul SK, et al. Effect of teneligliptin vs metformin on glycemic control in Indian patients with newly-diagnosed, drug-naïve type 2 diabetes mellitus: A 12-week randomized comparative clinical study. Int J Adv Med. 2019;6:481-8.
18. Suryawanshi SY, Bhargava A, Agarwal P, et al. Evaluation of safety and efficacy of teneligliptin in newly diagnosed Indian type 2 diabetes mellitus patients. The 52nd Annual Congress of European Association of Study in Diabetes, Munich. 2016:753. PS067.
19. Katsuno T, Ikeda H, Ida K. Add-on therapy with the DPP-4 inhibitor sitagliptin improves glycemic control in insulin-treated Japanese patients with type 2 diabetes mellitus. Endocr J. 2013;60:733-742.
20. Tanaka S, Suzuki K, Aoki C, et al. Add-on treatment with teneligliptin ameliorates glucose fluctuations and improves glycemic control index in Japanese patients with type 2 diabetes on insulin therapy. Diab Technol Ther. 2014;16(12):840-5.
21. Monnier L, Mas E, Ginet C. Activation of oxidative stress by acute fluctuations compared with sustained chronic hyperglycemia in patients with type 2 diabetes. JAMA. 2006;295:1681-87.
22. Kadowaki T, Kondo K, Sasaki N, et al. Efficacy and safety of teneligliptin add-on to insulin monotherapy in Japanese patients with type 2 diabetes mellitus: a 16-week, randomized, double-blind, placebo-controlled trial with an open-label period, Expert Opinion on Pharmacotherapy. 2017;18(13):1291-300.
23. Narita T, Katsuura Y, Sato T. Miglitol induces prolonged and enhanced glucagon-like peptide-1 and reduced gastric inhibitory polypeptide responses after ingestion of a mixed meal in Japanese type 2 diabetic patients. Diabet Med. 2009;26:187-88.
24. Scheen AJ. DPP-4 inhibitors in the management of type 2 diabetes: a critical review of head-to-head trials. Diabetes Metab. 2012;38(2):89-101.
25. Kadowaki T, Inagaki N, Kondo K, et al. Long-term safety and efficacy of canagliflozin as add-on therapy to teneligliptin in Japanese patients with type 2 diabetes. Diabetes Obes Metab. 2018;20(1):77-84.

41 CHAPTER Future Therapies in Pipeline for Diabetes Management

RM Anjana, Praveen Gangadhara

INTRODUCTION

Diabetes management has seen a paradigm shift over the last decade with improved understanding of etiopathogenesis of type 2 diabetes (T2D) mellitus. The whole focus has shifted from the classical "triumvirate" to the "ominous octet" concept. With this advancement, the approach to diabetes management has also moved from being "glucose-centric" to being "patient-centric". This has led to the development of various novel drugs such as dipeptidyl peptidase-4 (DPP-4) inhibitors, glucagon-like peptide-1 (GLP-1) analogs, and sodium-glucose cotransporter-2 (SGLT2) inhibitors apart from the existing commonly used antihyperglycemic medicines such as metformin, sulfonylureas, and insulin.[1]

The previous 2 decades have witnessed the development of an extensive range of new therapeutic options for T2D treatment. But, more than one-third of all patients with diabetes do not achieve or maintain appropriate glycemic targets. Despite these advancements, there is, therefore, a major unmet need for more efficient and durable treatment for T2D. Additionally, the complications and comorbidities (e.g. cardiac and renal diseases) that typically come with advanced insulin resistance and pancreatic β-cell dysfunction limit the choice of current available medications.[2]

These issues entitle for development of newer drugs (that act at newer targets) which can potentially aid in solving the earlier limitations. Oral once a week GLP-1 receptor agonist (GLP-1RA), once-weekly tablets of DPP-4 inhibitors, newer SGLT2 inhibitors and combined SGLT1 and 2 inhibitors, small molecule insulin releasers, glucokinase (GCK) activators, fatty acid receptor agonists, and imeglimin are some of the promising therapies that are in the pipeline. Also, adiponectin receptor agonists, selective peroxisome proliferator-activated receptor modulators, cellular glucocorticoid inhibitors, analogs of fibroblast growth factor 21, 11β-hydroxysteroid dehydrogenase 1 (11β-HSD1), etc. are in the pipeline.[3]

DRUGS ACTING AT THE PANCREATIC BETA CELL

- *Small molecule insulin releasers*: Apart from the existing molecules like sulfonylureas and meglitinides, many other compounds which improve the β-cell function have been tried. Succinate esters, imidazolines, selective phosphodiesterase inhibitors, α2-adrenergic antagonists, and agents that close Kir6.2 potassium channels or open membrane calcium channels are included. Most of them do not have the specificity for β-cells, and hence have not been investigated further.[4]
- *Glucokinase activators*: They are activators of the glucose phosphorylating enzyme which increases both insulin secretion and hepatic glucose metabolism. Initial studies have shown modest glucose-lowering effects, but their efficacy decreases over a few months. Side effects include hypoglycemia and accumulation of hepatic triglycerides due to long-term GCK activation. Ongoing research is to make liver selective GCK activators to avoid this effect.[5,6]
- *Dual activator of GCK and peroxisome proliferator-activated receptor-γ (PPARγ)*: SHP289-03 is a dual activator which improves glucose metabolism by enhancing insulin sensitivity, improves islet cell function, and reduces dyslipidemia without causing

hypoglycemia or weight gain. It appears to be a novel and improved drug when compared to sole GCK or PPARγ activators alone.[7]

- *Imeglimin*: Imeglimin is a triazine derivative. It is also first in the class of drugs called the "glimins" that acts on three primary pathophysiologic defects related to T2D, viz. elevated hepatic glucose production, decreased glucose uptake in skeletal muscle, and β-cell dysfunction. Human studies were done by Pacini et al. and others, which showed that the agent was effective and well-tolerated. The most common adverse effects were headache and gastrointestinal (GI)-related symptoms. In spite of all of the promising data currently available, further evidence is required for supporting the long-term safety.[8]
- *Fatty acid receptor agonists*: G-protein coupled receptors (e.g. GPR40, GPR119, and GPR120) expressed by pancreatic β-cells are activated by fatty acids that result in increase in insulin secretion.

  GPR40 agonists lead to increased insulin secretion by increasing cytosolic calcium. A promising GPR40 agonist (TAK-875) was discontinued due to hepatic side effects. However, other GPR40 agonists are in development.[9]

  Agonists of another fatty acid receptor (GPR119) activate adenylate cyclase, thus leading to increased cyclic adenosine monophosphate and potentiated nutrient-induced insulin secretion similar to GLP-1. Both GPR40 and GPR119 are formed by enteroendocrine pancreatic cells and other cells (K cells, L cells, and I cells). The synthetic agonists for these receptors may enhance the glucose-dependent insulinotropic peptide (also known as gastric inhibitory polypeptide, GIP), GLP-1, peptide YY (PYY), and cholecystokinin secretion. They are also expressed in the pancreatic alpha cells and may enhance the secretion of glucagon.

  GPR120, which is a long-acting fatty acid receptor expressed majorly by adipose tissue, promotes adipogenesis. Glucose homeostasis is improved by the small molecule agonists of this receptor by increasing insulin sensitivity and decreasing ectopic fat in preclinical studies.[10,11]
- *Incretin-based therapies*: The GLP-1 concentrations in T2D are often decreased, but the biological potency is mainly maintained, making GLP-1 an attractive target for treatment development. Glucose-dependent insulin secretion is enhanced and glucagon secretion is suppressed, gastric emptying is slowed, and food intake is reduced leading to weight loss. Incretins are quickly inactivated by DPP-4. To conquer their short half-life, DPP-4-resistant GLP-1 analogs and highly-specific DPP-4 inhibitors have been developed which are available today but further research is ongoing for oral preparations of GLP-1 analogs and long-acting DPP-4 inhibitors.
  - *Glucagon-like peptide-1 receptor agonists*: Currently available injectables GLP-1 analogs include exenatide, liraglutide, lixisenatide, albiglutide, dulaglutide, and semaglutide. To discover and develop GLP-1RA for once-weekly dosing, several technologies have been explored. Sustained release was one of the initial approaches to be evaluated in clinical trials and led to the approval of exenatide encapsulated formulation (exenatide extended-release). Other methods have included limiting the renal clearance of GLP-1 or exendin-based compounds by covalent peptide fusion to big, stable plasma proteins like albumin (albiglutide) or immunoglobulin G (IgG) Fc (dulaglutide).[12] After successful trial with weekly once injectable semaglutide, oral tablets with higher solubility and protection from enzymatic degradation have been developed which appear to be as effective as the injectables. A study on oral semaglutide by Davies et al. found that reduction in hemoglobin A1c (HbA1c) from baseline was 0.7–1.9% (dose dependent). Weight reduction was greater with oral semaglutide (2.1–6.9 kg) as compared to placebo. This was significant for dosage of 10 mg or more. Mild-to-moderate GI adverse effects were noted in the semaglutide group. Recently concluded CVOT, PIONEER 6 re-established the cardiovascular safety and noninferiority of oral semaglutide when compared to placebo [hazard ratio, 0.79; 95% confidence interval (CI), 0.57–1.11].[13,14]
  - *Dipeptidyl peptidase-4 inhibitors*: There are several long-acting DPP-4 inhibitors in the pipeline which possess similar efficacy in glycemic control and adverse effects comparable to currently available gliptins. Evogliptin, melogliptin, and gosogliptin are dosed daily whereas omarigliptin and trelagliptin are once-weekly drugs.
    - *Omarigliptin*: The evidence of the efficacy and safety of omarigliptin in the treatment of T2D was provided by a meta-analysis of studies involving 8,276 participants. Patients treated with omarigliptin had a significantly greater reduction in HbA1c, fasting plasma glucose (FPG), and a considerably stronger increased

number of participants who achieved HbA1c < 7.0% than patients treated with placebo or other oral antidiabetic drugs (OADs). Pooled evidence shows that there was no distinction in serious adverse events or hypoglycemic events between omarigliptin and placebo.

The cardiovascular safety of omarigliptin in 4,202 patients with T2D was tested by Gantz et al. When compared with placebo, omarigliptin did not increase the risk of major adverse cardiovascular events. It was generally well-tolerated and results were similar to some of the once-daily DPP-4 inhibitors.[15]

- *Tumor growth rate (TGR)-5 agonists*: TGR-5 agonists are biliary acid receptors mostly expressed in the enteroendocrine cells of the GI tract that helps in GLP-1 release. It is also seen in brown adipose tissue and muscle where it leads to enhancement of the expression of deiodinase type 2, modulating energy expenditure. Several TGR-5 agonists have been assessed for their role in energy homeostasis, lipid metabolism, and their ability to increase GLP-1 secretion. The antidiabetic effect of colesevelam, a bile acid sequestrant, leads to rise in the possibility that the presence of bile acids more distally along the ileum can activate TGR-5 and thereby improve the GLP-1 levels.[16]
- *Combined SGLT1 and 2 inhibitors (Fig. 1)*: SGLT2 inhibitors mainly act on the high capacity low affinity SGLT2 receptors in the kidney from the early proximal tubule S1 segment. The reabsorption of glucose leading to increased urinary glucose secretion is blocked by the selective inhibitors.

  This mechanism of action results in better glycemic control with reduced risk of hypoglycemia, weight loss from glucosuria, and blood pressure reduction. They have redefined the approach for diabetes management for their favorable cardiovascular and renal gains. Currently available SGLT2 inhibitors include canagliflozin, dapagliflozin, and empagliflozin and newer ones are remogliflozin, ertugliflozin, ipragliflozin, luseogliflozin, and tofogliflozin.

  The main uptake mechanism for glucose and galactose in the intestine is SGLT1. It is also responsible for 10% of renal glucose reabsorption in segment S3 of the proximal renal tubule.

  Sotagliflozin (LX4211) is a new, orally delivered, and small-molecule dual inhibitor of SGLT1 and SGLT2. SGLT1 inhibition delays and decreases absorption of glucose in the proximal intestine, while SGLT2 inhibition decreases renal glucose reabsorption.

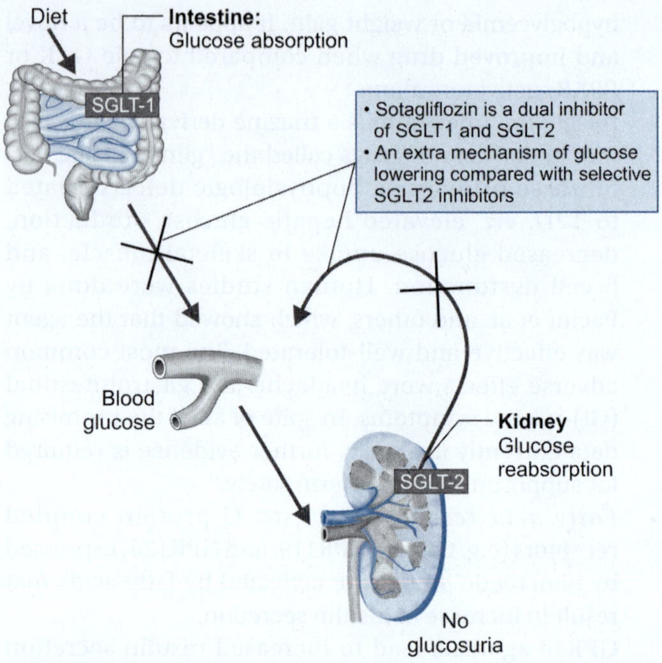

(SGLT1: sodium-glucose cotransporter-1)

Figure 1 Mechanism of SGLT1 and SGLT2 inhibitors.

Since inhibition of SGLT1 and SGLT2 is independent of β-cells, sotagliflozin provides a potentially unique, insulin-independent, therapeutic activity that comes with the additional anticipated therapeutic effects of improving postprandial glycemic control.

Studies have demonstrated that the SGLT1 inhibitor increased circulating levels of GLP-1 and PYY which play a role in insulin secretion and satiety. In patients with T2D not controlled with metformin alone, the efficacy, safety, and tolerability of four oral doses of sotagliflozin (75 mg once daily, 200 mg once daily, and 200 mg twice daily and 400 mg once daily) were tested. Sotagliflozin leads to better glycemic control by reducing HbA1c and FPG on a dose-dependent basis throughout the 12-week observation period (maximum efficacy was achieved with 400 mg once daily), with no corresponding elevation in urinary glucose excretion indicating that the improved efficacy observed with 400 mg once daily compared to the 200 mg daily dose is attained by clinically meaningful SGLT1 inhibition in the gut.

Various studies were also conducted to evaluate sotagliflozin effects added to insulin therapy in subjects with type 1 diabetes mellitus. In Tandem3, up to 28.6% of the sotagliflozin group achieved the primary endpoint (HbA1c < 7% at week 24, with no episodes of severe hypoglycemia or diabetic ketoacidosis), with a greater decrease in the glycated hemoglobin level from baseline in the sotagliflozin group than in the placebo group (difference, 0.46 percentage points; $P < 0.001$). The placebo-corrected declines from baseline in the mean daily total, bolus, and basal doses of insulin were—5.3 units per day (9.7%), 2.8 units per day (12.3%), and 2.6 units per day (9.9%), respectively ($P < 0.001$ for all comparisons) in the sotagliflozin group. The reduction in body weight and in systolic blood pressure from baseline to week 24 was considerably higher in the sotagliflozin group than in the placebo group (difference, 2.98 kg; $P < 0.001$; difference, 3.5 mm Hg; $P = 0.002$, respectively).

Though sotagliflozin addition to insulin in type 1 diabetes leads to reduction in the insulin dose, HbA1c, body weight, systolic blood pressure, and hypoglycemia, the study group in Tandem3 had higher incidence of ketoacidosis as compared to the placebo group (3.0% vs 0.6%). In fact, the Food and Drug Administration (FDA) issued a formal warning for the increased risk of diabetic ketoacidosis (DKA) with SGLTs.[17]

- *Adipokine-based treatments*: The adipocyte hormone adiponectin is generally low in patients with T2D, especially in overweight and obese individuals. It is known to exert several potentially beneficial effects including improved insulin sensitivity, improved endothelial function, and anti-inflammatory effects. ADIPOR1 and ADIPOR2 are the active small-molecule agonists of the adiponectin receptors that have demonstrated improved glycemic control and prolonged lifespan in insulin-resistant diabetic animals, raising expectations for clinical studies.

  Fibroblast growth factor 21 (FGF21) is a peptide that is secreted by adipose tissue, liver, and muscle, which cause increased fatty acid oxidation and hepatic gluconeogenesis during starvation. FGF21 levels are usually raised in obesity and T2D, possibly due to FGF21 resistance.

  Studies by Gaich et al. and Lin et al. have demonstrated that FGF21 analogs administration can improve lipid profile, decrease insulin resistance, and assist glucose-lowering, partly through increased adiponectin production.

  Leptin is known to cause loss in weight through centrally-mediated satiety and thermogenic effects. Insulin action is improved and glucagon action is suppressed. However, in obese patients with T2D, the glucose-lowering efficacy of leptin and leptin analogs was nominal during phase 3 trials, and benefits were seen only in individuals with leptin deficiency.[18,19]
- *Inhibitors of 11β-HSD1*: Individuals with glucocorticoid excess develop central obesity, insulin resistance, and dyslipidemia. Individuals with metabolic syndrome which mimics Cushing's syndrome have normal circulating glucocorticoid levels. The increased activity of 11β-HSD1 which converts inert cortisone to active cortisol within adipose tissues in humans may play a role in obesity. During a 12-week randomized phase 2 double blind placebo-controlled study in metformin-treated patients with T2D, it was observed that inhibitor of 11β-HSD1 *INCB13739* improved insulin sensitivity, lipid profile, HbA1c, and body weight. It was noted that there was lower efficacy and apart from reducing cortisol levels within adipose tissue and liver which leads to reduction in circulating cortisol levels, there can be compensatory rise in the adrenocorticotropic hormone.[20]
- *Selective peroxisome proliferator-activated receptor modulators*: PPARγ leads to improvement in insulin sensitivity, glycemic control, and several markers of vascular health while reducing inflammation. However, it increases retention of fluid and risk of heart failure, decreases bone mineral density, and often leads to excessive adipogenesis.

  Attempts are being made to develop selective PPAR modulators which will reduce these unwanted effects. SPPARM, INT131, a nonthiazolidinedione demonstrated similar glucose-lowering efficiency to pioglitazone but with less edema and less weight gain during phase 2A, 24-week randomized double-blind study in patients with T2D receiving a sulfonylurea with or without metformin.[21]

CONCLUSION

Reversal of the disease process and reinstatement of normal glucose homeostasis seem rarely possible despite the availability of various differently acting glucose-lowering drugs. Many developments are also going on in the existing group of drugs such as glitazones, gliptins, and SGLT2 inhibitors. The newer molecules have tried to address the various pathophysiologies that cause hyperglycemia and some of them have shown promise in clinical trials. Outcomes can be improved and the cost burden can be reduced by adding new options with new mechanisms of action to the treatment. It is prudent to remain hopeful as the research in this field is continuously evolving.

REFERENCES

1. Inzucchi SE, Bergenstal RM, Buse JB, et al. Management of hyperglycemia in type 2 diabetes, 2015: a patient-centered approach: update to a position statement of the American Diabetes Association and the European Association for the Study of Diabetes. Diabetes Care. 2015;38:140-9.
2. Tahrani AA, Bailey CJ, Del Prato S, et al. Management of type 2 diabetes: new and future developments in treatment. Lancet. 2011;378:182-97.
3. Bailey CJ, Tahrani AA, Barnett AH. Future glucose-lowering drugs for type 2 diabetes. Lancet Diabetes Endocrinol. 2016;4:350-9.
4. Bailey CJ. New drugs for the treatment of diabetes mellitus. In: DeFronzo RA, Ferrannini E, Zimmet P, Alberti GM (Eds). International Textbook of Diabetes Mellitus, 4th edition. Chichester: Wiley Blackwell; 2015. pp. 709-25.
5. Nakamura A, Terauchi Y. Present status of clinical deployment of glucokinase activators. J Diabetes Investig. 2015;6:124-32.
6. Erion DM, Lapworth A, Amor PA, et al. The hepatoselective glucokinase activator PF-04991532 ameliorates hyperglycemia without causing hepatic steatosis in diabetic rats. PLoS One. 2014;9:e97139.
7. Lei L, Liu Q, Liu S, et al. Antidiabetic potential of a novel dual-target activator of glucokinase and peroxisome proliferator activated receptor-γ. Metabolism. 2015;64:1250-61.
8. Vuylsteke V, Chastain LM, Maggu GA, et al. Imeglimin: A potential new multi-target drug for type 2 diabetes. Drugs R D. 2015;15:227-32.
9. Mancini AD, Poitout V. GPR40 agonists for the treatment of type 2 diabetes: life after 'TAKing' a hit. Diabetes Obes Metab. 2015;17:622-9.
10. Nunez DJ, Bush MA, Collins DA, et al. Gut hormone pharmacology of a novel GPR119 agonist (GSK1292263), metformin, and sitagliptin in type 2 diabetes mellitus: results from two randomized studies. PLoS One. 2014;9:e92494.
11. Oh DY, Walenta E, Akiyama TE, et al. A Gpr120-selective agonist improves insulin resistance and chronic inflammation in obese mice. Nat Med. 2014;20:942-7.
12. Knudsen LB, Lau J. The discovery and development of liraglutide and semaglutide. Front Endocrinol (Lausanne). 2019;10:155.
13. Davies M, Pieber TR, Hartoft-Nielsen ML, et al. Effect of oral semaglutide compared with placebo and subcutaneous semaglutide on glycemic control in patients with type 2 diabetes: A randomized clinical trial. JAMA. 2017;318:1460-70.
14. Husain M, Birkenfeld AL, Donsmark M, et al. Oral semaglutide and cardiovascular outcomes in patients with type 2 diabetes. N Engl J Med. 2019;381:841-51.
15. Wang X, Li X, Qie S, et al. The efficacy and safety of once-weekly DPP-4 inhibitor omarigliptin in patients with type 2 diabetes mellitus: A systemic review and meta-analysis. Medicine (Baltimore). 2018;97:e11946.
16. Duan H, Ning M, Zou Q, et al. Discovery of intestinal targeted TGR5 agonists for the treatment of type 2 diabetes. J Med Chem. 2015;58:3315-28.
17. Cefalo CM, Cinti F, Moffa S, et al. Sotagliflozin, the first dual SGLT inhibitor: current outlook and perspectives. Cardiovasc Diabetol. 2019;18:20.
18. Coppari R, Bjørbak C. Leptin revisited: its mechanism of action and potential for treating diabetes. Nat Rev Drug Discov. 2012;11:692-708.
19. Fisman EZ, Tenenbaum A. Adiponectin: a manifold therapeutic target for metabolic syndrome, diabetes, and coronary disease? Cardiovasc Diabetol. 2014;13:103.
20. Heise T, Morrow L, Hompesch M, et al. Safety, efficacy and weight effect of two 11 -HSD1 inhibitors in metformin-treated patients with type 2 diabetes. Diabetes Obes Metab. 2014;16:1070-7.
21. DePaoli AM, Higgins LS, Henry RR, et al. Can a selective PPAR modulator improve glycemic control in patients with type 2 diabetes with fewer side effects compared with pioglitazone? Diabetes Care. 2014;37:1918-23.

42 CHAPTER A Right Combination a Day: Keeps the Complications Away

Manoj Chawla, Purvi Chawla

INTRODUCTION

With an increase in the number of diabetes cases globally, it has emerged as an emergent public health problem. Type 2 diabetes (T2DM) is expected to reach 642 million by the year 2040, and it was estimated that nearly 400 million people were affected by diabetes in the year 2015.[1] It is accompanied by complications associated with retinopathy, blindness, cardiovascular (CV) disease, neuropathy, renal disease, amputation, and nonvascular complications.[1] Along with lifestyle interventions, pharmacotherapy is also required.[2,3] Evidences suggest that controlled glucose levels in blood would reduce the risk of developing complications.[1] Using appropriate drug could minimize the glucose variability, leading to manage the disease effectively resulting in a better quality of life.[1] A study by the UK Prospective Diabetes Study compared antihyperglycemic therapies in more than 5,000 newly diagnosed patients for 20 years. The outcome of the study showed considerable decrease in diabetic complications like retinopathy, nephropathy, and neuropathy with intensive glycemic control with sulfonylurea and insulin, or metformin in obese patients than conservative diet restriction.[1] The present guidelines recommend a solitary antihyperglycemic agent to treat initial T2DM; but the progressive nature of the disease necessitates two or more antihyperglycemic agents in most of the T2DM patients because of pancreatic beta (β)-cell functional decline[2] (Table 1).

TABLE 1: Approaches recommended in US guidelines for newly diagnosed T2D.[1]

	ADA	AACE

HbA1c target	Individualize goals:
	• HbA1c <7.0%
	• In some circumstances:
	  ○ HbA1c <6.5%
	  ○ HbA1c <80%
		Individualize goals:
		• ≤6.5% if low risk for hypoglycemia, no concurrent illness
		• >6.5% if high risk for hypoglycemia, concurrent serious illness

Treatment strategy	Depends on HbA1c levels at diagnosis:
	• **Monotherapy** (usually metformin) if **HbA1c <9.0%**, with stepwise addition of antihyperglycemic drugs to dual and triple therapy at 3 months intervals, until patient is at goal.
	• **Combination therapy if:**
	  ○ **HbA1c ≥9.0%** (dual therapy)
	  ○ **HbA1c ≥10%** (or blood glucose ≥300% mg/dL, or patient is symptomatic) [combination injectable therapy]
	• Lifestyle management to be emphasized along with any pharmacological therapy
		Depends on HbA1c levels at diagnosis:
		• **Monotherapy** (preferably with metformin), plus lifestyle therapy if **HbA1c <7.5%**, followed by therapy intensification to dual and triple therapy at 3 months intervals, until patient is at goal.
		• **Combination therapy if:**
		  ○ **HbA1c ≥7.5%** [dual therapy + lifestyle therapy]
		  ○ **HbA1c >9.0%** [insulin (± other drugs) or dual/triple therapy, if asymptomatic]

Specific therapeutic guidance provided	No preference provided, choice dependent on patient-and disease-specific factors	Yes, hierarchy of medication usage suggested

(HbA1c: glycated hemoglobin; ADA: American Diabetes Association; AACE: American Association of Clinical Endocrinologists; T2D: type 2 diabetes)

TREATMENT

For patients newly diagnosed with T2DM, stepwise approach and combination approach are the two approved management therapies. There are advantages and disadvantages for both the therapies.

Innovative therapeutic approaches like fixed-dose and fixed-ratio combinations focus on the complexity involved in the treatment and issues bothering the patient associated with combination therapy comprising individual drugs. The decision between the usage of stepwise and combination therapy, and the choice of drugs, purely depend on the individual.

Types of Therapy

They are mainly two types:
1. Stepwise therapy
2. Combination therapy.

Stepwise Therapy

This is one of the common approaches. Usually, patients are given metformin. If tolerated and not contraindicated, another oral agent, a GLP-1RA or a basal insulin, is provided. Therapy intensification is later suggested if there is no improvement. The American Diabetes Association (ADA) guidelines then suggest dual therapy with two non-insulin agents or with insulin itself for patients with glycosylated hemoglobin (Hb1Ac) of ≥10.0%, blood glucose level of 300 mg/dL or with symptoms of hyperglycemia, combination injectable therapy is recommended. In addition to this, additional treatments are designed in sequence with the patient's response. Insulin is only given when all the other treatments have failed.[1,2]

The advantages of the stepwise therapy may result in good patient adherence. Also, this allows for a greater and customized, focused individualization of therapy. This leads to minimal side effects and mitigation of the risks of the therapy. Stepwise therapy is best recommended for patients closer to achieving optimal glycemic results. However, there is a disadvantage of prolonging or impeding the therapy as it may take more time to achieve the goal; thus the patient is exposed to hyperglycemia for a longer duration.

In the recent VERIFY (Vildagliptin efficacy in combination with metformin for early treatment of type 2 diabetes) 5-year study published in Lancet in September 2019, it has been demonstrated that in newly diagnosed patients with type 2 diabetes, the recommended strategy of initiating treatment with metformin and then stepping up treatment with a second agent if monotherapy fails, would not be suited best and may not be ideal[4] (Table 2).

TABLE 2: Summary of the cellular mechanisms of action and physiological effects of the most commonly prescribed antihyperglycemic drugs (modified from Cersosimo et al.).[1]

Class	Compounds	Cellular mechanism	Primary physiological actions	
			Glycemic effects	Non-glycemic effects
GLP-1RAs	• Exenatide/Exenatide extended release • Liraglutide • Albiglutide • Lixisenatide • Dulaglutide	Activation of GLP-1 receptor	↑ insulin secretion (glucose dependent) ↓ glucagon secretion (glucose dependent)	↑ satiety ↓ gastric emptying ↓ body weight/↓ body-fat content ↓ blood pressure ↓ circulating lipids ↓ inflammatory markers
SGLT2 inhibitors	• Canagliflozin • Dapagliflozin • Empagliflozin	Inhibition of SGLT2 in proximal nephron	Increased glycosuria	↓ blood pressure ↓ body weight
Insulins	• Rapid-acting analogs • Short acting • Intermediate acting • Basal insulin analogs • Premixed	Activation of insulin receptor	↑ glucose disposal ↓ hepatic glucose production	

Contd...

Contd...

Class	Compounds	Cellular mechanism	Primary physiological actions	
			Glycemic effects	Non-glycemic effects
Biguanides	• Metformin	Activation of AMP-kinase	↓ hepatic glucose production	
Sulfonylureas	• Glyburide/glibenclamide • Glipizide • Gliclazide • Glimepiride	Closure of potassium-dependent ATP channels on β-cell plasma membranes	↑ insulin secretion	
Glinides	• Repaglinide • Nateglinide	Closure of potassium-dependent ATP channels on β-cell plasma membranes	↑ insulin secretion	
TZD	• Pioglitazone	Activation of PPAR-γ transcription factor	↑ insulin sensitivity	
DPP-4 inhibitors	• Sitagliptin • Saxagliptin • Linagliptin • Aloglipitin	Inhibition of DPP-4 activity increase in postprandial active incretin (GLP-1, GIP) concentrations	↑ insulin secretion (glucose dependent) ↓ glucagon secretion (glucose dependent)	

(AMP: adenosine monophosphate; ATP: adenosine triphosphate; DPP-4: dipeptidyl peptidase-4; GIP: glucose-dependent insulinotropic polypeptide; GLP-1 RA: glucagon-like peptide-1 receptor agonist; PPAR: peroxisome proliferator-activated receptor; SGLT2: sodium glucose co-transporter 2; TZD: thiazolidinediones)

Combination Therapy

The combination therapy may include two or more oral or injectable drugs for the treatment of T2DM. It is based on the idea that several defects contribute to the development of chronic hyperglycemia and other related complications, which further contribute to glucose intolerance (Box 1). The abnormalities could be reversed by using multiple drugs on different pathophysiological aspects. The introduction of multiple drugs is to be initiated from the beginning within 3–6 months from the diagnosis.

The combination therapy, in the recent past has emerged as an indispensable and an important therapeutic option. The benefits of combination therapy when compared with stepwise therapy are as follows:

- Decreased clinical inertia
- Parallel focus on multiple pathogenic mechanisms leading to faster and more recurrent HbA1c goal achievement
- Adequate delay of advancing disease.

The drawbacks of combinations therapy when compared to the stepwise therapy are as follows:

- Multidrug regimen seem complex for the patient resulting in less adherence to treatment
- The basis of poor efficacy of a drug and/or adverse effects cannot be ascertained easily
- Patient may not accept their disease
- Expensive treatment. (Table 3)

BOX 1	Pathological alterations that significantly cause the onset of glucose intolerance, referred to as "Ominous octet" of T2DM.[1]
1.	↓ insulin secretion by the pancreas
2.	↓ incretin effect in the gastrointestinal tract
3.	↑ lipolysis in fact cells
4.	↑ glucose reabsorption by the kidney
5.	↓ glucose uptake by muscle
6.	Neurotransmitter dysfunction
7.	↑ hepatic glucose production
8.	↑ glucagon secretion by islet α cells

The landmark INITIAL trial[5] published in 2018 evaluated the clinical effect of the combination vildagliptin/metformin in the relatively young age (mean age of approximately 50 years), drug-naïve 532 T2DM Asian subjects. The patients had a high baseline HbA1c (9.3%) and were often associated with CV risk factors. There was a significant and clinically relevant HbA1c reduction from baseline and effect observed at week 12 was maintained over 24 weeks, with good tolerability.

VERIFY study has been the largest long-term prospective trial to evaluate the durability of glycemic control in patients with diabetes who were initially treated with dual combination therapy of vildagliptin

TABLE 3: The potential advantages and disadvantages of stepwise and early combination therapy in newly diagnosed T2DM patients.[1]

Stepwise therapy	Combination therapy
Potential advantages • Good patient adherence • Cost • Easier to assess efficacy/side effects of new drug added (risk-to-benefit ratio) • Easier individualization of therapy	**Potential advantages** • Use of drug combination aimed at targeting multiple pathogenic mechanisms simultaneously, preferably by complementary mechanisms of action • Earlier and greater achievement of glycemic goals • Potential delay of disease progression and preservation of β-cell function • Reduction in clinical inertia
Potential disadvantages • Risk of prolonged hyperglycemia and subsequent complications • Increased risk of clinical inertia if not implemented properly • Little or no effect on disease progression	**Potential disadvantages** • Assessment of efficacy/side effects in individual patient more difficult • Long-term cost-effectiveness not easily assessed (in absence of comparative efficacy studies) • Patient adherence with complex, multidrug regimens

and metformin. The synergistic mechanisms have been found to be useful. The synergistic mechanisms work as metformin is known to increase the insulin sensitivity, and on the other hand, vildagliptin enhances β-cell function (Table 1).[5] The study enrolled 2,001 newly diagnosed across 254 centers from 34 countries. The patients were in the age group 18–70 years old and were diagnosed with T2DM in the previous 2 years. The range of HbA1c was between 6.5% and 7.5% and the BMI ranged across 22–40 kg/m^2. VERIFY enrolled 2,001 patients. The patients were randomly assigned either to the early combination treatment group (n = 998) or to the initial metformin monotherapy group (n = 1,003). The patients in the combination therapy group received metformin at a dose of 1,000 mg, 1,500 mg, or 2,000 mg per day, plus vildagliptin at a dose of 50 mg twice daily. The patients in the monotherapy arm received the same daily doses of metformin plus twice-daily placebo. If at any time from 6 months to 5 years from the initiation of the trial, the HbA_{1C} level was not maintained below 7.0% with initial treatment, patients in the metformin monotherapy group were given vildagliptin 50 mg twice daily in addition to metformin. 80% patients in each group completed the 5-year study. During the first phase of the study (before therapy was stepped up for any patients receiving monotherapy), 429 patients (43.6%) in the combination treatment group and 614 patients (62.1%) patients in the monotherapy group experienced treatment failure. The median time to treatment failure was 36 months in the monotherapy group; treatment failure had not occurred by 5 years in the combination therapy group. The risk for treatment failure was 49% lower with initial combination therapy than with initial monotherapy (hazard ratio, 0.51; $P<.0001$). Both treatment approaches were safe and well tolerated. There were no unexpected or new safety findings, and no deaths occurred that were related to study treatment.[4]

Combination therapy with GLP-1 receptor agonist and SGLT2 receptor

The sodium-glucose cotransporter-2 inhibitors (SGLT2i) and glucagon-like-1 receptor agonists (GLP-1 RAs) have different mechanisms in effectively reducing HbA1c. This makes them an effective combination therapy. Drugs have been shown to reduce CV events in both antidiabetic classes. SGLT2i use their CV protective actions by hemodynamic effects, while GLP-1 RAs work through antiatherogenic/anti-inflammatory mechanisms. The SGLT2i and GLP-1 RAs also reduced macroalbuminuria, decreased the time for doubling of serum creatinine, and slowed the time to end-stage renal disease.[6]

Diabetic dyslipidemia and combination therapy

There is a high residual risk of cardiovascular disease in T2DM patients though they are under maximum coverage of statins and other lifestyle modifications. A diabetic adult usually presents with increased levels of triglycerides, small dense LDL, and decreased high-density lipoprotein cholesterol (HDL). Combination therapy has been extensively tried with an additional drug like niacin, ezetimibe, fenofibrate, or n-3 fatty acids, though all the results were unsatisfactory. Trials where combination therapy is used to decrease the possibility of CV disease in cases with dyslipidemia are evaluated for benefits, if any. Though there is an improvement in lipid profile with combination therapy, clinical outcomes seem inconsistent. With all these results, combination therapy is not recommended by current guidelines in diabetic individuals. A recent study in high-risk patients, IMProved Reduction of Outcomes: Vytorin Efficacy International Trial (IMPROVE IT), confirmed that the addition of ezetimibe to statins showed advancement in clinical endpoints in high-risk patients. Though this study was not done with diabetic individuals in focus, the clinical outcome can affect the role of combination therapy in such people prospectively.[3]

REFERENCES

1. Cersosimo E, Johnson EL, Chovanes C, et al. Initiating therapy in patients newly diagnosed with type 2 diabetes: Combination therapy vs a stepwise approach. Diabetes Obes Metab. 2018;20(3):497-507.
2. Blonde L, Dipp S, Cadena D. Combination Glucose-Lowering Therapy Plans in T2DM: Case-Based Considerations. Adv Ther. 2018;35(7): 939-65.
3. Warraich HJ, Wong ND, Rana JS. Role for combination therapy in diabetic dyslipidemia. Curr Cardiol Rep. 2015;17(5):32.
4. Matthews DR, Paldánius PM, Proot P, et al. Glycaemic durability of an early combination therapy with vildagliptin and metformin versus sequential metformin monotherapy in newly diagnosed type 2 diabetes (VERIFY): a 5-year, multicentre, randomised, double-blind trial. VERIFY study group. Lancet. 2019;6736(19):32131-2.
5. Chawla Manoj, Kim TH, Mirasol RC, et al. Initial combination therapy with vildagliptin plus metformin in drug-naïve patients with T2DM: a 24-week real-life study from Asia. Curr Med Res Opin. 2018;34(9):1605-11.
6. DeFronzo RA. Combination therapy with GLP-1 receptor agonist and SGLT2 inhibitor. Diabetes Obes Metab. 2017;19(10):1353-62.

43 CHAPTER The Pursuit of Ultra-Fast Acting Insulin: Bridging the Barriers

Abdul Hamid Zargar

INTRODUCTION

In people without diabetes, pancreatic secretion of insulin is immediate in response to a meal.[1] In people with type 1 diabetes the postprandial insulin response is lacking, while in type 2 diabetes it is delayed and blunted.[2] Current rapid-acting mealtime insulin analogs approach the normal physiological insulin response but there is still a physiological gap.[3] Insulin aspart came closer to reducing the physiological gap compared to regular human insulin, which helped patients to achieve a quicker onset of insulin action and reduce the postprandial glucose (PPG). An even faster insulin than aspart, one that can approach physiological insulin responses even more, may help people with diabetes avoid prolonged time in an elevated glucose state.[4]

Epidemiological studies of both type 1 and type 2 diabetes suggest that it is challenging to achieve recommended glycemic targets, and current glycemic control is not adequate.[5] One reason for this is high PPG peaks. In people without diabetes, there is an immediate release of insulin in response to a meal, resulting in a normal glucose tolerance. For patients with type 1 diabetes, most or all insulin secretion is ceased. In patients with type 2 diabetes, there may still be some insulin production, but secretion is reduced, insulin resistance impairs its effects, and the hepatic glucose production is not appropriately suppressed.[2]

In type 2 diabetes, insulin resistance prevents the liver from reacting effectively to insulin, and liver glucose production does not slow after a meal. Therefore, hepatic glucose production accounts for a significant portion of postmeal glucose exposure in people with type 2 diabetes because of insulin resistance and inadequate suppression of hepatic glucose production.[6,7] The development of the first generation of rapid-acting insulin analogs was a significant advancement toward closing the physiological gap over regular human insulin.[3]

Rapid-acting insulin analogs were meant to better mimic *endogenous insulin* secretion. Despite the added benefits of the rapid-acting insulin analogs over regular human insulin, there is still a need for quicker absorption of mealtime insulins.[4] A faster-acting insulin would provide even earlier exposure of the liver to the insulin resulting in a greater suppression of hepatic glucose production, which would theoretically result in lower PPG excursions.[6] Additionally, a faster-acting insulin would more closely match the ideal physiological insulin secretion profile and further close the physiological insulin response gap (Fig. 1). A faster-acting insulin that could address these requirements is faster insulin aspart or Fiasp®.

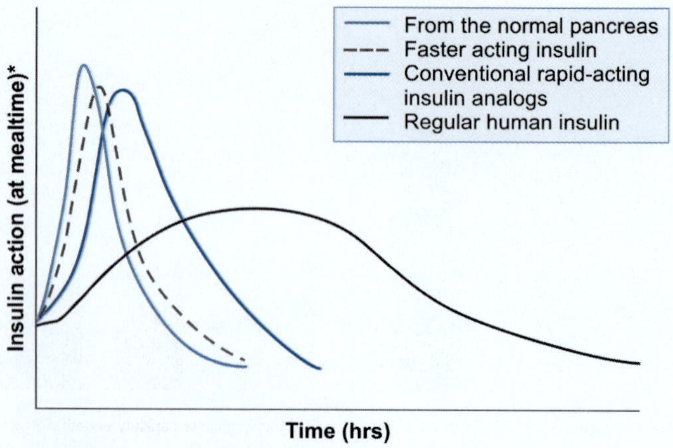

*Schematic representation

Figure 1 Schematic presentation of insulin action: Faster-acting insulin approaches the physiological insulin profile.

As seen in Figure 1, a faster insulin would better approach physiological insulin secretion in people with type 1 diabetes and replace early insulin secretion in people with type 2 diabetes. Additionally, a faster acting insulin would have a better profile for pump therapy because faster acting insulin has a decreased time to onset of action and a shortened duration of insulin action, which better mimics the insulin release in people without diabetes.

Fiasp® is the first insulin analog designed to fill this unmet need. Fiasp® has the same active substance, which is insulin aspart but the formulation includes two additional drug excipients, *niacinamide* and *L-arginine*, which accelerate absorption and stabilize the formulation, respectively. Additionally, both excipients are characterized as safe inactive ingredients for injectable drug products by the US FDA.[8] Although, innovative in formulation, Fiasp® does include insulin aspart—a molecule that has an established safety profile with more than 17 years of clinical experience.[9,10]

Niacinamide, or vitamin B3, is an absorption modifier.[11] One notable study sought to define the role of niacinamide in increased initial absorption of the insulin aspart after subcutaneous injection. This laboratory study analyzed absorption across a membrane comparing zinc to non-zinc formulations with and without niacinamide. The presence of niacinamide in the formulation containing zinc increased both the insulin aspart monomer fraction and the *transendothelial permeation* of the insulin aspart (Fig. 2). In the zinc-free formulations, which lack stable hexamer structures, the niacinamide had no notable effect on permeation rate. Therefore, niacinamide is concluded to increase rate of permeation of the insulin aspart by promoting the monomeric state.[12]

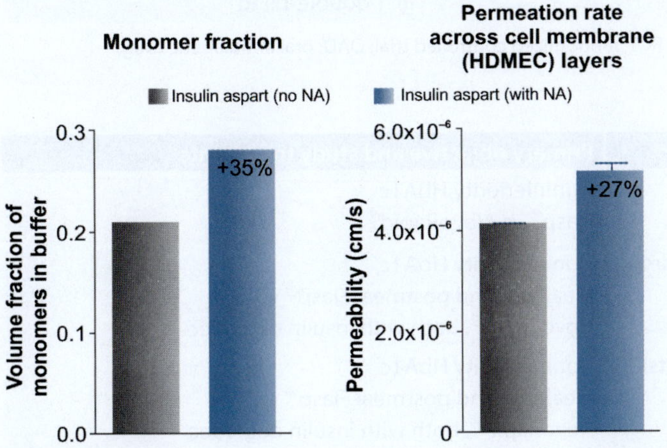

NA = niacinamide; HDMEC = human dermal-derived microvascular capillary endothelial cell

Figure 2 Niacinamide effect: Niacinamide increased both the insulin aspart monomer fraction and the transendothelial absorption of insulin aspart.[13,14]

The second excipient, L-arginine, is a naturally occurring amino acid. Arginine provides stability to insulin formulations and has been shown to effectively inhibit insulin aggregation. Aggregation of insulin may lead to loss of activity and even trigger an immune response.[15]

PHARMACOKINETIC RESULTS FOR FIASP

In a pooled analysis of six pharmacokinetic/pharmacodynamic (PK/PD) trials, the onset of exposure was earlier for Fiasp® compared with insulin aspart. Additionally, the time to early half maximal concentration was reduced by 10 minutes. Both insulin formulations had similar total and maximal exposures; however, Fiasp® has a shortened t_{Cmax} (approximately 7 minutes shorter). The onset of appearance in the bloodstream was reduced from 9 minutes to 4 minutes, demonstrating that Fiasp® is twice as fast as insulin aspart.[16]

Fiasp® also had a greater early insulin exposure than insulin aspart, approximately 2-fold greater within the first 30 minutes, based on the pooled analysis of six trials.[16] During the late phase, the left-shift in insulin exposure for the Fiasp® resulted in a shorter time to late half-maximal concentration (approximately 12 minutes shorter).[17]

PHARMACODYNAMIC ENDPOINTS FOR FIASP

In a pooled analysis of three trials using the euglycemic clamp technique, a graph of glucose infusion rate (GIR) versus time showed a noticeable left-shift in the curve representing Fiasp® compared to insulin aspart. The faster initial absorption of Fiasp® leads to an earlier onset of action. Fiasp® had an onset of action 5 minutes quicker than aspart, and the time to half-maximum GIR was approximately 10 minutes shorter with Fiasp®. The time to maximum GIR was approximately 11 minutes shorter with Fiasp® than aspart.[17] In the first 30 minutes after administration, Fiasp® had a glucose lowering effect 74% greater than that of aspart. The total and maximum glucose-lowering effects were comparable between the Fiasp® and aspart. Similarly, the time to late half-maximum effect was 14 minutes shorter for Fiasp® than aspart thus Fiasp® has a faster offset and shorter duration of action.[17]

FIASP CLINICAL TRIAL PROGRAM

The onset clinical trial program comprised four phase 3a clinical trials that enrolled more than 2,100 patients with type 1 and type 2 diabetes (Table 1).[18]

To supplement the clinical data from the onset clinical program, Novo Nordisk has designed a phase 3b program to explore a range of patient types and clinical settings, including combination therapies of Fiasp® and insulin degludec, and pediatric and pump patients (Table 2).[19-21]

Onset 1 Trial

Onset 1 is the pivotal randomized, parallel clinical trial examining the efficacy and safety of Fiasp® in type 1 diabetes. The primary objective of the trial was to show noninferiority of Fiasp® compared to insulin aspart in *glycated hemoglobin (HbA1c)* readings.[22]

The trial randomized a total of 1,143 patients with type 1 diabetes (1:1:1) into either one of two mealtime double-blinded treatment arms or a third postmeal, unblinded treatment arm. The two blinded treatment arms used either Fiasp® or insulin aspart as bolus mealtime insulins three times a day, in a basal-bolus regimen. The unblinded treatment arm tested postmeal administration of Fiasp® 20 minutes after the start of each meal in a basal-bolus regimen; all three treatment arms were coupled with insulin detemir once daily or twice daily. The treatment period lasted 26 weeks and double-blind arms were followed up by an additional 26-week treatment period to assess long-term safety and efficacy.[22]

TABLE 1: Overview of the onset clinical trial program.

	Patients enrolled	Primary objective and study treatments	Study design and randomized subjects
Onset 1 study 3852	T1D basal-bolus	Non-inferiority HbA1c Fiasp® (mealtime and postmeal) vs. NovoRapid®, all with insulin determir	n = 1143 26-week + 26-week extension RCT partially double-blind
Onset 2 study 3853	T2D basal + metformin +/– other OAD	Non-inferiority HbA1c Fiasp® vs. NonoRapid®, both with insulin glargine U100	n = 689 26-week RCT double-blind
Onset 3 study 4049	T2D basal + metformin +/– other OAD	Superiority HbAlc basal-bolus (Fiasp®) vs. basal (both with previous basal insulin)	n = 236 18-week RCT open-label
Onset 4 study 3931	T1D insulin pumps	Pump compatibility Fiasp® vs. NovoRapid®	n = 37 6-week RCT double-blind

(HbA1c: glycosylated hemoglobin; T1D: type 1 diabetes; T2D: type 2 diabetes; RCT: randomized controlled trial; OAD: oral antidiabetic drug)

TABLE 2: Summary of phase 3b program.

Trial	Patients enrolled	Primary objective and study treatments
Onset 5	T1D (CSII, adults)	Noninferiority HbA1c Fiasp® vs. NovoRapid®
Onset 7	T1D (MDI, combination with insulin degludec, children and adolescents)	Noninferiority HbA1c Mealtime and postmeal Fiasp® vs. NovoRapid®, both with insulin degludec
Onset 8	T1D (MDI, combination with insulin degludec, adults)	Noninferiority HbA1c Mealtime and postmeal Fiasp® vs. NovoRapid®, both with insulin degludec
Onset 9	T2D (MDI, combination with insulin degludec, adults)	Noninferiority HbA1c Mealtime Fiasp® vs. NovoRapid®, both with insulin degludec and metformin

(CSII: continuous subcutaneous insulin infusion; MDI: multiple daily insulin; T1D: type 1 diabetes; T2D: type 2 diabetes)

The mean HbA1c values decreased from approximately 7.6% (at randomization visits; for all treatment arms) to 7.3% (with mealtime Fiasp®), 7.4% (with mealtime insulin aspart), and 7.5% (with postmeal Fiasp®). Mealtime Fiasp® was noninferior to mealtime aspart in mean change from baseline of HbA1c levels after the 26-week treatment period, and the estimated treatment difference was statistically significant in favor of mealtime Fiasp®. One-third of the patients receiving mealtime Fiasp® achieved an HbA1c target value of 7% after the initial 26-week treatment period; a significantly higher proportion than among those patients receiving mealtime aspart.[22]

The PPG increment, or glucose spike, after the meal test at week 26 was the secondary endpoint in the study and showed that the estimated treatment differences in 2-hour and 1-hour PPG increments were significantly lower in patients taking mealtime Fiasp® compared to those taking mealtime aspart, –12.06 mg/dL and –21.24 mg/dL, respectively. The 2-hour PPG increment difference (confirmatory secondary endpoint) confirmed superior PPG control for Fiasp®. The estimated treatment differences in 3- and 4-hour PPG increments were not statistically significant.[22]

Change in body weight from baseline to week 26 was another secondary endpoint in onset 1. The mean body weight increase was similar for all three treatment arms and was less than 1 kg after 26 weeks.[22]

There were no clinically relevant differences in adverse event profiles between treatment arms. The rate of adverse events per patient-year of exposure was between 4.4 and 4.8 across treatment arms. The majority of adverse events were not serious and judged as unlikely to be related to the Fiasp®.[22]

Onset 2 Trial

Onset 2 was a randomized, parallel, double-blind trial in patients with type 2 diabetes designed to examine the efficacy and safety of Fiasp® compared with insulin aspart. The primary endpoint was the mean change from baseline in HbA1c levels.[22]

The mean HbA1c value at the time of randomization was 7.9%. Both Fiasp® and insulin aspart led to a decrease in the mean HbA1c value to 6.6% at the end of the 26-week treatment period.[22]

The PPG increment, at week 26 showed that the 1-hour PPG increment was significantly lower in patients taking Fiasp® compared to those taking insulin aspart. The treatment difference was approximately 10.8 mg/dL. The treatment differences for the 2-, 3-, and 4-hour PPG increments were not statistically significant.[16]

Change in body weight was comparable between insulin regimens with both groups gaining an average of 2.7 kg over 26 weeks of treatment.[22]

More than 50% of patients reported adverse events in both treatment groups, however most were nonserious. The overall rate of adverse events was comparable between the Fiasp® and insulin aspart treatment groups (0.1 and 0.2 events per patient-year of exposure, respectively). Major cardiovascular events were very few.[22]

CONCLUSION

The speed at which currently marketed, mealtime, rapid-acting insulins exert their effect does not match the natural physiological insulin response. Subsequently, there is a risk that people with diabetes are spending more time in an elevated glucose state, and require improved blood glucose control.

Through the clinical pharmacology trials and onset clinical program, Fiasp® has demonstrated advantages as a faster insulin formulation.

- *Speed:* Fiasp® enters into the bloodstream two times faster than insulin aspart.
- *Improved glycemic control:* Fiasp® versus Insulin aspart
  - Statistically significant HbA1c reduction in type 1 diabetes
  - Noninferior HbA1c reduction in type 2 diabetes
    - 1-hour PPG increment: Significantly lower with Fiasp® versus insulin aspart in type 1 and type 2 diabetes
    - 2-hr PPG increment: significantly lower with Fiasp® versus insulin aspart in type 1 diabetes but significant benefit in type 2 diabetes could not be confirmed
    - No significant difference in overall rate of severe and blood glucose confirmed hypoglycemia
- *Pump use:* A faster, more physiological option for pump users provides a 25% greater postmeal glucose-lowering effect versus insulin aspart.
- *Mealtime dosing:* Fiasp® should be injected up to 2 minutes before the start of a meal for improved PPG results. Fiasp® *can also be injected up to 20 minutes after starting a meal without compromising overall HbA1c* versus insulin aspart dosed at mealtime.
- *Novel, faster formulation:* Fiasp® is an insulin aspart formulation that includes niacinamide (vitamin B3) to speed up absorption and L-arginine to provide stability

- *Safety:* No significant differences in the overall rate of severe or blood-glucose confirmed hypoglycemia in people with type 1 and type 2 diabetes compared with insulin aspart.

Fiasp® aims to bridge the physiological gap and better mirror the insulin response of a healthy pancreas. In clinical studies to date, it has demonstrated success in achieving all trial primary endpoints. Additionally, Fiasp® contains the same insulin molecule (insulin aspart) that already has an established safety profile in addition to over 17 years of clinical experience.

REFERENCES

1. Wilcox G. Insulin and insulin resistance. Clin Biochem Rev. 2005;26:19-39.
2. Powers AC. Diabetes mellitus: diagnosis, classification, and pathophysiology. In: Kasper, DL, Fauci AS, Hauser SL (Eds). Harrison's Principles of Internal Medicine, 19th edition. New York, NY: McGraw-Hill; 2015. pp. 2399-407.
3. McKnight JA, Wild SH, Lamb MJE, et al. Glycaemic control of type 1 diabetes in clinical practice early in the 21st century: an international comparison. Diabet Med. 2015;32:1036-50.
4. Heinemann L, Muchmore DB. Ultrafast-acting insulins: state of the art. J Diabetes Sci Technol. 2012;6:728-42.
5. Polinski JM, Kim SC, Jiang D, et al. Geographic patterns in patient demographics and insulin use in 18 countries, a global perspective from the multinational observational study assessing insulin use: understanding the challenges associated with progression of therapy (MOSAIc). BMC Endocr Disord. 2015;15:1-9.
6. Bruttomesso D, Pianta A, Mari A, et al. Restoration of early rise in plasma insulin levels improves the glucose tolerance of type 2 diabetic patients. Diabetes. 1999;48:99-105.
7. Woerle HJ, Szoke E, Meyer C, et al. Mechanisms for abnormal postprandial glucose metabolism in type 2 diabetes. Am J Endocrinol and Metab. 2006;290:E67-E77.
8. Food and Drug Administration. Inactive ingredient search for approved drug products. [online] Available from http://www.accessdata.fda.gov/scripts/cder/iig/index.cfm. [Last Accessed October, 2019].
9. NovoLog® [insulin aspart (rDNA origin) injection]: Prescribing Information. Bagsvaerd, Denmark: Novo Nordisk A/S; 2015.
10. NovoRapid®: Summary of Product Characteristics. Bagsvaerd, Denmark: Novo Nordisk A/S; 2016.
11. New Fiasp® Summary of Product Characteristics. 2017.
12. Buckley ST, Jeppesen CB, Olsen HB, et al. Faster-acting insulin aspart: towards an understanding of the mechanism(s) of action of niacinamide. Diabetes. 2015:1024.
13. Buckley ST. Advanced Technologies and Treatments for Diabetes (ATTD 2016). Milan; 2016.
14. Buckley ST, Kildegaard J, Høiberg-Nielsen R, et al. Mechanistic analysis into the mode of action of niacinamide in faster-acting insulin aspart. Diabetes. 2015;64:(Suppl 1):1-9.
15. Gibson TJ, Murphy RM. Inhibition of insulin fibrillogenesis with targeted peptides. Protein Science. 2006;15:1133-41.
16. Heise T, Pieber TR, Danne T, et al. Faster onset and greater early exposure and glucose-lowering effect with faster-acting insulin aspart versus insulin aspart: a pooled analysis in subjects with type 1 diabetes. Presented at the American Diabetes Association, 76th Annual Scientific Sessions, 10–14 June 2016, New Orleans, Louisiana, USA.
17. Heise T, Pakseresht A, Haahr H, et al. Faster onset and greater early exposure and glucose-lowering effect with faster-acting insulin aspart vs. insulin aspart: a pooled analysis in subjects with type 1 diabetes. Can J Diab. 2016;65(Suppl 1):929.
18. Novo Nordisk. Faster-acting insulin aspart showed a statistically significant reduction in HbA1c in type 1 diabetes and a comparable HbA1c in type 2 diabetes versus NovoRapid® (insulin aspart). 2016.
19. Clinical Trials. Efficacy and safety of continuous subcutaneous insulin infusion of faster-acting insulin aspart compared to NovoRapid® in adults with type 1 diabetes (onset 5). [online] Available from https://clinicaltrials.gov/ct2/show/NCT02825251. [Last Accessed October, 2019].
20. Clinical Trials. Efficacy and safety of faster-acting insulin aspart compared to NovoRapid® both in combination with insulin degludec in children and adolescents with type 1 diabetes (onset 7). [online] Available from https://clinicaltrials.gov/ct2/show/NCT02670915. [Last Accessed October, 2019].
21. Clinical Trials. Efficacy and safety of faster-acting insulin aspart compared to NovoRapid® both in combination with insulin degludec in adults with type 1 diabetes (onset 8). [online] Available from https://clinicaltrials.gov/ct2/show/NCT02500706. [Last Accessed October, 2019].
22. Russell-Jones D, Bode BW, De Block C, et al. Fast-Acting Insulin Aspart Improves Glycemic Control in Basal-Bolus Treatment for Type 1 Diabetes: Results of a 26-Week Multicenter, Active-Controlled, Treat-to-Target, Randomized, Parallel-Group Trial (onset 1). Diabetes Care. 2017;40(7):943-50.

44 CHAPTER Initial Combination Therapy versus Traditional Stepwise Approach

Urman A Dhruv

INTRODUCTION

As per estimates of International Diabetes Federation, 415 million people are already diagnosed with type 2 diabetes (T2DM) and the figure is likely to rise to more than 600 million in next 25 years.[1] It is known that T2DM is a progressive disease and the control is gradually worsening over years as beta cells of pancreas are gradually becoming dysfunctional.[2] Due to multiple barriers on the part of patients and on the part of physicians, it is already difficult to maintain normoglycemia, which is essential to prevent complications, mainly microvascular and to a certain extent even macrovascular complications.[3] When we consider that the beta-cell function is reduced to 50% at the time of diagnosis of disease and is likely to worsen with advancing age, it becomes imperative that the therapy used at the initiation of treatment will not be enough as the time passes and to maintain the same level of glycemia, we will need to intensify therapy. The UK Prospective Diabetes Study (UKPDS) nicely illustrated that after 9 years of monotherapy with diet, sulfonylurea, or insulin, only 9%, 24%, and 28% of study subjects, respectively, attained an HbA1c level of less than 7% (53 mmol/mol) whereas in the subset of obese patients who were randomized to metformin only 13% attained an HbA1c of less than 7% (53 mmol/mol) after 9 years.[4]

One can increase the doses of existing therapy gradually or add some drugs to the existing therapy as the disease progresses. However, this creates a notion in patient's mind that his disease is not well controlled and works as a barrier to successful therapy. Recent studies have also shown that the risk of complications get increased with the extent of time spent in a hyperglycemic state.[5] Hyperglycemia can leave an early imprint in cells of the vasculature and of target organs, which can create a negative "metabolic memory" and favor the development of complications in future. This also means that achieving normoglycemia early in the course of disease is of paramount importance and one can say that management of diabetes has a window of "power play" of 5–6 years. Failure to intensify during this period may expose the patient to future macrovascular complications.

Alternatively, one may initiate therapy with combination of drugs. This should reduce clinical inertia and also improve compliance and may preserve beta cells for a longer duration.[6]

In this article, we will try to analyze these two strategies of managing T2DM with an eye on evidences available.

WHAT IS ALREADY CLEARLY KNOWN TO US FOR T2DM

1. Type 2 diabetes is a progressive disease.
2. Tight glycemic control decreases complications.
3. The issues are adherence and compliance.
4. Clinical needs remain unfulfilled, such as hypoglycemia, weight gain, etc.
5. Postprandial hyperglycemia is not properly controlled by most therapies.
6. Long-term glycemic control is not maintained by most of the therapies.
7. Clinical inertia is one of the factors in failure for intensifying therapy.

Improved Efficacy

The last decade has given insights into multiple pathophysiological mechanisms of T2DM.[6,7] Utilizing a single drug at the initial diagnosis is not enough to target most of these pathophysiological mechanisms. In most of the cases, the first line of treatment is metformin which can address only two out of eight pathophysiological mechanisms understood so far. Initiating treatment with more than one drug (fixed-dose combination or two separate drugs) can help targeting multiple pathophysiological mechanisms and this results in achievement of glycemic targets in more number of patients.[7] Therefore, addressing various metabolic pathways at the same time results in an increase in hypoglycemic effect.

Clinical Inertia

Clinical inertia is described as a failure in initiating or intensifying treatment in a timely manner among people in whom it is expected that health will improve with this intensification.[8] Despite knowing the significance of attaining the glycemic goals, there exists a gap between the targets achieved and targets set. As per findings of an online patient–physician survey, insufficient patient–physician communication and inadequate adherence to "goal setting" were suggested[8] to be contributors to clinical inertia. In 2015, newer recommendations by two of the largest academic societies across the globe, suggested for the first time to initiate treatment with more than one drug, if HbA1c was more than 7.5%[9] or more than 9%.[10] This was the first time that the world saw a proactive approach with a view to reduce clinical inertia.

However, the rate of progression of diabetes varies between individuals and cannot be accurately predicted at diagnosis. So it is likely that if sequential therapy is added in short burst of periods as recommended, clinical inertia may not be a valid reason to initiate therapy with combination therapy. Initial combination therapy with metformin, pioglitazone, and exenatide was compared with add-on therapy to metformin with a sulfonylurea and then insulin at 1 month, 2 months, and 3 months sequentially, if fasting plasma glucose did not reach 110 mg/dL. In this study,[11] sequential therapy was used aggressively and appropriately. Looking at the time-related change in HbA1c, it seems that both the sequential therapy and the initial triple therapy worked towards decreasing the levels of HbA1c during the first 6 months, although initial correction of HbA1c was faster with triple drug combination therapy due to action and mechanism of agents and not due to timing of agents. So initial combination therapy is not the preferred method when the intent is to reduce clinical inertia.

Beta-cell Preservation

The β-cell failure to compensate for increased insulin resistance was identified as the hallmark of T2DM and the rate of deterioration of glycemic control was parallel to that of deterioration of β-cell function and/or decrease in mass.[12] So ultimate goal for prolonging normoglycemia is to preserve beta cells for a longer time. However, at present, all efforts to fulfill this goal has not yielded optimal results. Multiple drugs have been tried with varying results but none has given sustainable results. It is universally accepted that such efforts to preserve beta cells must begin early in the course of disease as the attempts at a later stage will be futile.

Early striving for normoglycemia by intensive insulin therapy at the onset of disease has been demonstrated to cause a remission that has been shown to last up to 2 years.[13] Insulin, started very early in the course of disease, will yield more chances of remission.

In A Diabetes Outcome Progression Trial (ADOPT),[2] thiazolidinedione rosiglitazone was shown to have superior glycemic durability than glyburide and metformin. Incretin-based therapy showed much promise in animal models but could not transfer the beta-cell preserving effect in human beings.

Administration of dipeptidyl peptidase (DPP)-4 inhibitors like saxagliptin[14] in T2DM has demonstrated a positive impact on β-cell function in clinical studies. Other molecules from the same group also showed the similar results but these effects were ill sustained.

So far, the methods to successfully preserve the beta-cell function pharmacologically, are ill understood. Rather than the molecules, it is the maintenance of normoglycemia by any available and successful method seems to preserve beta-cell function. Whether the user of a particular drug or class has advantages beyond that of others is still unexplained. A dedicated study evaluating the advantages of bariatric surgery, metformin, or glucagon-like peptide 1(GLP-1) receptor agonists on β-cell function in early diabetes is ongoing and hopefully it will shed some light on the advantages of these strategies.[15]

It appears that the most significant contributor to β-cell preservation is the alleviation of hyperglycemia, irrespective of the means. Probably, striving for normaoglycemia early at the onset of disease or even during prediabetes stage and retaining normaoglycemia safely via combination therapy as needed may alter the natural history of the disease.[16,17] This once again brings into focus the use of combination therapy early in the course of disease.

Sustainability of Response

Sustainability of response is a function of agent used and its pathophysiological mechanism rather than timing of agent used. All of the studies to date have reported differences based on specific agent used, not the timing.

Individual Response to a Drug may vary

With the expanding knowledge about the genetic basis of T2DM, nearly 80 susceptibility loci have been identified. Attempts have been made to correlate phenotype of glucose disposition with particular genotypes.[17] The individual response to the medications, therefore varies from patient to patient. It is therefore of paramount significance to evaluate the advantage of antidiabetic medications on a one-to-one basis by adding each medication sequentially, or not, after mono/dual treatment failure.

Cost-effectiveness

Initial combination treatment may minimalize the amount of time taken in hyperglycemia secondary to progressive β-cell failure or clinical inertia, yet it stands to be confirmed in validated economic models that the extra time spent in hyperglycemia is more costly as compared to the initial combination of two drugs, one of which is generally comparatively expensive. So using initial combination therapy may not be always cost-effective.

Cost-effectiveness of any drug or drug combination will depend on multiple factors, especially the durability of response, efficacy, and its impact on long-term prevention of microvascular and macrovascular complications. The newer agents like sodium-glucose cotransporter-2 (SGLT2) inhibitors may be expensive per se but when one considers its impact on reducing, reversing or preventing diabetic complications, cost-effectiveness will be acceptable when combined with other agents.

Risk-to-Benefit Ratio

Addition of each agent exposes the patient to additional side effects as almost all medicines used in the management of T2DM has one or the other side effects. As far as metformin is considered, it is safe in clinical trials and epidemiological studies and is therefore, a reasonable first-line therapy.[9,10] As the patient with diabetes is vulnerable to multiple complications due to associated high comorbidities and possible risks of renal and cardiovascular complications, risk–benefit ratio becomes important.

Initial combination therapy may be a cause of unnecessary overtreatment of an individual who could have probably been controlled with monotherapy for a prolonged period of time.

Impact on Weight Gain and Hypoglycemia

Till date, there is no evidence that a change in timing of the similar agents as early combination versus sequential titration of therapy will have any favorable benefits on weight. Hypoglycemia will be a significant problem of individual agent, regardless of timing.

Impact on Adherence and/or Compliance

Although logic says that combination therapy should improve the compliance and adherence to therapy, but no evidence exists to prove this logic.

WHAT ARE THE PREFERRED INITIAL COMBINATIONS?

Nearly all the classes of drugs may be used in combination with each other, the exception being DPP-4 inhibitors and GLP-1 receptor agonists. However, there are certain combinations which have been studied extensively, especially because of their complementary actions.

Dipeptidyl peptidase 4 inhibitors and metformin were the most commonly used combinations. However, metformin–pioglitazone and metformin–sulfonylureas as combination therapies were also commonly used.[18]

Metformin has been the first line of treatment suggested by most of the guidelines of September 2019 and therefore, the highest number of combinations has been studied with metformin. Most of the combinations of metformin have shown better efficacy in reducing HbA1c. The combinations involving metformin also result in more number of patients achieving target HbA1c results.[19] When one excludes combination of metformin with sulfonylureas or glinides, combinations involving metformin do not increase the incidence of hypoglycemia also. Thus, initial combination therapy, which includes metformin as one of the molecules that are more efficacious and safe as compared with stepped-care approach.

Where cost is a constraint, sulfonylureas are reasonable second agents because they are inexpensive, effective, universally available, and have a long-term track record, including demonstration of reduced risk of microvascular complications. These benefits are offset by risks of hypoglycemia and weight gain. Sulfonylureas can be used safely and effectively with dose adjustment, even in people at risk of hypoglycemia, but this requires a bit more attention. The shorter-acting forms, glipizide or glimepiride are preferred since longer-acting glyburide is associated with a higher risk of hypoglycemia, especially in the older, frail patients.

In several trials, combination of metformin and thiazolidinediones has been studied. Although these trials reported positive findings such as better reduction in HbA1c with these fixed-dose combinations, safety issues related to the drug class have significantly restricted its usage.[20]

A novel class of antidiabetic medications is SGLT2 inhibitors, which exert their effect via inhibiting reabsorption of renal glucose and by producing glucosuria. The initial combination therapy of metformin and dapagliflozin has been demonstrated to be more effective in reduction of HbA1c as compared to metformin monotherapy or dapagliflozin monotherapy.

Combination of SGLT 2 inhibitors with DPP-4 inhibitors is commercially widening the scope because of their complementary actions. However, at higher doses of SGLT2 inhibitors, the combination may not be efficacious because of increased glucosuria, which is noted with high dose of SGLT2 inhibitors, especially when it is prescribed to patients having high baseline HbA1c, can result in a reciprocal increase in production of endogenous glucose that is beyond the capacity of DPP-4 inhibitors to overcome.[21]

Nowadays, combination tablets of metformin and all oral agents are available in different doses. The combination tablets provide the convenience of taking fewer pills for patients who are doing well on these specific doses. However, if an individual needs to change the dose of either drug independently of the other drug, then it is not helpful to have a fixed combination. Furthermore, the price of brand name combinations is significantly higher than individually taking the generic components.

CONCLUSION

The dilemma of initial combination therapy or sequential addition of medications as treatment fails is yet unresolved. Initial combination has high propensity to preserve beta-cell function and may be more efficacious than monotherapy but contrary to belief, it does not reduce clinical inertia but just delays it. Cost-effectiveness may not be always better for the combination. It is likely that a small number of patients may be over treated and also may be exposed to unnecessary side effects.

Newer guidelines based on robust evidences suggest starting dual therapy among patients who have been recently diagnosed with type 2 diabetes with HbA1c greater than 1.5% (12.5 mmol/mol) more than their glycemic target. A gray area exists for patients having baseline HbA1c closer to targets.[23,24] Aggressive sequential therapy may be equally effective for this group of patients.

It is recommended by a comparative effectiveness meta-analysis that each novel class of noninsulin agents added to the initial therapy usually reduces HbA1c by nearly 0.7–1.0%. In case the HbA1c target is not attained after around 3 months and the patient *does not have* chronic kidney disease or atherosclerotic cardiovascular disease, then combination of metformin along with any one of the preferred six treatment options should be considered—thiazolidinedione, sulfonylurea, SGLT2 inhibitor, DPP-4 inhibitor, basal insulin, or GLP-1 receptor agonist.[22–24]

It must be remembered that when one starts with dual or triple drug combination therapy, all attempts must be positively made to de-escalate the therapy, once the target HbA1c is achieved.

The use of initial combination therapy is perfectly justified for efficacy and safety but not for the sake of avoiding clinical inertia or as a measure to improve compliance and/or adherence to a therapy. Combination therapies enable patients to be treated with submaximal doses of a drug, with potentially less number of side effects and the capability to affect several aspects of the pathophysiology of disease.

REFERENCES

1. International Diabetes Federation. (2015). IDF Diabetes Atlas, 7th edition. [Online]. Available from http //www.idf.org/diabetesatlas. [Last accessed October, 2019].
2. Kahn SE, Haffner SM, Heise MA, et al. ADOPT Study Group. Glycemic durability of rosiglitazone, metformin, or glyburide monotherapy. N Engl J Med. 2006;355(23):2427-43.
3. Holman RR, Paul SK, Bethel MA, et al. A 10-year follow-up of intensive glucose control in type 2 diabetes. N Engl J Med. 2008;359(15):1577-89.
4. Turner RC, Cull CA, Frighi V, et al. Glycemic control with diet, sulfonylurea, metformin, or insulin in patients with type 2 diabetes mellitus: progressive requirement for multiple therapies (UKPDS 49). JAMA. 1999;281(21): 2005-12.
5. Stratton IM, Adler AI, Neil HA, et al. Association of glycaemia with macrovascular and microvascular complications of type 2 diabetes (UKPDS 35): prospective observational study. BMJ. 2000;321:405-12.
6. DeFronzo RA, Eldor R, Abdul-Ghani M. Pathophysiologic approach to therapy in patients with newly diagnosed type 2 diabetes. Diabetes Care. 2013;36(Suppl 2):S127-38.
7. Defronzo RA. From the triumvirate to the ominous octet: a new paradigm for the treatment of type 2 diabetes mellitus. Diabetes. 2009;58(4): 773-95.

8. Strain WD, Cos X, Hirst M, et al. Time to do more: addressing clinical inertia in the management of type 2 diabetes mellitus. Diabetes Res Clin Pract. 2014;105(3):302-12.
9. Handelsman Y, Bloomgarden ZT, Grunberger G, et al. American Association of Clinical Endocrinologists and American College of Endocrinology-clinical practice guidelines for developing a diabetes mellitus comprehensive care plan-2015. Endocr Pract. 2015;21(Suppl 1):1-87.
10. American Diabetes Association. (7) Approaches to glycemic treatment. Diabetes Care. 2015;38(Suppl):S41-8.
11. Abdul-Ghani MA, Puckett C, Triplitt C, et al. Initial combination therapy with metformin, pioglitazone and exenatide is more effective than sequential add-on therapy in subjects with new-onset diabetes. Results from the Efficacy and Durability of Initial Combination Therapy for Type 2 Diabetes (EDICT): a randomized trial. Diabetes Obes Metab. 2015;17(3): 268-75.
12. Meier JJ, Bonadonna RC. Role of reduced β-cell mass versus impaired β-cell function in the pathogenesis of type 2 diabetes. Diabetes Care. 2013;36(Suppl 2):S113-9.
13. Kramer CK, Zinman B, Retnakaran R. Short-term intensive insulin therapy in type 2 diabetes mellitus: a systematic review and meta-analysis. Lancet Diabetes Endocrinol. 2013;1(1):28-34.
14. Leibowitz G, Cahn A, Bhatt DL, et al. Impact of treatment with saxagliptin on glycaemic stability and β-cell function in the SAVOR-TIMI 53 study. Diabetes Obes Metab. 2015;17(5):487-94.
15. RISE Consortium. Restoring Insulin Secretion (RISE): design of studies of β-cell preservation in prediabetes and early type 2 diabetes across the life span. Diabetes Care. 2014;37(3):780-8.
16. Phillips LS, Ratner RE, Buse JB, et al. We can change the natural history of type 2 diabetes. Diabetes Care. 2014;37(10):2668-76.
17. Kleinberger JW, Pollin TI . Personalized medicine in diabetes mellitus: current opportunities and future prospects. Ann N Y Acad Sci. 2015; 1346(1):45-56.
18. Hampp C, Borders-Hemphill V, Moeny DG, et al. Use of antidiabetic drugs in the U.S., 2003-2012. Diabetes Care. 2014;37(5):1367-74.
19. Phung OJ, Sobieraj DM, Engel SS, et al. Early combination therapy for the treatment of type 2 diabetes mellitus: systematic review and meta-analysis. Diabetes Obes Metab. 2014;16(5):410-7.
20. Perez A, Zhao Z, Jacks R, et al. Efficacy and safety of pioglitazone/ metformin fixed-dose combination therapy compared with pioglitazone and metformin monotherapy in treating patients with T2DM. Curr Med Res Opin. 2009;25(12):2915-23.
21. Lewin A, DeFronzo RA, Patel S, et al. Initial combination of right and linagliptin in subjects with type 2 diabetes. Diabetes Care. 2015;38(3): 394-402.
22. Bennett WL, Maruthur NM, Singh S, et al. Comparative effectiveness and safety of medications for type 2 diabetes: an update including new drugs and 2-drug combinations. Ann Intern Med. 2011;154(9):602-13.
23. Cahn A, Cefalu WT. Clinical Considerations for Use of Initial Combination Therapy in Type 2 Diabetes. Diabetes Care. 2016;39(Suppl 2):S137-45.
24. AACE/ACE Comprehensive type 2 diabetes management algorithm 2019.

45 CHAPTER When Insulin is not an Option

Vijay P Panikar, Harshpreet Singh Tuteja

INTRODUCTION

Many patients with type II Diabetes Mellitus eventually need insulin, as their ability to produce their own insulin from pancreatic beta cells declines progressively [the United Kingdom Prospective Diabetes Study (UKPDS)].[1] Studies suggest that 30–60% of type 2 diabetes mellitus (T2DM) patients may be unwilling to initiate insulin therapy.[1,2] Various patient-related factors may lead to development of resistance in the patients to initiate insulin therapy. These include patient's lack of accurate knowledge and understanding about diabetes and use of insulin, feeling overwhelmed and incapable to manage the complexity and daily self-management needs of insulin administration, embarrassment to use syringes in the public places.[1,3]

Fear of injecting insulin may also be lying within individuals with concerns about incapability to self-administer injections or about pain related with injections. Fear of physiological side effects of hypoglycemia and weight gain have been commonly cited problems. Patients may also have concerns about the lifestyle changes imposed by insulin therapy, and the inconvenience and complexity it brings with it. Most guidelines suggest that when combinations of multiple oral agents (i.e. up to triple combination therapy) are no longer effective at controlling blood glucose, insulin should be added initially as a single injection of basal insulin. If this becomes ineffective in controlling glycated hemoglobin (HbA1c) and postprandial hyperglycemia then adding rapid-acting insulin as meal-related boluses ("basal-bolus" insulin therapy) would be required to control mealtime glycemic excursions.

Insulin therapy is a highly effective treatment to achieve tight glycemic control.[3] Physicians tend to delay insulin therapy primarily because of patient's reluctance to initiate insulin therapy and poor adherence to insulin related regimens.[4]

The most important question is:

- Can insulin initiation be postponed and still have good glycemic control?
- And if yes, for how long can it be postponed?
- What are the therapy options available for the treatment of type 2 diabetes when insulin therapy is denied or implausible?

Over the years, our understanding of pathophysiology of diabetes, lipid and blood pressure management, introduction of new insulin's, and newer oral antidiabetic drugs (OADs) having different and synergistic actions have improved glycemic control.

FROM THE TRIUMVIRATE TO THE OMINOUS OCTET

Insulin resistance in the muscle and liver and failure of beta-cells to produce not enough insulin characterize the core pathophysiologic defects in T2DM.[5] It is now renowned that the beta-cell failure occurs much earlier and with much more severity than previously thought. Subjects falling under the upper tertile of impaired glucose tolerance (IGT) are insulin resistant to maximal extent and have lost over 80% of their beta-cell function. The ominous octet of that includes muscle, liver and beta-cell (triumvirate), the fat cell (accelerated lipolysis), alpha-cell (hyperglucagonemia), gastrointestinal tract (incretin deficiency/resistance), kidney (increased reabsorption of glucose), and brain (insulin resistance) all play significant roles in the development of glucose intolerance in the T2DM individuals.[5]

- Multiple drugs used in combination will be required to correct the multiple pathophysiological defects
- Treatment should not be based simply on decreasing the A1c but based upon reversal of recognized pathogenic abnormalities
- Therapy must be initiated early for prevention or slowing of the progressive beta-cell failure that already is well-established in the subjects with IGT.

In other words, the elucidation of the ominous octet suggests that treatment algorithms are aimed to reverse pathophysiological defects, thereby offering a high probability of achieving durable glycemic control.[5]

THE PROBLEM WITH TREATMENT ALGORITHMS

There are eight therapeutic classes of hypoglycemic agents currently available:

- *Orals*:
  - Metformin
  - Sulphonylureas (including glinides)
  - α-glucosidase inhibitors
  - Thiazolidinediones (TZDs)
  - Dipeptidylpeptidase-4 (DPP4) inhibitors
  - Sodium-glucose cotransporter type 2 (SGLT2) inhibitor.
- *Injectables*:
  - Glucagon-like peptide 1 (GLP-1) agonists
  - Insulin.

Each of these drugs has a unique target and mode of action; a judicious and rational combination of these drugs can possibly and significantly delay the initiation of insulin therapy for a very long time.

Today six oral drugs and two injectable drugs are available for use. Treatment algorithms allow a permutation and combination of two or more agents from different classes. If the treatment is started with 1 of the 6 classes of oral agents and sufficient glycemic control is not achieved, the next therapeutic option would involve a selection between five classes. If a third agent is needed, there are four classes of agents to choose from, and if a fourth agent is contemplated, then there are another three classes of options available.

This then suggests that there are 150 therapeutic options (5 × 6 × 5) for triple therapy and 600 options (5 × 6 × 5 × 4) for quadruple therapy, and 1800 options (5 × 6 × 5 × 4 × 3) for quintuple drug therapy!!

Moreover, the treatment algorithms cannot be truly evidence based. This is because of lack of studies that compare all of the existing combination of treatment options.

Until 2000, the treatment approach included initiation with metformin. A sulphonylurea was added, when metformin failed as monotherapy. When glycemic control could not be achieved with the combination, insulin therapy was initiated.

THE ERA OF THIAZOLIDINEDIONES

The thiazolidinediones or "glitazones" were introduced in 2000. TZDs decrease insulin resistance in the adipose tissue, muscle, and the liver.[6] They also improvise insulin secretory capacity, preserving beta-cell mass and islet structure, and defending beta-cells from the oxidative stress. Additionally, intervention studies also suggested that the onset of diabetes can be delayed in the high-risk individuals by the TZDs.[7]

TZD Combined with Metformin

Clinical studies have shown that treatment with the TZDs—rosiglitazone and pioglitazone—significantly decreases insulin resistance and improves beta-cell function in people with type 2 diabetes [as estimated by Homeostasis Model Assessment (HOMA)]. Thus, a combination of a TZD such as pioglitazone and metformin coadministration addresses the dual defects of beta cell function and insulin resistance. Improvement in glycemic control, insulin sensitivity, and lipid profiles that remain the cardinal points of diabetes care, has been seen with the use of this combination.[8]

In addition, the combination could achieve long-term glycemic control and a "pharmacological remission" suggesting the benefits of the addition of insulin sensitizers such as pioglitazone.[9]

Moving to Triple Therapy with TZDs

Studies have revealed that when a sulfonylurea-metformin combination is failing to achieve the glycemic control, adding a TZD is effective for long-term management of diabetes. Moreover, in those patients in whom this triple oral antidiabetic therapy has become successful, the glycemic control is superb and there is an increase in the production of endogenous insulin.[10,11]

Suggestive of early shift to triple therapy, Charpentier et al.[12] showed that in patients with not well-controlled with dual combination therapy, the early addition of pioglitazone could improve HbA1c, fasting plasma glucose, and surrogate measures of β-cell function. Panikar et al.[13] assessed the effects of pioglitazone while combining with sulphonylurea and metformin on diabetes control in patients getting treated with insulin due to secondary failure of the oral antidiabetic agents. The study suggested that with proper selection of patients, pioglitazone with a sulphonylurea and metformin can be safely used in patients who are receiving insulin with good results. In the study, 124 patients with T2DM for 5 years or more were switched and put on to triple drug combination of glibenclamide 5 mg, metformin 500 mg, and pioglitazone 15 mg along with insulin.

A significant decrease can be seen with the combination as the glycated hemoglobin (HbA1c) level shifts from 11.5% to 7.32% ($P < 0.001$), average fasting blood glucose from 194.8 mg/dL to 124.06 mg/dL ($P < 0.01$), average postprandial blood glucose from 256.24 mg/dL to 162.32 mg/dL ($P < 0.01$). About 43.35% of patients did not need to be continued on insulin at 6 months. The total insulin requirement in 124 patients was reduced by 71.81%. No significant side effects were noticed, liver enzymes were within acceptable levels, average weight gain was 2.23 kg, significant hypoglycemia was seen in 28 patients with two needing hospitalization, these patients were those who did not stick to the follow-up schedules.

In another study including a triple-drug combination of glitazone, (rosiglitazone), sulfonylurea (glibenclamide), and metformin was found to be effective and well tolerated in T2DM patients receiving insulin with significantly improved metabolic control.[14]

THE INTRODUCTION OF DPP4 INHIBITORS (LAUNCHED IN INDIA IN 2008)

Dipeptidylpeptidase-4 inhibitors works in a way that is different from other oral glucose-lowering agents. The DPP-4 inhibitor class of oral antidiabetic agents selectively inhibits the DPP-4 enzyme. This would have otherwise rapidly degraded two major incretin hormones, GLP-1 and glucose-dependent insulinotropic polypeptide.[15]

The DPP-4 inhibitors have negligible risk of hypoglycemia, and do not cause weight gain.[15]

Efficacy of DPP4i as the Fourth Drug in the Management of T2DM

A retrospective analysis of 7,858 T2DM patients was done by Panikar et al.,[16] who received a DPP-4 inhibitor (sitagliptin, vildagliptin, teneligliptin, linagliptin, and saxagliptin) as the fourth drug to achieve glycemic control, adding up of the fourth drug was found to be effective in achieving the desired glycemic control within 8 weeks of therapy initiation. At the end of the monitoring period, there was significant decline in mean FPG by –28.1 ± 16.1 mg/dL ($P = 0.001$), mean post prandial plasma glucose by –55.3 ± 17.0 mg/dL ($P = 0.001$), and mean HbA1c by –1.2 ± 0.7 ($P = 0.001$). There was no major difference between the groups with respect to reduction in PPG and HbA1c.

Dipeptidylpeptidase-4 inhibitor offers an important addition to the armamentarium of treatment options for patients with T2DM by providing another mechanism to address the multiple pathophysiologic defects present in this disease. This data also shows the efficacy of a four-drug regime to effectively achieve glycemic control and delay insulin initiation.[16]

WHEN QUADRUPLE THERAPY FAILS? ROLE OF SGLT2 INHIBITORS (LAUNCHED IN INDIA IN 2012)

The importance of how the kidneys play a role in glucose homeostasis has gained wider considerations in the recent years.[17] Consequently, the development of a new pharmacological class of antidiabetes agents that targets the kidney has provided new treatment options for the T2DM management. SGLT2 inhibitors, such as dapagliflozin, canagliflozin, and empagliflozin, reduce reabsorption of renal glucose, which results in improved urinary glucose excretion and subsequent decrease in plasma glucose and HbA1c concentrations. Modest decrease in body weight and blood pressure has also been observed following treatment with the SGLT2 inhibitors. SGLT2 inhibitors appear to be generally well-tolerated and have been used safely when given as monotherapy or in combination with other oral antidiabetes agents and insulin. The risk of hypoglycemia is small with the SGLT2 inhibitors.[17]

SGLT2 as Fifth Drug to Delay Insulin Use

In the retrospective analysis published by Panikar et al. in the JAPI,[18] the efficacy of SGLT2 inhibitors as an add-on therapy along with stricter, lifestyle changes in 808 Asian Indian T2DM patients with insufficient glycemic control despite receiving an optimum dose of at least 4 OADs, was assessed.

A total of 87.4% cases responded to addition of SGLT2 inhibitors during a mean follow-up period of 6 months. The fasting plasma glucose was reduced by -63.65 ± 19.93 mg/dL to a mean FBS of 134.57 ± 33.65 mg/dL ($P = 0.001$).

The post prandial plasma glucose was reduced by -79.28 ± 23.57 mg/dL to a mean PPBS of 184.94 ± 38.34 mg/dL (P = 0.001). There were significant reductions in the mean HbA1c by -1.63 ± 0.99% (P = 0.001). The mean weight reduction at 6 months of therapy was -3.03 ± 01.84 kg that is 3.8% decrease from baseline (P = 0.001). The males responded more (91.0%) compared to females. Those with body mass index (BMI) < 23.5 kg/m^2 had marginally higher but insignificant response of 93.0% as compared to 87.1% in patients with a high BMI (≥23.5 kg/m^2) (P = 0.253). Patients with less than 5 years of duration of diabetes responded better (91.8%) as compared to patients with a more than or equal to 5 years of diabetes (85.4%).

Patients with type 2 diabetes who look forward to the further enhancement in glycemic control despite being on four OADs, and SGLT2 inhibitor as a fifth drug can be considered. They are highly efficacious when added as fifth drug along with sticking to strict lifestyle regime and can effectively reduce HbA1c and weight. They act likewise in obese and nonobese patients. They can be efficiently used at any stage of diabetes and can delay insulin initiation in type 2 diabetes patients not controlled on multiple OADs.

CONCLUSION

- When insulin is not an option, it is not the end of the road.
- Customized, intensive, and everyday disease state management of diabetes is an effective strategy.
- Many noninsulin treatment options exist and can be combined cleverly to attain the blood glucose targets.
- Newer, innovative drugs provide us a variety of potential combinations to help delay insulin initiation in patients who are reluctant to use injectable therapy.

REFERENCES

1. Allen NA, Zagarins SE, Feinberg RG, et al. Treating psychological insulin resistance in type 2 diabetes. J Clin Transl Endocrinol. 2016;7:1-6.
2. Mirahmadizadeh A, Delam H, Seif M, et al. Factors Affecting Insulin Compliance in Patients with Type 2 Diabetes in South Iran, 2017: We Are Faced with Insulin Phobia. Iran J Med Sci. 2019;44(3):204-13.
3. Hussein A, Mostafa A, Areej A, et al. The perceived barriers to insulin therapy among type 2 diabetic patients. Afr Health Sci. 2019;19(1): 1638-46.
4. Kim SG, Kim NH, Ku BJ, et al. Delay of insulin initiation in patients with type 2 diabetes mellitus inadequately controlled with oral hypoglycemic agents (analysis of patient- and physician-related factors): A prospective observational DIPP-FACTOR study in Korea. J Diabetes Investig. 2017;8(3):346-53.
5. Defronzo RA. Banting Lecture. From the triumvirate to the ominous octet: a new paradigm for the treatment of type 2 diabetes mellitus. Diabetes. 2009;58(4):773-95.
6. Hauner H. The mode of action of thiazolidinediones. Diabetes Metab Res Rev. 2002;18 (Suppl 2):S10-5.
7. Campbell IW, Mariz S. Beta-cell preservation with thiazolidinediones. Diabetes Res Clin Pract. 2007;76(2):163-76.
8. Derosa G, Salvadeo SA. Pioglitazone and metformin fixed-dose combination in type 2 diabetes mellitus: an evidence-based review of its place in therapy. Core Evid. 2008;2(3):189-98.
9. Panikar V, Joshi SR, Bukkawar A, et al. Induction of long-term glycemic control in type 2 diabetic patients using pioglitazone and metformin combination. J Assoc Phys India. 2007;55:333-7.
10. Bell DS, Ovalle F. Long-term efficacy of triple oral therapy for type 2 diabetes mellitus. Endocr Pract. 2002;8(4):271-5.
11. Dorkhan M, Magnusson M, Frid A, et al. Glycaemic and nonglycaemic effects of pioglitazone in triple oral therapy of patients with type 2 diabetes. J Intern Med. 2006;260(2):125-33.
12. Charpentier G, Halimi S; F-PIO-100 Study Investigators. Earlier triple therapy with pioglitazone in patients with type 2 diabetes. Diabetes Obes Metab. 2009;11(9):844-54.
13. Panikar V, Chandalia HB, Joshi SR, et al. Beneficial effects of triple drug combination of pioglitazone with glibenclamide and metformin in type 2 diabetes mellitus patients on insulin therapy. J Assoc Phys India. 2003;51:1061-4.
14. Panikar V, Chandalia HB, Joshi S, et al. Beneficial effects of Triple Drug Combination of Rosiglitazone with Glibenclamide and Metformin Type 2 diabetes mellitus patients on insulin therapy. IJDDC. 2003;23(4): 124-9.
15. Craddy P, Palin HJ, Johnson KI. Comparative effectiveness of dipeptidylpeptidase-4 inhibitors in type 2 diabetes: a systematic review and mixed treatment comparison. Diabetes Ther. 2014;5(1):1-41.
16. Panikar V, Joshi S, Tiwaskar M, et al. Efficacy of DPP4i as the Fourth Drug in the Management of Type 2 Diabetes Mellitus in Asian Indians Poorly Controlled by Use of at least 3 Oral Antidiabetic Drugs. JAPI. 2019;67.
17. Nauck MA. Update on developments with SGLT2 inhibitors in the management of type 2 diabetes. Drug Des Devel Ther. 2014;8: 1335-80.
18. Panikar V, Joshi SR, Deogaonkar N, et al. Efficacy of SGLT2 Inhibitors as the Fifth Drug in the Management of Type 2 Diabetes Mellitus in Asian Indians not Controlled with at least 4 Oral Antidiabetic Drugs. J Assoc Physicians India. 2018;66(12):46-9.

46

CHAPTER

How do We Cope with the Expectations of Young Patients? How Clinician can Achieve?

Vinod Mittal

INTRODUCTION

Diabetes is one of the most significant global public health challenges with young people constituting an important group. It has been estimated that young people of today will grow up to constitute the estimated 642 million living with diabetes worldwide in 2040. Younger diabetes patients require early intervention with good self-management practices in order to reduce the risk of lifetime complications, prevent early mortality, and lower costs for the health service.1

In India, the burden of diabetes has steadily increased over the past quarter century contributing to a major part of the global burden. The crude prevalence of diabetes in adults aging 20 years or above in India has seen an increase of 39.4% from 5.5% (4.9–6.1) in 1990 to 7.7% (6.9–8.4) in 2016,[2] with an increase in every state of India in the same period.

In India, an exponential increase in the prevalence of type 2 diabetes mellitus (T2DM) in the last 30 years has played a significant role in contributing to the increased burden of diabetes in the young adults. T2DM in Indian diabetics is characterized by increased body fat, lower body mass index (BMI), increased clinical and biochemical measures of insulin resistance and systemic inflammation, which is coupled with one of the highest global rates of progression of pre-diabetes to T2DM. This highlights a more aggressive diabetes phenotype in Indians. The onset of T2DM in Indians is almost two decades earlier than in the west, thus explaining the high prevalence of T2DM in young Indians.[3]

The incidence of various complications reported in numbers/1000 person years of follow-up showed that young T2DM patients had a 2.11 times greater risk of developing complications (of retinopathy, nephropathy, neuropathy and ischemic heart disease) compared to patients with T1DM.[4]

BARRIERS TO TREATMENT ADHERENCE IN DIABETES

Studies have investigated the barriers of adherence to treatment among patients with T2DM. A study by Rezaei et al. showed that lack of trust in the medical team, patients' false beliefs, and patients' unique experiences and daily challenges prevented complete adherence to treatment (Table 1).[5]

The study found that despite the recommendations provided by the medical team, the participants did not have enough trust in them, and in most cases, they did what they themselves considered appropriate. The authors of this study suggested that to try and gain the patient's trust, the medical team should focus on designing a particular care program for each patient based on their lived experiences and unique roles and challenges in life to increase their adherence to treatment.[5]

Another study in young at-risk patients emphasized the largely preventable and potentially reversible nature of early diabetes. The study suggested introduction of lifestyle modification programs that foster internal motivation, enhance key health knowledge, and modify health beliefs and risk perception could help better manage the condition (Flowchart 1).[6]

GUIDELINE RECOMMENDATIONS FOR OPTIMIZING PATIENT CARE

Online resources such as those that are part of The National Diabetes Education Program (NDEP) help healthcare

TABLE 1: Categories and subcategories formed during the data analysis on the barriers to treatment adherence in the diabetics.[5]

Main category	Subcategory	Primary category
Lack of trust in medical explanatory/ prescriptive knowledge	• Folk beliefs • Nonadherence to therapeutic regimen	• Misconceptions about diabetes • False beliefs • Ignorance • Self-medication • Voluntary disorganization of drug use consumption based on self-perception
Knowledge, lived experiences of the disease	Medication side effects; Physical challenges	• Mouth bitterness • Blurred vision • Tremor • Itching • Knee pain • Arthritis • Dyspnea • Obesity
Challenges of everyday life	Mental/psychological stress; Preoccupations of the everyday life	• Sadness • Discomfort • Disappointment • Fear of the future • Nervousness • Heavy homework • Housekeeping affairs • Daily activities
Interactive/economic challenges	Lack of empathy/behavioral affiliation; Weakness/financial dependence	• Being ignored by family members • Lack of support from family • Marital conflicts • Lack of skills • Financial strain • Impoverishment • Financial dependence

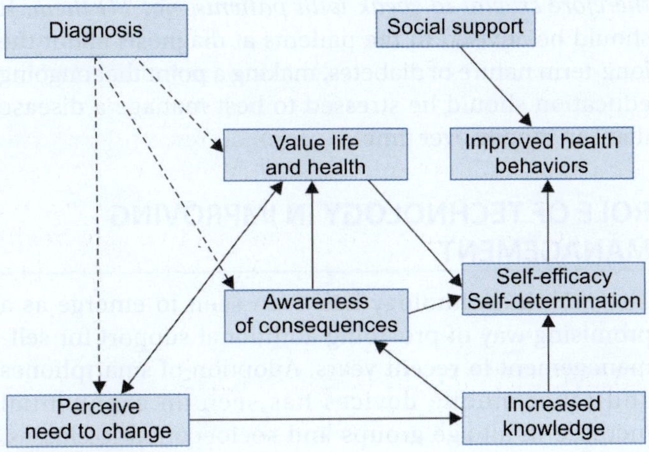

Flowchart 1 Factors influencing change.[6]

professionals to design and implement more effective healthcare delivery systems for those with diabetes through online resources such as www.betterdiabetescare.nih.gov.

The American Diabetes Association (ADA) highlights three themes to be kept in mind, while managing a patient with diabetes:

1. *Patient-centeredness*: Patients with diabetes are also at significantly higher risk of developing cardiovascular disease, a patient-centric approach should include a comprehensive plan to decrease cardiovascular risk by addressing issues of blood pressure, control on lipid levels, smoking cessation, weight management, and healthy changes in the lifestyle that include adequate physical activity.
2. *Diabetes management across the lifespan*
3. *Advocacy for patients with diabetes*

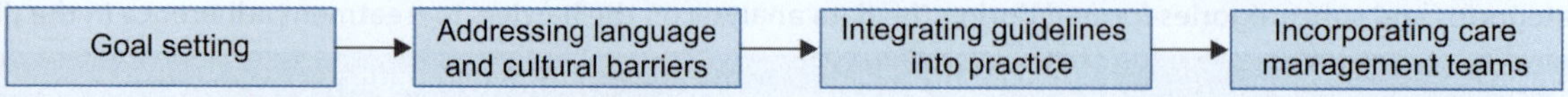

Figure 1 Strategies in optimizing provider and team behavior.

The ADA outlines the following specific objectives through practical strategies:[7]

Objective 1: Optimize Provider and Team Behavior

A timely and suitable intensification of lifestyle and/or pharmaceutical therapy should be prioritized by the care team for patients who have not achieved beneficial levels of blood glucose, blood pressure, and lipids.

Following strategies are included (Fig. 1):

- Detailed goal setting with patients
- Recognizing the barriers to diabetes care (language, numeracy, or cultural) and addressing each of them individually
- Integrating evidence-based guidelines and clinical information tools into the care process
- Incorporating different members of the care management teams, which include nurses, pharmacists, and other providers, has been shown to enhance provider and team behavior and thereby catalyze decrease in HbA1c, blood pressure, and LDL cholesterol levels.

Objective 2: Support Patient Behavior Change

As indicated in the ADA Standards of Care, an effective diabetes care needs a systematic approach that can support patients' behavior change efforts. This includes:

- Lifestyle modifications (increased physical activity, healthy diet, smoking cessation, weight management, and effective coping)
- Disease self-management (taking and managing medicines and self-monitoring of blood glucose and blood pressure, when clinically appropriate)
- Preventing complications of diabetes (self-monitoring of foot care; actively participating in the screening for eye, foot, and renal complications; and immunizations).

Self-management, satisfaction, and glucose control in the patients has been improved by the high-quality diabetes self-management education (DSME), as has providing ongoing diabetes self-management support (DSMS), so that gains achieved during DSME are sustained.

Objective 3: Change the Care System

Changes that have been shown to boost diabetes care quality include the following:

- The care is based on the evidence-based guidelines
- Role expansion of teams and staff and implementation of more intensive disease management strategies.

WINNING WAYS IN DIABETES MANAGEMENT

In a recent article,[8] experts shared best strategies for counseling newly diagnosed patients with diabetes. Helping patients feel in control of their disease and achieve meaningful change *requires both the patient and the healthcare professional to take on partner roles in long-term disease management.*

In this partnership, the patient needs to feel empowered. The patient empowerment philosophy, which involves patients' involvement and engagement in their diabetes care versus giving them purely fact-based information about the underlying disease in the form of a strict, regimented lecture has gained much attention recently and has proven rewarding in diabetes management.

Diabetes-related distress needs to be addressed. A patient who has been newly diagnosed often exhibits guilt feelings for "causing" a disease that can be delayed or prevented in some cases. The patient also exhibits fear from memories of loved ones who faced diabetic complications. It is important to address these feelings from the very beginning of a patient's disease journey and help patients understand that they are not alone.

Diabetes goals need to be made measurable. Goals should be motivating, specific, measurable, attainable, practical, relevant, and time-specific.

Type 2 diabetes is a disease in which lifestyle behavior is a big determinant of disease course. Many healthcare providers who deal with patients with type 2 diabetes note patient resistance to change as a big barrier. *It is therefore crucial to speak with patients, not TO them.* It should be advised to the patients at diagnosis about the long-term nature of diabetes, making a point that ongoing education should be stressed to best manage a disease that can modify over time.

ROLE OF TECHNOLOGY IN IMPROVING MANAGEMENT

The mobile technology has been seen to emerge as a promising way of providing additional support for self-management in recent years. Adoption of smartphones and other mobile devices has seen an exponential increase in all age groups and socioeconomic classes. This has enabled applications for diabetes and wellness to flourish. The available smartphone applications for diabetes are varied. They allow individuals to track their activities or diet, reminding medicines as well as to visualize the outcomes as graphic presentation. These types of applications propose novel ways of supporting the challenge of diabetes self-management.[9]

A meta-analysis of 22 trials that assessed the impact of mobile phone interventions on glycemic control demonstrated HbA1c reduction of 0.5% over a median of 6 months' follow-up duration. This effect was shown to be greater in T2DM patients than in T1DM. Early work on using mobile phones for diabetes management studied the use of telephonic calls or text messaging. Newer studies have focused on tracking applications (diet, blood glucose, weight, insulin, for example), educational content, or integrating with other systems, such as personal health records and social media. The use of secure messaging with providers resulted in improved HbA1c results by 0.7%. Combining mobile device and provider support, a randomized controlled trial with WellDoc Diabetes Manager™ (a FDA-approved application), showed a 1.2% reduction in the HbA1c with web- and mobile-based tools compared to usual care over a year. This application offers automated clinical coaching based on the data that patients track and supports sharing of that information with care providers. These results have suggested that mobile technology might be even more efficient as an element of a comprehensive suite of technological tools.[9]

REFERENCES

1. Papoutsi C, Hargreaves D, Colligan G, et al. Group clinics for young adults with diabetes in an ethnically diverse, socioeconomically deprived setting (TOGETHER study): protocol for a realist review, co-design and mixed methods, participatory evaluation of a new care model. BMJ Open. 2017;7(6):e017363.
2. India State-Level Disease Burden Initiative Diabetes Collaborators. The increasing burden of diabetes and variations among the states of India: The Global Burden of Disease Study 1990-2016. Lancet Glob Health. 2018;6(12):e1352-62.
3. Dutta D, Ghosh S. Young-onset diabetes: An Indian perspective. Indian J Med Res. 2019;149(4): 441-2.
4. Amutha A, Anjana RM, Venkatesan U, et al. Incidence of complications in young-onset diabetes: Comparing type 2 with type 1 (the young diab study). Diabetes Res Clin Pract. 2017;123:1-8.
5. Rezaei M, Valiee S, Tahan M, et al. Barriers of medication adherence in patients with type-2 diabetes: a pilot qualitative study. Diabetes Metab Syndr Obes. 2019;12:589-99.
6. Seear KH, Lelievre MP, Atkinson DN, et al. 'It's Important to Make Changes.' Insights about Motivators and Enablers of Healthy Lifestyle Modification from Young Aboriginal Men in Western Australia. Int J Environ Res Public Health. 2019;16(6). pii:E1063. doi:10.3390/ijerph1606103.
7. American Diabetes Association. Strategies for improving care. Sec. 1. In Standards of Medical Care in Diabetes 2015. Diabetes Care. 2015;38 (Suppl. 1):S5-S7.
8. Schaeffer J. Winning ways in diabetes management—best strategies for counseling newly diagnosed patients. Today's Dietitian. 2010;12(11):36.
9. Klasnja P, Kendall L, Pratt W, et al. Long-Term Engagement with Health-Management Technology: a Dynamic Process in Diabetes. MIA Annu Symp Proc. 2015;2015:756-65.

47 CHAPTER

Aligning Therapeutic Options with Management Goals in Elderly Patients with Diabetes

Supratik Bhattacharyya

INTRODUCTION

There is a rapid growth in the population of elderly patients with diabetes, with significant impact on global health and economics. The self-reported prevalence of diabetes among the elderly in India was 6.9% in 2007, and the prevalence is likely to double in the next 20 years.[1,2] In comparison with other age groups, the elderly with diabetes are at a higher risk for associated acute and chronic microvascular and macrovascular complications. The average annual expenditure for the elderly with diabetes was about twice more than that for younger patients, and ~61% of all costs attributed to diabetes were incurred by the elderly.[3] Due to extensive variability in clinical presentation, physiological profiles, functional capabilities, life expectancy, psychosocial environment, and resource availability within the population, management of diabetes in elderly patients can be challenging. Treatment goals must be adjusted by taking into account presence of comorbidities, patients' living conditions, and available resources.

GUIDELINES FOR DIABETES MANAGEMENT IN ELDERLY PATIENTS

The European Diabetes Working Party for Older People (2011) recommend an hemoglobin A1c (HbA1c) goal of 7–7.5% and a fasting glucose target range of 117–135 mg/dL in patients without major comorbidities, and an HbA1c goal of 7.6–8.5% and a fasting glucose target range of 137–162 mg/dL for patients with major comorbidities.[4] The recommendations by the American Diabetes Association (ADA, 2012) and International Diabetes Federation (IDF) are summarized in Table 1.[5–7]

TABLE 1: American Diabetes Association and International Diabetes Federation framework for treatment goals of diabetes in elderly patients.

Patient category	HbA1c goal (%)	Fasting glucose target range (mg/dL)	Bedtime glucose target range (mg/dL)	Rationale for the goal
Healthy (functionally independent)	<7.5	90–130	90–150	Significant life expectancy
• Few comorbidities • Functionally/cognitively intact	7–7.5 (IDF)			Goal is to prevent future macrovascular/microvascular complications
Complex/intermediate (functionally dependent)	<8	90–150	100–180	Intermediate life expectancy
• Multiple chronic comorbidities or	7–8 (IDF)			High treatment burden
• Two or more IADL impairments or				At risk for hypoglycemia and falls

Contd...

Contd...

Patient category	HbA1c goal (%)	Fasting glucose target range (mg/dL)	Bedtime glucose target range (mg/dL)	Rationale for the goal
• Mild to moderate cognitive impairment				
Very complex/poor health (end-of-life)	<8.5	100–180	110–200	Limited life expectancy
• Residency in a long-term care facility or	Avoid specific HbA1c goal (IDF)			Benefit uncertain
• End-stage chronic illnesses or				High risk of hypoglycemia and falls
Two or more IADL impairments or				
• Moderate to severe cognitive impairment				

(ADL: activities of daily living (e.g. bathing, toileting, transferring from place to place, dressing, and eating); IADL: instrumental ADL (e.g. using the telephone, managing medications, handling finances, performing housework, cooking, and arranging transportation); IDF: International Diabetes Federation)

(*Source*: Adapted from American Diabetes Association. Older adults: standards of medical care in diabetes 2018. Diabetes Care. 2018;41(Suppl 1):S119-25;[6] Cho N, Colagiuri S, Distiller L, et al. Managing older people with type 2 diabetes: Global Guideline. Brussels, Belgium: International Diabetes Federation; 2013.[7])

In patients with a life expectancy of <10 years due to advanced age (≥80 years), residents in a nursing home, or those with chronic comorbidities, a specific target HbA1c level should be avoided, as the harms in this population are more severe.[8]

SPECIAL CONSIDERATIONS IN MANAGEMENT OF DIABETES IN ELDERLY PATIENTS

Presence of Age-related Conditions

The risk of certain comorbidities, including vision and hearing impairments, cognitive dysfunction, depression, functional disabilities, falls and fractures, polypharmacy, chronic pain, and urinary incontinence, increase with age (geriatric syndromes).[9] Additionally, the risk of interactions between drugs can increase with polypharmacy; quality of life (QoF) can be directly affected by pain and incontinence. If clinicians are unaware of these coexisting conditions, a therapeutic regimen, that is, too complex for a patient with cognitive dysfunction may be unintentionally prescribed, and untreated depression may lead to treatment nonadherence and social isolation.[9] Strategies for optimizing care in such situations are outlined in Table 2.

TABLE 2: Comorbid geriatric conditions.

Condition	Strategies for optimizing care
Depression	Recognize, evaluate, and treat as needed
Cognitive dysfunction	• Avoid rigid glycemic control, complex diabetes prescription regimens and treatment programs • Educate caregivers • Avoid medications with high risks of hypoglycemia • Suggest alarms and pill boxes for medication reminders
Medication nonadherence	• Advise patients to carry all medications including all bottles, tablet strips during consultation and review them at every visit • Also ask to bring over-the-counter medications • Stop any medications that did not show benefit
Physical disabilities	• Patients with, hearing loss, visual impairment, and gait abnormalities should be advised to use hearing aids, glasses, canes, and walkers as needed • Suggest a safe exercise depending on physical capacity and need of patient

(*Source*: Adapted from Leung E, Wongrakpanich S, Munshi MN. Diabetes management in the elderly. Diabetes Spectr. 2018; 31(3):245-53.[9])

Balancing the Risk of Hypoglycemia against Poor Outcomes

Elderly patients have a higher risk with poor outcomes due to altered adaptive physiological responses to low glucose levels.[9] Moreover, several elderly patients are unaware of symptoms of hypoglycemia; hence, the risk of silent hypoglycemia remains unrecognized. Hypoglycemia can precipitate cardiovascular events, worsen cognitive function, and lead to poor outcomes, including an increase in falls and fractures, fear of falling, confusion, delirium, fatigue, dizziness, and a decline in QoL.[9] Hence, early recognition and management of hypoglycemia are crucial for elderly patients.[9]

Evaluating HbA1c in Elderly Patients

Hemoglobin A1c is the gold standard test to assess long-term glycemic control in the management of diabetes. Because the value of HbA1c depends on the time red blood cells (RBCs) spend in the blood circulation, several conditions that prolong RBC circulation time (Table 3) can falsely elevate HbA1c levels.[9] Moreover, HbA1c is a poor marker of glucose variability or risk of hypoglycemia. In addition, relaxing HbA1c goals in elderly patients does not rule out the risk of hypoglycemia. Hence, dependence on HbA1c as a sole parameter for glycemic goals in frail elderly patients with multiple comorbidities must be avoided. The best available option when HbA1c is deemed unreliable is to use finger-stick blood glucose testing to guide therapy.[9]

Physical Activity and Prevention of Diabetes in the Elderly

Physical activity and a lower consumption of fat- and sugar-rich diet can prevent obesity and insulin resistance. According to ADA, all overweight adults (BMI ≥ 25 kg/m^2 or ≥ 23 kg/m^2 in Asian Americans) with risk factors and all adults aged >45 years should be screened for prediabetes and diabetes every 1–3 years as it is frequently unnoticed in the elderly due to asymptomatic or nonspecific symptoms.[5] The benefits of screening in elderly patients depend upon life expectancy, estimated time frame of benefits, and aggressiveness of the intervention. However, for very elderly patients with several comorbidities and a short life expectancy, it is advisable to implement an intervention that inhibits the exacerbation of their complications that could further impair their functional status.[9] Extremely restrictive diets are not recommended; however, avoiding large carbohydrate loads can lower glucose excursions. The physical abilities of the patients must be determined before developing an appropriate exercise plan. Elderly patients who are slow and at risk of falls should be urged to walk for 5–10 min, 2–3 times/day, inside the house, which can be increased gradually as tolerated.[9]

TABLE 3: Factors that can falsely elevate or lower HbA1c.

Factors	Mechanism	False alteration in HbA1c
Patient age	Increased insulin resistance	Increase
Anemia of chronic diseases	Not known	Increase or decrease
Erythropoietin therapy	Increased premature RBCs/smaller RBC life span	Decrease
Hemodialysis	Short life span of RBCs	Decrease
Hemoglobinopathies	Different hemoglobin variants	Decrease
Hemolytic anemia, sickle cell anemia, or thalassemia	Augmented RBC turnover	Decrease
Iron deficiency anemia	Reduced RBC turnover with longer glycation exposure	Increase
Metabolic acidosis/uremia	Hemoglobin carbamylation	Increase
Polycythemia	Longer RBC life span	Increase
Race	Not known	Increase
Recent transfusion	Elevated RBC turnover	Decrease

(RBC: red blood cells)

(*Source*: Adapted from Leung E, Wongrakpanich S, Munshi MN. Diabetes management in the elderly. Diabetes Spectr. 2018;31(3):245-53.[9])

APPROACH TO PHARMACOTHERAPY IN ELDERLY PATIENTS

Since lifestyle modifications alone are unable to maintain target treatment goals, pharmacological interventions, including oral and injectable agents that are well-tolerated in elderly patients should be considered. In elderly patients on multiple medications, contraindications due to drug-drug interactions and risk of hypoglycemia are important considerations when selecting medications (Table 4).[9]

If the complexity of the therapeutic regimen is not overwhelming, insulin can be used safely. Overtreatment of diabetes in the elderly patients is common as several clinicians are unclear about how to de-intensify complex insulin regimen. Multiple daily insulin regimen can be simplified by changing to once-daily basal insulin with noninsulin agents, which lowers the risk of hypoglycemia without affecting glycemic control, and also improves diabetes-related distress.[10] The timing of injections should be moved to morning, if patients who are already on basal

TABLE 4: Antidiabetic agents for use in elderly patients.

Class of antidiabetic agent	Factors to be considered	
Biguanides	Benefits	Considered first-line treatment unless contraindicated, low risk of hypoglycemia, inexpensive
	Risks	Unsafe, if there are contraindications, gastrointestinal disturbances, weight loss in frail elderly patients, risk of vitamin B12 deficiency
	Remarks	Extended-release formulations are available which may reduce gastrointestinal side effects
Sulfonylureas	Benefits	Inexpensive
	Risks	Known for hypoglycemia risk, drug-drug interactions with frequently used geriatric drugs (e.g. warfarin)
	Remarks	Short-acting agents reduce the risk of hypoglycemia. Gliclazide is proven to have lesser risk of hypoglycemia, gliclazide is metabolized by liver to inactive metabolites and can be used without dose adjustments in mild to moderate renal dysfunction, however it should be avoided in severe impairment
Meglitinides	Benefits	Skip doses if meals are infrequent/skipped, low rate of hypoglycemia, useful in elderly patients with variable eating habits
	Risks	Multiple doses increasing the pill burden, expensive
	Remarks	Take before one large meal to control postprandial hyperglycemia
Glucagon-like peptide 1 receptor agonists	Benefits	Advantage of weight reduction, particularly for overweight patients; low hypoglycemia risk
	Risks	*Side effects*: Nausea, vomiting, diarrhea, and increased satiety; expensive and injectable formulation
	Remarks	May lead to unintended weight loss in frail elderly patients, associated with high risk in elderly patients
Dipeptidyl peptidase 4 inhibitors	Benefits	Low risk of hypoglycemia and weight-neutral
	Risks	*Side effects*: Nausea, vomiting, stomach discomfort, and diarrhea; expensive and has low efficacy
	Remarks	Once-daily pill formulation is well tolerated in frail elderly
Thiazolidinediones	Benefits	Low risk of hypoglycemia; in patients with reduced glucose tolerance, it can improve insulin secretion in response to glucose; can be used in impaired renal function
	Risks	*Side effects*: Edema and congestive heart failure, risk of bone loss and fractures and bladder cancer; expensive
	Remarks	Several contraindications in elderly including congestive heart failure, edema, and high risk of falls and fractures); less concerns for bladder cancer in elderly patients with limited life expectancy; well-tolerated and effective in reversing insulin resistance

Contd...

Contd...

Class of antidiabetic agent	Factors to be considered	
Sodium glucose cotransporter 2 inhibitors	Benefits	Low risk of hypoglycemia; useful in patients with atherosclerotic cardiovascular disease or congestive heart failure; useful to decrease progression of renal disease
	Risks	High risk for genital yeast infections and urinary tract infections, dehydration, weight loss, hyperkalemia, and elevated LDL cholesterol; high risk of euglycemic diabetic ketoacidosis, hypotension, dizziness, renal function worsening
	Remarks	Limited safety profile in elderly patients
Insulin	Benefits	Basal insulin, once-daily is effective with low complexity
	Risks	High risk of hypoglycemia
	Remarks	Complex regimen must be avoided; basal insulin doses should be used in the morning for the control of fasting blood glucose and noninsulin agents for the control of postprandial hyperglycemia in elderly patients; long-term sliding-scale insulin regimen must be avoided

(LDL: low-density lipoprotein)

(*Source*: Adapted from Leung E, Wongrakpanich S, Munshi MN. Diabetes management in the elderly. Diabetes Spectr. 2018;31(3):245-53.[9])

insulin are receiving it at bedtime. Basal insulin, when administered in the morning, with adjunctive noninsulin agents are well-tolerated. For patients on premixed insulin, 70% of the dose should be managed as basal insulin and 30% as mealtime insulin. The dose of basal insulin should be increased by 2–3 units every 5–7 days until fasting glucose lies within the individualized target range (90–150 mg/dL is a reasonable range). However, these goals should be adjusted based on overall health and presence of other comorbidities. While adding noninsulin agents, mealtime insulin should be discontinued.

Metformin is the first-line therapy for elderly patients due to its low risk of hypoglycemia. The choice of additional noninsulin agents should be individualized and noninsulin agents with a low hypoglycemia risk are preferred. A high frequency of renal insufficiency among elderly patients frequently prevents the use of several newer agents. Hence, it is advisable to titrate the dosage of these agents depending upon postmeal finger-stick blood glucose test results.[9]

CONCLUSION

Management of diabetes in elderly patients requires critical assessment of clinical, functional, and psychosocial factors and specific care. The overall health of a patient, comorbid medical conditions, personal preferences, coping capabilities, and factors affecting QoL should be considered before developing glycemic goals and treatment strategies. Treatment should be based on individualization to avoid complications, particularly hypoglycemia.

REFERENCES

1. Arokiasamy P, Parasuraman S, Sekher TV. Study on global AGEing and adult health (SAGE), Wave 1: India National Report. International Institute for Population Sciences. Geneva: World Health Organization; 2013.
2. Animaw W, Seyoum Y. Increasing prevalence of diabetes mellitus in a developing country and its related factors. PLoS One. 2017;12(11): e0187670.
3. American Diabetes Association. Economic costs of diabetes in the U.S. in 2017. Diabetes Care. 2018;41(5):917-28.
4. Sinclair AJ, Paolisso G, Castro M, et al. European diabetes working Party for Older People 2011 clinical guidelines for type 2 diabetes mellitus. Executive summary. Diabetes Metab. 201;37 Suppl 3:S27-38.
5. Kirkman MS, Briscoe VJ, Clark N, et al. Diabetes in older adults. Diabetes Care. 2012;35(12):2650-64.
6. American Diabetes Association. Older adults: standards of medical care in diabetes 2018. Diabetes Care. 2018;41(Suppl 1):S119-25.
7. Cho N, Colagiuri S, Distiller L, et al. Managing older people with type 2 diabetes: Global Guideline. Brussels, Belgium: International Diabetes Federation; 2013.
8. Qaseem A, Wilt TJ, Kansagara D, et al. Hemoglobin A1c targets for glycemic Control with pharmacologic therapy for nonpregnant adults with type 2 diabetes mellitus: A guidance statement update from the American College of Physicians. Ann Intern Med. 2018;168(8):569-76.
9. Leung E, Wongrakpanich S, Munshi MN. Diabetes management in the elderly. Diabetes Spectr. 2018;31(3):245-53.
10. Munshi MN, Slyne C, Segal AR, et al. Simplification of insulin regimen in older adults and risk of hypoglycemia. JAMA Intern Med. 2016;176(7): 1023-5.

48 CHAPTER Glycemic Pentad: A Holistic Approach to Diabetes Management

Rajesh Rajput

INTRODUCTION

We are well aware of diabetes being a metabolic disease affecting lifestyle of an individual which is characterized by decreased insulin sensitivity and hyperglycemia ultimately causing aberrant glucose homeostasis. Many guidelines have talked about diabetes management strategies that aim at maintaining and controlling the three factors, fasting plasma glucose (FPG), postprandial plasma glucose (PPG), and glycated hemoglobin (HbA1c), which are conventionally referred as glycemic triad.[1]

According to the American Diabetes Association recommends, HbA1c levels were targeted to be at <7.0% (53 mmol/mol), PPG levels to 80–130 mg/dL (4.4–7.2 mmol/L) and peak PPG levels to <180 mg/dL (10.0 mmol/L) in order to achieve better glycemic control.[2] Nevertheless, the guidelines talk about how the management of diabetes is not associated with the concept of "one size fits all". It is therefore recommended that treatment should be individualized based on the patient's status.[2]

SIGNIFICANCE OF POSTPRANDIAL HYPERGLYCEMIA IN DIABETES

Many evidences highlight the fact that reducing postprandial glucose excursions is equally or perhaps more important for achieving HbA1c goals.[1] When the HbA1c levels are below 7.5% in people with type 2 diabetes mellitus (T2DM), PPG levels contribute to fasting glycemia and this process decreases progressively with increasing HbA1c levels.[3]

There is a significant involvement of diet as well in maintaining the HbA1c levels of individuals. In a normal Indian diet, the carbohydrate content constitutes about 65% and this content is seemingly more than what is recommended for diabetic patients.[4] Carbohydrates are the main influencers of blood glucose levels in a person's diet and there has always been an association between the type of carbohydrate intake and PPG levels.[5] Consecutively, the overall glycemic control and postprandial glucose control in Indian diabetic population is of real concern since the major portion of an Indian diet contains high glycemic index and load.

GLYCEMIC PENTAD: A RISING IDEA

Conventionally, the goal of any diabetes control strategy is to reduce the levels of FPG, PPG and HbA1c (triad). However, there have been reports from the UKPDS and ADVANCE trials that failed to prevent macrovascular events and death while optimizing glucose levels.[6,7] This has brought light to the reality that there are factors other than blood glucose levels that cause diabetes complications and much advances in research have ushered in the inclusion of two more factors, i.e. glycemic variability and quality of life, to the existing components. This group of five elements are collectively termed as "glycemic pentad". Figure 1 displays different components of glycemic pentad.

GLYCEMIC VARIABILITY

The term "Glycemic Variability (GV)" can be explained as the degree of daily blood glucose fluctuations observed in an individual.[8] The fluctuations are due to both postprandial glucose spikes as well as hypoglycemic episodes.

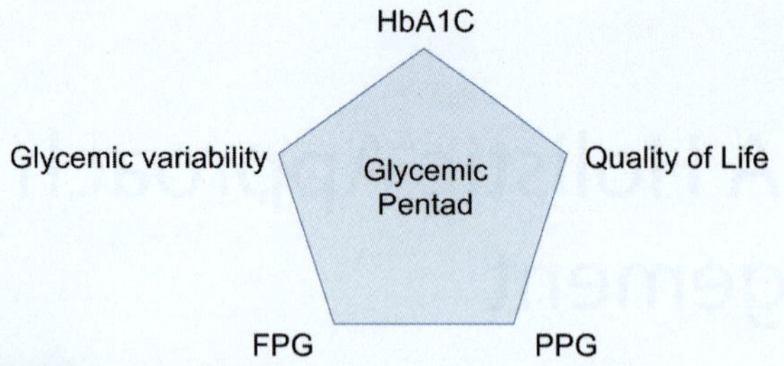

Figure 1 Representation of a glycemic pentad.

(HbA1c: glycated hemoglobin; FPG: fasting plasma glucose; PPG: postprandial plasma glucose)

Further, there are two types of glycemic variations. The first one is termed as "intraday glycemic variations", i.e. the variations measured within a day and the second type is termed as "Interday glucose variations", i.e. glucose variations measured at the same time on two consecutive days. The causative factors of glycemic variability are defective glycemic regulation and reduced insulin availability. It can be observed that even though certain degree of glycemic variations is common in normal individuals; it increases in people with diabetes and impaired blood glucose tolerance.[8]

Various studies report that hyperglycemia and deglycation are the key reasons in the occurrence of various microvascular and macrovascular complications in diabetes.[9] Hypoglycemia along with glycemic variations can influence the onset and progression of diabetes complications. However, there are several methods to effectively measure glycemic variability. One such method is called as Ambulatory glucose profiling (AGP) technique which retrospectively analyses blood glucose levels from the data collected with flash glucose monitoring (FGM).[10]

Eventually, there are appropriate biological evidences and rationale that enlighten the significance of GV as a risk factor in the pathogenesis of vascular complications in diabetes. Consecutively, it can be inferred that regulating glycemic variability is necessary to achieve proper glycemic control in patients with T2DM. Thus, it can be comprehended that GV and continuous glucose monitoring system (CGMS) have a role in redefining reasonable interventions in the healthcare environment in India.

QUALITY OF LIFE

Another important factor in the disease management routine is quality of life (QOL). The QOL is defined as a multidimensional construct incorporating an individual's subjective perception of physical, emotional, and social well-being, including two components of satisfaction and happiness.[11] Generally, in a diabetic patient, the QOL is low and it remains this way till the duration of the disease. In addition to this, complications associated with diabetes affects the QOL of patients.[12]

Consequently, these troublesome side effects and lifestyle restrictions demotivate the patients to comply with the treatment. Therefore, therapeutic protocols should aim at decreasing the complications thereby improving treatment adherence and compliance.

As far as India is concerned, its diversity with plethora of cultural and socioeconomic differences, the measurement tools for QOL created generally for other population might not elicit complete information. Hence, it is necessary to develop a specific QOL assessment tool for India. In this regard, Nagpal J, et al. has developed Quality of Life Instrument for Indian Diabetics (QOLID), to assess the QOL of Indian diabetes patients.[13] This tool comprises of eight domains and 34 questionnaires that evaluate the physical health, socioeconomic and psychological status of a diabetic patient. The first three domains are termed as health-related quality of life (HRQOL) that comprises of physical health, physical endurance, and general health as they evaluate the general health and well-being of an individual.

The remaining five factors, treatment satisfaction, symptom botherness, financial worries, emotional/mental health, and diet advice tolerance reflect the Diabetes Specific Quality of Life (DSQOL).[13] Thus, it can be inferred that QOL should be considered en route to achieve optimal glycemia in diabetes.

CONCLUSION

The glycemic pentad is regarded as a new concept that deserves to have its position in the diabetes management course. It is imperative that a global antidiabetic strategy should be aimed at reducing the four components of glycemic pentad, i.e. FPG, PPG, HbA1c, and glucose variability and improving the fifth element, quality of life.

REFERENCES

1. Ceriello A. The glucose triad and its role in comprehensive glycaemic control: current status, future management. Int J Clin Pract. 2010;64(12): 1705-11.
2. American Diabetes Association. 6. Glycemic targets: standards of medical care in diabetes—2019. Diabetes Care. 2019;42(1):S61-70.
3. Monnier L, Lapinsk iH, Colette C. Contributions of fasting and postprandial plasma glucose increments to the overall diurnal hyperglycemia of type 2 diabetic patients. Diabetes Care. 2003;26(3):881-5.

4. Joshi SR, Bhansali A, Bajaj S, et al. Results from a dietary survey in an Indian T2DM population: a STARCH study. BMJ Open. 2014;4(10):e005138.
5. Schultz WM, Varghese T, Heinl R, et al. Natural approaches in diabetes management: A review of diet, exercise, and natural products. Curr Pharm Des. 2018;24(1):84-98.
6. ADVANCE Collaborative Group. Intensive blood glucose control and vascular outcomes in patients with type 2 diabetes. N Engl J Med. 2008;358(24):2560-72.
7. UK Prospective Diabetes Study (UKPDS) Group. Intensive blood-glucose control with sulphonylureas or insulin compared with conventional treatment and risk of complications in patients with type 2 diabetes (UKPDS 33). The Lancet. 1998;352(9131):837-53.
8. Kovatchev B. Glycemic Variability: Risk Factors, Assessment, and Control. J Diab Sci Tech. 2019;13(4):627-35.
9. Akirov A, Shochat T, Dotan I, et al. Glycemic variability and mortality in patients hospitalized in general surgery wards. Surgery. 2019;166(2): 184-92.
10. Rodbard D. Continuous glucose monitoring: a review of successes, challenges, and opportunities. Diabetes Technol Ther. 2016;18(2):S3-13.
11. Raina SK. State of The Globe: Health-related quality of life as health status measure: Time to move on. J Glob Infect Dis. 2019;11(3):89-90.
12. Wieringa TH, de Wit M, Twisk JWR, et al. Does hypoglycaemia affect the improvement in QoL after the transition to insulin in people with type 2 diabetes? J Endocrinol Invest. 2018;41(2):249-58.
13. Nagpal J, Kumar A, Kakar S, et al. The development of quality of life instrument for Indian diabetes patients (QOLID): a validation and reliability study in middle and higher income groups. J Assoc Physicians India. 2010;58:295-304.

CHAPTER 49 Challenges in Indian Patients with Diabetes: Combination Insulins a Way Out

Ajay Kumar

INTRODUCTION

Globally, the number of people suffering from diabetes mellitus (DM) has gone up to 425 million in 2017. India ranks second with 72.9 million diabetic patients.[1] Progressive dysfunction of the beta-cells and their ultimate failure are elementary pathogenic features of type 2 diabetes mellitus (T2DM). The United Kingdom Prospective Diabetes Study (UKPDS) trial showed that only 50% of beta-cell function remains at the time of clinical diagnosis of T2DM.[2] Disturbance in fasting plasma glucose (FPG) and postprandial glucose (PPG) occurs during the progression of hyperglycemia in T2D (Type 2 diabetes). What is intriguing to note is that the disturbance in PPG control occurs a lot prior and is more contrasted with that of FPG.[3] Smart and judicious use of antidiabetic drugs is significantly dependent on a sound understanding of the natural history of diabetes as well as the underlying pathophysiologic defects. A paper published by Monnier and colleagues in Diabetes Care in 2007 showed that worsening of glucose homeostasis in T2DM patients progressed from postprandial to fasting hyperglycemia following a three-step process:

1. *First step*: Associated with the three diurnal postmeal periods considered as a whole
2. *Second step*: Happens during the morning period
3. *Third and final step*: Corresponded to continuous hyperglycemia over the night-time fasting periods.[4]

The evidences on the significance of fasting and postprandial plasma glucose, and their association with glycated hemoglobin (HbA1c) have been summarized in a systematic review and meta-analysis published in 2015. The pooled correlation coefficient (r) between PPG and HbA1c was 0.68 ($P < 0.001$) more than pooled correlation coefficient of FPG ($r = 0.61$ ($P < 0.001$)).[5] The DECODE study also showed that within each fasting-glucose classification, mortality noticed an increase with increasing 2 hour glucose.[6]

UNIQUE CHALLENGES IN TREATING INDIAN PATIENTS WITH DIABETES MELLITUS

There are few important Indian realities which need to be addressed in effectively managing our Indian T2D patients. They are mainly low doctor-to-population ratio, high carbohydrate diet, higher contribution of PPG to HbA1C, delayed insulin initiation and suboptimal insulin dosing, and need for a simple insulin regimen. The first reality is that Indian doctors are overstressed, overburdened and achieved WHO recommended doctor to population ratio of 1:1,000. According to Ministry of Health and Family Welfare, Government of India report released on February 2019 revealed that the doctor population ratio in India is 0.679/1,000 population which is less than that recommended by WHO.[7] In addition to this, the Government doctor population ratio is 0.09/1,000 population. There is a huge deficiency in terms of the number of doctors to the population especially in rural area where 70% of the Indian population reside. Because of this discrepancy there is a huge patient load for individual doctor in our country. In a systematic review of literature from 1946–2016 published in BMJ showed that the average consultation time in India varies from 1.5–2.3 minutes compared to 15–20 minutes in US and Sweden. Secondly, Indian diet has high carbohydrate content which leads to high PPG levels.[8] In both Rural and Urban India, carbohydrate is responsible for more than 70% of energy contribution. This is much higher when compared to western population where only 40% of the energy contribution comes from carbohydrates.

Thirdly, unlike the western population, PPG contribution to hyperglycemia is much higher in Asian population. In addition, no difference was seen even in the elevated quintiles of HbA1c for the PPG contribution to either 24-hour hyperglycemia or 4-hour hyperglycemia postmeals, in comparison to FG and preprandial glucose contribution.[9] Fourth, baseline characteristics of real-world evidence from India has shown poor glycemic control in patients who were on multiple OADs. Thus, despite fully leveraging oral antidiabetic drugs (OADs), HbA1c levels are high due to underutilization and delayed use of insulin.[10-11] Numerous options for initiating insulin are available but there is a need for simplicity and convenience for insulin therapy considering the above-mentioned unique challenges in Indian patients with diabetes mellitus.

INITIATION OF INSULIN THERAPY—WHEN?

For patients who suffer from T2DM along with other acute complications, it is almost imperative to use an intensive insulin therapy either as a monotherapy or in adjunct with other OADs. Insulin therapy should be initiated for any patient where the HbA1c levels are consistently above target for around 6 months.[12-13] The same has also been observed in the DURABLE study where patients on OADs failed to achieve their glycemic target were initiated on basal or premix insulins.[14,15] It was shown in the results that patients who had a lower baseline HbA1c were more likely to attain and maintain their glycemic target.[14,15] This study reinstates that early initiation of insulin holds significance in maintaining HbA1c targets. This fact is further armored by the understanding that intensive therapies not only have a favorable effect on the HbA1c, but also in delaying the complications onset.

HOW TO CHOOSE BETWEEN BASAL AND PREMIXED INSULIN THERAPIES TO START TREATMENT?

While choosing the type of insulin suited for a patient, the physician needs to not only take his choice of regimen in account but also the lifestyle of the patient. The usual regimens in which insulin is initiated are:

- Basal only
- Premix or self-mix (consisting both basal and prandial insulin)
- Insulin coformulation—insulin degludec/insulin aspart (IDegAsp).

In the early stages of treatment, either of the regimens will enable the patients to achieve their glycemic targets, the difference sets in at the later stages because of diabetes being a progressive disorder. In the later stages, both basal and a prandial insulin is required to achieve and maintain the glycemic target of the patient. For patients who predominantly suffer from meal-related insulin secretory defects, a prandial insulin (used either alone or as part of a premix insulin) should be used to address the concern (as observed in the DURABLE trial). This leads to another criterion which should be considered while deciding the insulin regimen-elevated PPG.

One of the simplest and convenient regimens is basal only. The pros of the regimen are that it requires the patient to take one insulin injection daily and limits the monitoring of blood glucose, hence the patient is more willing to adhere to the regimen. The cons of the regimen include patients failing to achieve and maintain their glycemic target during the progressive course of the disease when more intensive treatment with multiple insulins remains the only option.[16]

Till date, a lot of premixed analog insulins are available in different proportions of basal insulin: prandial insulin (30:70, 50:50) available in the market which makes it easier to use for the patient. These insulins provide the convenience of both meal time and basal insulin in a single pen, hence offer better PPG control which is of prime importance in achieving a HbA1c target <7%.[17] Premixed insulin analogs come with the advantage of meal-time flexibility without the risk of hypoglycemia. Premix insulin analogs offer multiple benefits to patients who do not want to use a complex regimen like basal-bolus for the management of hyperglycemia.[18] Premixed insulins are ideal for patients who have a consistent eating habit and lifestyle, high baseline HbA1c values, and elevated PPG levels. Premixed insulins can be used as an adjunct to other insulins in the management of severe hyperglycemia. As found and stated by various studies, greater HbA1c reductions are possible with premixed insulins and short-acting insulins as compared to basal insulin alone, incidence of hypoglycemia also remained the same.[12]

Coformulations

The recently developed coformulation of IDegAsp offers a unique advantage of combining an ultra-long-acting basal insulin namely insulin degludec with a short-acting prandial insulin aspart. The coformulations are different from the conventional premixed insulin in the sense that each of the components of the coformulation insulin maintain their individual pharmacokinetic and pharmacodynamic properties and tend to exist as a separate entity both in the insulin formulation (in the cartridge/vial) as well as after being injected in the subcutaneous tissue. Attempts to develop coformulation by mixing long-acting basal insulins (such as insulin glargine or insulin detemir) with short-acting prandial insulins has been made previously, however the attempts were futile due to incompatible pharmacokinetic and pharmacodynamic properties of these insulins. All the short-acting insulins are soluble at a neutral pH of 7.4, while insulin glargine is soluble at an acidic pH of 4. Hence, the coformulation could not be made. On the other hand, hybrid hexamers with unpredictable PK-PD profile of both the long-acting and short-acting component were formed when insulin detemir was mixed with insulin aspart.

Options for Insulin Initiation: Coformulation versus Basal–Clinical Evidence

A 26-week, open label, treat-to-target trial was performed to investigate the effectiveness and safety of IDegAsp vs. insulin glargine in insulin-naive [illegible]nese adults with type 2 diabetes. Patients meeting [illegible] inclusion criteria were randomized 1:1 to once-daily injections of IDegAsp or insulin glargine U100 (IGlar U100), both ±≤2 oral antidiabetic treatments. IDegAsp was administered before the largest meal at the discretion of each subject, and also maintained throughout the trial; IGlar U100 was dosed as per label. Both insulins were titrated to achieve a target pre-breakfast self-measured plasma glucose of 3.9 to <5.0 mmol/L. The mean HbA1c was 7% with IDegAsp and 7.3% with IGlar post 26 weeks; superiority of IDegAsp to IGlar was shown [estimated treatment difference, ETD; IDegAsp–IGlar: –0.28% points (–0.46; –0.10) 95% CI, p<0.01]. At the end-of-trial, mean fasting plasma glucose (FPG) was comparable for IDegAsp and IGlar [5.7 vs. 5.6 mmol/L; ETD IDegAsp–IGlar: 0.15 mmol/l (–0.29; 0.60) 95% CI, p = NS]. IDegAsp was related with numerically lesser rates of overall confirmed (27%) and night-time confirmed hypoglycemia (25%) vs. IGlar [estimated rate ratio IDegAsp/IGlar: 0.73 (0.50; 1.08) 95% CI, p = NS, and 0.75 (0.34; 1.64) 95% CI, p = NS, respectively]. At end-of-trial, mean daily insulin doses were similar between groups (both: 0.41 U/kg) as were the body weight increases from baseline (both: 0.7 kg). Adverse event profiles were also similar between the groups. It was concluded that IDegAsp provided superior long-term glycemic control compared to IGlar, with similar FPG and doses and numerically lower rates of overall and night-time hypoglycemia.[19] IDegAsp can be started at 10 units daily with dose titration of 2 units increment or decrement if the blood glucose is above or below target, respectively.

Options for Insulin Intensification

- Basal–bolus regimen
- Premix twice daily or thrice daily
- IDegAsp twice daily.

An individualized approach is always used to determine whether to use basal-bolus therapy or premix therapy in patients who have failed to achieve glycemic target on either OADs alone or in combination with basal insulin.[16] Premix insulin analogs can be given to either insulin-naïve patients or to patients who were previously on basal insulin but have high levels of PPG or to patients who find self-monitoring and titration of insulin dose in a basal–bolus regimen difficult and cumbersome.

Of all the existing insulin regimes, basal–bolus is the most physiological approach to insulin intensification. This regimen provides the physician the opportunity to provide a complete basal and prandial coverage; nevertheless it requires both strict and frequent self-monitoring of blood glucose (SMBG) along with the patient being capable of self-management. Since this approach requires multiple injections throughout the day, the patient should be more than willing to accept this regimen.

Options for Insulin Intensification: Coformulation versus Basal–Bolus Therapy

A recent trial was published in 2019 comparing coformulation vs. basal-bolus therapy as options for insulin intensification. This was a multinational trial with subjects' recruitment from India, US, Russia, Czech Republic, Serbia, Turkey and Algeria. More subjects achieved target HbA1c without hypoglycemia with IDegAsp (22.5%) than with IGlar U100 + IAsp (21.1%) at the end of 38 weeks, with considerably fewer nocturnal episodes [W0–W38, estimated rate ratio: 0.61 (95% CI: 0.40; 0.93)]. There was a similarity in the safety profiles across the treatment groups throughout.[20]

Overview of the Effects of Premix Insulins over Basal Insulin: Efficacy and Safety

BiAsp 30/70: Studies which evaluated the safety and efficacy of BiAsp 30 BD vs. insulin glargine OD revealed more patients achieved lower values of HbA1c that those on insulin glargine. Minor hypoglycemia, weight gain, and daily dose of insulin was higher in BiAsp vs. glargine.[21] When BiAsp 30 was evaluated against biphasic human insulin (BHI) in a long-term efficacy and safety study, there was seen no difference in hypoglycemic episodes and HbA1c reductions. Moreover, there was a reduction in major hypoglycemic events in the second year of treatment with BiAsp 30. BiAsp 30 when compared against LM25 was found to be noninferior in terms of HbA1c reduction and hypoglycemia events according to Niskanen et al. in a 12-week cross-over study.[22] Moreover there are additional studies which compare the PPG control of both BiAsp 30 vs. BHI OD or BD and revealed that BiAsp was more efficacious in reducing PPG as compared to BHI, despite the injection time.[14,15]

CONCLUSION

Newer insulin coformulation or premixed insulin analogs represent an attractive option for initiating and intensifying insulin therapy as they appropriately address the unique challenges in Indian diabetes patients with high carbohydrate load in diet, markedly elevated PPG levels and less doctor-patient interaction time. These newer insulin formulations are simplified and take lesser amount to time for clinicians and patients to comprehend and likely to improve adherence to insulin therapy in a developing country like India.

REFERENCES

1. International Diabetes Federation. (2017). IDF Atlas 8th edition. [online] Available from https://idf.org/e-library/epidemiology-research/diabetes-atlas.html [Last accessed September, 2019].
2. DeFronzo RA. Intensive blood-glucose control with sulphonylureas or insulin compared with conventional treatment and risk of complications in patients with type 2 diabetes (UKPDS 33). UK Prospective Diabetes Study (UKPDS) Group. Lancet. 1998;352(9131):837-53.
3. Kendall DM, Cuddihy RM, Bergenstal RM. Clinical application of incretin-based therapy: therapeutic potential, patient selection and clinical use. Am J Med. 2009;122(6 Suppl):S37-S50.
4. Monnier L, Colette C, Dunseath GJ, et al. The loss of postprandial glycemic control precedes stepwise deterioration of fasting with worsening diabetes. Diabetes Care. 2007;30(2):263-9.
5. Ketema EB, Kibret KT. Correlation of fasting and postprandial plasma glucose with HbA1c in assessing glycemic control; systematic review and meta-analysis. Arch Public Health. 2015;73:43.
6. Glucose tolerance and mortality: comparison of WHO and American Diabetes Association diagnostic criteria. The DECODE study group. European Diabetes Epidemiology Group. Diabetes Epidemiology: Collaborative analysis Of Diagnostic criteria in Europe. Lancet. 1999;354(9179):617-21.
7. Minister of State for Health. (2017). Less than one doctor for 1000 population in India. [online] Available from https://economictimes.indiatimes.com/industry/healthcare/biotech/healthcare/less-than-one-doctor-for-1000-population-in-india-government-to-lok-sabha/articleshow/59697608.cms. [Last Accessed October, 2019].
8. Mohan V, Radhika G, Sathya RM, et al. Dietary carbohydrates, glycaemic load, food groups and newly detected type 2 diabetes among urban Asian Indian population in Chennai, India (Chennai Urban Rural Epidemiology Study 59). Br J Nutr. 2009;102(10):1498-506.
9. Wang JS, Tu ST, Lee IT, et al. Contribution of postprandial glucose to excess hyperglycaemia in Asian type 2 diabetic patients using continuous glucose monitoring. Diabetes Metab Res Rev. 2011;27(1):79-84.
10. Mohan V, Shah SN, Joshi SR, et al. Current status of management, control, complications and psychosocial aspects of patients with diabetes in India: Results from the Diab Care India 2011 Study. Indian J Endocrinol Metab. 2014;18(3):370.
11. Baruah MP, Kalra S, Bose S, et al. An audit of insulin usage and insulin injection practices in a large Indian cohort. Indian J Endocr Metab. 2017;21(3):443-52.
12. Rodbard HW, Jellinger PS, Davidson JA, et al. Statement by an American Association of Clinical Endocrinologists/American College of Endocrinology Consensus Panel on type 2 diabetes mellitus: An algorithm for glycemic control. Endocr Pract. 2009;15(6):540-59.
13. Handelsman Y, Mechanick JI, Blonde L, et al. American Association of Clinical Endocrinologists Medical Guide lines for Clinical Practice for developing a diabetes mellitus comprehensive care plan. Endocr Pract. 2011;17 (Suppl. 2):S1-53.
14. Buse JB, Wolffenbuttel BH, Herman WH, et al. DURAbility of basal versus lispro mix 75/25 insulin efficacy (DURABLE) trial 24-week results: Safety and efficacy of insulin lispro mix 75/25 versus insulin glargine added to oral antihyperglycemic drugs in patients with type 2 diabetes. Diabetes Care. 2009;32:1007-13.
15. Buse JB, Wolffenbuttel BH, Herman WH, et al. The DURAbility of Basal versus Lispro mix 75/25 insulin Efficacy (DURABLE) trial: Comparing the durability of lispro mix 75/25 and glargine. Diabetes Care. 2011;34(2):249-55.
16. International Diabetes Federation. (2012). Glucose Control Therapy. Global Guideline for Type 2 Diabetes. Brussels, Belgium, 2012. pp. 55-64. [Online] Available from https://www.iapb.org/wp-content/uploads/Global-Guideline-for-Type-2-Diabetes-IDF-2012.pdf [Last accessed September, 2019].
17. Woo V, Shestakova MV, Orskov C, et al. Targets and tactics: The relative importance of HbA, fasting and postprandial plasma glucose levels to glycaemic control in type 2 diabetes. Int J Clin Pract. 2008;62:1935-42.
18. Garber AJ. Premixed insulin analogues for the treatment of diabetes mellitus. Drugs. 2006;66:31-49.
19. Onishi Y, Ono Y, Rabøl R, et al. Superior glycaemic control with once-daily insulin degludec/insulin aspart versus insulin glargine in Japanese adults with type 2 diabetes inadequately controlled with oral drugs: a randomized, controlled phase 3 trial. Diabetes Obes Metab. 2013;15(9):826-32.
20. Philis-Tsimikas A, Astamirova K, Gupta Y, Haggag A, Roula D, Bak BA et al. Similar glycaemic control with less nocturnal hypoglycaemia in a 38-week trial comparing the IDegAsp co-formulation with insulin glargine U100 and insulin aspart in basal insulin-treated subjects with type 2 diabetes mellitus. Diabetes Res Clin Pract. 2019;147:157-65.
21. Ismail-Beigi F, Moghissi E, Tiktin M, et al. Individualizing glycemic targets in type 2 diabetes mellitus: Implications of recent clinical trials. Ann Intern Med. 2011;154:554-9.
22. Liebl A, Jones S, Benroubi M, et al. Clinical outcomes after insulin initiation in patients with type 2 diabetes: 6-month data from the INSTIGATE observational study in five European countries. Curr Med Res Opin. 2011;27:887-95.

50 CHAPTER Changing Diabetes Care: From Glycemia to Cardiovascular Disease

Jothydev Kesavadev

INTRODUCTION

Diabetes mellitus (DM) is a chronic metabolic disorder which is characterized by hyperglycemia, and is a consequence of insulin defect.[1] The burden of diabetes has steadily increased over the past years in India, as well as across the globe.[1] Globally, prevalence of diabetes is approximately 415 million, and is expected to increase to 642 million in the next 25 years.[2] India has the highest prevalence of diabetes, with around 69.2 million affected individuals in 2015, and this number is expected to rise to 123.5 million by 2025.[3] According to the Global Burden of Disease Study (1990–2016) India, there is a rapid increase in age-standardized diabetes prevalence (7.7% in 2016 vs 5.5% in 1990) in every state, with highest increase in prevalence percentage among the lower-middle epidemiological transition level (ETL) state groups.[3] Chronic hyperglycemia results in long-term damage and subsequently leads to associated microvascular and macrovascular complications.[4] Studies have reported that among microvascular complications, nephropathy (32.5%) is the most frequent, followed by neuropathy (30.1%), and retinopathy (28.9%). Among macrovascular complications, cardiovascular complications are more common and hypertension is significantly associated with all complications (Fig. 1).[5]

Einarson et al. (2018) reported the prevalence data for cardiovascular diseases (CVD) in patients with diabetes, and it was found that in Indian population, the prevalence is as high as 42.6%.[6] CVD events and comorbidities have demonstrated a complex inter-relationship of macro- and microvascular complications in diabetes patients.[7] Glycemic index generally remains the main focus in diabetes management, although its pathological imprint involves the vasculature with both

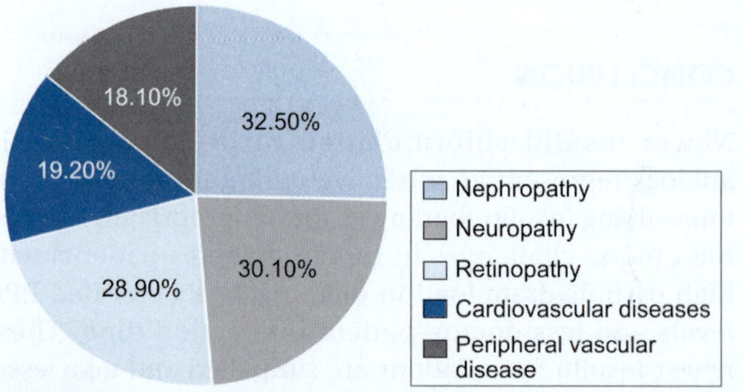

Figure 1 Prevalence of microvascular and macrovascular complications.[5]

(*Source*: Adapted from George B, Cebioglu M, Yeghiazaryan K. Inadequate diabetic care: global figures cry for preventive measures and personalized treatment. EPMA J. 2010;1(1):13-18.)

micro- and macrovascular complications.[5,8] It has been well-established, that the legacy effect begins as early as in the first year after diagnosis, and depends on the level of glycemic/HbA1c exposure as well.[8] A strong correlation exists between diabetes control during initial years after diagnosis and future risk for diabetic complications and mortality rates.[8] Thereby, the treatment of patients with type 2 diabetes (T2D) is not only directed toward treating hyperglycemia, or minimizing hypoglycemia risk, but also aids in preventing microvascular and macrovascular complications.[8,9] Glucagon-like peptide-1 receptor agonists (GLP-1RAs) and sodium-glucose cotransporter 2 inhibitor (SGLT2-i) drugs have demonstrated the potential of improving prognosis, and they also help in reducing macrovascular complications or multiple cardiovascular risk factors in type 2 diabetes mellitus (T2DM) patients.[9] Recent cardiovascular outcome trials (CVOTs) have demonstrated that GLP-1RA and SGLT2-i drug classes exhibit promising data on cardiovascular morbidity and mortality in T2DM patients.[9,10] Following a review of the latest published clinical evidences—including a range of trials dealing with drug and lifestyle interventions—the European Association for the Study of Diabetes (EASD) and the American Diabetes Association (ADA) have put forth an updated consensus statement for management of patients with T2D. The present chapter focuses on the overall concept on treatment paradigm shift from glycemic index to reducing microvascular complications.

CARDIOVASCULAR OUTCOME TRIALS AND ITS ROLE IN CHANGING DIABETES TREATMENT GUIDELINES

The concerns raised about the cardiovascular safety of T2D medications such as rosiglitazone (a thiazolidinedione) prompted the US Food and Drug Administration (FDA) to issue a draft guidance in 2008. This has made large CVOTs for all new T2D therapies mandatory.[6,11] Since this guidance was issued, several prospective CVOTs have been carried out and reported. The completed trials demonstrated the noninferiority of their respective test drugs when compared with the placebo in major adverse cardiac events (MACE). The nine completed trials examined three dipeptidyl peptidase 4 (DPP-4) inhibitors, four GLP-1RAs, and two SGLT2-i.[12]

Based on the evidence reporting benefits of diabetic medications on reducing mortality, heart failure (HF), and progression of renal disease in the setting of established CVD, their use was considered compelling in this patient group. Thus, the ADA and the EASD recommendations reported that the providers should consider patient history very early in the process of initiating treatment selection (Flowchart 1).[13]

The previously conducted long-term, noninterventional, follow-up trials such as DCCT (Diabetes Control and Complications Trial), UKPDS (the UK Prospective Diabetes Study), and VADT (Veterans Affairs Diabetes Trial) suggested a "legacy" CV benefit of initially tighter glycemic control.[12] In addition to these, four of the recently completed trials, viz. *LEADER, SUSTAIN-6, EMPA-REG OUTCOME*, and the *CANVAS* program demonstrated clinically relevant relative risk reductions of MACE outcomes in patients with high CV risk (Table 1).[14-20] This information has built a strong foundation of evidence that has transformed diabetes care and the treatment guidelines thereof. Subsequently, there was considerable revision in clinical treatment recommendations, given that cardio-protection is an added benefit.

GLYCEMIC CONTROL AND INTENSIFICATION: A STEP FROM HBA1C TO CARDIOVASCULAR PERSPECTIVES

It has been found that complications due to poor glycemic control and clinical inertia start developing in nascent stage even prior to disease establishment, when the glucose concentration is low. Studies have demonstrated the prevalence of microalbuminuria even at 8.3% and 9.9% with impaired fasting glucose and impaired glucose tolerance. It is also evident that frequency of diabetic neuropathy increases with disease progression, from normal glucose tolerance to the active disease stage. New diabetes drug classes have emerged, which target multiple risk factors, variably lower cardiovascular outcomes, new-onset HF, and slow decline of renal function. These can meaningfully increase the diabetes armory that helps in maintaining glycemic control, and reducing the associated complications.[8] Therefore, overcoming clinical inertia and early glycemic control is beneficial for minimizing the chance of macro and microvascular events and mortality.[8,18] Several clinical trials have helped in establishing treatment guidelines, which focus not only on HbA1c reduction, but also on cardiovascular perspectives.

EVIDENCE SUMMARY FROM CLINICAL TRIALS (EMPA-REG, DECLARE TIMI, CANVAS, LEADER, CAROLINA, CARMELINA, DAPA HF, ETC.)

Metformin remains the first-line therapy in individuals with diabetes with and without HF, with second-line options including SGLT2 inhibitors. GLP-1RAs provide another second-line option but require further focused HF trials to establish safety. Through different CV trials, we now have a better understanding on novel therapies and how to individualize treatment in diabetic populations at high risk for HF (Fig. 2).[19]

The advent of two new classes of antihyperglycemic agents, the SGLT2-i and GLP-1R and their respective large CVOTs, has led to a treatment paradigm shift in how cardiologists and healthcare practitioners conceptualize T2DM treatment.

ESTABLISHMENT OF TREATMENT AND MANAGEMENT APPROACH FOR REDUCING DIABETES DISEASE BURDEN

Current diabetes treatment guidelines and algorithms recommend an individualized approach along

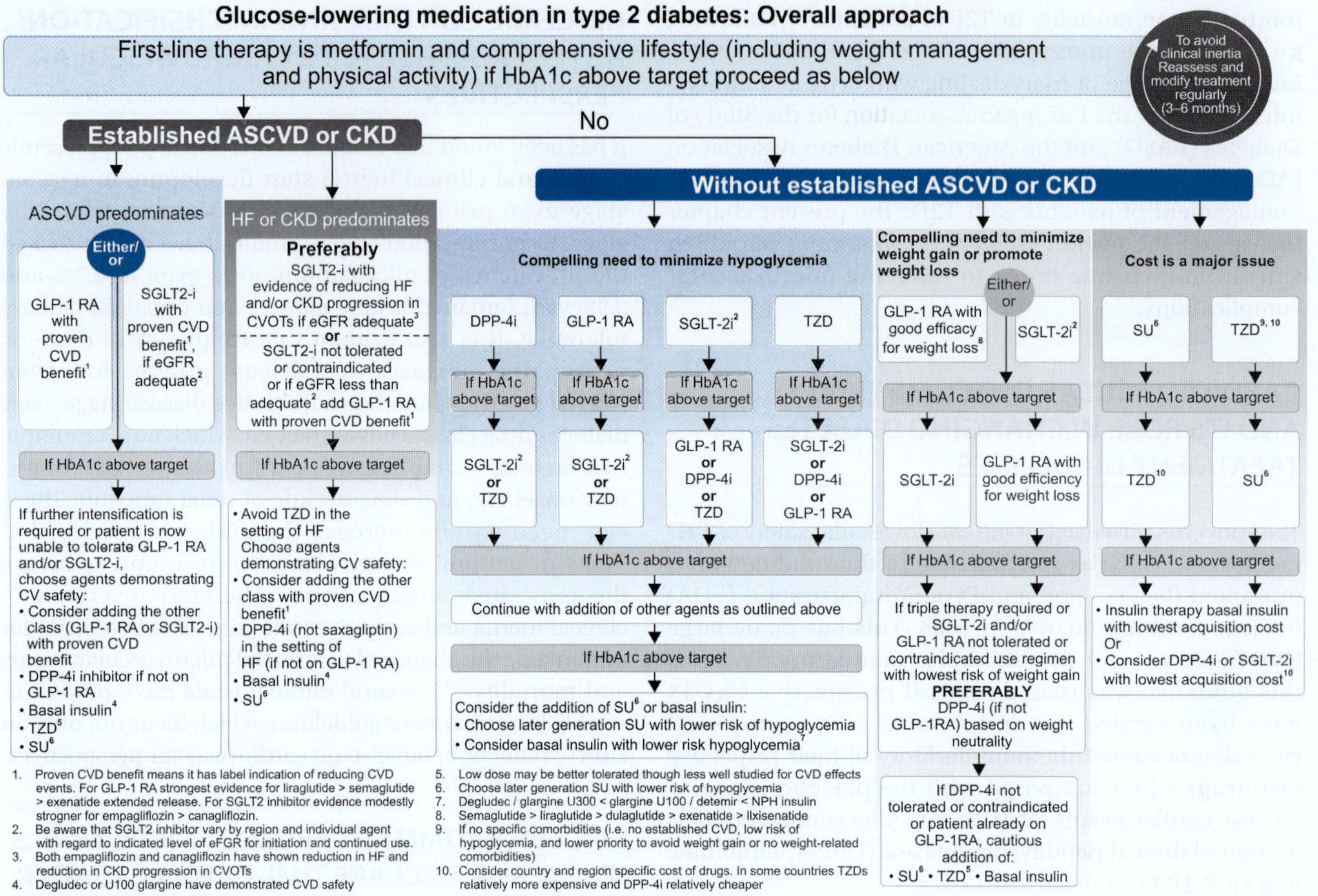

(ADA: American Diabetes Association; EASD: European Association for the Study of Diabetes; T2DM: type 2 diabetes mellitus)

Flowchart 1 Glucose lowering medication in T2DM (ADA and EASD consensus report).[13]

(*Source*: Adapted from Davies MJ, D'Alessio DA, Fradkin J, Kernan WN, Mathieu C, Mingrone G, et al. Management of hyperglycaemia in type 2 diabetes, 2018. A consensus report by the American Diabetes Association (ADA) and the European Association for the Study of Diabetes (EASD). Diabetologia. 2018 1;61(12):2461-98.)

with combination therapy for setting glycemic goals, minimizing micro-/macrovascular events and selecting treatment (Fig. 3).[19,13]

The new recommendations from the expert panel of ADA and EASD includes the following major pointers for choice of antidiabetic therapy based on presence or absence of established CVD, renal disease, etc. (Fig. 4).[13]

CONCLUSION

Type 2 diabetes mellitus is a major risk factor for developing micro-/macrovascular complications such as CVD, chronic kidney disease (CKD), retinopathy, etc. Despite improved risk factor control, adults with T2DM continue to experience substantial CVD risk. In earlier diabetes management setting, antidiabetic drugs were used primarily for glucose lowering, requiring titration, and monitoring of therapy. Until recently, improved glycemic control has not been associated with robust macrovascular benefits. Since the US FDA regulatory guidance in 2008, newer glucose-lowering therapeutic agents have been evaluated in several CVOTs. These trials have offered better understanding of benefits and risks of available antihyperglycemic agents.[19,21,22] Revision of the diabetes management guidelines was largely based on outcomes of different cardiovascular trials, and has led to a paradigm shift in T2DM treatment. The antihyperglycemic therapy should be combined with evidence-based treatment of cholesterol and blood pressure for cardiovascular risk reduction. The ADA and the EASD

TABLE 1: Risk reduction incompleted trials showing evidence of CV benefit.[12,14-20]

Trials	Diabetes duration (years)*	3-point MACE RRR (%)	CV death RRR (%)	HF hospitalization RRR (%)	Worsening nephropathy RRR (%)
LEADER	12.8	13	22	13	22
SUSTAIN-6	13.9	26	2	+11	36
EMPA-REG OUTCOME	57% > 10	14	38	35	39
CANVAS program	13.5	14	48; 13	33	40
DECLARE TIMI	11.0	22.6	4.9	6.2	3.7^
DAPA HF	Mean age: 66; diabetes percentage: 42	-	0.82 Hazard ratio	16.2	1.2

(*Reported as mean in all trials except EMPA-REG OUTCOME, which reported percentage of population with diabetes duration >10 years; DECLARE: Dapagliflozin Effect on Cardiovascular Events–Thrombolysis in Myocardial Infarction 58; ^: ≥40% decrease in eGFR to <60 mL/min/1.73 m^2, ESRD, or death from renal cause; RRR: relative risk reduction; DAPA HF: Dapagliflozin and prevention of adverse-outcomes in heart failure)
(*Source*: Adapted from References 12, and 14 to 20.)

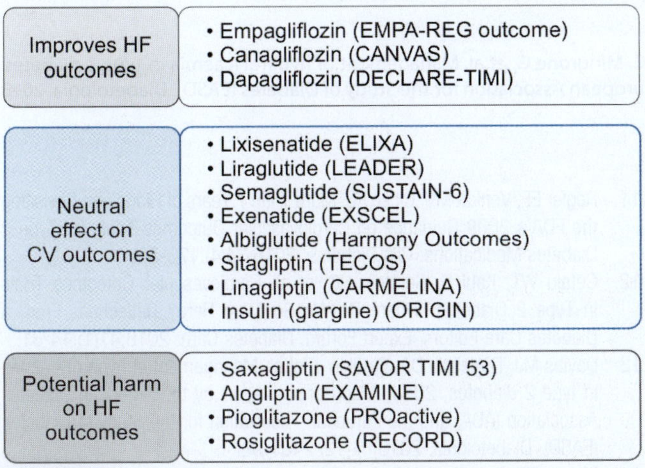

Figure 2 Heart failure (HF) outcomes with select glucose-lowering therapies.

(*Source*: Adapted from Bowes CD, Lien LF, Butler J. Clinical aspects of heart failure in individuals with diabetes. Diabetologia. 2019;62(9):1529-38.)

have proposed a set of patient and disease characteristics that has utility in guiding a patient-centered management approach for diabetes treatment. Thereby, the current therapies are rightly directed at addressing multiple risk factors comorbid with T2D for the prevention and progression of future micro-/macrovascular diseases. The ADA and EASD have highlighted that diabetes treatment require control of glycemia as well as cardiovascular risk factor management, a patient-centered approach for individualizing treatment goals and strategies. The recommendations address the approaches to glycemic management with the goal of reducing complications and

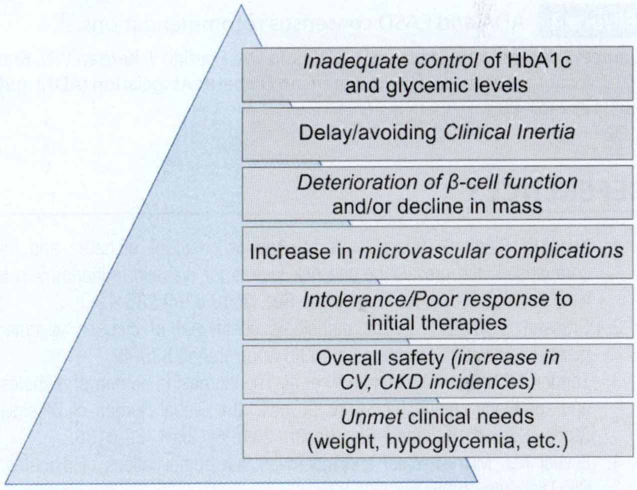

(The revised (ADA: American Diabetes Association; EASD: European Association for the Study of Diabetes) guidelines aimed at reducing diabetes burden and improving quality of life in patients with diabetes)

Figure 3 Setting guideline parameters for diabetes management.

(*Source*: Adapted from Davies MJ, D'Alessio DA, Fradkin J, Kernan WN, Mathieu C, Mingrone G, et al. Management of hyperglycaemia in type 2 diabetes, 2018. A consensus report by the American Diabetes Association (ADA) and the European Association for the Study of Diabetes (EASD). Diabetologia. 2018 1;61(12):2461-98.)[13]

maintaining quality of life in the context of comprehensive cardiovascular risk management and patient-centered care. Further, more large-scale clinical trials are required to evaluate the comprehensive risk/benefit ratio of different antihyperglycemic agents for better diabetes management and reduction of associated complications.

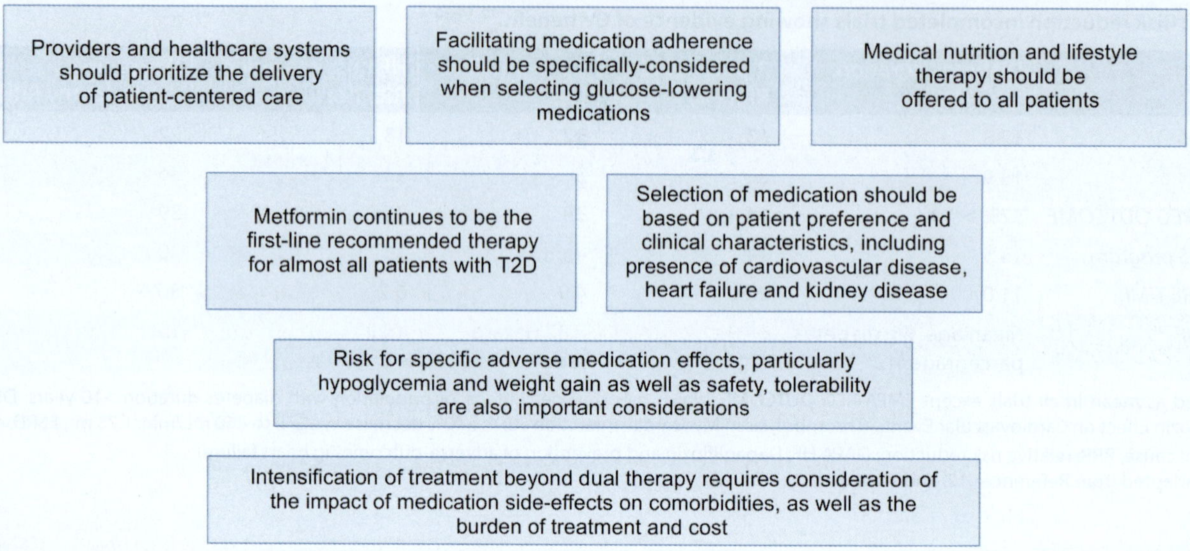

(ADA: American Diabetes Association; EASD: European Association for the Study of Diabetes; T2D: type 2 diabetes)

Figure 4 ADA and EASD consensus recommendations.[13]

(*Source*: Adapted from Davies MJ, D'Alessio DA, Fradkin J, Kernan WN, Mathieu C, Mingrone G, et al. Management of hyperglycaemia in type 2 diabetes, 2018. A consensus report by the American Diabetes Association (ADA) and the European Association for the Study of Diabetes (EASD). Diabetologia. 2018 1;61(12):2461-98.)

REFERENCES

1. Khan R, Singh S, Surya J, et al. Age of onset of diabetes and its comparison with prevalence and risk factors for diabetic retinopathy in a rural population of India. Ophthalmic Res. 2019;61(4):236-42.
2. Orasanu G, Plutzky J. The pathologic continuum of diabetic vascular disease. J Am Coll Cardiol. 2009;53(5 Supplement):S35-42.
3. Tandon N, Anjana RM, Mohan V, et al. The increasing burden of diabetes and variations among the states of India: the Global Burden of Disease Study 1990-2016. Lancet Glob Health. 2018;6(12):e1352-e1362.
4. Fowler MJ. Microvascular and macrovascular complications of diabetes. Clin Diabetes. 2008;26(2):77-82.
5. George B, Cebioglu M, Yeghiazaryan K. Inadequate diabetic care: global figures cry for preventive measures and personalized treatment. EPMA J. 2010;1(1):13-18.
6. Einarson TR, Acs A, Ludwig C, et al. Prevalence of cardiovascular disease in type 2 diabetes: a systematic literature review of scientific evidence from across the world in 2007-2017. Cardiovasc Diabetol. 2018;17(1): 83.
7. Chawla A, Chawla R, Jaggi S. Microvasular and macrovascular complications in diabetes mellitus: distinct or continuum? Indian J Endocrinol Metab. 2016;20(4):546-51.
8. Laiteerapong N, Ham SA, Gao Y, et al. The legacy effect in type 2 diabetes: impact of early glycemic control on future complications (the Diabetes & Aging Study). Diabetes Care. 2019;42(3):416-26.
9. Røder ME. Major adverse cardiovascular event reduction with GLP-1 and SGLT2 agents: evidence and clinical potential. Ther Adv Chronic Dis. 2018;9(1):33-50.
10. Goncalves E, Bell DSH. Combination treatment of SGLT2 Inhibitors and GLP-1 receptor agonists: Symbiotic effects on metabolism and cardiorenal risk. Diabetes Ther. 2018;9(3):919-26.
11. Regier EE, Venkat MV, Close KL. More Than 7 Years of Hindsight: Revisiting the FDA's 2008 Guidance on Cardiovascular Outcomes Trials for Type 2 Diabetes Medications. Clin Diabetes. 2016;34(4):173-80.
12. Cefalu WT, Kaul S, Gerstein HC, et al. Cardiovascular Outcomes Trials In Type 2 Diabetes: Where Do We Go From Here? Reflections From a Diabetes Care Editors' Expert Forum. Diabetes Care. 2018;41(1):14-31.
13. Davies MJ, D'Alessio DA, Fradkin J, et al. Management of hyperglycaemia in type 2 diabetes, 2018. A consensus report by the American Diabetes Association (ADA) and the European Association for the Study of Diabetes (EASD). Diabetologia. 2018;61(12):2461-98.
14. Marso SP, Daniels GH, Brown-Frandsen K, et al. Liraglutide and cardiovascular outcomes in type 2 diabetes. N Engl J Med. 2016;375:311-22.
15. Marso SP, Bain SC, Consoli A, et al. Semaglutide and cardiovascular outcomes in patients with type 2 diabetes. N Engl J Med. 2016;375:1834-44.
16. Wanner C, Inzucchi SE, Lachin JM, et al. Empagliflozin and progression of kidney disease in type 2 diabetes. N Engl J Med. 2016;375:323-34.
17. Neal B, Perkovic V, Mahaffey KW, et al. Canagliflozin and cardiovascular and renal events in type 2 diabetes. N Engl J Med. 2017;377:644-57.
18. Stolar M. Glycemic control and complications in type 2 diabetes mellitus. Am J Med. 2010;123(3 Suppl):S3-11.
19. Bowes CD, Lien LF, Butler J. Clinical aspects of heart failure in individuals with diabetes. Diabetologia. 2019;62(9):1529-38.
20. American College of Cardiology. (2019). Dapagliflozin in Patients With Heart Failure and Reduced Ejection Fraction - DAPA-HF. [online] Available from https://www.acc.org/latest-in-cardiology/clinical-trials/2019/08/30/21/33/dapa-hf [Last accessed September, 2019].
21. Reusch JE, Manson JE. Management of Type 2 Diabetes in 2017: Getting to Goal. JAMA. 2017;317(10):1015-6.
22. Newman JD, Vani AK, Aleman JO, et al. The Changing Landscape of Diabetes Therapy for Cardiovascular Risk Reduction: JACC State-of-the-Art Review. J Am Coll Cardiol. 2018;72(15):1856-69.

51 CHAPTER

BE-SMART: Basal Early Strategies to Maximize A1C Reduction with Oral Therapy

Mangesh Tiwaskar, Shilpa Tiwaskar

INTRODUCTION

Diabetes—the fear and apprehensions connected to this word are many, both in the mind of patients and their healthcare providers. This is mainly because diabetes is a life-crippling condition and a global health crisis which affects 425 million adults worldwide, out of whom 327 million are in the age group of 20–64 years. This global diabetic population is expected to soar by 48% to 629 million by 2045. Diabetes enhances cardiovascular disease (CVD) risk, is the 11th common cause of disability in the world and contributes to 1 death every 8 seconds. We represent the world's 2nd largest diabetic population (73 million) which translates to nearly every 6th diabetic being an Indian. One in every 10 adults in India is diabetic with another 42 million remaining undiagnosed. Type 2 diabetes (T2D) is the most prevalent form of diabetes and accounts for 90–95% of all diabetes cases. An analysis of the Global Burden of Disease 2016 data with respect to India found that, over the past ~3 decades, deaths and disability-adjusted life years (DALYs) attributed to diabetes have increased by three-fold with high fasting plasma glucose being the 5th largest cause of the total DALYs in India. Diabetes, in turn, played a significant role in increased risk for other disease conditions such as ischemic heart disease, stroke, chronic kidney disease (CKD), specific cancers, peripheral artery disease and tuberculosis. Key risk factors for diabetes were high body mass index (BMI), unhealthy diet (low in fruits, nuts and seeds, and whole grains) and tobacco use. Additionally, due to its chronic nature and associated complications, diabetes places enormous physical and economic burden on its sufferers with medical costs incurred being 2–5 times greater than for those without diabetes.[1-4] The fears associated with this condition are compounded by the high prevalence of uncontrolled diabetes nearly 1 out of every 2 diabetic individuals in India do not achieve their glycemic goal.[5] Ensuring effective glycemic control will need a clearly demarcated strategy, in fact a *SMART* strategy.

THE SMART WAY TO EFFECTIVE DIABETES MANAGEMENT

S: Swift Achievement of Targets

Studies show that early achievement of glycemic control, in newly diagnosed patients as well as in uncontrolled patients, had a durable positive impact and reduced the incidence of future complications.

In the newly diagnosed: Though the picture of diabetes prevalence and control is grim, effective control of glycemia can help to reduce both the microvascular and macrovascular complications of diabetes. The landmark United Kingdom Prospective Diabetes Study (UKPDS; n = 5,102 newly diagnosed diabetic patients) showed that tight glycemic control reduced the overall microvascular complication rate by 25%. Further analysis of the UKPDS data showed that every 1% drop in glycated hemoglobin (HbA1c) reduced microvascular complications by 35%, diabetes-related deaths by 25%, all-cause mortality by 7% and combined fatal and nonfatal myocardial infarction (MI) by 18%.[6]

The benefits seen in the intensive group of UKPDS persisted after 10 years wherein even after loss of between-group HbA1c differences over time, early and intensive glycemic control had a significant long-term impact denoted as the legacy effect (Fig. 1).[7] Similarly, in the

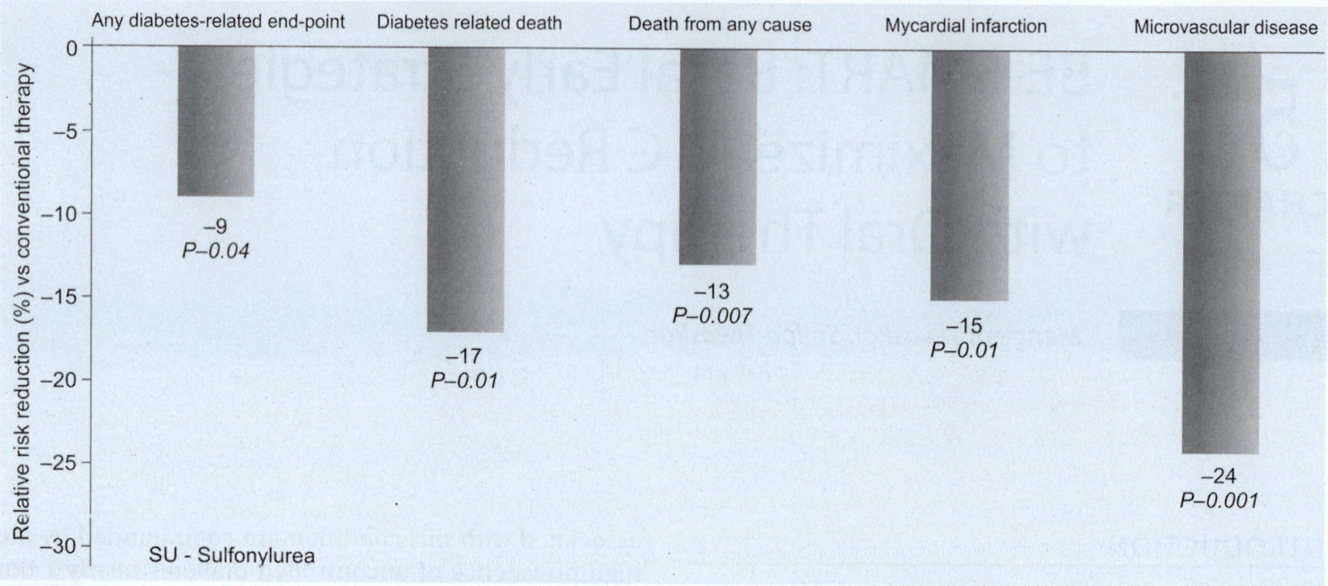

Figure 1 Impact of intensive vs conventional therapy with SU-insulin on 10 years outcome measures.
(*Source*: Adapted from Holman RR et al.[7])

Diabetes and Aging Study, newly diagnosed patients with T2D and 10 years of survival (n = 34,737) were followed up for a period of 13 years. When associations between HbA1c levels at various periods of early exposure (0–1, 0–2, 0–3, 0–4, 0–5, 0–6, and 0–7 years) and incident future microvascular and macrovascular events and death were sought, it was seen that HbA1c levels of <6.5% during the 1st year after diagnosis had maximal beneficial impact on the diabetic complications. Both the duration and the intensity of glycemia played an important role in incident complications, in fact, the longer the HbA1c levels remained ≥8%, greater were the associated microvascular and mortality risks.[8] Control achieved during the initial postdiagnostic period thus had maximal beneficial impact.

In uncontrolled patients: Early achievement of glycemic control had a significant impact even in uncontrolled patients as shown by another study which used the physiologically-based Archimedes model to simulate a clinical trial amongst a randomly selected United States population who had uncontrolled diabetes (HbA1c >7%). The projected effects of four programs were used to predict the 20-year impact of glycemic control: (1) *status quo*, where no change was made to the existing levels of compliance and control, (2) controlling HbA1c to <7% over a 6-month period, (3) controlling HbA1c to <7% over a year (12 months) and (4) controlling HbA1c to <7% over 2 years (24 months). The model predicted that getting patients to target earlier was more beneficial than delaying the glycemic control (Fig. 2). This model also predicted that swift glycemic control reduced MI and coronary heart disease risk by 11 and 17%, respectively. Moreover, greater the baseline HbA1c (e.g. HbA1c >9%), greater was the predicted beneficial impact on microvascular complications.[9] Thus, in uncontrolled patients, irrespective of the baseline HbA1c, prompt achievement of glycemic control had a wide-ranging positive impact.

M: Multilevel Management with Pharmacological Options

Both nonpharmacological and pharmacological therapies play a significant role in lowering HbA1c levels in diabetes. Lifestyle management includes diabetes self-management education and support (DSMES), appropriate physical activity, medical nutrition therapy (MNT), smoking cessation counseling and psychosocial care.[10] DSMES, MNT, weight loss and structured physical activity help reduce HbA1c levels by 0.3–2%.[10-14] Since lifestyle management alone often proves insufficient, pharmacological therapy is needed in most diabetic patients to achieve glycemic control.[9] Initiation of drug therapy is normally done after taking several factors into consideration such as presence of comorbidities like atherosclerotic cardiovascular disease (ASCVD), chronic kidney disease (CKD) and heart failure (HF), associated hypoglycemic risk, impact on body weight,

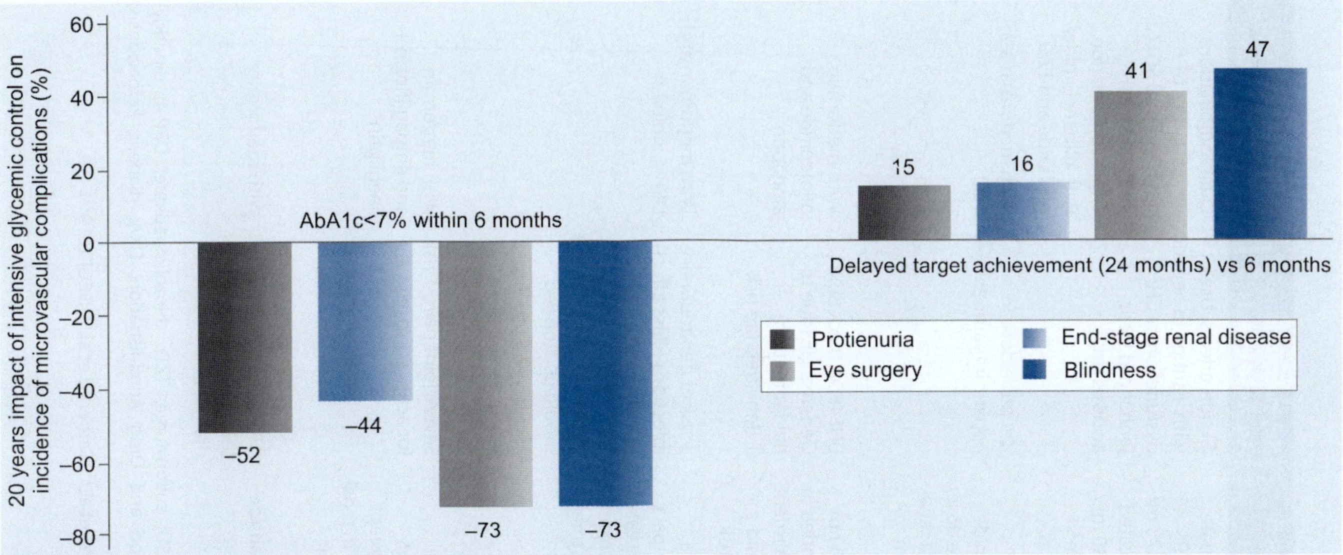

Figure 2 20 years projected impact of early vs delayed glycemic control.

(*Source*: Adapted from Bailey CJ et al.[9])

side effect profile, cost and patient preferences. Some of the key oral antidiabetic agents available for use include metformin, Sulfonylureas (SUs), thiazolidinediones (TZD), alpha-glucosidase inhibitors (AGIs), sodium glucose cotransporter 2 (SGLT2) inhibitors and dipeptidyl peptidase 4 (DPP-4) inhibitors or gliptins.[15] The overall profile of each drug class is detailed in Table 1.

A meta-analysis which compared the efficacy and safety of most antidiabetic medications showed that there was an overall reduction of 1% in HbA1c with most agents. Evidence proved that metformin was an able agent to treat T2D[21] and remains the recommended first-line of therapy along with lifestyle modifications in most T2D patients (unless contraindicated).[15]

However, one of the lessons from UKPDS was the progressive deterioration of glycemic control over the years with monotherapy. It was seen that over 3 years and 9 years only about half and quarter of the patients, respectively, on monotherapy were able to achieve HbA1c<7%.[24] The loss of glycemic control was linked to the progressive loss of β-cell function, which began much before the patient was diagnosed.[9] Earlier use of combination therapy may help mitigate these effects to achieve sustained glycemic control.

Early use of combination therapy: Since Metformin remains the mainstay of antidiabetic treatment for most patients, use of a combination of metformin with another drug with a complementary mechanism of action may help preserve β-cell function and achieve sustained glycemic control vis-à-vis a stepwise addition of agents.[25] The American Diabetes Association (ADA) and the American Association of Clinical Endocrinologists/ American College of Endocrinology (AACE/ACE) 2019 guidelines also advocate the initiation of dual therapy in patients with HbA1c ≥8.5% and ≥7.5%, respectively.[15,26]

The benefits of early combination therapy on glycemic control were assessed in a study involving patients who had failed to achieve glycemic targets on metformin alone (n = 5,870). The impact of early (within 3 months) versus late addition (10–15 months) of a 2nd drug in these patients was analyzed over 1.5–2 years. The proportion of patients who achieved HbA1c <7% was 47.2% versus 41.7% (p = 0.039) in the early and late add-on groups, respectively. Thus early use of combination therapy helped in better achievement of glycemic goals. Though treatment intensification is essential in patients who do not respond within the first 3 months of monotherapy, delay in addition of other drugs is mainly attributed to "clinical inertia" which needs to be overcome to achieve glycemic goals faster and in an effective manner.[27] Some of the common fixed dose combinations available for use are given in Table 1.

In addition to metformin, SUs have remained a crucial part of antidiabetic therapy for the past several decades. Though glibenclamide was plagued with safety issues, newer SUs such as glimepiride, glipizide and gliclazide combine efficacy with an enhanced safety profile. Combinations of metformin with these

TABLE 1: Key attributes of commonly availabe antidiabetic medications.

Drug class	Agents	Cost	Impact on weight	Hypoglycemia	CV effects	Renal effects	Key precautions/ Ad verse effects	Available fixed-dose combinations
Biguanides	Metformin	Economical	↓ or ↔	No	May reduce CV events and mortality	Do not initiate when eGFR < 45 mL/min/1.73 m^2; Conraindicated if eGFR < 30 mL/min/1.73 m^2	GI side-effects. Use with caution in hepatic dysfunction or CHF (enhanced lactic acidosis risk)	Dual combinations with SU, TZD, DPP-4, inhibitors and SGLT2 inhibitors Triple combination with glibenclamide/ gliclazide and TZD
SUs	Glibenclamide, Glimepride, Gliclazide, Glipizide	Economical	↑ Lesser with Glimepiride, Gliclazide, Glipizide	High with Glibenclamide, Lesser with others (combinations can even be used in the elderly)	↔	↔, Avoid glibenclamide and reduce dose of others in renal impairment	Decrease dose in hepatic impairment	With metformin and TZD
TZDs	Pioglitazone, Rosiglitazone	Economical	↑	No	Pioglitazone-potential benefit in ASCVD; ↑CHF risk with both	↔, though not recommended in renal impairment due to ↑fluid retention risk	CHF (FDA Black Box) Oedema, HF (due to fluid retention) ↑ Bone fracture risk	With metformin, glimepiride and alogliptin
SGLT2 inhibitors	Empagliflozin, Canagliflozin Dapagliflozin	High	↓	No	Empagliflozin, Canagliflozin beneficial in ASCVD, all 3 beneficial in CHF	All 3 have a positive impact on renal disease progression; renal dose adjustment needed	↓ risk of genitourinary infections (class effect) and amputation (FDA Black Box)/skeletal fractures (Canagliflozin) should be stopped 24–48 hours before surgeries/stressful activities (↑ DKA risk)	With metformin and DPP-4 inhibitor
DPP-4 inhibitors	Sitagliptin, Saxagliptin, Alogliptin, Linagliptin	High	↔	No	CV neutral; ↑HF risk (Saxagliptin and Alogliptin), more in those with pre-existing cardiac or renal conditions	Renal dose adjustment needed (except langliptin) in renal impairment	Severe joint pain; ↑ risk for acute pancreatitis	With metformin and empagliflozin + linagliptin
α-glucosidase inhibitors	Acarbose, Voglibose, Miglitol	Intermediate	↔	No	Some ASCVD benefit	Use with caution in CKD	GI side-effects (bloating, flatulence, diarrhea)	With metformin

(CV: cardiovascular; GI: gastrointestinal; eGFR: estimated glomerulor filtration rate: CHF: chronic heart failure; SU: sulfonylurea; TZD: thiozolidinedione; DPP-4: dipetidyl peptidose 4; SGLT2: sodium-glucose co-transportation 2; ASCVD: atherosclerosis cardiovascular disease; FDA: Food and Drug Administration; DKA: diabetic ketoacidosis; CKD: chronic kidney disease)

(*Source*: Adapted from ADA 2019[15,16], Kalra S et al.[18], Lupsa BC et al.[18], Diabetes Medicines[19], van de Laar FA et al.[20], Bennett WL et al.[21], Garber AJ et al.[22], DCGI 2019[23])

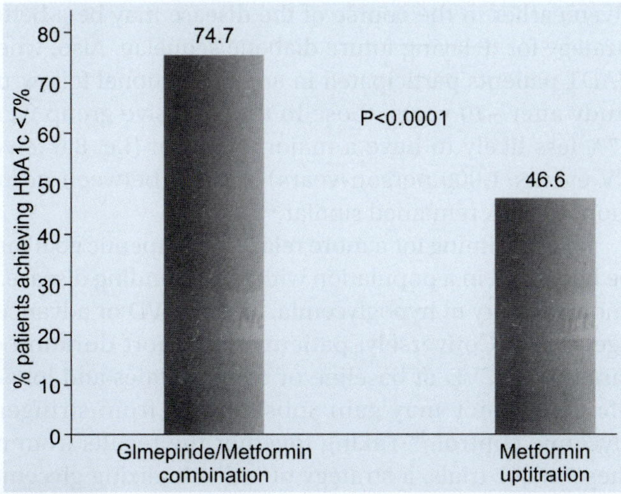

Figure 3 Glycemic target achievement with monotherapy vs combination therapy.
(*Source*: Adapted from Kim HS et al.[28])

TABLE 2: Efficacy and safety comparison of oral metformin combinations vs Metformin alone

Oral combinations	OR for the outcome of patients achieving HbA1c goal	OR for patients having hypoglycemic events
SU + Metformin	4.06	3.95
DPP-4 inhibitors + Metformin	3.13	1.19
TZDs + Metformin	2.3	1.59
Alpha-glucosidase inhibitors + Metformin	2.92	3.24
Meglitinides + Metformin	2.42	3.25

(OR: odds ratio; HbA1c: glycosylated hemoglobin; SU: sulfonylurea; DPP-4: dipeptidyl peptidose; TZD: thiozolidinedione)
(*Source*: Adapted from Zintzaras E et al.[29])

SUs are widely available and have been used in several countries worldwide.[17] A 24-week study compared the early use of combination therapy with glimepiride/metformin with metformin uptitration in T2D patients (n = 209) uncontrolled on metformin monotherapy (for 3 months). At the end of the study, HbA1c levels were more significantly reduced in the combination group than in the metformin uptitration group (–1.2 vs. 0.8%, P <0.0001). HbA1c <7% was also achieved in a significantly greater proportion of patients in the combination group (Fig. 3). Moreover, the dosage of the drugs used in the combination were lower with a shorter period of titration showing that suboptimal doses of individual drugs, when given in combination, continue to have a beneficial impact with better tolerability and safety.[28]

In a meta-analysis of 15 randomized clinical trials, the effect of metformin in combination with several other agents such as TZDs, SUs, DPP-4 inhibitors or SGLT-2 inhibitors was evaluated. Compared to metformin alone, combination therapy significantly reduced HbA1c levels by an average of 0.43%, enhanced HbA1c <7% goal achievement by 40% and decreased fasting plasma glucose (FPG) by a mean of 14.30 mg/dL, though the risk of hypoglycemia increased by 56%. However, when SUs and glinides were excluded from the analysis, this risk was no longer significant. Insulin sensitivity was also improved in some studies with one study showing that initial combination of metformin with DPP-4i improved β-cell function versus metformin monotherapy.[25]

A larger network meta-analysis included 277 studies and extrapolated data from >100,000 patients over 3 decades with 69 treatments with 173 direct comparisons for efficacy and 71 treatments with 180 direct comparisons for tolerability. Metformin when used in combination with either SUs, DPP-4 inhibitors, TZDs, meglitinides, AGIs and glucagon-like peptide-1 agonists (GLP-1a) had a 3-11 fold greater likelihood of achieving the HbA1c goal compared to its monotherapy (Table 2). An indirect analysis across the 2-drug regimens that superseded metformin monotherapy showed that 5 combinations (metformin + SU/DPP-4 inhibitors/TZD/meglitinide/GLP-1a) yielded similar results. In the analysis for hypoglycemic risk, an impact similar to metformin monotherapy was seen with combination of metformin with DPP-4 inhibitors/TZDs/GLP-1, whereas combinations with SUs, meglitinides and AGIs resulted in higher risk (Table 2).[29]

Choosing the right combination of agents is thus essential to obtain maximum benefit with minimal adverse impact. Moreover, availability of fixed dose combinations of several appropriate agents (Table 3) has helped simplify drug regimens, improving compliance and adherence.[30]

A: Assigning "Achievable" Glycemic Targets

Since the impact of intensive glycemic control was positive in the UKPDS, three other landmark trials, the Action to Control Cardiovascular Risk in Diabetes (ACCORD), Action in Diabetes and Vascular Disease: Preterax and Diamicron MR Controlled Evaluation (ADVANCE) and the Veterans Affairs Diabetes Trial (VADT), sought to determine its impact on microvascular and macrovascular diabetic complications.[31-35] However, unlike UKPDS,

TABLE 3: Commonly available fixed dose antidiabetic combinations

Drug class	Drug names
SU + Biguanide	Glipizide/Glimepiride/Glipizide/ Glibenclamide + Metformin
DPP-4 inhibitors + Biguanide	Sitagliptin/Saxagliptin/Alogliptin/ Linagliptin + Metformin
SGLT2 inhibitors + Biguanide	Canagliflozin/Dapagliflozin + Metformin
TZD + Biguanide	Pioglitazone/Rosiglitazone + Metformin
TZD + SU	Pioglitazone/Rosiglitazone + Glimepiride
TZD + DPP-4 inhibitor	Pioglitazone + Alogliptin
SGLT2 inhibitor+ DPP-4 inhibitor	Empagliflozin + Linagliptin

(SU: sulfonylurea; DPP-4: Dipeptidyl peptidase-4; SGLT2: sodium glucose contransporter 2; TZD: thiazolidinedione)
(*Source*: Adapted from Kalra S et al.[17], Diabetic Medicine 2018.[19])

participants in these three trials were nearly 10 years older, had long-standing diabetes (8–11 years) and presented with established CVD or cardiovascular (CV) risk factors. The intensive group in the ACCORD trial showed a 29% reduction in development of macroalbuminuria and decrease in some measures of eye complications and neuropathy. However, the study was terminated at 3.5 years due to excessive mortality risk in the intensive group. The tight glycemic control group of the ADVANCE study showed a 10% relative reduction in the combined outcome of major macrovascular and microvascular events, mainly due to 21% relative reduction in nephropathy over a period of 5 years. The VADT study did not show any positive impact of intensive control, though significant reduction in deterioration in albumin excretion and progression to macroalbuminuria was observed, over a median of 5.6 years. There was no reduction in CV events in these trials. On the other hand, the participants in the intensive group showed higher incidence of hypoglycemia and weight gain. These trials were also of too short a duration to exhibit the macrovascular impact of intensive glucose control.

Some interesting aspects in these trials emerged upon further study. Increased mortality in ACCORD was observed only in the group that remained at HbA1c >7% even after intensive control.[22] Moreover, an analysis of subgroups in ACCORD showed reduction in the primary outcome (CV event or CV-related mortality) in the groups with HbA1c <8% at baseline and in those with no previous CV event.[34] This reiterates the fact that intensive treatment given earlier in the course of the disease may be a better strategy for delaying future diabetic sequelae. Also, when VADT patients participated in an observational follow-up study after ~10 years, those in the intensive group were 17% less likely to have a major CV event (i.e. 8.6 fewer CV events/1,000 person-years), though between-group mortality risk remained similar.[22]

Hence, aiming for a more relaxed therapeutic goal may be beneficial in a population with long-standing disease, a known history of hypoglycemia, known CVD or advanced age/frailty. Conversely, patients with short duration of disease, no CVD at baseline or comorbidities and longer life expectancy may gain substantially from stringent glycemic control.[36] Taking together the results from all these major trials, a strategy of individualizing glycemic targets to suit the patient profile might prove beneficial to achieve optimal glycemic control without any adverse impact (Table 4).

R: Reconfiguring Oral Therapy to Suit the Patient's Needs and Preferences

Since diabetes commonly coexists with other metabolic disorders, customization of the antidiabetic regimen to the patient profile will ensure optimal protection against diabetic complications. Metformin is considered the first-line of therapy along with lifestyle management strategies. After therapy initiation, detailed and repeated assessments at 3-month intervals of all factors which may have an impact on glycemic control [e.g. HbA1c, self-monitoring blood glucose records, suspected hypoglycemic events, lipid and BP values, side effects/adverse events (if any), etc.] is essential to enhance patient care. Once glycemic targets are achieved, review periods can be less frequent.[22] If metformin and lifestyle strategies are not successful in achieving glycemic goals, subsequent therapy can be customized in certain key categories of patients in the manner outlined here.[15,16,22]

- In *patients without any specific comorbidities, for whom cost is a limiting factor*, SUs or TZDs can be added to the regimen. Subsequent lack of control might necessitate the addition of the most economical option amongst DPP-4 inhibitors or SGLT2 inhibitors.
- *Patients without comorbidities but at increased risk for hypoglycemia* can be further treated with either DPP-4 inhibitors, SGLT2 inhibitors or TZDs as second-line therapy. Subsequent therapy can involve the drug class not utilized before. Lastly, if glycemic control has not been achieved, newer SUs (with lower hypoglycemic impact) can be utilized. Enhancing patient awareness

TABLE 4: Recommended glycemic targets.

Organization	Glycemic targets (HbA1c)	Diabetic patient profile
ADA 2019	<7%	Most non-pregnant patients
	<6.5%, if achievable without adverse impact	Longer life expectancy, without CVD, short duration of diabetes, managed on metformin and lifestyle modifications alone
	<8%	H/O of severe hypoglycemia, presence of severe complications, longer disease duration, several comorbidities, limited life expectancy, difficult to treat to target in spite of appropriate medications
	<7.5%	Reasonably healthy older adults with fewer coexisting conditions and intact cognitive and functional capabilities
	<8–8.5%	In older adults with several comorbidities, cognitive and functional impairment
AACE/ACE 2019	≤6.5%	No coexisting serious illness, low hypoglycemic risk
	>6.5%	With coexisting serious illness, at risk for hypoglycemia
NICE 2019	<6.5%	Managed by either by lifestyle and diet alone or along with a single drug not associated with hypoglycemia
	<7%	Managed by drug causing hypoglycemia
	Relax target	Older/frail, reduced life expectancy, significant comorbidities, at risk for hypoglycemia
SIGN 2017	<7%	Most patients
	<6.5%	Newly-diagnosed patients
	Customise target	Evaluatie risk vs benefit ratio, especially hypoglycemia and weight gain

(ADA: American Diabetes Association; AACE/ACE: American Association of Clinical Endocrinologists/American College of Endocrinology; NICE: National Centre for Health and Care Excellence; SIGN: scottish intercollegiate guidelines network; CVD: cardiovascular disease; H/O: history of)

(*Source*: Adapted from ADA 2019[16,36], AACE/ACE 2019[26], NICE 2019[37], SIGN 154[38])

about hypoglycemia, its signs and symptoms, is the key to avoiding detrimental consequences. This is especially true in the elderly and in those with erratic eating patterns. Emphasizing the benefits of compliance and ensuring regular self-monitoring of glucose (whenever needed) in this class of patients will also help in enhancing glycemic control.

- For *obese patients without established coexisting conditions*, in whom weight loss is to be promoted or weight gain minimized, based on their weight-neutrality, either SGLT2 inhibitors or DPP-4 inhibitors can be used. If these prove insufficient, one of the newer SUs can be added to the regimen. Moreover, if these adults are newly diagnosed and present without any complications, prompt and effective treatment and frequent reassessments will help in reducing periods of hyperglycemia and thus delay appearance of diabetic complications.
- In *older adults*, the patients' characteristics or health status—healthy, intermediate (with one or more coexisting conditions, some amount of functional/cognitive impairment) or severe (requiring long-term care, significant cognitive/functional decline) should be taken into account while prescribing antihyperglycemic medications. Some precautions to be observed include preference for medication classes with low risk of hypoglycemia, avoidance of overtreatment and usage of simplified treatment regimens. A careful balance must be maintained between glycemic control and risk of hypoglycemia, with repeated monitoring of the treatment regimen to assess risk of decline in glycemic control and functional abilities. Metformin should be avoided in those with severe hepatic/renal dysfunction, TZDs should be used with caution (especially in those at risk for HF or fractures/falls) and newer SUs with low hypoglycemic risk should be preferred. DPP-4 inhibitors, on the other hand, may prove expensive whereas long-term effects of SGLT2 inhibitors have not been sufficiently studied, hence these drugs should be used with caution, if at all.
- In *patients with established ASCVD or CKD*, SGLT2 inhibitors if estimated glomerular filtration rate (eGFR) is adequate can be added. If glycemic control is not achieved at 3–6 months, DPP-4 inhibitors can be included followed by newer SUs such as glimepiride or gliclazide. For patients with ASCVD on SGLT2 inhibitors, CVD benefit is slightly more with empagliflozin than canagliflozin. TZDs can be included

in the regimen if ASCVD is the predominant condition, but both TZDs and saxagliptin should be avoided in the setting of HF. Intensive management of CVD risk in these patients is essential. Since these patients may have a higher pill burden, evaluating contraindications vis-à-vis the current treatment regimen is a must. If glycemic control remains poor, other factors such as excessively conservative management, poor adherence to antidiabetic regimens or unsuitable choice of agents must be reviewed.

The above categories are by no means a comprehensive list since diabetic patients present with wide-ranging profiles with varying comorbidities. Effective achievement of glycemic targets without detrimental impact remains the basic tenet of antidiabetic treatment and all therapeutic options (whether used alone or in combination) are aimed towards this goal. Extensive patient-doctor interaction and repeated review of the treatment will help in maintaining this delicate balance to ensure optimal benefit.

T: Targeting Comprehensive Care (Holistic Approach to Diabetes Management)

Type 2 diabetes often occurs in the setting of dyslipidemia and hypertension and these comorbidities also need to be simultaneously and effectively treated along with achievement of glycemic control.[39] Both hypertension and dyslipidemia contribute to enhanced CV risk in diabetic patients. A blood pressure target of <130/80 mmHg is generally recommended for diabetic patients with concomitant hypertension. Along with lifestyle modifications, treatment with appropriate antihypertensive medications, based on the patient profile, such as angiotensin-converting enzyme inhibitors (ACEIs), angiotensin II receptor blockers (ARBs), beta blockers, calcium channel blockers (CCBs) and thiazide diuretics, can be carried out.[22] In fact, early use of combination therapy has proven effective in achieving blood pressure goals.[9] In case of dyslipidemia, lifestyle changes will need to be combined with statin monotherapy or with add-on nonstatin lipid-lowering therapies to ensure appropriate reduction in low-density lipoprotein cholesterol (LDL-C) levels to minimize risk.[22]

CONCLUSION

India is the second largest contributor to the growing epidemic of diabetes worldwide. The heavy burden of morbidity and mortality associated with this condition make optimal glycemic control essential. Despite the availability of several medications, mainly oral in nature, the HbA1c goal of <7% remains elusive. Early achievement of the glycemic goal has been found to have a significant positive impact on subsequent diabetic complications. Intensive control earlier in the course of the disease, preferably with combination therapy, also may go a long way in avoiding future complications. Since patient profiles in diabetes are wide-ranging, customization of therapy and targets help tremendously in achieving optimal control without causing harm. Since diabetes rarely occurs alone, control of other coexisting disorders such as hypertension and dyslipidemia is warranted to enhance overall patient care (Box 1). Stringent application of these SMART ideas may aid in augmenting therapy and preventing the more severe complications associated with diabetes.

BOX 1 Strategies to enhance glycemic control.

- Aim for HbA1c <6.5–7% in most patients, without adverse impact
- Customize targets in specific patient populations after weighing the risk to benefit ratio
- Initiate combination therapy with agents having complementary modes of action to derive maximum benefit
- Tailor antidiabetic regimen according to patient profile
- Target other concomitant conditions to maximize impact
- Review response to therapy at intervals of 3–6 months and modify/intensify as needed

(*Source*: Adapted from ADA 2019.[36,37], AACE/ACE 2019.[26], Bailey CJ et al.[9], Del Prato S et al.[35,39])

REFERENCES

1. Diabetes Atlas. (2017). IDF Diabetes Atlas, 8th edition. [online] Available from https://diabetesatlas.org/resources/2017-atlas.html. [Last Accessed October, 2019].
2. American Diabetes Association. Classification and diagnosis of diabetes: Standards of Medical Care in Diabetes 2019. Diabetes Care. 2019;42(Suppl 1):S13-28.
3. Tripathy JP. Burden and risk factors of diabetes and hyperglycemia in India: findings from the Global Burden of Disease Study 2016. Diabetes Metab Syndr Obes. 2018;11:381-7.
4. Pradeepa R, Mohan V. Prevalence of type 2 diabetes and its complications in India and economic costs to the nation. Eur J Clin Nutr. 2017;71(7):816-24.
5. Venkataraman K, Kannan AT, Mohan V. Challenges in diabetes management with particular reference to India. Int J Diabetes Dev Ctries. 2009;29(3):103-9.
6. Genuth S, Eastman R, Kahn R, et al. Implications of the United kingdom prospective diabetes study. Diabetes Care. 2002;25(Suppl 1):S28-32.
7. Holman RR, Paul SK, Bethel MA, et al. 10-year follow-up of intensive glucose control in type 2 diabetes. N Engl J Med. 2008;359(15):1577-89.
8. Laiteerapong N, Ham SA, Gao Y, et al. The Legacy Effect in Type 2 Diabetes: Impact of Early Glycemic Control on Future Complications (The Diabetes & Aging Study). Diabetes Care. 2019;42(3):416-26.

9. Bailey CJ, Del Prato S, Eddy D, et al. Earlier intervention in type 2 diabetes: the case for achieving early and sustained glycaemic control. Int J Clin Pract. 2005;59(11):1309-16.
10. American Diabetes Association. Lifestyle management: Standards of Medical Care in Diabetes 2019. Diabetes Care. 2019;42(Suppl. 1): S46-60.
11. Norris SL, Lau J, Smith SJ, et al. Self-management education for adults with type 2 diabetes: a meta-analysis of the effect on glycemic control. Diabetes Care. 2002;25(7):1159-71.
12. Chrvala CA, Sherr D, Lipman RD. Diabetes self-management education for adults with type 2 diabetes mellitus: A systematic review of the effect on glycemic control. Patient Educ Couns. 2016;99(6):926-43.
13. Franz MJ, MacLeod J, Evert A, et al. Academy of Nutrition and Dietetics Nutrition Practice Guideline for Type 1 and Type 2 Diabetes in Adults: Systematic Review of Evidence for Medical Nutrition Therapy Effectiveness and Recommendations for Integration into the Nutrition Care Process. J Acad Nutr Diet. 2017;117(10):1659-79.
14. Standl E, Erbach M, Schnell O. Glycemic control: a combination of lifestyle management and the use of drugs. Cardiol Ther. 2013;2(1):1-16.
15. American Diabetes Association. Pharmacologic approaches to glycemic treatment: Standards of Medical Care in Diabetes 2019. Diabetes Care. 2019;42(Suppl 1):S90-102.
16. American Diabetes Association. Older adults: Standards of Medical Care in Diabetes 2019. Diabetes Care. 2019;42 (Suppl 1):S139-47.
17. Kalra S, Bahendeka S, Sahay R, et al. Consensus recommendations on sulfonylurea and sulfonylurea combinations in the management of Type 2 diabetes mellitus – International task force. Indian J Endocr Metab. 2018;22:132-57.
18. Lupsa BC, Inzucchi SE. Use of SGLT2 inhibitors in type 2 diabetes: weighing the risks and benefits. Diabetologia. 2018;61(10):2118-25.
19. Diabetes Medicines. FDA Office of Women's Health. [online] Available from https://www.fda.gov/media/119148/download. [Last Accessed October, 2019].
20. van de Laar FA, Lucassen PL, Akkermans RP, et al. Alpha-glucosidase inhibitors for patients with type 2 diabetes: results from a Cochrane systematic review and meta-analysis. Diabetes Care. 2005;28(1): 154-63.
21. Bennett WL, Maruthur NM, Singh S, et al. Comparative effectiveness and safety of medications for type 2 diabetes: an update including new drugs and 2-drug combinations. Ann Intern Med. 2011;154(9):602-13.
22. Garber AJ, Abrahamson MJ, Barzilay JI, et al. Consensus Statement By The American Association Of Clinical Endocrinologists and American College of Endocrinology on The Comprehensive Type 2 Diabetes Management Algorithm—2019 Executive Summary. Endocr Pract. 2019;25(1):69-100.
23. Central Drugs Standard Control Organization. Fixed dose combinations approved by DCG (I) since 1961 to 13th September 2019. [online] Available from https://cdsco.gov.in/opencms/opencms/system/modules/CDSCO.WEB/elements/download_file_division.jsp?num_id=NDk2NQ. [Last Accessed October, 2019].
24. Turner RC, Cull CA, Frighi V, et al. Glycemic control with diet, sulfonylurea, metformin, or insulin in patients with type 2 diabetes mellitus: progressive requirement for multiple therapies (UKPDS 49). UK Prospective Diabetes Study (UKPDS) Group. JAMA. 1999;281(21):2005-12.
25. Phung OJ, Sobieraj DM, Engel SS, et al. Early combination therapy for the treatment of type 2 diabetes mellitus: systematic review and meta-analysis. Diabetes Obes Metab. 2014;16(5):410-7.
26. American Association of Clinical Endocrinologists/American College of Endocrinology. AACE/ACE comprehensive type 2 diabetes management algorithm. [online] Available from https://www.aace.com/pdfs/diabetes/AACE_2019_Diabetes_Algorithm_FINAL_ES.pdf. [Last Accessed October, 2019].
27. Rajpathak SN, Rajgopalan S, Engel SS. Impact of time to treatment intensification on glycemic goal attainment among patients with type 2 diabetes failing Metformin monotherapy. J Diabetes Complications. 2014;28(6):831-5.
28. Kim HS, Kim DM, Cha BS, et al. Efficacy of glimepiride/metformin fixed-dose combination vs metformin uptitration in type 2 diabetic patients inadequately controlled on low-dose metformin monotherapy: a randomized, open label, parallel group, multicenter study in Korea. J Diabetes Investig. 2014;5(6):701-8.
29. Zintzaras E, Miligkos M, Ziakas P, et al. Assessment of the relative effectiveness and tolerability of treatments of type 2 diabetes mellitus: a network meta-analysis. Clin Ther. 2014;36(10):1443-53.
30. Pan F, Chernew ME, Fendrick AM. Impact of fixed-dose combination drugs on adherence to prescription medications. J Gen Intern Med. 2008;23(5):611-4.
31. Duckworth W, Abraira C, Moritz T, et al. Glucose control and vascular complications in veterans with type 2 diabetes. N Engl J Med. 2009;360(2):129-39.
32. Patel A, MacMahon S, Chalmers J, et al. Intensive blood glucose control and vascular outcomes in patients with type 2 diabetes. N Engl J Med. 2008;358(24):2560-72.
33. Ismail-Beigi F, Craven T, Banerji MA, et al. Effect of intensive treatment of hyperglycaemia on microvascular outcomes in type 2 diabetes: an analysis of the ACCORD randomised trial. Lancet. 2010;376(9739):419-30.
34. Gerstein HC, Miller ME, Byington RP, et al. Effects of intensive glucose lowering in type 2 diabetes. N Engl J Med. 2008;358(24):2545-59.
35. Del Prato S, LaSalle J, Matthaei S, et al. Tailoring treatment to the individual in type 2 diabetes practical guidance from the Global Partnership for Effective Diabetes Management. Int J Clin Pract. 2010;64(3):295-304.
36. American Diabetes Association. Glycemic targets: Standards of Medical Care in Diabetes 2019. Diabetes Care. 2019;42(Suppl 1):S61-70.
37. NICE. Type 2 diabetes in adults: management. NICE guideline [NG28]. [online] Available from https://www.nice.org.uk/guidance/ng28/resources/type-2-diabetes-in-adults-management-pdf-1837338615493. [Last Accessed October, 2019].
38. SIGN. Pharmacological management of glycaemic control in people with type 2 diabetes. [online] Available from https://www.sign.ac.uk/assets/sign154.pdf. [Last Accessed October, 2019].
39. Del Prato S, Felton AM, Munro N, et al. Improving glucose management: ten steps to get more patients with type 2 diabetes to glycaemic goal. Int J Clin Pract. 2005;59(11):1345-55.

52 CHAPTER Therapeutic Inertia and Poor Glycemia: Our Way Out

Shashi Panicker

INTRODUCTION

Diabetes is the worst epidemic in the history of human diseases. There were 31.7 million people with diabetes in India in 2000, but that number has increased to over 75 million[1] and is likely to double to 150 million in the next 15 years. The age of onset of type 2 diabetes (T2D) in Asian Indians is about a decade earlier because they progress faster from prediabetes to diabetes, and on to earlier complications compared to Europeans.[2] Diabetes doubles the risk of cardiovascular (CV) events in Asian Indians who are already 3 times more prone to coronary artery disease (CAD) compared to the US population.[3] One-fifth of all global deaths due to CAD occurs in the Asian Indian population. Therapeutic inertia (TI) leads to suboptimal control of hyperglycemia resulting in irreversible complications. The ICMR-INDIAB study showed that only 31% patients with diabetes in India had hemoglobin A1c (HbA1c) below 7%.[4] Only 53.6% of patients succeeded in achieving an HbA1c below 7% in Europe.[5] Alarmingly, recent reports have revealed that control of hyperglycemia has worsened globally. In USA there was a decline of well-controlled patients from 69.8% to 63.8%, and an increase from 12.6% to 15.5% in people with HbA1c > 9% between 2007 and 2014.[6] In India, the TIGHT study recently reported that only 23.4% of patients were well-controlled,[7] compared to 31.0% in 2014.[4]

CLINICAL IMPACT OF THERAPEUTIC INERTIA

Therapeutic inertia is defined as "the failure of healthcare providers to follow guidelines to initiate or intensify therapy", measured as the period of time taken from recognition of a risk factor to initiation of a corrective therapeutic intervention. The term "clinical inertia" is a broader term which includes failure to screen, assess for risk factors, initiate measures for prevention of complications, and refer when appropriate for management of risks and complications. Intensification of treatment can be achieved by increasing the dosage of the current drugs, adding newer drugs with different mechanisms of action, or by starting an appropriate type of insulin.

Therapeutic inertia also applies to failure to discontinue or reduce therapy if it is no longer beneficial. A "frail patient phenotype" has been described which includes diabetic patients who are older, underweight and have had diabetes for a long duration, with underlying CV and renal dysfunction. Frail patients require reduction in the intensity of therapy to reduce morbidity or mortality.

Therapeutic inertia has been reported at all levels of healthcare. In an analysis of 7389 patients from a tertiary hospital in USA, two-thirds of patients on treatment for diabetes had uncontrolled hyperglycemia and no intensification of treatment was done in over 44% of patients, even when the HbA1c was ≥ 9%.[8] A recent systematic review found that intensification of therapy when HbA1c was >7% took a median time of more than 1 year, and in many cases even more than 7 years.[9] The probability of intensification with insulin after oral antidiabetic drug (OAD) failure was 5.1–12.0% in a large study of over 81,000 people with T2D in the UK.[10] The A1chieve study from India showed that only 18% of T2D adults were on insulin and initiation occurred only when the mean HbA1c was 9.2%. Multiple complications were already present in over one-fifth of the patients studied.[11]

Up to 80% of CV events in T2D have been attributed to TI. Complications which were significantly increased within 1 year due to lack of treatment intensification were: myocardial infarction (MI) 67%, stroke 51%, heart failure (HF) 64% and composite CV events 62%.[12] The timing of intensification of therapy was the critical factor which dictated long-term outcomes. Delayed initiation of insulin therapy may explain adverse CV outcomes in the ACCORD and VADT trials in patients who received intensive glycemic control after over 10 years of poorly controlled hyperglycemia with OADs.

CAUSES

All the stakeholders—patients, healthcare providers, healthcare systems, insurance, and the pharmaceutical industry, contribute to TI. The physician becomes helpless when the patient cannot access newer, expensive drugs due to cost concerns and barriers raised by payers. However, true TI exists if a physician does not intensify therapy when no barriers exist and access to drugs is unhindered. True TI amounts to medical malpractice and is prone to litigation.

Box 1 shows the characteristics of physicians which lead to TI.

A global survey of eight countries including India for assessing causes of TI revealed that physicians expected low compliance from patients and patients lacked comprehension of the consequences of poor control, in spite of adequate patient education. Most patients did not believe that lifestyle modifications were important and many did not follow them.[13]

The burden of self-care in diabetes, progressive metabolic deterioration, inability to procure medicines and occurrence of complications—all result in the patient feeling overpowered and defeated, and this condition can aptly be called "diabetes overwhelms". Therapeutic inertia sets in at this stage and all the stakeholders are responsible for the aftermath of increasing complications, morbidity and mortality.

BOX 1 Role of physicians in therapeutic inertia (TI).

- Inadequate time with patient
- Reactive rather than proactive care
- Not recognizing patient's needs
- Lack of knowledge of the benefits of new treatments
- Poor understanding of guidelines for management
- Reluctance to prescribe costly drugs for fear of losing patients
- Believes adherence to treatment will be lost if more medicines are added
- Fear of hypoglycemia with insulin
- Does not believe patients can manage complicated regimens
- Inability to individualize treatment

CHALLENGES IN INTENSIFICATION OF THERAPY

Therapeutic inertia should be addressed as a challenge rather than as a failure. The age of the patient, the duration of diabetes, the HbA1c level, the specialization of the physician and the level of the medical institution affect intensification of therapy. Intensification of treatment may be difficult in patients with multiple comorbidities, very young or older patients, those taking several medications and those who are financially weak. Individualizing targets is important, especially in patients with high risk. The physician's wisdom in not intensifying treatment should not be mistaken for TI.

THE WAY OUT—STRATEGIES FOR OVERCOMING THERAPEUTIC INERTIA

A patient-centered approach for individualized and personalized treatment is recommended.[14]

- *The patient*
  Structured Education Programs like the following need to be implemented:
  - The Diabetes Self-Management, Education and Support Program (DSMES) is implemented in the USA at four critical points—at the time of diagnosis of T2D, annually for health maintenance and prevention of complications, when complications arise, and when transitions in care arise.
  - The DESMOND is an evidence-based, self-management program for people with T2D, successfully used in the UK and Australia. There are two half-day sessions of 3 hours each.
  - The X-PERT Program (UK) imparts training for 2.5 hours every week for 6 weeks.
  - The ROMEO Program (Italy) consists of a 1-hour session of training every month.
- *The physician*
  - Must be fully updated and knowledgeable about the objectives of therapy, the guidelines for treatment, and the options for appropriate control.
  - Must maintain belief in reliable evidence-based guidelines. Doubts created by observational studies and frequent "expert views" propagated in the media create uncertainty in the mind, and goals of therapy are sidelined.

    - Must remember that if initial HbA1c is >7.5%, metformin plus a second drug must be started together and if >9%, two drugs plus insulin may be initiated.[15]
- *The team*
  Collaboration within a multidisciplinary team provides individualized, patient-focused management. Such a Structured Management Program prevents TI and vastly improves diabetes care.
- *The healthcare system*
  An electronic record-keeping system with an in-built method for flagging abnormal values and providing reminders, and assessment of performance to the clinician can effectively trigger timely intervention. Feedback on efficacy of treatment by physicians, visit planning, outreach programs and a central registry of patients can improve outcomes in diabetes management.
- *Re-addressing HbA1c*
  Guidelines which advocate reappraisal of treatment with HbA1c testing after 3 months may delay intensification and contribute to TI.[16] The first 6 months are lost in the slow process of initiation of therapy in a stepwise manner, according to the guidelines. This is unsuitable for Indian patients who are diagnosed late with high HbA1c, have a more rapid deterioration in beta-cell function and develop complications earlier than their Western counterparts.

  Clinical studies have shown that 50% of the HbA1c is formed in the month prior to the test, 25% in the month before that and the remaining in the 2–4 months before the test.[17] HbA1c measurement at 2 months adequately reflects the result of treatment intensification. Patients with high fasting and post-prandial glucose levels at 1 month and 2 months after intensification of oral therapy cannot achieve an HbA1c of ≤ 7% at the end of the third month.
- *Telemedicine and web-based tools*
  Telemedicine and health-related mobile apps can significantly improve monitoring and intensification of therapy to improve outcomes and quality of life.[18] An Artificial Intelligence software combined with telemedicine has been successfully used for real-time screening of diabetic retinopathy in peripheral India.[19] A new web-based clinical tool called KALMOD has been tested in the UK. Based on an online questionnaire, the software algorithm analyses patients' responses and provides a result sheet which guides discussion. It has been shown to successfully improve patient–physician interactions to overcome several barriers.[20]

CONCLUSION

Suboptimal control of hyperglycemia due to delayed intensification of therapy leads to irreversible complications and doubles the risk of CV events in T2D. Target HbA1c is reached in only 30–50% of patients. This failure is due to TI for which all stakeholders are responsible. Strategies for overcoming TI must aim to improve the physician's knowledge and training and focus on therapeutic goals. Structured education programs for patients with improved communication and collaboration with a multidisciplinary team can improve outcomes. Combining HbA1c at 2 months with fasting and postprandial glucose tests can alert the patient and physician for early intensification of therapy.

Upgradation of the healthcare system to ensure availability of electronic data for individualized care, provision for reminders and evaluation of physician's performance will reinforce intensification of therapy. Use of telemedicine, mobile health apps and web-based analytical software for better patient–physician interactions can vastly improve clinical outcomes.

REFERENCES

1. International Diabetes Federation. (2017). IDF DIABETES ATLAS—8th Edition. [online] Available from https://diabetesatlas.org/resources/2017-atlas.html [Last accessed September, 2019].
2. Gujral UP, Pradeepa R, Weber MB, et al. Type 2 diabetes in South Asians: similarities and differences with white Caucasian and other populations. Ann N Y Acad Sci. 2013;1281(1):51-63.
3. Misra A, Khurana L. Obesity-related non-communicable diseases: South Asians vs White Caucasians. Int J Obes. 2011;35(2):167-87.
4. Unnikrishnan R, Anjana RM, Deepa M, et al. Glycemic Control Among Individuals with Self-Reported Diabetes in India—The ICMR–INDIAB Study. Diabetes Technol Ther. 2014;16(9):596-603.
5. Stone MA, Charpentier G, Doggen K, et al. Quality of Care of People With Type 2 Diabetes in Eight European Countries. Diabetes Care. 2013;36(9):2628-38.
6. Carls G, Huynh J, Tuttle E, et al. Achievement of Glycated Hemoglobin Goals in the US Remains Unchanged Through 2014. Diabetes Ther. 2017;8(4):863-73.
7. Borgharkar SS, Das SS. Real-world evidence of glycemic control among patients with type 2 diabetes mellitus in India: the TIGHT study. BMJ Open Diabetes Res Care. 2019;7(1):e000654.
8. Pantalone KM, Misra-Hebert AD, Hobbs TM, et al. Clinical Inertia in Type 2 Diabetes Management: Evidence From a Large, Real-World Data Set. Diabetes Care. 2018;41(7):e113-4.
9. Khunti K, Gomes MB, Pocock S, et al. Therapeutic inertia in the treatment of hyperglycaemia in patients with type 2 diabetes: A systematic review. Diabetes. Obes Metab. 2018;20(2):427-37.
10. Khunti K, Wolden ML, Thorsted BL, et al. Clinical Inertia in People With Type 2 Diabetes: A retrospective cohort study of more than 80,000 people. Diabetes Care. 2013;36(11):3411-7.

11. Mohan V, Shah S, Saboo B. Current glycemic status and diabetes related complications among type 2 diabetes patients in India: data from the A1chieve study. J Assoc Physicians India. 2013;61(1 Suppl):12-5.
12. Paul SK, Klein K, Thorsted BL, et al. Delay in treatment intensification increases the risks of cardiovascular events in patients with type 2 diabetes. Cardiovasc Diabetol. 2015;14:100.
13. Strain WD, Blüher M, Paldánius P. Clinical Inertia in Individualising Care for Diabetes: Is There Time to do More in Type 2 Diabetes? Diabetes Ther. 2014;5(2):347-54.
14. American Diabetes Association. Standard of Medical Care in Diabetes. 2019;42(Suppl. 1):S1-194.
15. Garber AJ, Abrahamson MJ, Barzilay JI, et al. Consensus Statement By The American Association Of Clinical Endocrinologists And American College Of Endocrinology On The Comprehensive Type 2 Diabetes Management Algorithm – 2019 Executive Summary. Endocr Pract. 2019;25(1):69-100.
16. Pimazoni-Netto A, Zanella MT. Diabetes Guidelines May Delay Timely Adjustments During Treatment and Might Contribute to Clinical Inertia. Diabetes Technol Ther. 2014;16(11):768-70.
17. Tahara Y, Shima K. Kinetics of HbA1c, glycated albumin, and fructosamine and analysis of their weight functions against preceding plasma glucose level. Diabetes Care. 1995;18(4):440-7.
18. Cafazzo JA. A Digital-First Model of Diabetes Care. Diabetes Technol Ther. 2019;21(S2):S252-S258.
19. Pradeepa R, Rajalakshmi R, Mohan V. Use of Telemedicine Technologies in Diabetes Prevention and Control in Resource-Constrained Settings: Lessons Learned from Emerging Economies. Diabetes Technol Ther. 2019;21(S2):S29-216.
20. Barnard-Kelly K. Utilizing eHealth and Telemedicine Technologies to Enhance Access and Quality of Consultations: It's Not What You Say, It's the Way You Say It. Diabetes Technol Ther. 2019;21(S2):S241-S247.

53 CHAPTER Next Evolution in Diabetes Treatment: Evogliptin

Ashu Rastogi

INTRODUCTION

In the 21st century, diabetes is a leading global health issue. In 2017, there were 73 million Indian adults with diabetes; it is estimated that this number will increase by 85%, increasing to 134 million by 2045, making India the world's diabetes capital. Additionally, there is an increase in the diabetes-related DALYs rate by 40% in the past two decades.

Taking into consideration the huge epidemic of type 2 diabetes mellitus (T2DM), it is always required and preferred to use novel therapies that can improve tolerability, efficacy, long-term compliance, and prevent complications related to T2DM. A new inhibitor of dipeptidyl peptidase-4 (DPP-4-i), evogliptin, has recently been released in India. This review emphasizes the place of evogliptin therapy in T2DM management.

ROLE OF DIPEPTIDYL PEPTIDASE-4 INHIBITORS IN MANAGEMENT OF TYPE 2 DIABETES MELLITUS

Dipeptidyl peptidase 4 inhibitors are associated with a lower risk of hypoglycemia because the insulin-stimulation effect of DPP-4 inhibitors is dependent on glucose, and no inhibitory activity takes place at low levels of glucose (less than 80 mg/dL). Furthermore, it is suggested by the evidence that DPP-4 inhibitors show neutral effects on cardiovascular outcomes. Therefore, DPP-4 inhibitors are an important therapeutic option for T2DM.

Presently, eight DPP-4 inhibitors are available for management of T2DM, which are: alogliptin, anagliptin, gemigliptin, linagliptin, saxagliptin, sitagliptin, teneligliptin, and vildagliptin. Mechanism of action and safety profile of all of these DPP-4 inhibitors are similar. Despite similar mechanism of action, there is difference in DPP-4 inhibitors in some of the important pharmacokinetic and pharmacodynamic parameters, which may have clinical significance in real-life settings.

Dipeptidyl Peptidase-4-Inhibitor: Current Place of Therapy

- Favorable clinical efficacy
- Low risk of hypoglycemia
- Weight neutral
- Rare chances of side effects
- Backed by extensive scientific evidence.

EVOGLIPTIN IN MANAGEMENT OF TYPE 2 DIABETES MELLITUS: AN EVOLVING LANDSCAPE

Evogliptin is a new potent and selective DPP-4 inhibitor. In both the preclinical and clinical studies, it has been demonstrated to have glucose-lowering efficacy. Evogliptin received the first global approval in 2015 in South Korea for use among T2DM patients who are not adequately controlled by diet and exercise along with those with uncontrolled T2DM on the metformin monotherapy.

Evogliptin: Binding and Selectivity

- Binds to S1, S2, and S2 extensive binding sites
- It has noncovalent binding
- It has 6,000 times higher selectivity than human DPP-VIII and DPP-IX
- It has 20,000 times greater selectivity in comparison to human DPP-I and DPP-II.

Evogliptin: Pharmacokinetics

- Evogliptin's absolute bioavailability was 50.24%
- After a single oral dose, plasma concentration of evogliptin reached its peak at 3.0–5.5 hours
- Inhibition of plasma DPP-4 rapidly surpassed 80% in less than an hour following administration
- Evogliptin showed a terminal elimination half-life (t1/2) of 32.5–39.8 hours
- Food intake had no effect on pharmacokinetics of evogliptin
- Within 3 days, Evogliptin reached a steady-state concentration and accumulated a small amount with an accumulation index of 1.38–1.50
- As per in vitro studies, evogliptin is neither an inducer of cytochrome P450 (CYP) 3A4 nor an inhibitor of CYP1A2, 2C9, 2C19, 2D6, or 3A4, though its metabolism is mainly mediated by CYP3A4
- Renal clearance of 15.0–16.8 L/hour and fraction excreted unchanged in urine of 27–34%
- There is no requirement of dose adjustment in renal impairment as for the elimination of evogliptin urinary excretion is not the major pathway
- Dosage and administration adjustment is not needed in patients with mild to moderate hepatic impairment.

Evogliptin: Pharmacodynamics

- It increases the postprandial levels of GLP-1 by 1.5- to 2.4-fold
- It decreases the levels of postprandial plasma glucose (PPG) by 20–35%
- Inhibition of DPP-4 increased in a dose-dependent manner, and persisted more than 80% in 24 hours.

Evogliptin: Animal Data

- Improved insulin sensitivity
- Delayed the onset of DM
- Increased β-cell replication and neogenesis
- Renal protective effect
- Improved hepatic steatosis.

Clinical Efficacy and Safety

Efficacy and Safety of Evogliptin Monotherapy in Patients with Type 2 Diabetes and Moderately Elevated Glycated Hemoglobin Levels after Diet and Exercise

Aims: This study aimed to assess the efficacy and safety of evogliptin, which is a newly developed DPP-4 inhibitor, among patients having T2DM that is not adequately controlled by diet and exercise.

Materials and methods: This was a randomized, double-blind, placebo-controlled, parallel-group, multicenter, phase III study. Total 160 T2D patients were randomized to either evogliptin 5 mg or placebo for duration of 24 weeks. The primary endpoint considered in the study was mean change in values of glycated hemoglobin (HbA1c) from baseline to 24th week (Fig. 1).

Results: There was no significant difference in the mean baseline HbA1c levels in the evogliptin and the placebo groups (7.20% ± 0.56% vs 7.20% ± 0.63%, respectively). At 24th week, evogliptin significantly reduced levels of HbA1c from baseline as compared to placebo (–0.23% vs 0.05%, respectively, $P < 0.0001$). In addition, the proportion of patients achieving HbA1c less than 6.5% was found to be significantly higher in the evogliptin group as compared to the placebo group (33.3% vs 15.2%; $P = 0.008$). In both the groups, the overall incidence of adverse events, including hypoglycemia, was comparable.

Conclusion: In this study, once daily evogliptin monotherapy showed a significant improvement in glycemic control and it was well tolerated among T2DM patients.

Efficacy and Safety of Adding Evogliptin versus Sitagliptin for Metformin-treated Patients with Type 2 Diabetes: A 24-week Randomized, Controlled Trial with Open Label Extension

Aims: In this trial, a 24-week multicenter, randomized, double-blind, double-dummy, active-controlled study and a 52-week open label extension study included for assessing the efficacy and safety of evogliptin, which is a new DDP-4 inhibitor, compared to sitagliptin among

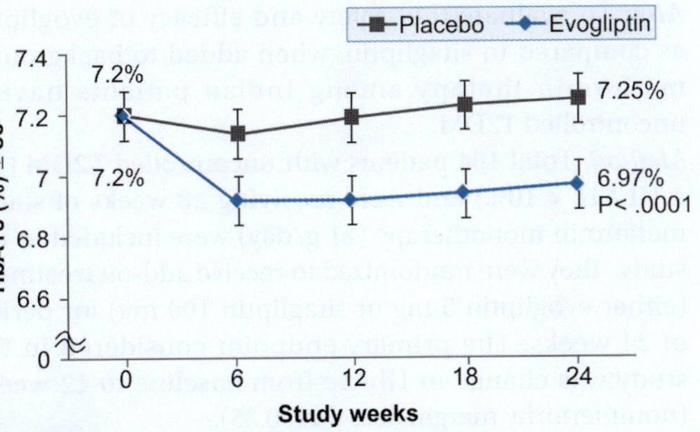

Figure 1 Changes of glycated hemoglobin (HbA1c) from baseline to 24th week.

T2DM patients who have insufficient glycemic control with metformin alone.

Methods: Total 222 adult patients with T2DM were included in the study. These patients had HbA1c 6.5–11% and were receiving stable doses of metformin (1,000 mg/day or more). They were randomized 1:1 to add-on evogliptin 5 mg (n = 112) or sitagliptin 100 mg (n = 110) once daily for period of 24 weeks. The primary efficacy analysis included comparison of the change from baseline HbA1c at week 24. Noninferiority was concluded if the upper limit of the two-sided 95% confidence interval (CI) for the HbA1c difference between treatments was less than 0.35% (Fig. 2).

Results: Mean changes in HbA1c after addition of evogliptin was –0.59% and after sitagliptin was –0.65%. The between-group difference was 0.06% (two-sided 95% CI, –0.10 to 0.22), demonstrating non-inferiority. Evogliptin caused a persistently reduced HbA1c level after the 52-week treatment (–0.44% ± 0.65%, P < 0.0001). Both treatments were well tolerated among patients; incidences and types of adverse events were similar between the two groups. Hypoglycemic events, which were mostly mild, were observed in 0.9% of the patients who were treated with evogliptin and in 2.8% of the patients treated with sitagliptin for 24 weeks.

Conclusion: Evogliptin 5 mg added to metformin therapy showed effective improvement in the glycemic control; it was noninferior to sitagliptin and well tolerated among T2DM patients, which was insufficiently controlled by metformin alone.

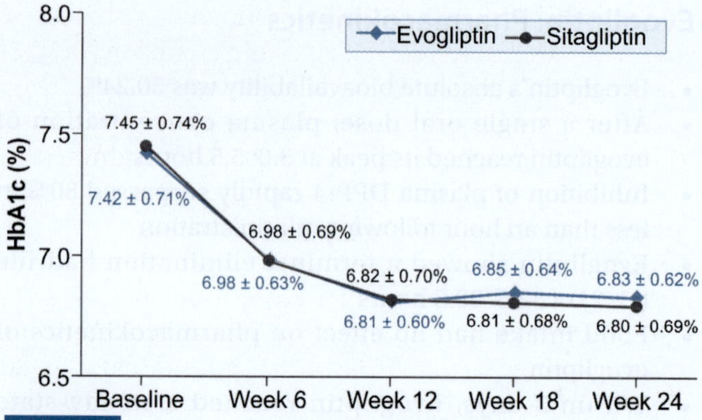

Figure 2 Changes of glycated hemoglobin (HbA1c) from baseline to week 24.

Efficacy and Safety of Evogliptin versus Sitagliptin as an Add-On Therapy in Indian Patients with Type 2 Diabetes Mellitus Inadequately Controlled with Metformin: A 24-week Randomized, Double Blind, Non-inferiority, EVOLUTION India Study

Aim: To evaluate the safety and efficacy of evogliptin as compared to sitagliptin, when added to background metformin therapy among Indian patients having uncontrolled T2DM.

Method: Total 184 patients with uncontrolled T2DM (7% ≤ HbA1c < 10%) and were receiving ≥8 weeks of stable metformin monotherapy (≥1 g/day) were included in the study. They were randomized to receive add-on treatment (either evogliptin 5 mg or sitagliptin 100 mg) for period of 24 weeks. The primary endpoint considered in the study was change in HbA1c from baseline to 12 weeks (noninferiority margin, less than 0.35).

Results: At 12 weeks, mean reduction in HbA1c in evogliptin-treated patients was –0.37 ± 1.06 and in sitagliptin-treated patients was–0.32 ± 1.14, respectively. The adjusted mean difference between the two treatment groups was –0.022 (95% CI, –0.374, 0.330; P = 0.901), which showed non-inferiority. At 12 and 24 weeks, reductions in FPG and PPG were comparable between evogliptin and sitagliptin. There was no significant difference in the changes in body weight between the treatment groups. The patients who achieved target HbA1c less than 7.0% (evogliptin, 26.7% vs sitagliptin, 20%) was almost equal in both treatment groups. Treatment-emergent adverse events were observed in 52 patients (evogliptin, 25% and sitagliptin, 31.5%) and were usually mild.

Conclusion: In HbA1c reduction, evogliptin was noninferior to sitagliptin. It effectively improved glycemic control. It was well tolerated among T2DM patients insufficiently controlled by metformin alone.

Recent Clinical Trials with Evogliptin

Efficacy and Safety of Evogliptin in Patients with Type 2 Diabetes: A Multicenter, Active-controlled, Randomized Study with Open Label Extension (EVERGREEN Study)

Background and aims: Evogliptin is a novel DPP-4 inhibitor. This study was aimed at investigating the safety and efficacy of evogliptin as compared to linagliptin in T2DM patients.

Materials and methods: Total 207 naïve patients with T2DM with HbA1c 7.0–10.0% were included in the study. Mean age of the patients was 56.1 ± 10.4 years; mean body mass index was 26.1 ± 3.4 kg/m^2. Patients were randomized 1:1 for either 5 mg evogliptin (n = 102) or 5 mg linagliptin (n = 105) once daily for 12 weeks. Primary efficacy endpoint considered in the study was the change from baseline

HbA1c at 12th week. The secondary endpoint included the change in mean amplitude of glycemic excursion (MAGE) assessed by 72-hour continuous glucose monitoring. In the extended study for another 12 weeks, open-label treatment with evogliptin 5 mg qd was conducted in both groups; evogliptin/evogliptin group (n = 95) and linagliptin/evogliptin group (n = 92).

Results: The mean change in HbA1c of evogliptin group was −0.85% and in linagliptin group was −0.75%, after 12 weeks of treatment. The between-group difference was −0.10% (95% CI, −0.32 to 0.11%), which showed noninferiority, meeting the prespecified margin of 0.40%. In the evogliptin group, the changes in MAGE were −24.6 mg/dL and that in the linagliptin group was −16.7 mg/dL, which were significantly lower as compared to baseline values in both groups. At week 24, in the evogliptin/evogliptin group, the mean change from baseline in HbA1c was −0.94%, attaining HbA1c less than 7.0% in 80.2% of the patients. There was no difference in the incidence and types of adverse events, including hypoglycemic events, between the two groups for 24 weeks.

Conclusion: In this study, once-daily evogliptin 5 mg treatment significantly reduced levels of HbA1c by 0.94% at 24th week and improved glycemic variability without causing any serious adverse events in Korean T2DM patients.

Efficacy and Safety of Evogliptin in a Brazilian T2DM Population: A Bridging Study

Ethnicity is a known factor for DPP-4 inhibitors (DPP-4i) response in T2DM. A bridging study was conducted to confirm the approved dosage of evogliptin (EVO), in Korea (once daily 5 mg) and the safety for the Brazilian population. In this randomized, double-blind, double-dummy, parallel trial, 146 T2DM patients (male: 50.7%; age: 51.5 ± 10.2 years; time from T2DM diagnosis: 1.7 ± 3.5 years; baseline HbA1c: 8.9 ± 0.9%) with inadequate glycemic control on diet and exercise were randomly assigned to a 12-week once daily treatment with EVO 2.5 mg, EVO 5 mg, EVO 10 mg or sitagliptin (SITA) 100 mg. In this study, patients with T2DM in the age range of 20–75 years, with 7.5% ≤ HbA1c ≤ 10.5% at screening, and who have not been using hypoglycemic agent within 12 weeks before screening were included. Subjects with fasting plasma glucose ≥ 300 mg/dL at screening in the presence of severe signs/symptoms of T2DM were excluded. Sample size was estimated for identifying a clinically relevant HbA1c mean reduction 0.5% or more within each treatment group. Change from baseline to week 12 (mean; 90% CI) in HbA1c (%) and, fasting plasma glucose levels (mg/dL) was calculated. Treatment effects on HbA1c and fasting glucose levels adjusted by baseline HbA1c, fasting plasma glucose, and BMI were also estimated. The results confirmed the clinical benefit of a daily EVO 5 mg regimen in the Brazilian population.

CLINICAL TRIAL PLANS

See Tables 1 to 3.

CONCLUSION

- Evogliptin (DA-1229) is a piperazine derivative.
- It is a selective, potent, and reversible inhibitor of DPP-4.
- It was widely studied in vitro and in vivo animal models for its efficacy and safety and two Phase III studies, among T2DM patients.
- Drugs have low potential for interaction with other coadministered drugs
- *Indication*: It is indicated for treatment of T2DM as an addition to diet and exercise for improving glycemic control, when it is used as a monotherapy or in combination with metformin

TABLE 1: Clinical evidence: on-going (SIT = sponsor initiated trial).

Type	Full name	Participant	Period	Remarks
Phase 1 (completed)	A study to evaluate the PK and safety of Evogliptin in subjects with hepatic dysfunction and in healthy control volunteers (DA1229_HI_I)	Hepatic dysfunction group: 12 • Mild (Child-Pugh A): 6 • Moderate (Child-Pugh B): 6 • Healthy control group with normal hepatic function: 12	2016. 09-2018.01	• Aim to reflect to an approved NDA and publication within 2019 • Prof. Park min sco. Yonsei University medical school, Severance Hospital and another 1 hospital • 19/01 CSR completed

Contd...

Contd...

Type	Full name	Participant	Period	Remarks
Phase 1 (on-going)	A randomized, open-label, multiple-dose crossover study to investigate the PK and PD drug-drug interaction of Evogliptin 5 mg and Empagliflozin 25 mg or Dapagliflozin 10 mg after oral administration in healthy male adults (DA1229_DIS_I)	N=40 (10 per each sequence group)	2018, 11-2019.01	Aim to publication within 2019 • Prof. Park Min Soo, Yonsel University Medical School, Severance Hospital • 19/01 study completed
Phase IV (Complete/Be presented)	Amulticenter, randomized, double blind, active controlled, phase IV clinical trial to evaluate the efficacy and safety of Evogliptin vs Linagliptin in patients with inadequately controlled type 2 diabetes, using continuous glucose monitoring system (DA1229_DM_IV. EVERGREEN)	Type 2 diabetes patients N=207 Evo: 102 Lina: 105	2016. 09-2018.05	18/10/13, Oral PT-2018 ICDM (Seoul) • 18/11/25, Oral PT-2018 IDF-WPR (Kuala Lumpur) • Prof. Moon Kyu Lee, Samsung Medical Center • 18/12 CSR completed
Phase IV (Onging)	A multicenter, randomized, double-blind, active controlled, parallel comparison, phase IV clinical trial to evaluate the efficacy and safety of Evogliptin in patients with NAFLD (DA1229_NAFLD_IV)	N=50 Evo:25 Pio: 25	2019. 03-2020.06	Aim to publication in 2021 • Prof. Lee Byung Wan, Yonsai University Medical School, Severance Hospital and another 7 hospitals • 19/01 Study protocol completed

TABLE 2: Clinical evidence: planned (SIT = sponsor initiated trial).

Type	Full name	Participant	Period	Remarks
Phase 1 (Planned)	Phase 1 clinical trial to evaluate the PK and safety profile of Evogliptin in renal dialysis patients (tentative)	N= about 12 to 16 • Hemodialysis patients subject group: about 6 to 8 • Healthy subject group: about 6 to 8	2019, 06-2020.05	Aim to reflect to an approved NDA and publication within 2021 • *Study sites:* Prof. Young Chul Kim, MD, PhD, Seoul National University college of Medicine and Hospital
Phase III (Planned)	A Phase III clinical study to investigate the efficacy and safety of Evogliptin after co-administration in patients with T2DM with insufficient blood glucose control with Metformin and SGLT-2i (Tentative)	N=about 280	2019. 12-2022.07	Aim to be granted a new indication and publication in 2023 (to be granted a new indication of EVO and develop combination therapy) • Study sites: About 30 to 35 sites
Observational study (Planned)	A retrospective observation study to investigate the efficacy and safety of switching from other DPP-4i to Evogliptin (tentative)	N= about 5000	2019-2021	Evidence for switching effect of EVO • Aim to publication in 2022 • Study sites: Prof. Jong Chul Won, Inje Univesity Sanggye Paik Hospital and including another HP, Clinic
Cardiovascular outcome (Planned)	A retrospective observation study to determine the effect of Evogliptin on cardiovascular risks using public data from Korean Health insurance Review and Assessment Service center, (Tentative)		2021	Evidence for cardiovascular safety effect of EVO • Aim to publication in 2022 (Data analysis of cardiovascular disease patients who are hospitalized and hospital visit)

TABLE 3: Clinical evidence: planned (IIT = investigated initiated trial).

Type	Full name	Participant	Period	Remarks
IIT (On-going)	A multi-center, randomized, double-blind, active-controlled, phase II non-inferiority, investigator-initiated clinical trial to investigate the effect on kidney and diabetes of Evogliptin after oral administration in patients with impaired renal function and type 2 diabetes (DA1229_RP_ST)	In patients with chronic renal failure with T2DM (7.0% <HbA1c < 10.0% • N= 210 • Evo: 105 • Lina: 105	2018.04-2019.4	• Evidence for renal protective effect • Aim to publication in 2020 (patients recruitment completed) • Study sites: Prof. Jae Hyun Kim, MD, PhD, Samsung Medical Center and another 12 Hospitals
IIT (On-going)	Effect of evogliptin on coronary calcium scoring using CT in patients with type 2 diabetes mellitus	In patients with diabetic Nephropathy with T2DM • N 210 • Evo: 40 • Convnl. Treat: 40	• 2019–TBD	• To confirm improvement of vascular calcification • Study sites: Prof. In-Kyu Lee, Kyungpook National University Hospital and another 2 hospitals
IIT (On-going)	In patients with chronic hepatitis B with T2DM and significant hepatic fibrosis, compared to administration of metformin vs. ploglitazone vs evogliptin and to evaluate the effect on liver fibrosis (PREVENT trial)	In patients with chronic hepatitis B with T2DM and significant hepatic fibrosis • N= 54 • Evo: 18 • Pio: 18 • Met: 18	2019-2020	• To confirm improvement of hepatic fibrosis with chronic hepatitis B patients • Study sites: Prof. Seung Up Kim, Yonsei University College of Medicine Severance Hospital

- It has similar efficacy to sitagliptin and linagliptin
- It is weight neutral
- Once daily dosing regardless of meal timing
- Low risk of hypoglycemia
- Adjustment of dose is not needed in patients with renal dysfunction.

SUGGESTED READING

1. International Diabetes Federation. (2017). IDF Diabetes Atlas. International Diabetes Federation: Brussels, Belgium; 2017. [online] Available from http://www.diabetesatlas.org [Last accessed October, 2019].
2. Pathak R, Bridgeman MB. Dipeptidyl peptidase-4 (DPP-4) inhibitors in the management of diabetes. PT. 2010;35:509-13.
3. Nauck MA. Unraveling the science of incretin biology. Am J Med. 2009;122:S3-S10.
4. Gu N, Park MK, Kim TE, et al. Multiple-dose pharmacokinetics and pharmacodynamics of evogliptin (DA-1229), a novel dipeptidyl peptidase IV inhibitor, in healthy volunteers. Drug Des Devel Ther. 2014;8:1709-21.
5. Tan X, Hu J. Evogliptin: a new dipeptidyl peptidase inhibitor for the treatment of type 2 diabetes. Expert Opin Pharmacother. 2016;17:1285-93.
6. McCormack PL. Evogliptin: First Global Approval. Drugs. 2015;75:2045-9.
7. Park J, Park SW, Yoon KH, et al. Efficacy and safety of evogliptin monotherapy in patients with type 2 diabetes and moderately elevated glycated haemoglobin levels after diet and exercise. Diabetes Obes Metab. 2017;19:1681-7.
8. Hong SM, Park CY, Hwang DM, et al. Efficacy and safety of adding evogliptin versus sitagliptin for metformin-treated patients with type 2 diabetes: a 24-week randomized, controlled trial with open label extension. Diabetes Obes Metab. 2017;19:654-63.
9. Lim S, Kim G, Kwonada HS, et al. 1140-P: Efficacy and Safety of Evogliptin in Patients with Type 2 Diabetes: A Multicenter, Active-Controlled, Randomized Study with Open Label Extension (EVERGREEN Study). Diabetes. 2019; 68(Supplement 1).
10. Forti AC, Felício JS, Russo LA, et al. 1005-P: Efficacy and Safety of Evogliptin in a Brazilian T2DM Population—A Bridging Study. Diabetes. 2019;68(Supplement 1).

54 CHAPTER

PPG Challenges in Indian Type 2 Patient

Sanjay Agarwal, Akshita Gokhale, Swara Pendse

INTRODUCTION

Postprandial or post-meal hyperglycemia refers to the glucose concentration in plasma after a meal. The American Diabetes Association (ADA) and the International Diabetes Federation (IDF) define it as blood glucose levels more than 200 mg/dL (11.1 mmol/L) following a 75 g oral glucose tolerance test, measured at 2 hours post-meal.

It is a highly widespread condition in Asia, especially in India and is often underdiagnosed.

It is the earliest markers of an aberration from the normal glucose homeostasis, one of the first steps that lead to the deterioration of glucose homeostasis and loss of postprandial control, ultimately resulting in a sustained hyperglycemia overnight. If uncontrolled, it can be the rate-limiting step for achieving optimal glycemic control.

Due to the absorption of dietary carbohydrates, the glucose concentration in blood starts increasing approximately 10 minutes after the start of a meal. The plasma glucose concentration peaks at approximately 60 minutes after the start and reaches its sustained plateau at 2 hours, following which there is a drop in the plasma glucose concentration and it reaches its original pre-prandial levels by roughly 3 hours after the meal (Fig. 1).

This sustained increase in the blood glucose levels occurs as a result of the actual amount of carbohydrate absorbed and the homeostasis between the insulin and glucagon secretion. This is aided by the glucose metabolism occurring in the liver and other organs.

The aforementioned phenomenon is witnessed in nondiabetic individuals.

On the other hand in diabetic individuals, the insulin peaks are typically delayed and as a result of the fault in glucose homeostasis, there is inadequate control of postprandial hyperglycemia.

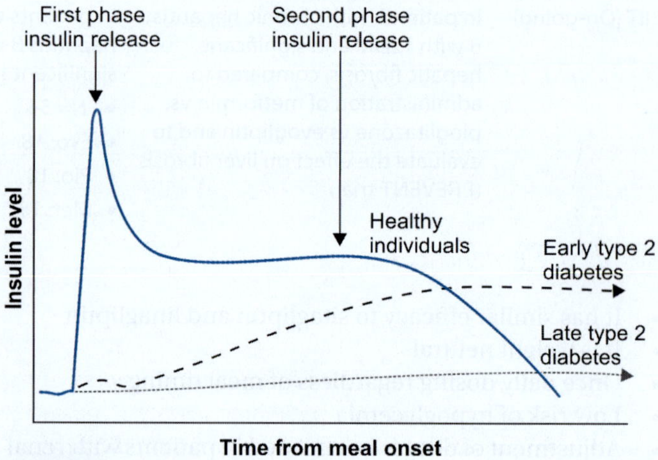

Figure 1 Insulin levels at different time periods from meal onset.

In patients with type 1 diabetes mellitus (DM), the control of postprandial hyperglycemia poses to become an even bigger obstacle owing to the complete lack of insulin secretion from the minimally or nonfunctioning pancreas.

Studies by Monier et al. assessed the importance of postprandial and fasting plasma glucose in over 290 patients and proved that lack of postprandial control was the cause of 70% of day long hyperglycemia in patients with glycosylated hemoglobin levels <7.3% and for 40% in patients with levels >9.3%. Similar studies undertaken by Woerle et al. corroborate these findings. A study by Riddle et al. showed that controlling postprandial glucose levels bought about better glycemic control in patients on poor control with basal insulin therapy.

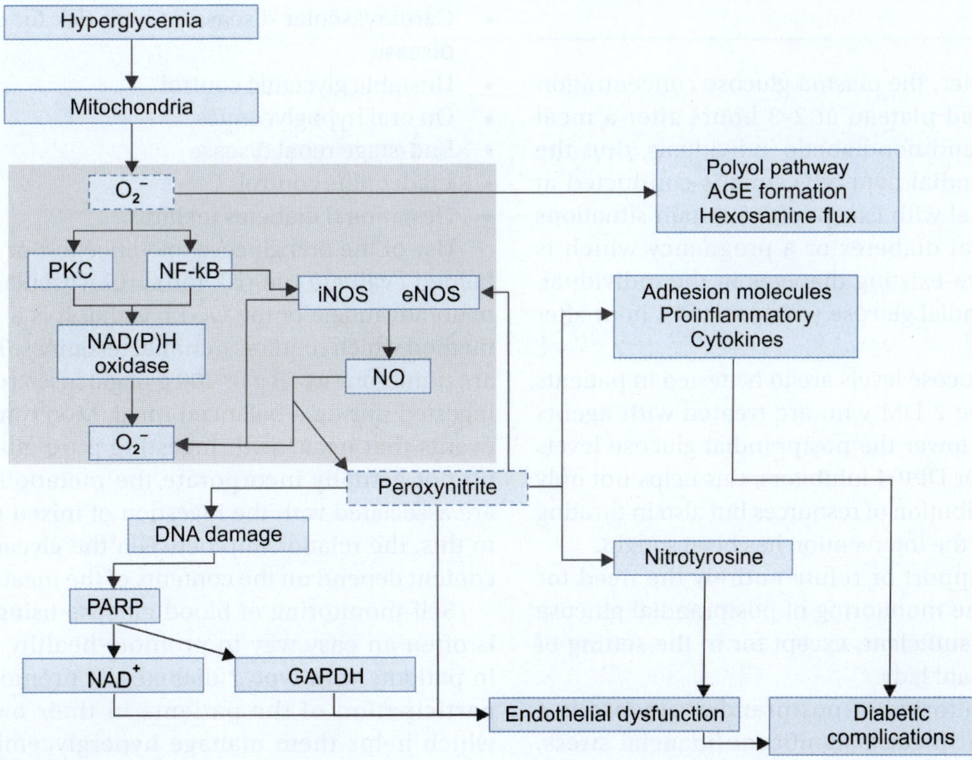

Flowchart 1 Pathogenesis.

Even so, there is evidence that with controlled fasting sugars of a patient, they may have increased postprandial sugars—this phenomenon is commonly referred to as isolated postprandial hyperglycemia and is more common than one can expect to see. In a study with 90 patients of type 2 DM, isolated postprandial glucose was shown to be present in 24.4% patients.

PATHOGENESIS

In nondiabetic individuals, there is an increase in the beta cell output after a meal, which inhibits glucagon secretion and helps in tissue glucose uptake. In diabetic individuals, due to poor pancreatic function, the insulin release is not only delayed, but the peak is also smaller, leading to a "hyperglycemic spike". There is also a decrease in the tissue glucose clearance and oxidation, with an increase in the nonoxidative glycolysis and glycogen cycling.

Hence, hyperglycemia-induced oxidative stress is proposed as the link between postprandial glucose and cardiovascular disease. It leads to an increase in superoxide production in the mitochondria resulting in an increase in endothelial nitric oxide, nitric oxide synthase, and reactive oxygen species, such as peroxynitrite. This causes DNA damage and acute vascular endothelial dysfunction, which is now known to be the key step in the development of cardiovascular disease at an early age. The endothelial dysfunction sets into motion a variety of proinflammatory responses which lead to the development of atherosclerosis (Flowchart 1).

Hence, the association between postprandial glucose and markers of cardiovascular diseases like oxidative stress, endothelial dysfunction, inflammation and carotid intima-media thickness (CIMT) puts into perspective the importance of postprandial glucose.

Furthermore, postprandial glucose has also been connected with cognitive dysfunction in elderly and an increase in the incidence of carcinomas in patients with type 2 DM.

FACTORS DETERMINING POSTPRANDIAL HYPERGLYCEMIA

- Timing
- Quantity
- Composition of a meal.

TESTING

As mentioned earlier, the plasma glucose concentration reaches a sustained plateau at 2–3 hours after a meal in both diabetics and nondiabetic individuals, thus the testing of postprandial hyperglycemia is conducted at 2 hours after a meal with exception of certain situations such as gestational diabetes or a pregnancy which is complicated by pre-existing diabetes in the individual, where the postprandial glucose will be tested 1 hour after a balanced meal.

Postprandial glucose levels are to be tested in patients with type 1 or type 2 DM who are treated with agents which specifically lower the postprandial glucose levels such as incretins, or DPP-4 inhibitors, this helps not only in the judicial distribution of resources but also in titrating the treatment after the intervention has been sought.

The data to support or refute entirely the need for extensive or routine monitoring of postprandial glucose in diabetes is not sufficient, except for in the setting of diabetes in a pregnant lady.

Since the monitoring of postprandial glucose is a process that might incur a significant financial stress, it must be used judiciously and based on the needs of individual patients. This testing plan must also include specific patient education and a pro-active healthcare team must guide the patient in each step of the way.

SCREENING TESTS

Postprandial glucose testing is to be done in all individuals with BMI >25 kg/m^2 and with additional risk factors such as:

- Recommended in individuals with impaired glucose tolerance/impaired fasting glucose/glycosylated hemoglobin ≥5.7%
- With a high risk for cardiovascular disease/known coronary artery disease
- History of gestational diabetes mellitus
- Hypertensive individuals—on/off treatment
- Dyslipidemia
- Polycystic ovary syndrome
- Sedentary lifestyle
- Strong family history of diabetes.

In prediabetics or patients with impaired glucose tolerance, screen patients with:

- Fasting plasma glucose >100 mg/dL
- 2-hour oral glucose tolerance test suggestive of impaired glucose tolerance
- Glycosylated hemoglobin between 5.7% and 6.4%.

In overt diabetic individuals, particularly in:

- Cardiovascular disease/at high risk for cardiovascular disease
- Unstable glycemic control
- On oral hypoglycemics
- End-stage renal disease
- Inadequate control
- Gestational diabetes mellitus.

Use of the oral glucose tolerance test or the OGTT has helped evaluate the risk for cardiovascular disease. The main advantage of the OGTT is that it is a simple testing method which requires minimal resources. The drawbacks are numerous as 75 g or 100 g of glucose are almost never ingested during a balanced meal. More importantly, the events that occur with ingesting pure glucose solution do not actually incorporate the metabolic events that are associated with the ingestion of mixed meals. To add to this, the relationship between the glycemic and meal content depend on the contents of the meal.

Self-monitoring of blood glucose using glucometers is often an easy way to promote healthy eating habits in patients with type 2 diabetes. It promotes the active participation of the patients in their own treatment which helps them manage hyperglycemic excursions through diet as well as physical activity. Various studies by Schwedes et al., Muchmore et al., etc. have further strengthened this fact.

Newer modalities of testing such as the automated glucose monitor or continuous glucose monitor help in profiling patients with postprandial hyperglycemic excursions and can show real-time changes in the glucose levels after active interventions have been sought.

COMPARISON BETWEEN GLYCOSYLATED HEMOGLOBIN AND POSTPRANDIAL GLUCOSE LEVELS

While postprandial glucose level is a dynamic way of testing for glycemic control, testing the glycosylated hemoglobin levels helps with a snapshot view of glycemic control over the last 3 months and hence takes into account both the pre- and post-meal glucose levels of the patient. While the fasting plasma glucose of patients is shown to have an adequate dominance over the glycated hemoglobin values, those of postprandial glucose show a poorer correlation with glycosylated hemoglobin.

COMPLICATIONS

There is enough evidence to suggest that postprandial hyperglycemia can pose to be an independent risk factor macrovascular complications such as stroke, renal failure, and neurological complications, but most importantly it can pose to be the most deleterious in case of cardiovascular disease. Hence, postprandial glucose control can help mitigate the imminent cardiovascular injury.

Studies show an increase in systolic and diastolic blood pressure in patients with postprandial glucose excursions. This may occur as acute hyperglycemia increases the underlying vascular tone via a glutathione pathway which maybe mediated through free radicals.

As is evidenced clearly in studies such as the Hoorn Study, the Honolulu Heart Study, the Chicago Heart Study, and, more recently, the DECODE (Diabetes Epidemiology: Collaborative Analysis of Diagnostic Criteria in Europe) study. Multiple meta-analysis have also been conducted to prove these facts—studies by Cioutinho et al. and a study that pooled data from the Whitehall study, Paris Prospective Study, and Helsinki Policeman study.

Carotid initima-medial thickness correlates not only with postprandial glucose but also particularly with the glycemic spikes during OGTT.

Nephropathy

Postprandial glucose has a stronger correlation with the incidence of diabetic microangiopathy when compared to glycated hemoglobin. Postprandial hyperglycemic excursion has been demonstrated as an independent risk factor in diabetic nephropathy, as proven in the Kumamoto study which followed up patients of type 2 DM for 8 years and found that in fact postprandial hyperglycemia was an independent and a strong risk factor for nephropathy as well as retinopathy.

Retinopathy

The National Health and Nutrition for Nutrition Examination Survey data demonstrated that patients with a 2-hour postprandial glucose level of 194 mg/dL, had a three times increase in the incidence of retinopathy, even in patients of normal fasting glucose levels. Studies from Japan showed that post-meal hyperglycemia is a more accurate predictor of retinopathy as compared to glycated hemoglobin levels. Multiple studies from Egypt, India, and Pima further revealed that despite normal fasting glucose levels, high postprandial glucose levels (>200 mg/dL) lead to increased retinal deterioration.

Cancers

Epidemiological evidence along with meta-analyses showed that type 2 DM increases the risk of tumor-specific mortality of certain cancers. A study in Sweden, which included a cumulative of over 60,000 participants, demonstrated the increase in the relative risk for tumors when there was an increase in the levels of both fasting as well as post prandial glucose levels. Relative risk for cancer in women was 1.31 in postprandial glucose group as compared to 1.26 in the fasting group. Further studies revealed a strong correlation between pancreatic cancer mortality and postprandial glucose levels. Risk for developing pancreatic cancer was 2.15 in patients with postprandial glucose of over 200 mg/dL.

MANAGEMENT

The first line of preventive therapy remains patient education, creating awareness about the harmful effects postprandial hyperglycemic excursions.

Goal

- International Diabetes Federation (2011)—levels less than 9.0 mmol/L (160 mg/dL)
- American College of Endocrinology—levels less than 140 mg/dL
- American Diabetes Association—levels less than 180 mg/dL
- European Association for the Study of Diabetes—levels less than 7.5 mmol/L (135 mg/dL).

Nonpharmacological Therapy

- *Physical activity*: Exercising in the postprandial state causes better reduction in the blood glucose levels when compared to exercising in the fasting state.
  High intensity exercise after a substantial caloric intake causes reduction in the glucose concentration and gives an impetus to the insulin secretion.
- *Diet modification*: Decreasing the dietary glycemic load (GL) by reducing the carbohydrate intake helps reduce postprandial excursions. GL is used as an estimate of insulin requirement and post-meal glycemia. Higher carbohydrate load also causes greater increase in glucosidase and incretin levels, in turn causing higher glycemia peaks and jeopardizing the cardiovascular well-being.

- *Medical nutrition therapy (MNT)*: 45–65% of daily caloric intake must come from carbohydrates, with a minimum of 130 g/day for adults. Low glycemia index foods must be encouraged and saturated fat should replace unsaturated fat.

Pharmacological Therapy

Drugs targeting postprandial hyperglycemias can be used as monotherapy or in combination with others. Evidence shows maximal postprandial control with repaglinide and glyburide, especially on carotid intima-media thickness. Along with these, alpha-glucosidase inhibitors, glinides, short-acting sulfonylureas, and insulin help cover postprandial hyperglycemias.

Oral Antidiabetic Drugs

Metformin

- Reduces postprandial glycemia, triglycerides, and free fatty acids.
- Better control on postprandial cholesterolemia and insulinemia when compared with repaglinide.

Sulfonylureas and glinides

- Repaglinide is a short-acting meglitinide
- More relevant when β cell function is sufficient
- Do not produce hypoglycemia
- Glinides—attenuate post-meal glucose excursions thus reducing the risk of post-meal hypoglycemia.

Alpha-glucosidase inhibitor

- Delay absorption of carbohydrates
- Acarbose—reduces postprandial glucose with a reduction in HbA1c levels by 0.8%.

  First line in newly diagnosed T2DM with high postprandial blood glucose.
- Acarbose can be combined with metformin, sulfonylureas or insulin; leads to a better reduction in HbA1c, fasting blood glucose as well as postprandial glucose
- Acarbose has better cardiovascular outcome when compared with voglibose and miglitol.

DDP-4 inhibitor

- Teneligliptin, linagliptin, saxagliptin, sitagliptin, and vildagliptin
- Effective in early stages of T2DM
- Monotherapy or combination with metformin or other oral agent—demonstrates better blood glucose control
- No change in body weight
- Minimal risk of hypoglycemia.

Injectable agents

- *GLP-1 based therapy*:
  - Induces weight loss
  - Stimulates insulin secretion, inhibits glucagon, decreases gastric emptying and in turn induces satiety
  - "Incretin effect"—reduced insulin secretion in response to a meal
  - GLP-1 analogs overcome the incretin effect
  - Exenatide and liraglutide
  - Exenatide—lowers HbA1c in patients failing on metformin and/or sulfonylurea.

    It requires twice daily administration.
  - Liraglutide—LEAD trails

    Improves β-cell function, reduces systolic pressure, and induces weight loss.
- *Rapid-acting insulin analogs*:
  - Mimics physiological insulin response
  - Lispro, Aspart, Glulisine
  - Faster absorption and peak at 1 hour after injection
  - Higher peak insulin concentration around high postprandial glucose values
  - Lower risk of late hypoglycemia and weight gain
  - Feinglos et al. demonstrated combination of insulin Lispro with a sulfonylurea reduced postprandial glucose along with fasting plasma glucose and HbA1c along with cholesterol concentrations
  - Compared to regular human insulin, better postprandial glucose control has been demonstrated with the use of rapid-acting insulin.

FURTHER READING

1. American Diabetes Association. Postprandial Blood Glucose. Diabetes Care. 2001;24(4):775-8.
2. Bonora E, Muggeo M. Postprandial blood glucose as a risk factor for cardiovascular disease in type II diabetes: the epidemiological evidence. Diabetologia. 2001;44(12):2107-14.
3. Vinik AI, Jenkins DJ. Dietary fiber in management of diabetes. Diabetes Care. 1988;11(2):160-73.
4. Kearney ML, Thyfault JP. Exercise and postprandial glycemic control in type 2 diabetes. Curr Diabetes Rev. 2016;12(3):199-210.
5. Gerich J. Pathogenesis and management of postprandial hyperglycemia: role of incretin-based therapies. Int J Gen Med. 2013;6:877-95.
6. de Vegt F1, Dekker JM, Ruhé HG, et al. Hyperglycaemia is associated with all-cause and cardiovascular mortality in the Hoorn population: the Hoorn Study. Diabetologia. 1999;42(8):926-31.
7. Donahue RP, Abbott RD, Reed DM, et al. Postchallenge glucose concentration and coronary heart disease in men of Japanese ancestry: Honolulu Heart Program. Diabetes. 1987;36(6):689-92.
8. Lowe LP, Liu K, Greenland P, et al. Diabetes, asymptomatic hyperglycemia, and 22-year mortality in black and white men: the Chicago Heart Association Detection Project in Industry study. Diabetes Care. 1997;20(2):163-9.
9. The DECODE Study Group, the European Diabetes Epidemiology Group: Glucose tolerance and mortality: comparison of WHO and American Diabetes Association diagnostic criteria. Lancet. 1999;354:617-21.

55 CHAPTER Treatment of Type 2 Diabetes Mellitus after Metformin Failure

Hemraj B Chandalia

INTRODUCTION

Preferred modality of treatment after metformin failure is the most crucial part of the current algorithm of treatment of type 2 diabetes mellitus (T2DM). At this level, there are six available options and presently, a large number of studies available have advocated the preference of one over the other in varied situations. This chapter examines these issues critically and additionally discusses the use of combination therapy with metformin or use of an alternative monotherapy in place of metformin at the time of treatment initiation. The treatment modalities with triple drug therapy or with insulin and sensitizing agents at the next tiers of treatment does not attract as much discussion as that evoked by therapeutic considerations after metformin failure and is beyond the scope of this chapter.

INITIAL TREATMENT OF TYPE 2 DIABETES MELLITUS

Classically, lifestyle intervention is considered the basic first step in controlling T2DM. An important issue is to identify those who would need immediate addition of an oral antidiabetic drug or even an injectable therapy. The guidelines are not clear in this regard and no study has exclusively addressed this issue. However, if hemoglobin A1c (HbA1c) is >8%, it would indeed be difficult to achieve a target of 6% or 6.5% HbA1c with lifestyle intervention alone. In those individuals who can apply lifestyle measures vigorously and sustain the same, we follow a strategy of introducing at least one oral antidiabetic drug (OAD) when the HbA1c at entry point is >8%. However, we look for an earliest opportunity to omit the OAD in about 2–3 months' time in such subjects.

INERTIA IN THE MANAGEMENT OF TYPE 2 DIABETES MELLITUS

In a patient with an initial HbA1c of 7.5%, if it is decided to use lifestyle intervention alone how long is it necessary to wait before considering introduction of an OAD? Similar questions are recurring themes in the algorithms of treatment of T2DM. How much time-lag is ideal in between the treatment escalations? For want of adequate number of diabetes-care personnel, the prevailing routing practice is to schedule the follow-up visits at quarterly intervals, probably based on the calculation that the time HbA1c is down after 3 months will reflect faithfully the status of glycemic control and adequacy of treatment modality. It is important to note that the HbA1c is a 90% reflection of ambient blood glucose in the past 2 months; hence, waiting for 3 months is not a good strategy. Another important consideration is to use self-monitoring of plasma glucose (SMPG) to decide upon the need for escalation of treatment. Table 1 gives the appropriate time interval required for each treatment modality to exert its full effect. Thus, a failure of treatment as revealed by SMPG can be used far more quickly than waiting to see the reduction in HbA1c. The follow-up at short intervals can be used to complete the process of treatment escalations as well as education, which in a newly diagnosed patient, cannot be completed at one visit. At Diabetes Endocrine Nutrition Management and Research Center (DENMARC) about 2 hours are devoted to each new patient at the first visit, one hour for medical evaluation, and one hour for education. Furthermore, patient education continues during the 2–3 subsequent visits, or even at many future visits. In case it is difficult for a patient to physically report with such increased

TABLE 1: Earliest time interval needed before evaluating glycemic control with varied therapies.

Therapy	Time interval	Comments
Lifestyle intervention	2 weeks	Use SMPG
Metformin	2 weeks	Use SMPG
Sulfonylureas	1 week	Use SMPG
Pioglitazone	6 weeks	Use SMPG and/or HbA1c
Insulin	Each dose shows its full effect in 4 days. Arriving at final dose may take 2–4 weeks	Use SMPG and HbA1c
DPP- 4 inhibitor	2 weeks	Use SMPG
SGLT-2 inhibitor	2 weeks	Use SMPG
GLP-RA	2weeks for dose escalation, Additionally 4 weeks for full effect	Use SMPG and HbA1c

(DPP-4: dipeptidyl peptidase 4; SGLT-2: sodium-glucose cotransporter-2; GLP-RA: glucagon-like peptide receptor agonist; SMPG: self-monitoring of plasma glucose)

frequency, changes in treatment should be undertaken at appropriate intervals on e-mail or phone. What is needed is a rationalization of timing the follow-up visits, based upon the time taken by each treatment modality to exert its significant or full effect.

INITIAL TREATMENT WITH ALTERNATIVE MONOTHERAPY OR COMBINATION THERAPY WITH METFORMIN

Metformin is the most widely used drug initially, except in patients exhibiting metformin intolerance. There are no clear data on the prevalence of metformin intolerance. From a large number of studies, it is extrapolated that it probably occurs in about 10% of patients. No clear differences have been observed between immediate release and slow release form, although the latter is considered to be better tolerated. Interestingly, metformin intolerance occurring from drug interactions has not been fully appreciated. A large number of commonly used drugs like tricyclic antidepressants, proton-pump inhibitors, verapamil, doxazosin, spironolactone, clopidogrel, and tramadol alter the absorption and excretion of metformin and increase concentration of the drug in the gut lumen, thus producing intolerance. The intolerance may be related to genetic polymorphism of genes responsible for the hepatic or enterocyte uptake of metformin or its transport across the gut lumen to serosal side. Organic cation transporters 1 and 2 (OCT-1 and OCT-2) are encoded by the genes *SLC22AI* and *SCL22A3*, respectively and their genetic polymorphism has been reported. Metformin intolerance caused by other drug interactions may also operate through these genetic polymorphisms. Metformin intolerance can be dose related. In general, dose of 1,500 mg of metformin is well tolerated in most Indian subjects and doses higher than this dose must be watched carefully.

In case of metformin intolerance, it is advisable to consider an alternative monotherapy. Both dipeptidyl peptidase 4 (DPP-4) inhibitors and sodium-glucose cotransporter-2 (SGLT-2) inhibitors have been proposed in this situation. We use DDP-4 inhibitors in recently diagnosed and SGLT-2 inhibitors in T2DM of more than 10-year duration or with cardiovascular-renal complications. The rationale for this approach has been discussed in detail subsequently in this article. For cost considerations, one could use a sulfonylurea (SU) or thiazolidinedione (TZD) here. With clear evidence of benefits in patients of atherosclerotic vascular disease, especially with obesity, glucagon-like peptide receptor agonist (GLP-RA) should be considered. Criteria used in choosing an alternate drug in this situation or subsequently in the downstream algorithm are discussed subsequently in this article.

Initial combination therapy has also been proposed, mostly by American Association of Clinical Endocrinologists based on the HbA1c level at entry. It is advocated that if initial HbA1c >9%, a two-drug combination should be used. There are some advantages in this approach. As most modalities of treatment, specifically metformin has been shown to lower HbA1c at best by 1.5%. Therefore, an HbA1c of >9% is not likely to reach the target by monotherapy. This approach also avoids loss of time involved in exhibiting these drugs sequentially. The two drugs used together are most likely to lower HbA1c by 2–2.5%, as they work through different mechanisms and thus demonstrate synergism. The dosage used may also be low, especially that of metformin, thus avoiding dose-related metformin intolerance.

Second-Tier Treatment Modalities

Presently, there are six different treatment modalities available after metformin failure. It must be made clear that the word "metformin failure" is a misnomer, as metformin is continued with the addition of a new drug or drugs. This concept is unusual, but accepted in diabetology. This implies that metformin continues to exert some antihyperglycemic effect. In this context, a word like "partial failure" or "partial efficacy" may be more appropriate.

Each of these six options is discussed here individually mainly from the angle of their efficacy, propensity to cause weight gain, hypoglycemia and major adverse side effects, and potential for cardiovascular-renal protection. Following this discussion, a critical analysis of algorithm is presented.

DIPEPTYL PEPTIDASE-4 INHIBITORS

This group of drugs is in extensive use for the past 8 years. They act by increasing GLP-1 levels, which stimulate endogenous insulin secretion. Metformin also increases GLP-1 levels and has an insulin sensitizing effect operating through a peroxisome proliferator-activated receptor α and not by increasing DPP-4 activity. Thus, a combination of metformin and DPP-4i is synergistic. DPP-4 inhibitors work through several mechanisms, thus covering several etiopathological aspects of T2DM. The antihyperglycemic effect of DPP-4i is durable over more than 4 years. The lowering of Hb1Ac by DPP-4i was somewhat lesser than SGLT-2i (0.7% vs. 0.9% respectively) in a head-on study of sitagliptin vs. empagliflozin in subjects with average baseline HbA1c of 8%. It is important to note that the absolute lowering of HbA1c with all OAD depends upon the initial HbA1c.

There are two very important aspects of the action of DPP-4 inhibitors: a very low incidence of hypoglycemia and a side effect profile, which almost resembles the side effect profile of placebo. Hypoglycemia with these drugs is seen only when they are used in combination with other hypoglycemic agent like insulin, glinides or SUs. The side effects include nasopharyngeal congestion or a skin rash, both of which are rare. There is a very small increase in the incidence of acute pancreatitis, which is estimated to be 0.13%. These drugs are weight neutral. They have no adverse or favorable effect on cardiovascular-renal systems, with a few exceptions. In the SAVOR-TIMI 53 trial, saxagliptin had shown an increased hospitalization with heart failure. Linagliptin has been shown to have reduced urinary albumin/creatinine ratio without any improvement in eGFR.

SODIUM-GLUCOSE COTRANSPORTER-2 INHIBITORS

This class of drugs has emerged as a very import modality of treatment of T2DM for the past 5 years. These drugs increase urinary excretion of glucose by inhibiting SGLT-2, an enzyme responsible for the absorption of excreted urinary glucose in proximal renal tubules. On an average, almost 75 g of glucose is excreted daily, resulting in the blood glucose lowering effect. The average HbA1c lowering with the use of these drugs is 0.9% or more. The effect is durable beyond 4 years. Originally, their use was not advised in patients of reduced eGFR as the therapeutic efficacy in this situation was in doubt. Subsequently, these drugs have not only been shown to be efficacious, but considered beneficial with reduced eGFR, as low 30–45 mL/min/1.7 m^2.

The main side effect of SGLT-2i is genital fungal infections in about 5–10% of subjects. The urinary tract infections are increased in less than 1% of subjects, hence they are contraindicated in patients with active urinary infection or history of recurrent urinary tract infections. There is possibility of hypovolemia and dehydration, especially in elderly and frail individuals. Concomitant use of loop diuretics may produce hypotension. There is rare possibility of acute kidney injury. In insulin-deficient subjects, there is possibility of euglycemic ketoacidosis, again a rare side effect. There is possibility of increased fractures due to an increase in the phosphate resorption leading to secondary hyperparathyroidism. These drugs do not cause significant hypoglycemia. They cause an average weight loss of about 2–3 kg. Rarely, some patients complain of more weight loss and loss of muscle mass, a side effect not fully investigated.

The most important aspect of SGLT-2i is the fact that they offer significant cardiovascular and renal protection. This was first brought out in the EMPA-REG trial. The patients recruited were average 63 years old, all patients had documented cardiovascular disease although 35% had no cardiovascular event. The average duration of diabetes in this study was 10 years. This study showed reduction of a composite (death due to CV disease, myocardial infarction, and stroke) 3-point MACE by 14%. It further showed a reduction in hospitalization for heart failure by 35%. An analysis of a subgroup of 643 patients, so labeled "credence-like group" with established renal disease also showed improvement in renal outcomes and hospitalization for heart failure.

Data from the studies of canagliflozin and dapagliflozin also show similar effects on the CV outcomes of these drugs with minor differences. These differences emerge from the type of patients recruited in these studies. For example, the component of recruited patients without cardiovascular disease was nil in EMPA-REG study, 34% in Canvas program and 60% in the Declare study. The Canvas program as well as Declare Timi58 studies showed a reduction in 3-point MACE but no clear reduction in both, the CV or all-cause mortality. Thus, reduction in CV death was significant only in the EMPA-REG study, although seen in Credence study, as a secondary end-point. The statistical design of these studies is robust yet confusing for the clinicians. However, a common thread of CV risk reduction, renal protection, and reduction in heart failure appears to be the class effects of these drugs. The Credence study which recruited patients with established renal disease brought out the renoprotective effect as well as reduction in hospitalization for heart failure. The renoprotective effect as well as a reduction in hospitalization for heart failure was robust and highly significant in all these studies. In Credence Study, a reduction in CV mortality was seen as a secondary end-point. DAPA-HF study, reported in the 2019 EASD meeting, has shown benefits in heart failure with reduced ejection fraction, both in diabetics as well as nondiabetics.

A few disturbing side effects of these drugs need to be discussed. For example, the increased incidence of toe amputations seen in Canvas program was not brought out in the Credence study. Increased fracture risk, seen in Canvas program needs further studies in patients on canagliflozin, as well as other SGLT-2i. However, it was not seen in credence study. Mechanistic studies are also called for, because that supports the causality by using an alternate route of scientific evidence. At present, increased phosphate reabsorption leading to secondary hyperparathyroidism is being advanced as one of the mechanisms. The increased incidence of stroke in EMPA-REG study was seen in most cases after the discontinuation of drug where the patients were being followed as a mandatory requirement of intention-to-treat studies. Thus, the increased gangrene in Canvas program and increased strokes in EMPA-REG study appear to be of accidental nature, a possibility difficult to eliminate in spite of a large number of subjects studied by a randomized controlled study design.

The side effect of euglycemic or classic diabetic ketoacidosis can occur with the use of these drugs in long-standing T2DM. It occurred in 0.1–0.3% of patients in the three (EMPA-REG, Canvas Program, and Declare-Timi58 CV) outcome studies. Based upon these facts, it is important to ensure that patients prescribed these drugs have adequate endogenous insulin production or are given adequate doses of exogenous insulin. If it is decided to add an SGLT-2i in a type 2 diabetic on insulin, the insulin dose reduction as a precaution to avoid hypoglycemia should not be more than 20%.

SULFONYLUREAS

Presently, only second and third generation SUs like glimepiride and gliclazide need to be considered, as older SUs like chlorpropamide is obsolete and glibenclamide and glipizide are rarely used except in a few special situations. Glibenclamide does not cross-placental barrier and hence can be considered in a pregnant gestational diabetic, where for important reasons, metformin or insulin therapy is not possible. Glipizide can be rarely considered as an oral drug in T2DM with renal failure as an inexpensive but effective drug option. Possibility of hypoglycemia is very high with the use of these potent drugs. Glimepiride is a long-acting SU and can be given once a day, though in practice, in combination with metformin, it is often given in twice a day regime. Although there are studies demonstrating safety of this drug in renal failure as well as hepatic disease, it is likely to produce severe hypoglycemia in these situations. This author uses gliclazide in small divided dosages like 20–40 mg, three times a day to achieve good control in difficult type 2 diabetics. SUs are excellent insulin sensitizers, a fact often not appreciated by clinicians after the advent of pioglitazone and metformin as sensitizing agents. There are numerous studies on the sensitizing effect of SUs in the literature. However, combining an SU with insulin needs to be undertaken cautiously, as possibility of hypoglycemia is enhanced. Moderate weight gain can also occur with the use of these drugs. This author does not use modified release and long-acting gliclazide for this purpose and uses only unmodified from of gliclazide in divided doses. This is effective in reducing post-prandial blood glucose and producing an excellent sensitizing effect. The most important fact in favor of the use of SUs is their low cost and great efficacy. These drugs can produce 0.75–2% lowering of HbA1c.

Thiazolidinediones

The molecule in use currently is pioglitazone. This drug is efficacious, the frequently used dose is 15–30 mg, although there are some Indian data describing effective use of 7.5 mg dose. This drug can produce 0.5–1.5% lowering of HbA1c. However, the hypoglycemic effect is manifest only after 4–6 weeks. The most common side effects are weight gain and water retention. The weight gain can be moderate, but at times can be huge; although insulin sensitivity is maintained. It has never been studied how long the insulin sensitivity post weight-gain with pioglitazone use is maintained after the drug discontinuation. This drug can also increase the incidence of bone fractures. Pioglitazone does not cause much hypoglycemia. This drug is very inexpensive.

Basal Insulin

Basal insulin used are NPH, levemir, glargine, glargine 300, and degludec. Of these, glargine is the most frequently used basal. Use of NPH in two doses a day is a cost-effective basal regime. It may also find its use in very young (<8 years of age) type 1 diabetic. The newer ones, glargine 300 and degludec insulin are long-acting basal insulins with less likelihood of hypoglycemia, nocturnal hypoglycemia, and severe hypoglycemia needing external assistance for recovery.

It must be noted that overall, all basal insulins are less likely to produce hypoglycemia and weight gain than prandial insulins. Hence, they can be used lot more widely than what is being done in current practice in India. The HbA1c lowering with properly planned insulin therapy can be 1–3%, resulting in full normalization.

Basal insulin must be considered in undernourished T2DM, when BMI is 18–20 kg/m^2 or when person is losing weight unintentionally and rapidly. Inertia in initiating basal insulin or if required, even a full scale basal-bolus insulin therapy has disastrous consequences as severe hyperglycemia is highly catabolic and leads to rapid loss of not only body fat but muscle mass. This is occurring frequent in India, because of inertia in initiating insulin therapy both at the level of patient or treating physician.

The lowering of fasting blood glucose by basal insulin is also accompanied by the lowering of postprandial glycemia to some extent. However, oral agents like metformin or metformin plus SUs or DPP-4i must be continued for added basal effect by metformin and prandial effect by DPP-4i and SU. This is key to successful basal insulin therapy.

GLP-1 Receptor Agonists (GLP-RAs)

These are injectable therapies, the molecules in use in India being liraglutide and dulaglutide. Liraglutide is injected once daily while dulaglutide is injected once a week. Lixisenatide and semaglutide are not in clinical use in India and hence, will be discussed briefly. Injectable semaglutide is more efficacious and can lower HbA1c by 1.4%. Durability of semaglutide and exenatide is better than liraglutide and lixisenatide. All GLP-RAs act by raising GLP-levels, which stimulates glucose-dependent insulin secretion and suppresses glucagon. They diminish gastric motility thus prolonging gastric emptying time. They suppress appetite by acting on the hypothalamic pathways. They induce considerable weight loss, in fact liraglutide has been approved for this purpose in nondiabetic obese subjects. These drugs lower the HbA1c by about 0.5–1%, but their effect is seen after about 6 weeks.

These drugs are indicated in obese (BMI >23 kg/m^2) type 2 diabetics. Additionally, patients with atherosclerotic cardiovascular disease show a reduction of 20% in the incidence of MACE and all-cause mortality. Average weight reduction of 4.3 kg was seen in the treated group as compared to placebo. These drugs do not improve renal outcomes or heart failure but can be used with any degree of renal compromise. However, with renal failure, undernutrition and gastrointestinal symptoms are frequently present, which limits the use of these drugs. The main side effects of these drugs are nausea, vomiting, epigastric fullness, and diarrhea. There are signals for increased incidence of pancreatitis. Long-term use needs monitoring calcitonin, as C-cell hyperplasia and tumors have been described in preclinical studies.

These drugs have been combined with basal insulin either in a premixed form (IDegLira) or in separate administration. This has provided good synergism, as basal insulin controls fasting blood glucose and GLP-RA controls postprandial blood glucose.

These drugs are expensive and although introduction of oral semaglutide is round the corner, the cost may continue to be an important factor in limiting their use.

CHOOSING TREATMENT MODALITY AFTER METFORMIN FAILURE

Based upon the knowledge of efficacy, durability of response, cost, and side effects, it is possible to choose optimum therapy. In 2018 and 2019, EASD and ADA issued combined guidelines where a clinical approach was suggested. It involved the following five clinical considerations: (1) Presence of atherosclerotic vascular disease or more than one CV risk factor, (2) propensity toward recurrent hypoglycemia or serious hypoglycemia necessitating hospitalization, (3) obesity and treatment-related weight gain, (4) cost considerations, and (5) none of the above issues.

For the first time, the clinical considerations were given the central position and cost issues were emphasized. Interestingly, the RSSDI treatment guidelines issued in 2017 had approached the treatment from the same angle. It appears that in both these situations, and obviously so in India, the guideline committee included a good number of practicing diabetologists.

It is important to examine each of these five issues further.

Atherosclerosis CV Disease and CV Risk Factors

The main controversy in this regard surrounds clinical criteria used for the recognition of atherosclerotic CV disease. In order to expand the use of SGLT-2 inhibitors for improving CV outcomes, a so-called primary prevention cohort was included in the recruited group in treatment and placebo arms. However, the average duration of diabetes in the major three randomized controlled CV trials was more than 10 years; hence, these so-called primary prevention groups were very likely to have suffered from significant atherosclerotic vascular disease. The first study, EMPA-REG contained all patients with documented CVD, except that 35% had not suffered a cardiovascular event. This design was found suitable to show a reduction in CV disease and mortality in a relatively short time of study period. The next two studies, Canvas program and Declare study increased the proportion of patients without cardiovascular disease to allow them to expand the indications for the use of these drugs.

An important question to answer is whether T2DM a CV risk factor at the time of diagnosis. We have visited this issue several times in the past two decades, since the publication of Steve Haffner's paper, showing that T2DM at the time of diagnosis carries a risk of myocardial infarction equivalent to the risk of a repeat myocardial infarction in a nondiabetic individual who has suffered a myocardial infarct earlier. It was appreciated that many newly diagnosed type 2 diabetics, who were well controlled by lifestyle interventions or monotherapy with metformin and did not have any other comorbidity or had a single, easily controlled comorbidity were indeed not at a myocardial infarction risk equivalent to that in a nondiabetic with history of myocardial infarction.

An interesting study reported by Kaiser Permanente Group of California throws some light into this issue. It included 1,586,061 subjects under follow-up on a long-term basis where diabetics were compared with nondiabetics. It was seen that at the time of diagnosis of diabetes, the CHD risk was about half that seen in the nondiabetic group with previous CHD but after 10 years of diabetes, the risk for myocardial infarction equaled the risk in nondiabetic with previous myocardial infarction. A recently diagnosed type 2 diabetic may not be a CV risk equivalent, while a long-standing (>10-year duration) is a CV risk equivalent. Based upon these premises, clinicians can individualize their approach. In any case of ambiguity, the clinicians are trained to take a safer course, based on the basic principle "First, do no harm".

As described above, SGLT-2 inhibitors have shown a CV protection and reduction in CV and all course mortality. They have also shown improvement in renal outcomes and hospitalization for heart failure. In fact, the protection in the last two situations is almost 30–40%, thus their use is almost mandatory in these situations, as recommended by the regulatory bodies (Table 2).

GLA-RA, liraglutide was shown to offer a reduction in atherosclerotic CV disease. If the main issue is atherosclerotic CV disease and not heart failure or renal failure, and more so if the person is obese, GLP-RA will

TABLE 2: T2DM with CV risk factors or CV disease.

Patient profile	GLP-RA Safety	GLP-RA benefits	SGLT-2i Safety	SGLT-2i benefits
Atherosclerotic CV disease	√	√	Permissible up to eGFR of 30–45 mL/min/1.7 m^2	—
>2 CV risk factors	√	√	√	√
>10-year duration of diabetes with or without clinical CV disease or CV risk factors	√	√	√	√
Renal failure (eGFR ≥30–45	√	—	Safe up to eGFR 30–45 mL/min/1.7 m^2	√
Cardiac failure	√	—	√	√

(SGLT-2i: sodium-glucose cotransporter-2i; GLP-RA: glucagon-like peptide receptor agonist; T2DM: type 2 diabetes mellitus; CV: cardiovascular; eGFR: estimated glomerular filtration rate)

be a preferred form of therapy. A combination of GLA-RA and SGLT-2i also may be considered, although data in this regard are not available.

Propensity to Develop Hypoglycemia

Hypoglycemia is a frequent occurrence with the use of insulin, SUs and glinides. These drugs have to be used cautiously in this regard.

Insulin therapy is the most common cause of hypoglycemia. Basal insulin is less likely to produce hypoglycemia than prandial insulin. Multiple doses of insulin are less likely to produce hypoglycemia than 1–2 doses. Hence, in difficult patients with history of hypoglycemia, use of premixed insulin in 1–2 doses is inadvisable. The dose of insulin should be kept low. This is achieved by using insulin sensitizers, like metformin and pioglitazone. DPP-4i and SGLT-2i also serve as sensitizers as they reduce the insulin dose. SUs are very potent sensitizers; however, combining them with insulin increases the risk of hypoglycemia. As described above use of unmodified gliclazide in small multiple doses is a good solution to this situation.

There are certain reasons why some patients are prone to hypoglycemia. Undernourished (BMI <18 kg/m^2) subjects are more prone to hypoglycemia. Renal failure makes patient susceptible to hypoglycemia due to reduced contribution of failing kidney toward the pool of glucose arising from gluconeogenesis, poor nutrition, anorexia, and poor food intake. Liver disease can also cause fasting hypoglycemia and occult liver disease may remain undiagnosed in T2DM. As nonalcoholic fatty liver disease (NAFLD) is common in diabetes, cirrhosis of liver in varying stages of progression can occur in T2DM and remain undiagnosed. Box 1 gives the approach toward successful avoidance of hypoglycemia in T2DM.

BOX 1 Avoidance of hypoglycemia in T2DM.

- Use metformin, GLP-RA, DPP4i, SGLT 2i, and pioglitazone as preferred drugs.
- Avoid sulfonylureas, glinides, and insulin.
- If insulin is introduced, usual small, multiple doses, adequate proportional dose of basal insulin and sensitize patient to insulin by using antidiabetic agents described in 1 above. If drugs listed in 2 above are used, exercise extreme caution.

(SGLT-2i: sodium-glucose cotransporter-2i; GLP-RA: glucagon-like peptide receptor agonist; T2DM: type 2 diabetes mellitus; DPP-4: dipeptidyl peptidase 4)

Obesity and Treatment-related Weight Gain

Obesity is present in about 50–60% of T2DM. Hence, this is an important consideration in choosing therapy (Box 2). Treatment-related weight gain is also an important issue, primarily seen with pioglitazone and insulin therapy. It is interesting to note that good part of weight gain with insulin therapy is due to reversal of weight loss that occurred due to uncontrolled diabetes prior to instituting insulin therapy.

Most drugs causing weight gain are also known to produce hypoglycemia, in fact the degree of weight gain is often proportional to their hypoglycemia potential. Pioglitazone is an exception; as it does not lead to hypoglycemia, yet causes severe weight gain. There is genetic polymorphism regarding the quantity of weight gain with the use of pioglitazone. Hence, rapid weight gain in the first 2 months of therapy should prompt the treating physician to withdraw the drug.

Cost of Treatment

GLP-RA, SGLT-2i, and DPP-4i are expensive form of therapies. Although we are likely to see in future less expensive options, and also see a cost reduction of these drugs when the patents expire, presently the cost of these drugs is prohibitive.

In India, teneligliptin and remogliflozin have been introduced in therapy. Their efficacy and potential for CV risk reduction remains to be seen. Considering class effect, the outcomes can be predicted to be favorable, but there are many examples of drugs, where the class affect does not hold true, for example, liraglutide has shown CV benefits but not exenatide. Preclinical studies, Real World Studies, and eventually RCTs are required to establish CV outcome benefits of these drugs.

BOX 2 Choice of treatment in obese T2DM.

- Preferably use drugs that induce weight loss:
  - GLP-1 RA
  - SGLT-2i
- Use drugs that are weight-neutral:
  - Metformin, DDP4 inhibitor
  - Nutrient blockers
- Aroid drugs causing weight gain:
  - Insulin therapy
  - Sulfonylureas
  - Pioglitazone
  - Glinides

(SGLT-2i: sodium-glucose cotransporter-2i; GLP-RA: glucagon-like peptide receptor agonist; T2DM: type 2 diabetes mellitus; DPP-4: dipeptidyl peptidase 4)

NONE OF THE ABOVE ISSUES

This has not been discussed clearly in the recent ADA/ EASD guidelines. In this situation, the main criterion should be duration of diabetes. It is well known that on an average there is 2–3 years delay in the diagnosis of T2DM. However, from the time of diagnosis, 10 years of disease has a potential of producing a state of myocardial infarct equivalence. In these subjects, GLA-RA or SGLT-2i must be considered. A combination of both has not yet been studied by a RCT.

CONCLUSION

Presently, six options are available to treat T2DM after metformin failure. The treatment is individualized, depending upon the duration of diabetes, presence of obesity, propensity to recurrent hypoglycemia and presence of cardiovascular and renal complications. GLP-RAs are drugs of choice in the presence of atherosclerotic cardiovascular disease. SGLT-2i also offers cardiovascular protection, but the renal and heart failure benefits are more prominent. It is possible to achieve good glycemic control without producing hypoglycemia. If there is unintended weight loss, basal insulin must be considered. Cost considerations are important, therefore metformin, SUs, and thiazolidinediones should be considered in appropriate situations.

CONFLICT OF INTEREST

Author is on the speaker bureau of advisory board of Novo Nordisk, Sanofi, Boehringer Ingelheim, MSD, Novartis, Lupin, USV, and Glenmark Pharmaceuticals.

56 CHAPTER Top 10 Clinical Papers Presented in American Diabetes Association/European Association for the Study of Diabetes 2019

NK Singh, Leena Singh, Richa Manaswita, Vaibhav Agnihotri

INTRODUCTION

The 79th American Diabetes Association (ADA) 2019 conference at San Francisco from June 7 to June 11 and the European Association for Study of Diabetes (EASD) and 59th Annual Conference from 16th to 20th September at Barcelona 2019 were very significant as many guideline changing clinical papers were presented, especially at ADA. These conferences are "Maha Kumbh of Diabetology" and usually attended by over 15,000 professional attendees from 115 countries.

Following top ten papers give an updated clinical insight. Some equally important papers presented at EASD have been summarized in Table 1. Needless to say hottest interest was related to cardiovascular outcome trials (CVOTs), renal effects of glucagon-like peptide-1 receptor agonist (GLP-1RA) and sodium-glucose co-transporter 2 (SGLT2) inhibitors. These results keep tremendous potential to change the way we treat diabetes (Table 2).

TRIALS IN RELATION TO CARDIOVASCULAR OUTCOME TRIALS/RENAL DISEASE

REWIND (Table 3)

This trial was a major attraction at ADA 2019 and findings appear to rewind the way we treat diabetes. REWIND, a very ambitious study, conclusively studied the once weekly injectable GLP-1 agonist dulaglutide. It significantly reduced the risk of major adverse cardiovascular event (MACE) by 12% in comparison to placebo primarily by reducing the risk of stroke. REWIND is one of the longest CVOT till date with a long median follow-up of 5.4 years with only 31.5% people with previous cardiovascular disease, and it is unmatched by showing that weekly injections of GLP1-RA dulaglutide reduces cardiovascular outcomes in both with or without cardiovascular disease and in both sexes.[1,2]

PIONEER Program

PIONEER phage 3a development program is a very ambitious global development program for oral semaglutide. It has enrolled 9,543 people with type 2 diabetes across 10 clinical trials. From concept to successful oral semaglutide, which proves superior to empagliflozin, noninferior to liraglutide for lowering HbA1c, two PIONEER trials of peptide semaglutide were of main interest and reviewed at ADA and EASD. PIONEER 6 trial full results were presented at ADA. This trial demonstrated the noninferiority of cardiovascular safety profile of oral semaglutide compared to placebo but did not demonstrate superiority despite overall positive trend which was driven by cardiovascular death. PIONEER 8 presented at EASD, showed that semaglutide add-on lowers HbA1c in type 2 diabetes insulin users. Most important message, which these trials impart, is that this can lead to an early initiation of GLP-1RA therapy which is so justified in today's continuum of care.[3,4]

CAROLINA Trial (Table 4)

It was a major attraction at ADA as for the first time cardiovascular safety of compared drug glimepiride came out in limelight, although it was done to establish superiority of linagliptin. In one way, this trial has done great service to diabetes care providing robust proof that modern SU can be continued with persons with diabetes.

TABLE 1: Best of EASD.[9,11,12,18]

Top take home clinical messages from EASD	
Trial	**Take Home Message**
VERIFY:	
• Stated to be the largest long-term prospective trial to test the durability of glycemic control • Early combination of vildagliptin and metformin group over the 5-year study had significant reduction in relative risk for time to initial treatment failure. (HR 0.51; CI 0.45–0.58, P < 0.0001) • At most, we can say that this study validates off-label use of initial dual therapy	• In true sense this study has no potential to guideline changing impact. The results were not unexpected too because these medications have synergistic mechanisms • The message of this study is reassurance of combination treatment regarding its safety and effectiveness • It does not give us license that early combination treatment strategy will be needed to all patients with type 2 diabetes patients
***DEFINE-HF*:**	
• 263 patients with optimally managed HFrEF, received dapagliflozin 10 mg/day or placebo for 12 weeks • No significant difference in the average adjusted 6-week and 12-week NT-pro BNP levels (this was first of the two primary endpoints) • Odds ratio for the effect of dapagliflozin on end points: 0.95 (95% CI, 0.84–1.08); P = 0.43	• Even without affecting mean NT-proBNP over 12 weeks, dapagliflozin brought clinically meaningful improvements in HF-related health status which extends to patients without type 2 diabetes • Message is that dapagliflozin may have a favorable effect on improving disease-specific health status after 12 weeks of treatment • The benefits of this drug clearly represent a SGLT-2i class effect in the arena of HF prevention for people of diabetes. *Dapagliflozin does not really capture all that it may offer*
***DAPA-HF*:**	
• 5,000 patients • Having moderate heart failure and reduced ejection fraction with or without heart failure • Randomized for dapagliflozin 10 mg or placebo on top of contemporary therapy for HF	• DAPA cohort had 26% lower rate of the primary outcome of worsening HF or CVD (HR 0.74; 0.00001), with NNT of 21 • DAPA benefited consistently among the primary and secondary outcomes and pre-specified subgroups • Most stunning and impressive fact emerged that consistent benefit occurred in patients with HF, both with or without diabetes
Trial of Imeglimin for Efficacy and Safety (TIMES 1):	
• This new drug improves mitochondrial function, which in turn increases insulin secretion and insulin sensitivity in the muscle and also decreases hepatic glucose production	• In all phase 2 and phase 3 trials very robust efficacy has been documented • The safety and tolerability profile is very good. It could be the next blockbuster drug in type 2 diabetes therapy • The primary endpoint change from baseline in HbA1c at week 24 was significantly greater with Imeglimin (0.87% P < 0.0001)
***PRIORITY*:**	
• [Proteomic prediction and renin angiotensin aldosterone system inhibition prevention of early diabetic nephropathy in type 2 diabetes patients with normoalbuminuria]	• In type 2 diabetes and normoalbuminuria, the urinary proteomic classifier CKD273 predicts progression to microalbuminuria, independent of clinical characteristics • CKD273 predicts decline in renal function • Spironolactone did not prevent progression to microalbuminuria in high risk subjects
***CONCLUDE*:**	
• This was designed to compare the efficacy and safety of insulin degludec and insulin glargine 300 units/mL in type 2 diabetes patients inadequately treated with basal insulin and OHA	• The primary outcome failed as the rate of overall symptomatic hypoglycemia with degludec U200 was not significantly lower versus glargine U300 in the maintenance period • For all other hypoglycemia endpoints during the maintenance and total treatment periods, degludec U200 showed lower rates and proportions compared with glargine U300 • Too many uncertainties prevent drawing firm conclusion from the CONCLUDE trial—Dr Stefano Del Prato

(CI: confidence interval; CVD: cardiovascular disease; EASD: the European Association for the Study of Diabetes; HF: heart failure; HR: hazard ratio; OHA: oral hypoglycemic agent)

It is a paradox that after this trial glimepiride was more in news than linagliptin. No doubt CAROLINA is unique as the first CVOT which provides valuable information about both linagliptin and glimepiride.[5] The CAROLINA COGNITION study, presented at EASD, no difference in risk for cognitive decline was observed between linagliptin and glimepiride cohorts over 6.1 years.

TABLE 2: Top 10 clinical papers at ADA/EASD.

Trials in relation to CVOT/Renal disease
• REWIND and DECLARE-TIMI 58
• PIONEER program
• CAROLINA
• CREDENCE and CARMELINA
• DEFINE-HF and DAPA-HF
Medication study/Complication
• RISE and TODAY's
• VERIFY and CONCLUDE
• IMEGLIMIN TIME1
New therapeutic approach in type 1
• TRIALNET
Prevention
• D2d AND PREVIEW

(ADA: American Diabetes Association; CVOT: cardiovascular outcome trial; DAPA-HF: dapagliflozin and prevention of adverse-outcomes in heart failure; EASD: the European Association for the Study of Diabetes)

DECLARE-TIMI 58 Trial

It assessed patients with diabetes and risk factors for atherosclerotic cardiovascular disease receiving dapagliflozin. The session at ADA 2019 covered renal end points and other safety aspects. This trial showed that cardiorenal specific outcome was achieved across all subgroups analysis robustly. It imparts a message of potential kidney disease prevention in type 2 diabetes. It was the renal analysis by Mosenzon and colleagues who conducted in 17,160 participants with type 2 diabetes from the DECLARE-TIMI 58 trial. Median follow-up was for 4.2 years. This renal analysis showed a 40% reduction in eGFR to below 60 mL/min/1.73 m^2 threshold along with end-stage renal disease (ESRD) or renal or CV death. Primary cardiorenal outcome event rate was higher in the placebo group compared with the dapagliflozin group (5.3% vs 4.2%) and as was event rate for the renal-specific outcome (2.6% vs 1.5%; $p < 0.0001$) for both. It is worth to note that dapagliflozin treatment reduced the incidence of the primary outcome by 24% [hazard ratio

TABLE 3: REWIND Trial.[1,2]

What was cohort characteristics
• Total people: 9,901; Dulaglutide arm: 4,949, Placebo arm: 4,952
• Median follow-up period: 5.4 year
• People with low proportion with previous CVD: 31.5%
• High proportion of women: 46.3%
• Mean HbA1c: 7.3%
What was key outcomes
• The primary composite outcome occurrence 12% in dulaglutide arm versus 13.4% in placebo arm. (HR, 0.88, 95% CI: 0.79–0.99) P = 0.026.
• Renal benefits: Development of new microalbuminuria (HR, 0.77%; CI: 0.68–0.87) P = 0.0001 and sustained decline in eGFR of 30% or more (HR, 0.89; CI: 0.78–1.01) P = 0.066 in dulaglutide arm.
• Gastrointestinal adverse effect: 31.1% in dulaglutide arm (p < 0.0001)
What is unique about REWIND
• It prospectively tested the hypothesis for superiority in contrast to other trials
• Most of the participants did not have the previous CVD
• Longer median follow-up showed that CVD benefits of GLP-1RA extend much longer
• Showed safety and durability of dulaglutide on glucose, blood pressure and weight
Message
• Most important message knocks the door that dulaglutide can be in unique potion to use in middle-aged and older type 2 diabetes with either previous CVD or without CVD

(CI: confidence interval; CVD: cardiovascular disease; eGFR: estimated glomerular filtration rate; GLP-1RA: glucagon-like peptide-1 receptor agonist; HR: hazard ratio)

TABLE 4: CAROLINA Trial.[5]

What was cohort
• This is a pretty long CVOT trial, over a median of 6.3 years • 3,010 cohorts of linagliptin, 3,010 cohorts of glimepiride
Outcome
3 point MACE: • 11.8% of the linagliptin cohorts, 12% of the glimepiride cohorts (HR: 0.98; P = 0.7625); CV death (HR: 1.00; 5.6% vs 5.6%; P = 0.9863); Nonfatal MI (HR: 1.01; 4.8% vs 4.7%; P = 0.9060); Nonfatal stroke (HR: 0.87; 3.0% vs 3.5%; P = 0.3352) *Secondary end points*: • Hospitalization for heart failure (HR: 1.21; 3.7% vs 3.1%; P = 0.1761), CV death (HR: 1.00), non-CV death (HR: 0.82), all-cause mortality (HR: 0.91)
What was unique
• CAROLINA speaks in favor of linagliptin • In CAROLINA, a high proportion of patients within linagliptin group (16%) were able to achieve the secondary composite endpoint of treatment sustainability versus the glimepiride group (10. 2%) • Both demonstrated similar overall effects on HbA1c, relative risk for hypoglycemia was reduced by 77% by linagliptin (10.6% of patients treated with linagliptin experienced any hypoglycemic incident versus 37.7% for glimepiride) • Importantly the risk reduction was consistent and significant across all hypoglycemia categories • Linagliptin was also associated with a modest weight reduction of 1.5 kg versus glimepiride
Message
• This clearly indicates that there was no difference in overall composite endpoints of cardiovascular death • Even with individual component of CV death, nonfatal MI and nonfatal stroke, there was no significant difference • Secondary endpoints were also in the same direction • Secondary composite endpoint of treatment sustainability was much better with linagliptin • Risk of hypoglycemia was significantly less with linagliptin

(CI: confidence interval; CV: cardiovascular; CVOT: cardiovascular outcome trial; HR: hazard ratio; MACE: major adverse cardiovascular event; MI: myocardial infarction)

(HR) 0.76; 95% confidence interval (CI) 0.67–0.87] and the incidence of renal-only secondary outcome by 47% (HR 0.53; 95% CI: 0.43–0.66).[6,7]

CREDENCE and CARMELINA Trials (Tables 5 and 6)

At ADA, EASD key findings were reviewed and new data analyses presented. These major trials explored the effects of canagliflozin and linagliptin respectively, in patients with type 2 diabetes at high risk for renal and cardiovascular complications.

At ADA new linagliptin analyses was presented. It showed CV, renal safety across all age, and renal impairment groups. In established cardiovascular disease and renal impairment linagliptin did not increase risk for a new CV event. It also did not increase progression of renal disease regardless of age and level of renal impairment.

Although landmark CREDENCE trial was presented at International Society of Nephrology in April 2019 and made a big win showing with canagliflozin, there was 30% lower relative risk in composite of ESRD, doubling of serum creatinine level, or death from renal or cardiovascular causes. At ADA and EASD, CREDENCE again made highlights with primary and secondary subgroup analysis.[8]

DEFINE-HF and DAPA- HF (Table 1)

Both these trials attracted huge number of delegates at EASD. New metabolic and safety data were consistent with prior reports. Dapagliflozin now appears extremely safe, even in sickest group of patients.[9]

TRIAL IN RELATION TO ADULT MEDICATION STUDY

RISE

The RISE is a unique study in sense that it tested role of interventions to preserve or improve β-cell function

TABLE 5: CARMELINA Trial.[8]

New linagliptin analyses presented at ADA
What was cohort characteristics
• 6,979 type 2 diabetics with a history of vascular disease and a urinary albumin to creatinine ratio of at least 200 mg/g • 605 sites, 27 countries, mean diabetes duration—14.8 years
What is unique about CARMELINA
• It had highest proportion of individuals with reduced renal function compared with other DPP-4 inhibitors to date
What was key outcome
• Secondary renal outcome: 9.4% in linagliptin group, 8.8% in placebo group (HR, 1.04; 95% CI: 0.89–1.22) P = 0.62
Message
• Is linagliptin safe in high CV risk diabetics, including elderly—Yes • This trial showed no increase in risk for HF hospitalization in participants with high risk of HF including across renal function and age groups • As linagliptin reduced UACR over time including across UACR and renal function categories, improvement in albuminuria is likely • It proved categorically the CV and renal safety of linagliptin in those with type 2 diabetics at high cardiovascular risk when some degree of renal disease is associated

(CI: confidence interval; CV: cardiovascular; HF: heart failure; HR: hazard ratio; UACR: urine albumin-to-creatinine ratio)

TABLE 6: CREDENCE Trial.[8]

What was cohort characteristics
• No history of CVD, primary prevention cohort N = 2,181, 49.6% • With history of CVD or PVD, secondary prevention cohort: N, 2220, 50.5%
What was renal outcome
Canagliflozin reduced the risk of: • ESRD, doubling of serum creatinine, or renal or CV death by 30% • ESRD, doubling of serum creatinine and renal death by 34% • ESRD by 32% (exploratory outcome) (HR, 0.66, 95 CI: 0.53–0.81) P<0.001 • Dialysis, transplantation or renal death by 28% (post hoc outcome) (HR, 0.68, 95 CI: 0.54–0.86) P = 0.002 • Attenuated the slope of chronic eGFR decline by 2.7 mL/min/1.73 m^2/year (1.9 vs 4.6) • No risk of lower limb fractures, AKI or hyperkalemia
What was CV outcome
• Lower risk of MACE (HR, 0.80, 95% CI: 0.67–0.95) P = 0.01 • Lower risk of hospitalization with heart failure (HR, 0.61, 95% CI: 0.47–0.80) P<0.001
Message
• Deep dive into CV and renal outcomes and safety assurance, makes it the first antidiabetic to offer CV benefits in patients without a history of CVD • Well executed and clear-cut beneficial results keep the potential to change clinical practice

(AKI: acute kidney injury; CI: confidence interval; CV: cardiovascular; CVD: cardiovascular disease; eGFR: estimated glomerular filtration rate; ESRD: end-stage renal disease; HR: hazard ratio; PVD: peripheral vascular disease)

with medications in individuals with impaired glucose tolerance or early type 2 diabetes. In individuals with IGT or early type 2 diabetes, evaluating persistence of treatment-induced changes after a 3-month period of treatment withdrawal, it was shown that at the end of 12 months of treatment, significant increase in glucose-stimulated β-cell responses occurred and it was greatest in the liraglutide and metformin group but without persisting effects when interventions were withdrawn. So, current available strategies need to be continued to restore β-cell function in prediabetes.[10]

VERIFY (See Table 1)

It was presented for the first time at EASD, although gives a message of durability of metformin and vildagliptin combination as initiation therapy, it has no potential to change any guideline.[11]

Imeglimin (See Table 1)

Trial result of this new drug was presented at EASD and it was a major attraction. This drug has potential to change the landscape of therapy due to its robust efficacy and safety including elderly and chronic kidney disease (CKD) diabetic patients. It improves mitochondrial function.[12]

NEW THERAPEUTIC APPROACH IN TYPE 1

Trial Net Results: Game Changer

Teplizumab (Fc receptor-nonbinding anti-CD3 monoclonal antibody) is a drug that disrupts the immune system's destruction of β cells. It is known that relatives of people with type 1 diabetes are significantly more likely to develop the disease themselves. A randomized, placebo-controlled, double blind study, known as TrialNet, using Teplizumab, showed that at the end of the trial, individuals in the treatment group who developed type 1 diabetes did so an average of 2 years later in comparison with those who received placebo. Importantly median delay in the diagnosis of diabetes for 2 years is exciting. The percentage of diabetes free persons in teplizumab group was 57% and in the placebo group was 28%. This was a phase 2 trial and a single course of teplizumab significantly slowed progression to clinical type 1 disease in those who were at high risk, (nondiabetic relatives of patients with type 1 diabetes having at least two autoantibodies and abnormal glucose tolerance test). The message of the trial is that this drug could be promising prevention strategy for type 1 diabetes supporting the notion that type 1 diabetes is a chronic T-cell-mediated disease and immunomodulation could be an answer. This trial concludes stating that a 2-week course of teplizumab delays the diagnosis of clinical type 1 diabetes in high-risk participants. It is worth to note that for the first time such study to delay type1 diabetes was presented at ADA.[13]

TRIAL IN RELATION TO DIABETES PREVENTION

D2d Study (Table 7)

The mystery to prevent type 2 diabetes by supplementation of vitamin D is still not completely solved even after very important D2d study. At present message is that any

TABLE 7: D2d trial.[1,12]

What was cohort characteristics
• Total number of participants: 2,423; Vitamin D group N = 1,211; Placebo group N = 1,212 • Mean serum 25-hydroxyvitamin D in vitamin D group = 54 ng/mL from base line of 28.2 ng/mL
What was outcome
• Mean follow-up—2.5 years • Primary outcome of diabetes in vitamin D3 group—9.39 (HR: 0.88; 95% CI: 0.75–1.04, p = 0.12) and in placebo group; 10.66 events per 100 person-years
What is unique
• This trial is the largest of a number of randomized controlled trials which looked into role of vitamin D supplementation to prevent progression of type 2 diabetes and was long awaited
Message
• If there is no vitamin D3 insufficiency state among persons at high risk for type 2 diabetes, there is no need of supplementation of vitamin D3 at a dose of 4,000 IU per day as it does not significantly lower risk of diabetes • It will be erroneous to conclude from this trial that there is no role of vitamin D in diabetes prevention in those with very low vitamin D (<12 ng/mL) as this issue in unresolved • In post hoc analysis of D2d trial, vitamin D supplementation potentially had a benefit in those with very low vitamin D levels

(CI: confidence interval; HR: hazard ratio)

benefit of vitamin D for type 2 diabetes prevention, if present is modest and clearly does not signify to a vitamin D-sufficient population. Even targeting populations with levels below 12 ng/mL has got effect on β-cell function and progression remains unresolved. One important question this trial raised that whether BMI modifies the vitamin D effects. Also it must be appreciated that a longer intervention might have provided different findings. In this sense this well deigned and rigorously conducted trial was underpowered and missed the bus.[14,15]

PREVIEW Study

The PREVIEW was a much talked, largest multinational diet and exercise related study to understand effect of intensive weight loss, behavior change on prevention of diabetes in adults. In this trial an initial weight loss of at least 8% over 8 weeks with intervention of meal replacement products followed by lifestyle intervention of diet and physical activity to maintain weight for a 3-year period, markedly reduces the number of new diabetes cases. The message in simple way is that keeping the weight off after first achieving weight loss in initial 8 weeks, diabetes prevention is possible. In this study, only 50% participants achieved the initial weight loss in spite of a high-intensity program and this the other side of the story.[16]

COMPLICATIONS IN YOUNG ADULTS

TODAY-2 Study

This is told to be the first multicentric, multiethnic, randomized trial which examined youth-onset type 2 diabetes documenting the course of type 2 diabetes and its comorbidities like renal, eye, cardiac, nerve in the transition from youth to young adulthood. In the Longitudinal Outcomes in Youth with Type 2 Diabetes (TODAY-2) study, those young people diagnose with type 2 diabetes in their early teens were found having alarming high rate of diabetes associated complications. It occurred when they hit their mid-20s. CV risk factors are highly prevalent in these population and target organ damage is evident. Many kids in the study population had very rapid course in terms of loss of glycemic control and development of complications. This study suggests to adopt a more aggressive approach to control diabetes. The primary objective of this study is to track the progression of type 2 diabetes and related complication and comorbidities as the transition to young adulthood. The primary objective of TODAY-2 is to track the progression of type 2 diabetes and related comorbidities and complications as the participant's transition to young adulthood. This cohort study has given a very alarming signal.[17]

CONCLUSION

American Diabetes Association 2019, San Francisco brought very exciting and decision changing conclusive trials. It paves further new perspective ways for better care of diabetes patients. At EASD-Barcelona, three important new trials were presented, namely, VERIFY, CONCLUDE[18] and PRIORITY. Several new analyses and very fruitful review sessions were very useful and exciting.

REFERENCES

1. American Diabetes Association. Once-weekly dulaglutide and major cardiovascular events: results of the REWIND trial. Presented at American Diabetes Association 79th Scientific Sessions. San Francisco: American Diabetes Association; 2019.
2. Gerstein HC, Colhoun HM, Dagenais GR, et al. Dulaglutide and cardiovascular outcomes in type 2 diabetes (REWIND): a double-blind, randomised placebo-controlled trial. Lancet. 2019;394(10193):121-30.
3. Montanya E, Rosenstock J, Canani LH, et al. PIONEER – 2. Presented at American Diabetes Association. 79th scientific sessions 2019, June 7–11, San Francisco, CA. Abstract number 54—OR doi,org/10.2337/db19.
4. Pratley RE, Amod A, Hoff ST, et al: PIONEER 4. Presented at American Diabetes Association. 79th scientific sessions 2019, June 7–11, San Francisco, CA. Abstract number 55—OR doi,org/10.2337/db19
5. American Diabetes Association. CAROLINA: Cardiovascular safety and renal microvascular outcome with linagliptin in patients with T2D at high vascular risk. Oral presented at the American Diabetes Association 79th Scientific Sessions. San Francisco: American Diabetes Association; 2019.
6. Mosenzon O, Wiviott SD, Cahn A, et al. Effects of dapagliflozin on development and progression of kidney disease in patients with type 2 diabetes: an analysis from the DECLARE-TIMI 58 randomised trial. Lancet Diabetes Endocrinol. 2019;7(8):606-617.
7. Raz I. Effects of dapagliflozin on the urinary albumin-to-creatinine ratio in patients with type 2 diabetes: A predefined analysis from the DECLARE-TIME 58 randomised placebo-controlled trial. Presented at American Diabetes Association 79th Scientific Sessions. San Francisco: American Diabetes Association; 2019.
8. American Diabetes Association. CREDENCE AND CARMELINA: results from two major clinical trials in kidney and cardiovascular disease in diabetes Presented at: American Diabetes Association 79th Scientific Sessions. San Francisco: American Diabetes Association; 2019.
9. Nassif ME, et al. Dapagliflozin Effects on Biomarkers, Symptoms, and Functional Status in Patients With Heart Failure With Reduced Ejection Fraction The DEFINE-HF Trial Circulation. 2019; [Epub ahead of print] and Mikhil Kosiborod M. Background, design and results of DAPA-HF-key cardiovascular outcomes trial. Presented at 55th EASD congress. European Association for the Study of Diabetes: Barcelona; 2019.
10. American Diabetes Association. Results and comparisons from the RISE Clinical Trial: Adult Medication Study. Presented at: American Diabetes Association 79th Scientific Sessions. San Francisco: American Diabetes Association; 2019.

11. Mathews DR, Paldánius PM, Proot P, et al. Glycemic durability of an early combination therapy with vildagliptin and metformin monotherapy in newly diagnosed type 2 diabetes (VERIFY): a 5-year, multicentric, randomised, double-blind trial. Lancet. 2019; published online Sept18:https//doi.org/10.1016/S0140-6736(19)32131-2 and presented at 55th EASD congress 2019, Barcelona.
12. Dubourg J, DeFronzo R. Clinical evidence to support the safety of Imeglimin in type2 diabetes. Presented at 55th EASD congress. Barcelona: European Association for the Study of Diabetes; 2019.
13. Herold KC, Bundy BN, Long SA, et al. An Anti-CD3 Antibody, Teplizumab, in Relatives at Risk for Type 1 Diabetes. N Engl J Med. 2019;381(7): 603-13.
14. American Diabetes Association. The Vitamin D and Type 2 Diabetes (D2d) study: a multicentric randomised controlled trial for diabetes prevention. Presented at American Diabetes Association 79th Scientific Sessions. San Francisco: American Diabetes Association; 2019.
15. Wexler DJ. D2d—No Defense against Diabetes. N Engl J Med. 2019;381:581-2.
16. Macdonald I. Prevention of diabetes through lifestyle intervention: results from the multicenter PREVIEW study. Presented at American Diabetes Association 79th Scientific Sessions. San Francisco: American Diabetes Association; 2019.
17. Zeitler PS. Lead investigator of the TODAY studies. Press briefing ADA report. Very young T2DM high complication rate 20 years later, TODAY-2. 79th American Diabetes Association (ADA) 2019 Scientific Sessions. San Francisco: American Diabetes Association; 2019.
18. Philis-Tsimikas A, Pieber TR et al. CONCLUDE Trial, Presented at European Association for Study of Diabetes, Annual Meeting 2019, Sept 16–20, Barcelona, Spain.

57 CHAPTER The Clinical Recommendations for Measuring Lipoproteins to Manage ASCVD Risk

NK Agrawal, Ranjan Asha, Bharmal Vahid

INTRODUCTION

Atherosclerosis involves deposition of lipids and lipoproteins along with onset of chronic inflammation in large- and medium-sized arteries. The association of atherosclerosis and raised cholesterol levels has been widely studied and acknowledged. Circulating low-density lipoprotein (LDL) traverses endothelium and gets deposited in arterial intima where they undergo oxidation, and are taken up by the macrophages leading to atherosclerosis.[1] The major atherosclerotic cardiovascular disease (ASCVD) events include coronary artery disease (CAD) (myocardial infarction or acute coronary syndrome within 12 months), ischemic stroke, symptomatic peripheral arterial disease (PAD), history of claudication or ankle-brachial index (ABI) <0.85 or previous revascularization or amputation. According to a WHO report, one-third of CAD events and 4.5% of total deaths are attributable to high cholesterol worldwide. It is not only a concern in developed world but has widely affected people in developing countries also, especially diabetic individuals. Global prevalence of raised total cholesterol among adults was 39% (37% for males and 40% for females). The total cholesterol was highest in prevalence in the WHO Region of Europe (54% for both sexes), followed by WHO Region of the Americas (48% for both sexes), The WHO African Region (22.6%), and the WHO South East Asian Region (29%).[2]

LIPOPROTEINS

Lipoproteins are particles in circulation that help to transport hydrophobic lipids like cholesterol ester and triglycerides (TGs) from intestine and liver to the peripheral tissues by complexing them with more polar cholesterol (unesterified cholesterol and phospholipids) and apolipoproteins. Lipoproteins are categorized according to density gradient of ultracentrifugation (Table 1). Apolipoproteins are proteins that act as targeting molecules for lipid modifying enzymes, or receptors and transporters. Each lipoprotein has different composition and properties.

Chylomicron and very low-density lipoprotein (VLDL) contain predominantly triglycerides (TGs), intermediate-density lipoprotein (IDL) contains both TGs and cholesterol, and LDL and HDL are cholesterol-carrying particles with very little associated TGs. This knowledge allows physicians to identify the most likely lipoprotein abnormality with serum TGs and cholesterol values. VLDL transports the TGs produced in liver and intestine to muscle and adipose tissue for use. Excess is re-esterified to glycerol and fat in adipose tissue. IDL are formed after removal of TGs from VLDL and are further metabolized to LDL. VLDL also accepts cholesterol from HDL mediated by cholesteryl ester transfer protein enzyme. LDL is major carrier of cholesterol in humans and supply cholesterol to tissues with higher cholesterol demands like adrenals, gonads and is the main lipoprotein implicated in causing atherogenic plaque formation. The diabetic individuals have smaller, denser subform of LDL-C (sd-LDL) which is more atherogenic. Circulating LDL is high in people who consume high saturated fats and cholesterol. HDL is smallest of all and carries lipid from peripheral tissues to liver and gut for excretion. It decreases atherosclerosis because of reverse transport process and proteins with anti-inflammatory and anti-oxidant properties. Lipoprotein (a) produced in liver consists of LDL particles in which apolipoprotein apo (a) has been covalently linked to apo B100. Apo (a) has substantial protein homology to

TABLE 1: Properties of various lipoproteins.

S.No.	Lipoproteins	Density (g/mL)	Size (nm)	Sources	Apolipoproteins	Other constituents	Composition
1	Chylomicrons	<0.95	100–500	Intestine	B48, AI, AIV, E, CI, CII, CIII	Retinyl esters	85% TGs
2	Very-low density lipoproteins (VLDL)	<1.006	30–80	Liver	B100, E CI, CII, CIII	Vitamin E	55%TGs 20% CHE
3	Intermediate-density lipoproteins (IDL)	1.006–1.109	25–35	Derived from VLDL	B100, E	Vitamin E	35% CHE 25% TGs
4	Low-density lipoprotein (LDL)	1.019–1.063	18–25	Derived from IDL	B100	Vitamin E	60% CHE 5% TGs
5	High-density lipoproteins (HDL)	1.063–1.21	5–12	Liver, intestine, plasma	AI, AII, C1 C2, C3, E	LCAT, CETP Paroxonase	25% PL 20% CHE 5% TGs
6	Lipoprotein a [Lp(a)]	1.05–1.09	30	Liver	B100, apo(a)		60% CHE 5% TGs

(CETP: cholesteryl ester transfer protein; CHE: cholesterol; LCAT: lecithin cholesterol acyltransferase; TGs: triglycerides)

plasminogen required for the endogenous thrombolytic response. Higher levels increase the risk of myocardial infarction (MI) and aortic valve calcification.[3]

ASCVD RISK, RISK ASSESSMENT, AND LIPOPROTEIN MEASUREMENT

The dominant form of atherogenic cholesterol is LDL-C. VLDL, which is the chief carrier of triglycerides, is also atherogenic. Chylomicron atherogenicity is uncertain due to their inability to traverse endothelium secondary to their large size. There is adequate evidence from animal studies, genetic forms of hypercholesterolemia, epidemiological studies, and randomized controlled trials (RCTs) that cholesterol contributes to the risk of ASCVD and reduction in its levels gives a protective effect.[4-7]

In addition to cholesterol, other risk factors for ASCVD include age >65 years, heterozygous familial hypercholesterolemia, prior history of CAD, prior coronary artery bypass surgery, percutaneous coronary intervention outside of the major ASCVD event, presence of diabetes mellitus, hypertension, CKD (eGFR 15–59 mL/min/1.73 m^2), current habit of smoking, constantly increased LDL-C (>100 mg/dL) in spite of maximally tolerated statin and ezetimibe therapy and congestive heart failure. Combining the contributions of these major risk factors into a prediction equation, life time risk in an individual for ASCVD can be assessed and this helps clinicians and patients to start pharmacologic and nonpharmacologic measures of risk reduction and to intensify the cholesterol-lowering drug therapy. The Framingham Heart Study took the lead to create risk prediction equations. Risk prediction equations modified in the 2013 ACC/AHA cholesterol guidelines collecting data from five community-based cohorts, which were mostly representative of the US population.[8] These are called population cohort equations (PCE). They have been validated now and can also be accessed online. ASCVD risk assessment should be started after 20 years age and assessed every 4 to 6 years. Risk assessment is not required in patients with primary hypercholesterolemia, diabetics, and in secondary prevention of ASCVD. In addition to major risk factors, there are certain risk-enhancing factors which include additional lipid biomarkers Lp (a), apo B100, and elevated primary hypertriglyceridemia (≥175 mg/dL).[9]

A relative indication of Lp(a) measurement is family history of premature ASCVD, premature ASCVD or personal history of ASCVD not explained by major risk factors. A level ≥50 mg/dL is significant.[9,10] Apo B48 and apo B100 are derived forms by unique mechanism that involves RNA editing only in intestine. There is one copy of apo B100 in each VLDL, IDL, and LDL particle. Measurement of apo B100 in plasma reflects this particle number and is useful in determining whether hypertriglyceridemia is an atherogenic condition. The measurement of apo B100 is advised when triglycerides are above 200 mg/dL and a level ≥130 mg/dL corresponds to an LDL-C >160 mg/dL.[9,11] These factors that enhance the risk can help in patients with intermediate risk which is defined as 7.5% to ≤20% risk of ASCVD in 10 years in comprehending patient characteristics that cause an increase in the ASCVD risk, both short- and long-term. These factors also decide the therapy initiation.

The common lipid estimation technique involves estimation of triglycerides and total cholesterol by enzymatic processes and then calculating LDL by using Friedewald formula [LDL-C = (TC) - (triglycerides/5) - (HDL-C)]. This formula assumes that cholesterol content of VLDL is 20% of plasma TGs levels.[12] This equation is fairly accurate when TGs are elevated up to levels below 400 mg. But in case of profound hypertriglyceridemia or when TGs to cholesterol ratio of VLDL differs from usual 4:1 (dysbetalipoproteinemia) or when LDL is <70 mg/dL, this calculation can be erroneous. Hence, LDL should be measured by direct methods in these settings. LDL-C level differs minimally with fasting and nonfasting state after taking normal food and hence samples in nonfasting state can be used for risk assessment in primary prevention and for assessment of baseline LDL-C levels before start of statin in primary and secondary prevention. In adults above 20 years of age who are not on lipid-lowering therapy, it is recommended that measurement of either fasting or a nonfasting plasma lipid profile is effective to estimate an ASCVD risk and documenting baseline LDL-C. In those who present with an initial nonfasting triglyceride level above 400 mg/dL, fasting state lipid profile should be repeated on another day. Fasting lipid profile is required to evaluate those with family history of premature ASCVD or genetic hyperlipidemia. Additionally, if LDL-C is <70 mg/dL, measurement of direct LDL-C or modified LDL-C estimate is rational. In case an extremely high-fat meal in the preceding 8 hours has been taken by an individual, he/she should be counseled to shun such meals and get test repeated on another day.[9]

In children and adolescents with risk factors like obesity, family history of early CVD or significant hypercholesterolemia, fasting or nonfasting lipoprotein profile as early as age of 2 years can be done. This helps to identify both severe hypercholesterolemia and multifactorial lifestyle-related dyslipidemia. Only a portion of childhood lipid abnormalities could be identified by selective screening for lipid disorders on the basis of family history or lifestyle-related factors [9]. Hence, universal pediatric lipid screening has been advised to reduce cardiovascular risk and promote heart health in children and adolescents particularly focusing on ages 9 to 11 years and then ages 17 to 21 years since TC and LDL-C levels reduce by 10–20% during puberty.[13] Reverse-cascade screening of family members, which includes cholesterol testing for first-, second-, and third-degree biological relatives should be performed in children and adolescents with moderate or severe hypercholesterolemia, for detection of familial forms of hypercholesterolemia.

Chronic inflammatory disorders or HIV are also factors that enhance risk and fasting lipid profile and assessment of ASCVD risk factors is useful to guide to benefit of statin therapy and tracking or tuning lipid lowering drug therapy before and 4 to 12 weeks after initiating inflammatory disease-modifying therapy or antiretroviral therapy.[9] Inflammation promotes atherosclerosis and mediated progression, instability, erosion, and rupture of vulnerable atherosclerotic plaques.[12] In adults with RA who undergo ASCVD risk assessment with measurement of a lipid profile, lipid values have to be rechecked and other major ASCVD risk factors 2 to 4 months after controlling the patient's inflammatory disease.

MANAGEMENT

Atherosclerotic cardiovascular disease (ASCVD) risk assessment is not required in patients with known ASCVD events (secondary prevention), severe hypercholesterolemia (LDL-C >190 mg/dL), and diabetes mellitus. Treatment with statins and other nonstatin drugs is immediately required in addition to lifestyle medication (diet, weight reduction, exercise, quitting smoking) in these patients. In patients with known ASCVD event with age ≤75 years, high intensity statin therapy (≥50% LDL-C reduction) should be initiated to keep LDL-C <70 mg/dL target. Ezetimibe therapy should be added if target is not achieved.[14] In very high-risk individuals with clinical ASCVD (history of multiple major ASCVD events or 1 major ASCVD event and multiple high-risk conditions), PCSK9 inhibitors can be added if target is not achieved with maximally tolerated statin and ezetimibe doses. A moderate- or high-intensity statin therapy should be added in patients aged >75 years with clinical ASCVD, after evaluating the potential for ASCVD risk reduction, adverse effects, and drug–drug interactions, as well as patient frailty.

In patients of severe hypercholesterolemia between age of 20 years and 75 years, high-dose statin therapy should be initiated. Patients who do not achieve <50% reduction in LDL-C on maximally tolerated statin therapy and or whose LDL-C remains >100 mg/dL or higher, ezetimibe therapy should be added or bile acid sequestrants may be added if fasting TGs are 300 mg/dL or less. PCSK9 inhibitor may be considered in patients with heterozygous familial hypercholesterolemia between age of 30 years and 75 years and in patients between age of 40 years and 75 years with a baseline LDL-C level of ≥220 mg/dL or on-treatment LDL-C ≥130 mg/dL while receiving maximally tolerated statin and ezetimibe therapy.[9]

The diabetic individuals, between age of 40 years and 75 years, should be started on moderate intensity statin therapy (30–49% LDL-C reduction) regardless of 10-year ASCVD risk to keep target LDL-C <70 mg/dL. However, 10-year ASCVD risk should be calculated for first ASCVD event in patients with diabetes too. In diabetics with multiple ASCVD risk factors, high-intensity statin therapy may be started with an objective to decrease LDL-C levels by 50% or more or to <70 mg/dL. Ezetimibe may be added to maximally tolerated statin therapy for reducing LDL-C levels by 50% or more. In adults >75 years age, with diabetes mellitus, initiation of statin therapy after a clinician-patient discussion of potential benefits and risks should be done and those already on statin therapy should continue it. Diabetic adults, aging between 20 years and 39 years, may be started on statin therapy based on diabetic-specific risk enhancers [long duration (≥10 years of type 2 diabetes mellitus, ≥20 years of type 1 diabetes mellitus), albuminuria (≥30 μg of albumin/mg creatinine), estimated glomerular filtration rate (eGFR) <60 mL/min/1.73 m^2, neuropathy, retinopathy or ABI <0.9)], initiating statin therapy may be reasonable.

For primary prevention of ASCVD in adults between age of 40 years and 75 years, decision regarding statin therapy should be made using estimated ASCVD risk for 10 years. However, lifestyle modification is encouraged in all the patients. The calculated risk is categorized in four categories from low to high (low risk: <5%; borderline risk: 5% to <7.5%; intermediate-risk: ≥7.5% to <20%; and high-risk: ≥20%). Lifestyle modification is recommended for low-risk individuals. In addition to lifestyle modification, moderate intensity statin may be added for patients with borderline risk and intermediate risk if ASCVD risk-enhancing factors [familial history of premature ASCVD; persistently elevated LDL-C levels ≥160 mg/dL; history of preeclampsia or premature menopause (age <40 years); metabolic syndrome; chronic kidney disease; chronic inflammatory disorders (e.g. rheumatoid arthritis, psoriasis, or chronic HIV); high-risk ethnic groups (e.g. South Asian); persistent increase in triglycerides ≥175 mg/dL and, apolipoprotein B ≥130 mg/dL, high-sensitivity C-reactive protein ≥2.0 mg/L, ankle-brachial index <0.9 and lipoprotein (a) ≥50 mg/dL] are present. In case of intermediate-risk or selected borderline-risk adults, if the choice about statin use remains unsure, use of coronary artery calcium (CAC) score should be opted. If CAC score is 0, statin therapy should be withheld and reassessed in 5 to 10 years; if CAC score is 1 to 99, statin therapy should be initiated for patients ≥55 years. If CAC score ≥ 100 or ≥75th percentile, start statin therapy. Intermediate-risk adults requiring more aggressive LDL-C lowering and in whom high-intensity statin is not acceptable or tolerated, ezetimibe or bile acid sequestrant may be added. In high-risk individuals, high-intensity statin therapy should be initiated to lower LDL to <70 mg/dL. In adults ≥75 years with LDL-C level of 70 to 189 mg/dL, initiate moderate-intensity statin and CAC score may be used to reclassify to avoid statin therapy in those with score of 0.[9]

In children and adolescents (age 10–19 years) with lipid disorders related to obesity, it is recommended to intensify lifestyle therapy and if LDL-C level remains persistently ≥190 mg/dL or ≥160 mg/dL or higher with clinical presentation of familial hypercholesterolemia (FH) or who do not respond adequately to 3 to 6 months of lifestyle therapy, it is recommended to initiate statin therapy. In adults of age 20 to 39 years, lifestyle modifications are advised and statins are added if LDL is ≥160 mg/dL or family history of premature ASCVD is present.[9,15]

In moderate hypertriglyceridemia (fasting or nonfasting triglycerides 175 to 499 mg/dL), it is recommended to treat lifestyle factors (obesity and metabolic syndrome), secondary factors (diabetes mellitus, chronic liver or kidney disease, nephrotic syndrome, hypothyroidism), and medications that increase triglycerides in the patients of ≥20 years age, and in adults of age 40–75 years with moderate or severe hypertriglyceridemia and ASCVD risk of 7.5% or higher, the following measures should be considered—initiation or intensification of statin therapy, reduction of triglycerides by implementation of a very low-fat diet, avoiding refined carbohydrates and alcohol, consuming omega-3 fatty acids, and fibrate therapy, if necessary, to prevent acute pancreatitis.

Chronic kidney disease in adults 40–75 years of age with LDL-C 70–189 mg/dL and 10-year ASCVD risk of ≥7.5%, not treated with dialysis or kidney transplantation, is a factor that enhances the risk and initiating a moderate-intensity statin or moderate-intensity statins combined with ezetimibe is helpful. Statins should be continued in adults with advanced kidney disease requiring dialysis treatment on LDL-lowering therapy. In adults with advanced kidney disease who need dialysis treatment, it is not recommended to initiate a statin.[9,16] LDL apheresis is an option in selective patients with severe hypercholesterolemia whose LDL-C is not adequately controlled with drug therapy like FH homozygotes from age of 7 onward if their serum cholesterol cannot be reduced by >50% and or decreased to ≤350 mg/dL by drug therapy; patients with either heterozygous FH or a family history of premature cardiac death whose coronary artery disease progresses and where LDL cholesterol remains >/= 190 mg/dL or is decreased by <40% with maximal drug therapy. LDL apheresis should also be considered for patients with aggressive progressing coronary disease and Lp(a) > 60 mg/L whose LDL cholesterol remains >130 mg/dL despite maximal drug therapy.[9,17]

Repeat lipid measurements are recommended to be done in 4–12 weeks to assess for adherence to treatment and also to calculate percentage reduction in LDL-C with lifestyle changes and medications after statin initiation or dose adjustment, repeated every 3 to 12 months as needed.

CONCLUSION

Atherosclerotic cardiovascular disease (ASCVD) risk assessment and lipids measurement should start after 20 years of age in adults and earlier, if family history of premature CAD or hypercholesterolemia and lifestyle-related risk factors are present. Nonfasting lipid assessment is adequate for risk assessment and baseline LDL assessment for initiating statin therapy. Fasting lipid assessment is to be done in state of marked hypertriglyceridemia. Apo B100 and Lp (a) measurement in certain situation helps to decide lipid-lowering strategy. All patients with known ASCVD event, severe hypercholesterolemia, calculated ASCVD risk of ≥20% should receive high-intensity statin therapy and all patients with diabetes between 40 years and 75 years of age should receive moderate intensity statin therapy.

REFERENCES

1. Tabas I, Williams KJ, Bore´n J. Subendothelial lipoprotein retention as the initiating process in atherosclerosis: update and therapeutic implications. Circulation. 2007;116:1832-44.
2. World Health Organization. Global Health Observatory (GHO) data. [online] Available from https://www.who.int/gho/ncd/risk_factors/cholesterol_text/en/ [Last accessed September, 2019].
3. Jameson JL, De Groot LJ, Kretser DM, et al. Endocrinology: Adult and Pediatric, 7th edition. Philadelphia: Elsevier Saunders; 2016.
4. Ference BA, Ginsberg HN, Graham I, et al. Low-density lipoproteins cause atherosclerotic cardiovascular disease. 1. Evidence from genetic, epidemiologic, and clinical studies. A consensus statement from the European Atherosclerosis Society Consensus Panel. Eur Heart J. 2017;38(32):2459-72.
5. Nordestgaard BG, Chapman MJ, Humphries SE, et al. European Atherosclerosis Society Consensus Panel. Familial hypercholesterolaemia is underdiagnosed and undertreated in the general population: guidance for clinicians to prevent coronary heart disease. Consensus Statement of the European Atherosclerosis Society. Eur Heart J. 2013;34:3478-90.
6. Lewington S, Whitlock G, Clarke R, et al. Blood cholesterol and vascular mortality by age, sex, and blood pressure: a meta-analysis of individual data from 61 prospective studies with 55,000 vascular deaths. Lancet. 2007;370:1829-39.
7. Collins R, Reith C, Emberson J, et al. Interpretation of the evidence for the efficacy and safety of statin therapy. Lancet. 2016;388:2532-61.
8. Goff DC Jr, Lloyd-Jones DM, Bennett G, et al. 2013 ACC/AHA guideline on the assessment of cardiovascular risk: a report of the American College of Cardiology/American Heart Association Task Force on Practice Guidelines. J Am Coll Cardiol. 2014;63(25):2935-59.
9. Grundy SM, Stone NJ, Bailey AL, et al. Clinical Practice Guideline 2018 AHA/ACC/AACVPR/AAPA/ABC/ACPM/ADA/AGS/APhA/ASPC/NLA/PCNA Guideline on the Management of Blood Cholesterol. A Report of the American College of Cardiology/American Heart Association. Task Force on Clinical Practice Guidelines. J Am Coll Cardiol. 2019;73:e 285-350.
10. Klingel R, Heibges A, Fassbender C. Lipoprotein(a) and mortality—a high risk relationship. Clin Res Cardiol Suppl. 2019;14(1):13.
11. Robinson JG, Williams KJ, Gidding S, et al. Eradicating the Burden of Atherosclerotic Cardiovascular Disease by Lowering Apolipoprotein B Lipoproteins Earlier in Life. J Am Heart Assoc. 2018;7(20):e009778.
12. Smith AJ, Turner EL, Kinra S. Universal cholesterol screening in childhood: a systematic review. Acad Pediatr. 2016;16:716-25.
13. Mason JC, Libby P. Cardiovascular disease in patients with chronic inflammation: mechanisms underlying premature cardiovascular events in rheumatologic conditions. Eur Heart J. 2015;36(8):482-9.
14. Sabatine MS, Giugliano RP, Keech AC, et al. Evolocumab and clinical outcomes in patients with cardiovascular disease. N Engl J Med. 2017;376:1713-22.
15. Lozano P, Henrikson NB, Morrison CC, et al. Lipid screening in childhood and adolescence for detection of multifactorial dyslipidemia: evidence report and systematic review for the US Preventive Services Task Force. JAMA. 2016;316:634-44.
16. Cholesterol Treatment Trialists' (CTT) Collaboration; Herrington W, Emberson J, Mihaylova B, et al. Impact of renal function on the effects of LDL cholesterol lowering with statin-based regimens: a meta-analysis of individual participant data from 28 randomised trials. Lancet Diabetes Endocrinol. 2016;4:829-39.
17. Thompson GR. Recommendations for the use of LDL apheresis. Atherosclerosis. 2008;198(2):247-55.

58 CHAPTER Genetic Predisposition to Complications of Diabetes

Jalees Fatima, Mohd Talib

INTRODUCTION

Diabetes mellitus is a chronic metabolic disorder which exerts its effects over a period of time and manifests with multiorgan involvement leading to complications which are classified as either microvascular or macrovascular.

Microvascular complications of diabetes include diabetic retinopathy, diabetic nephropathy, and diabetic neuropathy, and macrovascular complications include coronary artery disease, peripheral vascular disease, and stroke.[1]

There is clear evidence that onset and progression of chronic complications is associated with duration and control of diabetes.[2–4]

The upcoming data, however, suggest profound variation in the occurrence of these complications, irrespective of the duration and degree of hyperglycemia and the presence of known risk factors. Thus, indicating a genetic basis for individual, familial or subgroup susceptibility to the complications of diabetes. Diabetic nephropathy along with other complications has been shown to be having strong familial association signaling possible genetic linkages.[5-7]

Population subgroups having either very low risk or high risk of developing complications are more likely to have genetic association because in others the conventional known risk factors such as hypertension, persistent poor glycemic control, dyslipidemia, and cigarette smoking play a key role in pathogenesis.

Therefore, the researchers have addressed these extreme subgroups at two ends of the spectrum for revealing genetic markers of predisposition to or protection from complications of diabetes, irrespective of known risk factors.

The results of these studies would pave way to detect genes, the presence of which may help protect an individual from complications of diabetes, despite being exposed to high risk factors. Focused research has also been done to recognize population groups having higher genetic linkages to microvascular complications despite absence of conventional risk factors.[7]

Genetic factors have been implicated in many complications of diabetes and this has been supported by results of many studies.

DIABETIC NEPHROPATHY

Among the patients developing diabetic nephropathy, approximately 50% have uncontrolled hyperglycemia and half of these develop this complication in spite of having good glycemic control.

Diabetic nephropathy has been seen to occur with high clustering in certain families in genetic studies. There is growing evidence in favor of genetic predisposition or protection of diabetic nephropathy which may not be explained by conventional risk factors. Research evidence on inheritance of diabetes complications has clearly demonstrated presence of albuminuria as one trait to which there is genetic predisposition.

Nearly one-third of genetic variance of albuminuria can be attributed to familial predisposition.[7]

Various genetic modalities have been applied to determine specific genes or loci that can possibly be implicated in progression of diabetic nephropathy.

Genetic linkage analysis along with genetic association analysis has led to identification of many genes or genetic variants responsible for susceptibility to diabetic nephropathy.

Many genetic loci have been identified by application of genetic linkage analysis in related individuals with use of rare variant hypothesis. These studies have been done on pairs of sibling or first degree relatives or families.[8]

Common variant hypothesis has been used in identification of genetic susceptibility pattern through dense marker map.[8]

Mitochondrial DNA mutations have also been implicated in progression of diabetic microvascular complications.

Better understanding of development and progression of diabetic nephropathy have been made possible using Mitochondrial DNA genome association studies and *copy number variation analysis.*[9]

Another hypothesis supports effect of *epigenetic factors*. According to this, environmental factors lead to variations in cellular chromatin thereby affecting transcription process of genes, in turn leading to development of diabetic nephropathy.[10]

Preventive measures can be planned for diabetic individuals with higher susceptibility to develop complication based on these genetic studies.

Multifactorial causation of diabetic nephropathy, thus involves extracellular matrix homeostasis in the background of a complex interaction between environment, epigenetic, and genetic factors.

Hyperglycemia in this context acts as a catalyst because it may cause increased synthesis of mitochondrial superoxide which thereby leads to overactivation of protein kinase C, overproduction of advanced glycation end products, and enhanced availability of glucose for hexosamine biosynthesis pathway.

Genetic variability in biochemical pathways along with environmental triggers leads to growth factor activation, thereby causing increased synthesis and deposition of extracellular matrix, which is the final pathophysiological pathway for progression to diabetic nephropathy.

Genetic polymorphisms within various specific (candidate) genes involved in various biochemical pathways have been implicated including bradykinin, renin-angiotensin-aldosterone-system (RAAS), nitric oxide synthase (NOS), aldose reductase, transforming growth factor alpha (TGF-α), and glucose transporter 1 (GLUT1).

Genomic mapping studies have not been done extensively for diabetic nephropathy and very few are available in literature. Chromosome 7 q was found to be strongly linked to diabetic nephropathy and retinopathy in a study done on Pima Indians.[9-11]

Angiotensin II type 1 receptor gene (*AGTR1*) linkages were found to be strongly associated in population involving type 1 diabetes with diabetic nephropathy.[12]

Strong linkage with chromosome 18 was found in genome scan of Turkish population with type 2 diabetes and significantly higher rates of consanguineous marriages.[13]

Familial associations of genetic locus for nephropathy involving chromosome 3, chromosome 7p, and chromosome 18q was found in 30%, 40%, and 65% families, respectively.

Angiotensin-converting enzyme (ACE), fatty acid binding protein 2 (FABP2), ectonucleotide pyrophosphatase/phosphodiesterase (ENPP1), and GLUT1 genes have been found to be linked with diabetic nephropathy in many gene association studies.

In GoKinD (Genetics of Kidneys in Diabetes) study involving diabetic subjects with or without diabetic nephropathy and characterized by long duration of diabetes, whole genome wide association scan was done and the results were used in Diabetes Control and Complications Trial (DCCT)/Epidemiology of Diabetes Interventions and Complications (EDIC) trial.[13]

Single nucleotide polymorphism located on chromosome 9p near FRMD3, showed strong genetic association and other SNPs having linkage were traced to CHN2 and CPVL on chromosome 7p, CARS on 11p, and on chromosome13q.[14] Single nucleotide polymorphism of 13q has also been found to be implicated with diabetic kidney disease in a Japanese meta-analysis.

DIABETIC CARDIOVASCULAR COMPLICATIONS

Presence of coronary calcium scoring and carotid artery intima media thickness (CIMT) as surrogate markers of cardiovascular disease variations of up to 40–50 % have been linked to familial factors amongst diabetes patients in various genetic analysis studies.

19q locus has been found to be having most significant genetic association in linkage study amongst Caucasians.[13]

Coronary artery disease (CAD) and stroke have been found to be strongly associated with polymorphisms in *APOE, APOB*, or *APOC genes.*

In subjects of type 2 diabetes selected from varying ethnicity, rs662, rs854560, and Q191R polymorphisms of paraoxonases (PON) gene have been strongly linked to development of cardiovascular disease.

Two fold risk of myocardial infarction is associated with polymorphism of *rs662 gene* harboring its G allele.

Polymorphisms in cholesteryl ester transfer protein (*CETP)* rs1800774 have strong association with CAD and

CVA risk in diabetic patients irrespective of presence or severity of dyslipidemia.

miRNA ASSOCIATION ANALYSIS

MicroRNAs are 22- nucleotide RNAs which are noncoding, may be regulated by epigenetic effects and can degrade normal RNAs. They exert significant effects on end organ tissues like heart, muscles, other viscera, and endothelium. They can regulate important metabolic pathways in individuals and may cause insulin resistance. Recent studies indicate their role in vascular complications of diabetes especially cardiac and endothelial dysfunction.

DIABETIC RETINOPATHY

Duration of diabetes, glycemic control, and hypertension has been implicated in development of diabetic retinopathy in many studies; however, these risk factors have not been found to have a consistent association in all patients. A number of patients develop diabetic retinopathy in absence of known risk associations.

With this view, genetic susceptibility analysis performed in a cohort study in Finland have found >50% inheritance of diabetic retinopathy.

Looker et al. performed genome wide linkage analysis for patients of diabetic retinopathy involving North American population and found strong association with chromosome 3 and 12.[14]

Association of HbA1c levels with diabetic retinopathy have been found in a study done on Caucasians which identified *RAGE* gene, the postulated mechanism being tissue injury as a result of direct tissue injury by advanced glycation end products.

Similar results have been found in other studies involving Asian Indians population.[15]

Polymorphism of the *VEGF gene* has been found to be associated in several candidate gene studies, done in subjects of different ethnic backgrounds with proliferative diabetic retinopathy especially with new vessel formation.[16]

Another gene *ALR 2* has been identified and its polymorphisms have been found to be reproducibly associated irrespective of ethnic variability.

CONCLUSION

Significant research and efforts have been put, focusing on finding relationship between complications of diabetes and genetic factors.

Several genetic loci have been found to be associated in diabetic nephropathy in various studies but no specific gene has been implicated as a single consistent determinant.

Angiotensin-converting enzyme, FABP2, ENPP1, and GLUT1, have been found to be associated with diabetic nephropathy in many gene association analysis studies; however, the results were not reproducible with ethnic variations. The link of *ALR2, VEGF,* and *RAGE* genes with proliferative diabetic retinopathy in genetic association analyses has been consistent to some extent.

Chromosome 9p21 links with CAD and diabetes mellitus have been proven suggesting significant genetic association between these two entities.

Role of miRNA in insulin metabolism and its association with diabetes onset and progression can be utilized for new advances in diabetes care.

Efforts need to be done to identify cardinal events in disease progression so as to provide better understanding of spectrum of disease ranging from reversible to irreversible and to thereby find ways to prevent the onset and reverse the progression of complications of diabetes and develop new therapeutic avenues.

A broader approach to study of genetic basis is required in order to establish specific genetic linkages which can be applied in management of complications of diabetes.

REFERENCES

1. Orasanu G, Plutzky J. The pathologic continuum of diabetic vascular disease. J Am Coll Cardiol. 2009;53(5 Suppl):S35-42.
2. Rewers M, LaPorte RE, King H, et al. Trends in the prevalence and incidence of diabetes: Insulin-dependent diabetes mellitus in childhood. World Health Stat Q. 1988;41(3-4):179-89.
3. Rewers MJ. The changing face of the epidemiology of insulin-dependent diabetes mellitus (IDDM): Research designs and models of disease causation. Ann Med.1991;23(4):419-26.
4. Pociot F, McDermott MF. Genetics of type 1 diabetes mellitus. Genes Immun. 2002;3(5):235-49.
5. Bell GI, Polonsky KS. Diabetes mellitus and genetically programmed defects in beta-cell function. Nature. 2001;414(6865):788-91.
6. Saltiel AR, Kahn CR. Insulin signalling and the regulation of glucose and lipid metabolism. Nature. 2002;414(6865):799-806.
7. Weijnen CF, Rich SS, Meigs JB, et al. Risk of diabetes in siblings of index cases with type 2 diabetes: Implications for genetic studies. Diabet Med. 2002;19(1):41-50.
8. Demenais F, Kanninen T, Lindgren CM, et al. A meta-analysis of four European genome screens (GIFT Consortium) shows evidence for a novel region on chromosome 17p11.2-q22 linked to type 2 diabetes. Hum Mol Genet. 2003;12(15):1865-73.
9. Imperatore G, Hanson RL, Pettitt DJ, et al. Sib-pair linkage analysis for susceptibility genes for microvascular complications among Pima Indians with type 2 diabetes. Pima Diabetes Genes Group. Diabetes. 1998;47(5):821-30.

10. Vardarli I, Baier L, Hanson JA, et al. Gene for susceptibility to diabetic nephropathy in type 2 diabetes maps to 18q22.3-23. Kidney Int. 2002;62(6):2176-83.
11. Pezzolesi MG, Poznik GD, Mychaleckyj JC, et al. Genome-wide association scan for diabetic nephropathy susceptibility genes in type 1 diabetes. Diabetes. 2009;58(6):1403-10.
12. Maeda S, Araki S, Babazono T, et al. Replication study for the association between four Loci identified by a genome-wide association study on European American subjects with type 1 diabetes and susceptibility to diabetic nephropathy in Japanese subjects with type 2 diabetes. Diabetes. 2010;59(8):2075-9.
13. Elbein SC, Hasstedt SJ. Quantitative trait linkage analysis of lipid-related traits in familial type 2 diabetes: evidence for linkage of triglyceride levels to chromosome 19q. Diabetes. 2002;51(2):528-35.
14. Looker HC, Nelson RG, Chew E, et al. Genome-wide linkage analyses to identify Loci for diabetic retinopathy. Diabetes. 2007;56(4):1160-6.
15. Lindholm E, Bakhtadze E, Sjogren M, et al. The -374 T/A polymorphism in the gene encoding RAGE is associated with diabetic nephropathy and retinopathy in type 1 diabetic patients. Diabetologia. 2006;49:2745-55.
16. Awata T, Inoue K, Kurihara S, et al. A common polymorphism in the 5-untranslated region of the VEGF gene is associated with diabetic retinopathy in type 2 diabetes. Diabetes. 2002;51(5):1635-9.

59 CHAPTER Hypoglycemia-associated Autonomic Failure

Meena Chhabra

INTRODUCTION

What is Hypoglycemia?

Hypoglycemia, or low blood sugar or low blood glucose, takes place when the glucose level in blood drops to lower than the normal range of 70 mg/dL or less. However, the glucose level that defines hypoglycemia is variable. This results in a variety of symptoms such as trouble in talking, clumsiness, confusion, feeling of hunger, and sweatiness.

What is Hypoglycemia-associated Autonomic Failure?

The concept of hypoglycemia-associated autonomic failure (HAAF) limits the ability of diabetic patients to attain target glycemia. This suggests that recent antecedent iatrogenic hypoglycemia leads to both defective glucose counter-regulation and hypoglycemia unawareness, and therefore a vicious cycle of recurrent hypoglycemia ensues. The most compelling support for HAAF is perhaps the fact that as little as 2–3 weeks of scrupulous avoidance of the hypoglycemia reverses hypoglycemia unawareness and leads to improvement in the reduced epinephrine component of defective glucose counter-regulation in most of the affected individuals. Insight into this pathophysiology has resulted in a wider view of the clinical risk factors for hypoglycemia to take into account the indexes of the compromised glucose counter-regulation and provided a framework for studying the mechanisms of iatrogenic hypoglycemia and, finally, its eradication from the lives of diabetic people.

In individuals with type I diabetes (Fig. 1) as well as in those with advanced type II diabetes, the clinical impact of HAAF is well known. In most of the affected patients, it is now considered to be mainly reversible, by as little as 2–3 weeks of scrupulous avoidance of hypoglycemia. However, the mechanisms of HAAF and its component syndromes are largely unknown. The loss of the glucagon secretory response, which is an important feature of defective glucose counter-regulation, is described by deficiency of insulin, particularly loss of the decrement in intraislet insulin that normally signals secretion of glucagon with a fall in the levels of glucose. Decreased neurogenic symptoms, which is an important feature of hypoglycemia unawareness, are mainly due to decreased sympathetic neural responses to falling levels of glucose. The process by which hypoglycemia shifts the glycemic

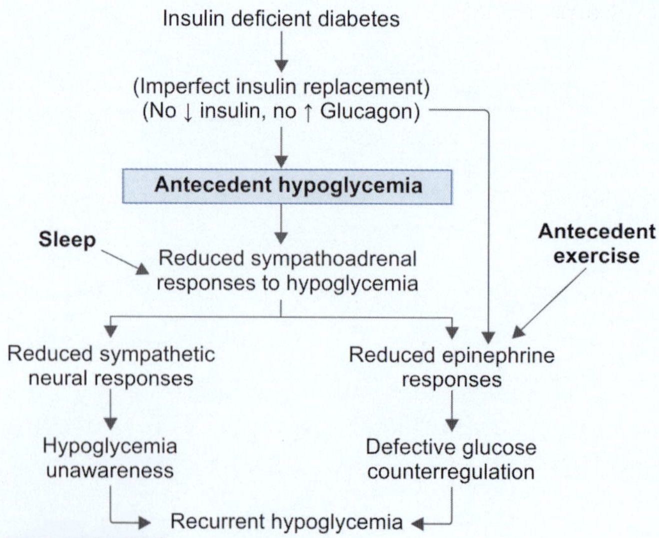

Flowchart 1 Hypoglycemia-associated autonomic failure in type 1 diabetes.

thresholds for the sympathoadrenal activation to lower concentrations of plasma glucose is still not known. It does not seem to be due to the release of a systemic mediator (such as epinephrine and cortisol) during antecedent hypoglycemia or due to enhanced blood-to-brain glucose transport, though increase in transport of optional fuels is conceivable. It is possibly due to changes of brain metabolism.

It also raised the probability that HAAF could result from posthypoglycemic brain glycogen supercompensation. Finally, various causes of HAAF seem to exist. These consist of exercise and sleep-related HAAF along with recent antecedent hypoglycemia.

CLINICAL SIGNIFICANCE

Iatrogenic hypoglycemia is the limiting factor in the glycemic management of diabetes. This happens because there is a mismatch between drugs given, food, and exercise that maintain the blood sugar level.

Effects of HAAF

- Episodes of hypoglycemia, even asymptomatic episodes, may prove to be fatal. Besides it can affect diabetes patients in the following ways:
  - Recurrent morbidity in type I/II diabetics
  - Impairs defenses against subsequent hypoglycemia
  - May lead to clinical syndromes related to defective glucose counter-regulation and hypoglycemia unawareness
  - May lead to a vicious cycle of recurrent hypoglycemia
  - Can prevent in maintaining euglycemia throughout the lifetime
  - Prevents complete realization of the advantages of glycemic control.

Although glycemic control short of euglycemia decreases (but does not eliminate) the microvascular complications of diabetes, in a large proportion of people with diabetes, long-term euglycemia may be important to reduce macrovascular complications.

In spite of the gradual improvements in glycemic management of diabetes and perhaps owing to the impetus for glycemic control arising from the positive results of the Diabetes Control and Complications Trial and the United Kingdom Prospective Diabetes Study, it is indicated by the population-based data that hypoglycemia remains a problem for people with both type I and type II diabetes.

Eliminating the risk of hypoglycemia from lives of diabetic people and maintaining euglycemia for long term will undoubtedly need glucose-regulated insulin replacement or secretion. Pending that final goal, there is an essential requirement of developing therapeutic strategies that minimize both hypoglycemia and hyperglycemia. It is a hypothesis that in type I and type II diabetes, these improved strategies will be on the basis of insight into the pathophysiology of glucose regulation, particularly glucose counter-regulation. In insulin-deficient (type I and advanced type II) diabetes, the integrated pathophysiology has been reviewed with the focus being on what is known and what is unknown, the concept of HAAF, and the mechanisms of the clinical syndromes of defective glucose counter-regulation and hypoglycemia unawareness.

PATHOPHYSIOLOGY OF GLUCOSE COUNTER-REGULATION IN DIABETES

The essential components of the physiology of glucose counter-regulation, which are the mechanisms normally preventing or rapidly correcting the hypoglycemia, are as follows:

- Reduction in pancreatic islet beta-cell insulin secretion
- Increase in pancreatic islet alpha-cell glucagon secretion and absence of the latter
- Increase in adrenomedullary epinephrine secretion.

In insulin-deficient type I and advanced type II diabetes, all the above three defenses against developing hypoglycemia are compromised.

It was found that iatrogenic hypoglycemia in such patients is due to the interplay of relative or absolute insulin excess that must take place from time to time owing to the pharmacokinetic imperfections of all therapeutic insulin regimens, in addition to the compromised glucose counter-regulation. With the fall in concentrations of plasma glucose, concentrations of plasma insulin do not decrease and those of plasma glucagon do not increase but the concentrations of plasma epinephrine increase, though the rise is typically attenuated; the glycemic thresholds for sympathoadrenal activation are typically shifted to lower plasma glucose concentrations. The latter, which is a critical feature of the pathophysiology of glucose counter-regulation, usually results from recent antecedent iatrogenic hypoglycemia, though sleep, and to some extent previous exercise, have the same effect.

Therefore, in the setting of absent beta-cell insulin and alpha-cell glucagon responses, an attenuated adrenomedullary epinephrine response to declining plasma glucose concentrations results in the clinical syndrome of defective glucose counter-regulation. The patients who are affected have 25-fold or more increased risk of severe iatrogenic hypoglycemia during aggressive glycemic therapy. An attenuated sympathoadrenal response results in the clinical syndrome of hypoglycemia unawareness. The patients who are affected are at nearly sixfold enhanced risk for severe iatrogenic hypoglycemia during the aggressive glycemic therapy.

MECHANISM OF THE LOSS OF THE GLUCAGON RESPONSE TO HYPOGLYCEMIA IN INSULIN-DEFICIENT DIABETES

In 1973, Gerich et al. were the first who reported the fact that type I diabetes patients do not secrete glucagon in response to hypoglycemia. In type I diabetes and advanced type II diabetes, loss of the glucagon secretory response to falling plasma glucose concentrations is an essential feature of defective glucose counter-regulation and, therefore, HAAF. It is a selective defect.

Thus, there is a correlation between loss of the glucagon response and the loss of endogenous insulin secretion, but no correlation exists with the presence of classical diabetic autonomic neuropathy. Though it is usually related to functional autonomic failure, the glucagon response is not present in some of the patients with a normal epinephrine response. Clearly, there is a difference in the mechanisms of these two features of defective glucose counter-regulation.

MECHANISM OF HYPOGLYCEMIA UNAWARENESS IN DIABETES: THE SYMPATHETIC NEURAL HYPOTHESIS

In 1922, with the beginning of insulin therapy of diabetes, the fact that some of the patients with insulin-treated diabetes tolerate low concentrations of plasma glucose with few symptoms was identified. In the mid-20th century, Lawrence described the clinical syndrome of hypoglycemia unawareness in diabetes, i.e. loss of the warning symptoms of developing hypoglycemia, which earlier allowed the patient to identify and abort the episode by eating.

Hypoglycemia unawareness, or impaired awareness of hypoglycemia, was usually considered to be a permanent long-term complication of the diabetes till the time it was discovered to be reversible, by scrupulous avoidance of iatrogenic hypoglycemia, in a large number of affected patients 70 years following the advent of insulin therapy.

Symptoms of hypoglycemia can be classified into neuroglycopenic, which means brain dysfunction that is attributable to central nervous system (CNS) glucose deprivation per se, or neurogenic. Neurogenic (or autonomic) symptoms are due to the perception of physiological changes that are caused by the CNS-mediated sympathoadrenal discharge, which is triggered by hypoglycemia. They comprise symptoms such as arousal or anxiety, palpitations, and tremor (which are mediated by catecholamines), and symptoms such as hunger, paresthesia, and sweating (which are mediated by acetylcholine released from sympathetic postganglionic neurons). Hypoglycemia awareness is mainly the result of the perception of neurogenic, instead of neuroglycopenic, symptoms among nondiabetic individuals. It is decreased by at least 70% by administrating antagonists of the classical endogenous autonomic agonists. Hence, it can be said that impaired awareness in hypoglycemia in diabetes must be mainly the result of decreased autonomic, particularly sympathoadrenal, activation by a given level of hypoglycemia.

DIVERSE CAUSES OF HAAF IN DIABETES

The presence of HAAF in diabetes can be attributed to antecedent events as well as hypoglycemia.

It has been observed that antecedent exercise reduces the sympathoadrenal responses to subsequent hypoglycemia. Galassetti et al. noted that exercise decreased the epinephrine and muscle sympathetic nerve activity, but not neurogenic symptom, which are responses to subsequent hypoglycemia. We also observed that by antecedent exercise there was a decrease in the epinephrine response to subsequent hypoglycemia. However, there was no reduction in neurogenic symptom responses to hypoglycemia. Hence, as antecedent exercise does not decrease symptoms, that is, produce impaired awareness of hypoglycemia, exercise-related HAAF seems to be a partial HAAF syndrome.

A more compelling example is sleep-related HAAF. Type I diabetic patients have substantially decreased sympathoadrenal responses to a given level of hypoglycemia; their sympathoadrenal responses are further decreased while sleeping. Possibly due to the marked reduction in sympathoadrenal responses, type I diabetic patients are much less likely to be awakened from sleep by hypoglycemia as compared to nondiabetic people.

CONCLUSION

There exists many causes of HAAF in diabetes including the originally identified exercise-related HAAF, sleep-related HAAF, and hypoglycemia-related HAAF. Clearly, a unifying mechanism of HAAF would require including the effects of antecedent exercise, sleep, and antecedent hypoglycemia.

SUGGESTED READING

1. Cryer PE. Diverse causes of hypoglycemia-associated autonomic failure in diabetes. N Engl J Med. 2004;350:2272-79.
2. Hirsch IB: Insulin analogues. N Engl J Med. 2005;352:174-83.
3. Leese GP, Wang J, Broomhall J, et al. The DARTS/MEMO Collaboration: Frequency of severe hypoglycemia requiring emergency treatment in type 1 type and 2 diabetes: a population-based study of health service resource use. Diabetes Care. 2003;26:1176-80.
4. Cryer PE. The prevention and correction of hypoglycemia. In Handbook of Physiology. Section 7: The Endocrine System. Volume II: The Endocrine Pancreas and Regulation of Metabolism. Jefferson LS, Cherrington AD, Eds. New York, Oxford University Press. 2001;1057-92.
5. White NH, Skor DA, Cryer PE, et al. Identification of type 1 diabetic patients at increased risk for hypoglycemia during intensive therapy. N Engl J Med. 1983;308:485-91.
6. Gold AE, MacLeod KM, Frier BM: Frequency of severe hypoglycemia in patients with type 1 diabetes with impaired awareness of hypoglycemia. Diabetes Care. 1994;17:697-703.
7. Segel SA, Paramore DS, Cryer PE: Hypoglycemia-associated autonomic failure in advanced type 2 diabetes. Diabetes. 2002;51:724-33.
8. Fritsche A, Stumvoll M, Grüb M, et al. Effect of hypoglycemia on β-adrenergic sensitivity in normal and type 1 diabetic subjects. Diabetes Care. 1998;21:1505-10.
9. Bolli G, De Feo P, Compagnucci P, et al. Abnormal glucose counterregulation in insulin dependent diabetes mellitus: interaction of anti-insulin antibodies and impaired glucagon and epinephrine secretion. Diabetes. 1983;32:134-41.
10. Samols E, Tyler J, Marks V. Glucagon-insulin interrelationships. In Glucagon: Molecular Physiology, Clinical and Therapeutic Implications. Lefebvre P, Unger RH, Eds. Elmsford, NY, Pergamon. 1972;151-74.

CHAPTER 60 Noninsulinoma Pancreatogenous Hypoglycemia Syndrome

Chandar Mohan Batra, Monika Goyal

INTRODUCTION

Noninsulinoma pancreatogenous hypoglycemia syndrome (NIPHS) is a rare syndrome characterized by endogenous hyperinsulinemic hypoglycemia not caused by insulinoma. Presents predominantly with postprandial hypoglycemia rarely fasting hypoglycemia. Pancreatic specimens in these patients are characterized by nesidioblastosis, a term that refers to neoformation of islets of Langerhans from pancreatic duct epithelium. Similar findings are seen in neonates and infants with persistent hyperinsulinemic hypoglycemia.

F John Service from Mayo clinic first described this syndrome.[1] They described five adults with neuroglycopenic episodes from hyperinsulinemic hypoglycemia within 4 hours of meal ingestion and negative 72 hour fast. The imaging done by transabdominal ultrasound, spiral CECT and coeliac axis angiography of the pancreas was negative but selective arterial calcium stimulation tests were positive indicative of beta cell hyperfunction. At pancreatic exploration, no insulinoma was detected by complete mobilization, palpation and intraoperative ultrasonography. The resected pancreata showed islet hypertrophy, enlargement of nucleus and budding of islet cells from the pancreatic ducts (nesidioblastosis). Gradient guided partial pancreatectomy relieved the hypoglycemic episodes in these patients.

This is a rare disorder with only 100 cases published so far. The prevalence is reported to be 0.5–5% of NIPHS among cases of hyperinsulinemic hypoglycemia but as bariatric surgery with Roux-en-Y gastric bypass is getting more popular the prevalence of NIPHS is increasing. The prevalence of NIPHS is 0.36% after Roux-en-Y gastric bypass surgery for obesity.[2]

ETIOPATHOGENESIS OF NIPHS

Exact etiology is not known but appears to have genetic origin. Abnormal overexpression of a protein called islet cell neogenesis associated protein (INGAP) has been found in the pancreatic ducts and islets in 3/5 patients of NIPHS. This protein, a human cytokine was first found in pancreatic neoplasia and is responsible for the regeneration of islet cells in the pancreas. This protein could be one factor responsible for islet cell neogenesis and ductal proliferation. INGAP was detected by double labeling immunofluorescence. In normal patients this protein is localized to periphery of the islets or not present at all but in these 3 NIPHS patients it was seen in the pancreatic ducts and the islets.[3]

In nesidioblastosis, the clinical equivalent to NIPHS, seen in children, mutations in 9 genes have been found of which the most common are autosomm recessive, inactivating mutations of the genes encoding the beta cell inwardly rectifying channel (Kir 6.2) and the sulfonylurea receptor 1 (SUR1) which control the KATP channel which is responsible for release of insulin from the beta cells, resulting in abnormal function of these channels and hypoglycemia. In adults no mutant genes have been found so far.[3]

Recently bariatric surgery for morbid obesity, involving gastric bypass Roux-en-Y, is emerging as the most common cause of NIPHS (0.36% of cases). The mechanisms which have been postulated are that the rapid transit of nutrients to the jejunum increases the amount of GLP1 secreted to 10 times normal. This increases secretion of insulin and causing postprandial hypoglycemic attacks. The fact that this is a late complication and occurs about a year after surgery indicates that excessive GLP1 hormone stimulates the hypertrophy of the islet cells and budding of new islet cells and the ductoinsular complexes formation (nesidioblastosis), which is found in the histopathology of these patients.[2]

HISTOLOGY OF RESECTED PANCREAS

The H&E sections show characteristic pancreatic tissue with area of hypertrophic islets in opposition to the small pancreatic ducts. The nuclei of the islet cells are enlarged. Immunostaining is positive for insulin, glucagon, somatostatin and chromogranin. Rare insulin staining cells associated with small pancreatic ducts and budding of islet cells from the pancreatic ducts called ductoinsular complex is also seen.[1] Figures 1A to H show the details of the histopathology and immunostaining in two of our patients.

CLINICAL FEATURES OF NIPHS

Clinically, patients present with postprandial spontaneous hypoglycemia in nondiabetic patient. The characteristic symptoms are neurogenic (palpitations, tremors, anxiety, sweating, hunger) and neuroglycopenic symptoms (behavioral changes), fatigue, confusion, seizures, loss of consciousness. These symptoms develop at a mean plasma glucose of <55 mg/dL). To avoid unnecessary workup and healthcare cost, recommendations are such, that only patients patient who fulfill the criteria for Whipple's triad, i.e. documented blood sugar below 55 mg/dL, symptoms of neuroglycopenic hypoglycemia and relief of the symptoms on carbohydrate ingestion should be subjective for further evaluation.[4]

WORKUP OF A PATIENT OF SPONTANEOUS HYPOGLYCEMIA

This needs a systemic approach. A complete history and physical examination and investigations are done to rule out the ingestion of any drug that could cause hypoglycemia and critical illness like renal, liver, cardiac failure and adrenocortical deficiency. In a seemingly well patient presenting with spontaneous hypoglycemia after above mentioned conditions have been ruled, work up is done to demonstrate endogenous hyperinsulinemia. This can be done by measuring serum insulin, c-peptide, proinsulin and beta-hydroxybutyrate levels during episode of hypoglycemia either spontaneous or induced by 72 hour fast or in some patients after a mixed meal test and then inject 1 mg of glucagon SC and blood sugar is measured after 1 hour of injection. The values that confirm hyperinsulinemic hypoglycemia are serum insulin >3 uU/mL, c-peptide >0.6 ng/mL, proinsulin >5 pmol/L and beta-hydroxybutyrate level of <2.7 nmol/L. A rise of blood sugar above 25 mg/dL after glucagon confirms that the glycogen stores are adequate. Insulin antibodies are done to rule out autoimmune insulin syndrome and screening for sulfonylureas is done.[4]

Role of Imaging

After the biochemical confirmation of hyperinsulinemic hypoglycemia imaging is done for insulinoma which is the most common cause of hyperinsulinemic hypoglycemia in adults. The tests are triple phase contrast enhanced CT abdomen, contrast enhanced MRI abdomen, endoscopic

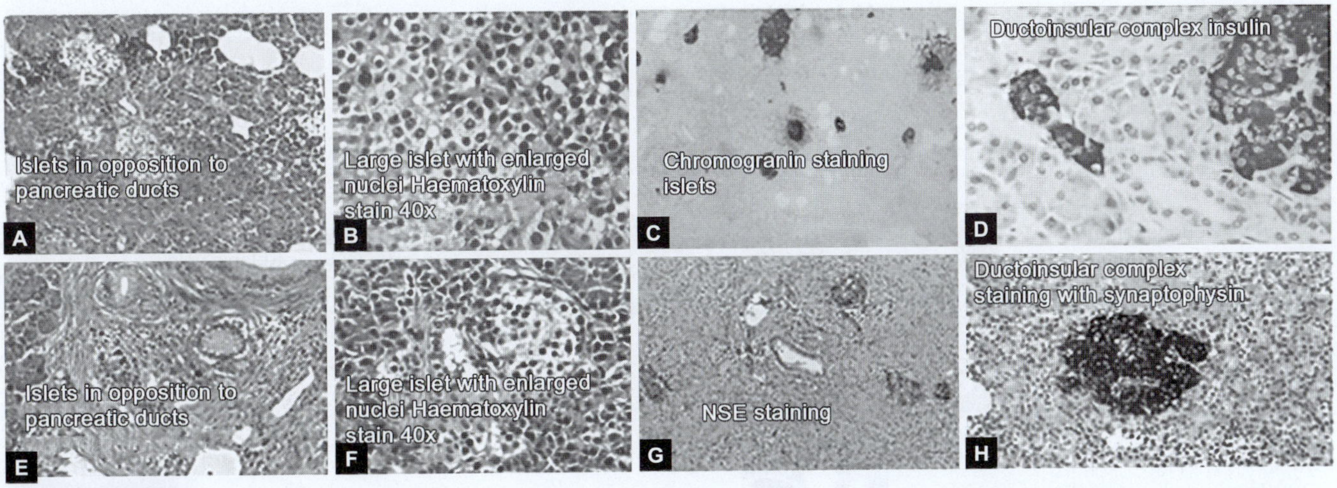

Figures 1A to H HPE findings of 2 patients showing histopathological features of NIPHS, (A to D) Patient 1; (E to H) Patient 2. *(For color version see color plate No. 7)*

ultrasonography are done. If the patient has postprandial hyperinsulinemic hypoglycemia, a negative 72 hours fast and the pancreatic tumor is not located by any of these radiological means then patient most probably has NIPHS.

Investigations for NIPHS

The investigation of choice of this syndrome is selective intra-arterial calcium injection and hepatic venous sampling based on the principle that calcium stimulation causes abnormal beta cell to produce excessive insulin while normal production by other cell. Right hepatic vein is canalized through femoral vein puncture. The coeliac axis angiography is done via the femoral artery. Splenic, gastroduodenal and superior mesenteric artery are canalized in turn with a gap of 15 minutes each and 0.025 mEq/kg body weight (1.0 mg/kg) of calcium is injected rapidly. Samples for serum insulin and c-peptide were taken at 0, 30, 60, 90, 120 sec after calcium injection from the right hepatic vein. Samples are stored on ice and assayed within 1 hour.[1] The pancreas is supplied by three main arteries. The superior pancreaticoduodenal artery supplies the head of the pancreas, the body and tail are supplied by the splenic artery and the superior mesenteric artery supplies the uncinate process. A doubling of the serum insulin values after calcium injection into an artery signifies abnormal beta cells in the part of the pancreas supplied by the artery (Fig. 2).

The results of this procedure in one of my patients are summarized in the Table1.

In this case the doubling of serum insulin was in the area supplied by the splenic artery indicating that the abnormal beta cells were in the body and tail of the pancreas. If the doubling of serum insulin occurs if after injection in the superior pancreaticoduodenal artery then the abnormal beta cells are in the head of the pancreas. And if occurs in territory supplied by the superior mesenteric artery then the uncinate process has abnormal beta cells. Sometimes the doubling of serum insulin is in all the three arteries indicating a diffuse disease all over the pancreas.[1]

TABLE 1: Selective pancreatic arterial stimulation and venous sampling in right hepatic vein.

Artery	Serum insulin and c-peptide	osec	30	60	90	120
Splenic	Insulin UIU/L	19.5	50	38.7	30.3	25.4
	c-pep ng/dL	*3.18*	*5.5*	*4.54*	*4.37*	*4.16*
Gastro-duodenal	Insulin	15.6	24.0	20.6	17.1	16.3
	c-pep	2.95	2.40	3.52	3..44	3.42
Superior mesenteric	Insulin	21.8	24.2	25.9	27.6	25.5
	c-pep	3.15	2.42	3.92	3.92	3.92

Role of PET SCAN for Diagnosis of NIPHS

F-18 DOPA PET Scan

Fluorine 18 L dihydroxyphenylalanine (18-F DOPA) positron emission tomography is the most sensitive imaging tool for detection of insulinoma and beta cell hyperplasia with a sensitivity of 90% compared to 30–40% in MRI and CT scan. Diazoxide, somatostatin analog or cortisone is stopped 24 hours before the study. The

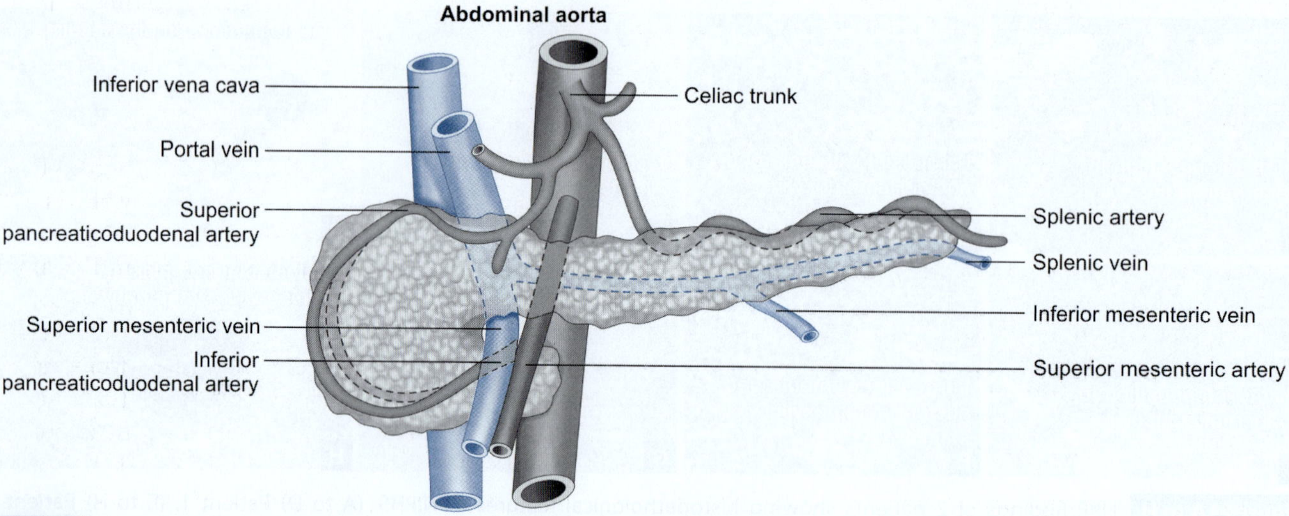

Figure 2 Arterial supply of the pancreas. (*For color version see color plate No. 7*)

average dose is 234 mEq given IV and scanning is done 60 minutes after injection. The blood sugar has to be kept between 80 mg/dL and 100 mg/dL.[5]

111In-GLP-1 SPECT CT

111In-labeled GLP-1R agonist, 111In-DOTA exendin-4 in localizing insulinomas using single photon emission computed tomography in combination with computed tomography images has a sensitivity of 95% in the detection of insulinomas and in nesidioblastosis. Method of choice when other conventional methods have failed.[6] *Ga-68 DOTATOC PET* scan was used to differentiate focal versus diffuse nesidioblastosis and to detect diffuse nesidioblastosis in infants. There are some case reports of it being used successfully in adults to diagnose NIPHS. 68-Ga DOTATATE specifically binds to the high affinity somatostatin receptors (SSTR type II) which are highly concentrated in the pancreatic islet cells.[7]

TREATMENT OF NIPHS

Treatment of Acute Hypoglycemic Attacks

If the attack is mild the treatment is 10–15 g of carbohydrates mixed with protein or fat but if the patient is on acarbose glucose alone is given. In case of severe hypoglycemic attack and inability to swallow give injection glucagon SC 1 mg stat.[2]

Diet Therapy

Drug therapy is the first line of treatment. It is a low carbohydrate, high protein diet in 5–6 meals/day. The carbohydrates given should be complex carbohydrates 90–130 g/day and fructose should be substituted for glucose. It reduces insulin hypersecretion and thus hypoglycemic attacks. Uncooked corn starch has delayed absorption in the intestine and is slowly hydrolyzed by pancreatic amylase and intestinal glucoamylase to provide a steady flow of glucose. This has been found useful to prevent hypoglycemia. Proteins and healthy fats can also slow down absorption of nutrients thus preventing glucose spikes and excessive insulin release.[2]

Medical Treatment

Acarbose

This drug is an alpha-glucosidase inhibitor which inhibits the absorption of carbohydrates from the gut by inhibition of intestinal alpha-glucosidase thus reducing the increase of insulin after a meal. The dose is 50–100 mg thrice daily premeals. This is effective but has the side effects of gaseous distention and flatulence.[2]

Diazoxide

This drug is an effective drug which activates the K-ATP channel preventing the gate closure and release of insulin. It is an effective drug used in doses of 50 mg twice daily or 100 mg twice daily orally and is effective but causes fluid retention, edema, nausea, hypotension, and headache. Chlorothiazide is used in combination with diazoxide to prevent edema.[2]

Somatostatin Analog

Somatostatin analog reduce insulin and GLP-1 secretion by binding to somatostatin receptor 2 and 5. Octreotide a somatostatin analog acts by similar mechanism but can also inhibit glucagon and growth hormone and can precipitate hypoglycemic attack and caution should be taken while using it. It is started subcutaneously in a dose of 50–100 µg thrice daily and if found effective, given as a long acting depot once a month intramuscularly. It is an effective drug in some patients. The side-effects are diarrhea, steatorrhea, and risks of cholelithiasis and QT prolongation. The other limitation is the high cost.[2]

Verapamil

This is a voltage gated calcium channel blocker that decreasing insulin release from beta cells. This is not an effective drug with very few case studies supporting it.[2]

New Drugs under Development

Pasireotide is a somatostatin analog which acts by somatostatin receptor1, 2 and 5 but the affinity of this drug for receptor 5 is much more than receptor 2. Pasircotide thus suppresses mainly insulin secretion and is much more powerful than octreotide.[2]

A new drug exendin (9-39) has been recently discovered which blocks the release of GLP1 from the gut resulting in decreased insulin production. It is a potent competitive antagonist of the GLP1 receptor. There are two studies which show that this drug is effective given IV or SC in preventing hypoglycemia and phase 2 trials are underway.[2]

Glucagon delivery by a pump at the time of impending hypoglycemia guided by a CGMS device is also in experimental phases. This works as the same way as an insulin pump.[2].

There is also a recent development of monoclonal antibodies that can block the insulin receptor and reduce hypoglycemic episodes in mice and human beings. This is IgG2 monoclonal antibody (XOMA358). It increases fasting and postprandial glucose levels in human studies.[2]

Role of Surgery

Patients are first treated by diet therapy and medical therapy. Cases resistant to diet and medical therapy and those with severe life threatening hypoglycemic episodes are treated by subtotal pancreatectomy guided by the findings of selective intra-arterial calcium injection and hepatic venous sampling. If the abnormal beta cells are in the region of the splenic artery a distal pancreatectomy is done to the right of the superior mesenteric vein. If the superior mesenteric artery is involved then a distal pancreatectomy is done to the left of superior mesenteric vein. If the territory supplied by the superior gastroduodenal is involved then the head of the pancreas is removed by a Whipple's operation. After surgery due to removal of the abnormal beta cells the hypoglycemic episodes do not occur. The patient may be euglycemic or become diabetic as is evident in the postoperative OGTT in one of our cases. The excessive serum insulin secretion after glucose ingestion does not occur (Table 2).[1]

NIPHS management following Bariatric Surgery with Roux-en-Y gastric bypass

- Feeding via a gastrectomy tube through the gastric remnant.
- Reversal of bypass
- Placing a silastic ring around the gastric pouch

TABLE 2: OGTT postoperative with 75 gm glucose.

	Blood sugar (mg/dL)	Serum insulin level (μIU/mL)
0 hour	124	9.20
1 hour	*232*	32.11
2 hours	*240*	33.85
3 hours	152	24.11
4 hours	138	13.87
5 hours	113	14.57

- Partial pancreatectomy guided by the findings of selective intra-arterial calcium injection and hepatic venous sampling

Feeding via a gastrectomy tube through the gastric remnant delays the entry of the gastric nutrients into the jejunum thus reducing GLP1 production. If this works then reversal of gastric bypass is likely to work though weight gain will occur. Placing a silastic ring around the gastric pouch also works by delaying the entry of nutrients into the jejunum reducing GLP1 production.[2] Enthusiasm for partial pancreatectomy for NIPHS following gastric bypass following for bariatric surgery has waned following studies showing immediate relief from hypoglycemia but recurrence of hypoglycemia in 90% of these patients.[2,8]

CONCLUSION

The dictum that a negative 72 fast rules out insulinoma, and postprandial hyperinsulinemic hypoglycemia even if severe and life threatening was labeled as reactive hypoglycemia and prescribed frequent low carbohydrate meals and acarbose, needs to be changed. Large series have now shown that upto 4% of pancreatic specimens from patients with hyperinsulinemic hypoglycemia, do not have insulinoma but have nesidioblastosis. Hypertrophic islets, beta cells with pleomorphic nuclei and ductuloinsular complexes are the key features of nesidioblastosis on histopathology.[9]

Diet therapy and medical treatment is the first choice but if patient is nonresponsive to medical treatment surgery needs to done. Gradient guided distal pancreatectomy is done to the right of superior mesenteric vein if the splenic artery territory is involved and to the left if superior mesenteric and a whipple surgery if the gastroduodenal artery territory is involved. It is associated with perioperative complications and development of diabetes. It is not done unless all other medical treatment has proved unsuccessful. Overall prognosis is good.

REFERENCES

1. Service FJ, Natt N, Thompson GB, et al. Noninsulinoma pancreatogenous hypoglycemia: a novel syndrome of hyperinsulinemic hypoglycemia in adults independent of mutations in Kir6.2 and SUR1 genes. J Clin Endocrinol Metabol. 1999;84:1582-9.
2. Salehi M, Vella A, McLaughlin T, et al. Hypoglycemia after gastric bypass surgery: current concepts and controversies. J Clin Endocrinol Metab. 2018;103(8):2815-26.
3. Won JG, Tseng HS, Yang AH, et al. Clinical features and morphological characterization of 10 patients with noninsulinoma pancreatogenous hypoglycaemia syndrome (NIPHS). Clin Endocrinol. 2006;65(5): 566-78.

4. Cryer PE, Axelrod L, Grossman AB, et al. Evaluation and management of adult hypoglycemic disorders: an Endocrine Society Clinical Practice Guideline. J Clin Endocrinol Metab. 2009;94(3):709-28.
5. Kauhanen S, Seppanen M, Minn H, et al. Fluorine-18-L-dihydroxyphenylalanine (18F-DOPA) positron emission tomography as a tool to localize an insulinoma or β-cell hyperplasia in adult patients. J Clin Endocrinol Metabol. 2007;92(4):1237-44.
6. Christ E, Wild D, Forrer F, et al. Glucagon-like peptide-1 receptor imaging for localization of insulinomas. J Clin Endocrinol Metabol. 2009;94(11):4398-405.
7. Arun S, Mittal BR, Shukla J, et al. Diffuse nesidioblastosis diagnosed on a Ga-68 DOTATATE positron emission tomography/computerized tomography. IJNM. 2013;28(3):163.
8. Yaqub A, Smith EP, Salehi M. Hyperinsulinemic hypoglycemia after gastric bypass surgery: what's up and what's down? Int J Obes. 2018;42(3):286.
9. Anlauf M, Wieben D, Perren A, et al. Persistent hyperinsulinemic hypoglycemia in 15 adults with diffuse nesidioblastosis: diagnostic criteria, incidence, and characterization of β-cell changes. Am J Surg Pathol. 2005;29(4):524-33.

61 CHAPTER Nonalbuminuric Renal Disease in Diabetes: Is it a Separate Entity?

Anuj Maheshwari, Jalees Fatima, Lekha L Pradhan

INTRODUCTION

In the developed countries, diabetes mellitus (DM) is considered to be the leading cause of end-stage renal disease (ESRD).[1] Worldwide, about 40% of diabetic people develop diabetic kidney disease (DKD), making it one of the most common complications of diabetes. It is very crucial to diagnose DKD early because it is also an indicator of increase in cardiovascular risk.

Presence of persistent albuminuria in urine is the initial clinical presentation and the pathological hallmark of DKD.[2] It is shown by mounting evidence that in a significant number of type 2 diabetes mellitus (T2DM) patients, there is a reduced glomerular filtration rate (GFR) without significant albuminuria; it is called nonalbuminuric renal disease (NADKD).

ALBUMINURIC (CLASSIC) DIABETIC NEPHROPATHY

It is since 1980s that renal disease in diabetes is classified in to stages by increase in proteinuria/albuminuria levels (normo-micro-macro). Typically, the development of overt proteinuria or macroalbuminuria marked the beginning of faster glomerular filtration ratio (GFR) declining.[1,3]

The main risk factors that are associated with the development of diabetic nephropathy (DN) comprise poor glycemic control, hypertension, dyslipidemia, and smoking. There are many genetic polymorphisms, which are also associated with development of DN, comprising angiotensin-converting enzyme (ACE) and angiotensin type 2 receptor. With the rise in DN, the number of patients requiring renal replacement therapy for ESRD has increased in the recent years.

Stages of Classic Diabetic Nephropathy

Diabetic nephropathy originates with renal hyperfiltration and glomerular hyperperfusion; then, it progresses to microalbuminuria and a reduced GFR. Four main criteria are used in current guidelines for defining DN: (1) a decline in renal function, (2) proteinuria, (3) diabetic retinopathy, and (4) a reduced GFR.[4] Overt nephropathy is particularly characterized by persistent proteinuria (>500 mg/24 hour), which generally precedes a fall in GFR. Diagnosis of DN is done by urinalysis and confirmed, if required, by a kidney biopsy. Monitoring of its progression is done by regular measurements of serum creatinine, calculated GFR, and microalbuminuria.

Histological criteria on biopsies that are diagnosed as DN are classified as following:

- *Class I*: Glomerular basement membrane thickening; isolated glomerular basement membrane thickening; only mild, nonspecific changes by light microscopy, which do not meet Classes II to IV criteria.
- *Class II*: Mesangial expansion—mild (IIa) or severe (IIb): Glomeruli is classified as mild or severe mesangial expansion, however without global glomerulosclerosis or nodular sclerosis (Kimmelstiel-Wilson lesions) in > 50% of the glomeruli.
- *Class III*: Nodular sclerosis (Kimmelstiel-Wilson lesions)
  At the minimum one glomerulus along with nodular increase in mesangial matrix (Kimmelstiel-Wilson) without changes that are described in class IV.
- *Class IV*: Advanced diabetic glomerulosclerosis
  Over 50% global glomerulosclerosis along with other pathological or clinical evidence that sclerosis is attributable to DN.[5]

By the histological analysis of biopsy samples, a correct estimate of damage in DN can only be attained. In diabetes, glomerular basement membrane thickening is the earliest structural abnormality. Significant hypertrophy is noted in cases of kidney with early diabetes. Occlusion of glomerular capillaries and mesangial expansion result in loss of available surface area for filtration and decline in function. The third stage (which is also called incipient nephropathy) is characterized by the microalbuminuria.[3,6] Persistent increase in urinary albumin excretion occurs most frequently during the second decade following the diagnosis of diabetes. In the absence of specific renal lesions, it reflects the existence of endothelial damage. It is also found to be associated with the initiation of advanced podocyte loss. The overt nephropathy is characterized by the persistent proteinuria, which generally accompanies a reduced GFR, and it is related with the typical diabetic kidney lesions.

NONPROTEINURIC DIABETIC NEPHROPATHY

As discussed previously, the presence of proteinuria represents a significant prognostic factor, which reflects damage to the glomerular filtration barrier. However, many studies have reported DN without significant proteinuria (more than 500 mg/24 hour) in more than 50% of the patients having diabetes with a varying percentage of patients in these reports suffering from advanced (stages 3–5) kidney disease.

The most important pathway in progression of DN is renin-angiotensin aldosterone system (RAAS); it is considered as the most important pathway as it has a central role in maintenance of glomerular pressure, blood pressure, and fluid and electrolyte balance through angiotensin II.[2]

Formation of angiotensin II is increased by the action of ACE, which enhances renal vascular constriction through activation of its receptor ATR1 (angiotensin receptor 1) during DN progression. Activation of ATR2 (angiotensin receptor 2), however, results in useful effects comprising vasodilation, antiproliferative, and anti-inflammatory actions.[2,7]

The natural history of patients with diabetes as well as renal impairment and reduced levels of proteinuria needs to be established. Majority of the patients having with chronic kidney disease (GFR less than 60 mL/minute) do not have albuminuria. The reasons for this changing pattern of renal disease in patients with diabetes are being investigated.

Reversal of Albuminuria and Relation of Diabetic Nephropathy with Traditional Risk Factors

Albuminuria was extensively believed to be the first clinical sign of DKD. Due to the increase in evidence of presence of nonalbuminuric DKD (NA-DKD), using albuminuria as an early marker of onset or progression of DKD needs a cautious interpretation as among patients with diabetes albuminuria has an immense tendency of regressing spontaneously to normal levels (about 18–51%).

In 1994, Tsalamandris et al. observed for the first time that some of the patients with T2DM showed no significant proteinuria, but they had renal insufficiency and DKD developed in them [i.e. estimated glomerular filtration rate (eGFR) less than 60 mL/min/1.73 m^2]. This was described as normoalbuminuric diabetic kidney disease (NADKD).[7,8]

Impact of changes in diabetes treatment like increasing use of RAAS blocking drugs should be considered a factor in increasing prevalence of NADKD.

Among patients having NADKD, risk factors comprise sex, hypertension, obesity, high levels of TG, poor glycemic control, and glomerular hyperfiltration, which may have a role in nephrosclerosis. There is variation in the prevalence of NADKD, i.e. from 14.29% to 56.6% in diabetic patients of different ethnicities.

The increase in the prevalence of nonalbuminuric chronic kidney diseases can be because of *macroangiopathic lesions that prevail over the microangiopathic alterations in T2DM*. This type of shift can also reflect changes in the treatment, specifically to decreased lipids levels and improved glycemic control, and levels of blood pressure that is being attained in patients with diabetes. This view is similar to the results of UKPDS, which shows that glycated hemoglobin (HbA1c) is an independent risk factor for increase in excretion of albumin, but not for impairment of GFR. Furthermore, nonproteinuric kidney disease was found to be less closely associated with other microvascular complication, i.e. retinopathy, as compared to the classic proteinuric DN.

Hypertension had better correlation with albuminuric DN than with nonalbuminuric DN, however there was a significant association between nonalbuminuric diabetic kidney diseae and major acute cardiac events. This is in accordance with the view that GFR < 60 mL/minute is a strong predictor of CVD mortality and morbidity among general population and among diabetic patients, independent of the traditional CVD risk factors and albuminuria.

Proposed Mechanisms

The studies involving renal biopsy and histopathological findings are limited in diabetic patients with nonproteinuric renal impairment, but it can be hypothesized that age-related sclerotic changes in glomeruli, interstitial fibrosis, and ischemia, may be significant factors.[2] Cholesterol emboli might also contribute to loss of renal function.[2,9]

It is suggested by latest research that there is a role of enhanced vascular resistance in renal interlobar arteries that can lead to damage of glomerular and nonglomerular nephron structures and play a role in the onset and progression of nonproteinuric diabetic nephropathy (NPDN).[2,5] In patients with NPDN, *elevation in arterial stiffness, which was measured by using aortic and brachial-ankle pulse wave velocity*, was found to be strongly associated with increase in atherosclerosis and cardiovascular morbidity and mortality and reduced renal function.[7] Therefore, NPDN patients are likely to have more atherosclerosis and enhanced vascular resistance. Many studies evaluating *NPDN observed increased levels of serum uric acid, which were found to be strongly associated with the development of kidney disease*. Uric acid is an antioxidant in the blood; however, uric acid is also a potent pro-oxidant and by stimulating NADPH oxidases it damages mitochondria. Increased levels of uric acid can also damage vascular elements and cause endothelial dysfunction by different mechanisms, comprising *activation of toll-like receptor* pathways. Uric acid causes vascular smooth muscle cell proliferation, activation of the renin-angiotensin system, and renal inflammation. In patients with NPDN, prolonged elevation of uric acid levels can cause significant vascular changes, which impair renal function resulting in NPDN. Thus, in NPDN patients, increased uric acid levels can cause more vascular damage as compared to DN patients.

In recent times, sodium-glucose cotransporter-2 (SGLT2) inhibitors were shown to enhance excretion of uric acid via the proximal tubule transporter, SLC2A9 (GLUT9), which enhanced glycemia control, blood pressure control, and weight loss in patients with DN. For investigating this mechanism, studies should comprise serial measurements of uric acid and uric excretion between DN and NPDN patients who were prescribed SGLT2 inhibitors.

Nonproteinuric diabetic nephropathy patients have increased concentrations of the serum tumor necrosis factor alpha (TNFα) and Fas-pathways. TNFα is a main mediator of inflammation via chemokines induction, intercellular adhesion molecule-1, vascular adhesion molecule-1, and IFN-γ inducible protein-10, which enhance albumin permeability and glomerular vasoconstriction. TNFα is involved in the regulation of blood pressure, acute kidney injury, inflammation within the renal vasculature, and blood flow. Fas and TNFα also play key roles in apoptosis. During immune and inflammatory responses, the FasL-Fas system regulates renal cell apoptosis by activating renal cell Fas receptors. Additionally, during ischemia-reperfusion experiments, murine models blocking the FasL-Fas system and prevent renal and tubular cell injury. Therefore, enhanced levels of Fas and TNFα in NPDN can modify renal vasculature and cause damage to the kidney.[2]

Patients with NPDN also have increased levels of *osteoprotegerin and vascular endothelial growth factor (VEGF)*, which function in inflammation and angiogenesis, respectively. There is an inverse relation between VEGF levels and proteinuria levels in patients with DN. VEGF signaling results in apoptosis and potentially cause the glomerular vascular atrophy. In diabetic patients, osteoprotegerin is associated with chronic kidney disease, which results in calcification of vascular tissue, glomerular damage, and proteinuria.[2]

Diagnostic and Therapeutic Implications

For improvement in early diagnosis and treatment of conventional NPDN and DN patients, there is a requirement for the development of safe and accessible diagnostic markers.

For examining and grading the progression of DN, ultrasonography is an inexpensive and noninvasive method. It has been demonstrated that *an increased renal resistive index* (RRI), which measures renal vascular resistance, reliably detect, differentiate, and monitor the progression of NPDN and DN.[4,9]

Onset of DN can be prevented before the appearance of proteinuria with pharmacological agents. There are only a few studies that have systematically compared the renal function, prognosis, as well as several blood and urine components in conventional NPDN and DN patients. More studies are needed for assessing changes in the levels of TNFα, TGF-β, endothelin as well as other interleukins in the blood and urine of NPDN and DN patients.

It seems that the pathogenesis of NPDN include vascular and soluble elements circulating in the blood. On comparing DN patients with NPDN patients, it was revealed that inflammation play a central role in NPDN.

A detailed analysis of renal disease of a patient can be provided by kidney biopsies. However, because of the complications, like bleeding, infection, and other vascular injuries, its wider use in limited in physicians.[5] Moreover, the vascular changes that occur in NPDN and DN patients may not be fully detected by kidney biopsies.

Drugs like heparin, antibodies and pentoxifylline as anti-inflammatory agent are still in experimental stage for renoprotection in diabetes.

CONCLUSION

Evidences reveal significant variability in patients with DN therefore, DN is now viewed as a spectrum of varying presentations.

Further clinical studies are required for examining the differences between proteinuric and NPDN in the pathogenesis, diagnosis, and treatment. Research that focus on the use of allopurinol for reducing levels of uric acid in NPDN patients would give an easy option of treatment for both patients and clinicians. With the increase in number of cases of NPDN, new diagnostic markers and treatment are required for understanding the pathogenesis of both DN and NPDN. For the prevention and treatment of DN and NPDN, novel therapies other than existing antihypertensive therapy regimens are an effective measure. More studies for the pathophysiology of NPDN needs recognition of new biomarkers and cardiovascular factors that influence renal function for early detection of diabetic kidney disease.

REFERENCES

1. KDOQI. KDOQI clinical practice guidelines and clinical practice recommendations for diabetes and chronic kidney disease. Am J Kidney Dis. 2007;49:S12-154.
2. Chawla V, Roshan B. Non-proteinuric diabetic nephropathy. Curr Diab Rep. 2014;14:529.
3. Tuttle KR, Bakris GL, Bilous RW, et al. Diabetic kidney disease: a report from an ADA Consensus Conference. Diabetes Care. 2014;37:2864-83.
4. Kopel J, Pena-Hernandez C, Nugent K. Evolving spectrum of diabetic nephropathy. World J Diabetes. 2019;10:269-79.
5. Tervaert TW, Mooyaart AL, Amann K, et al. Pathologic classification of diabetic nephropathy. J Am Soc Nephrol. 2010;21:556-63.
6. Madhu SV. Normoalbuminuric diabetic kidney disease: a distinct entity?. Int J Diabetes Devg Ctries. 2019;39:241-2.
7. Tsalamandris C, Allen TJ, Gilbert RE, et al. Progressive decline in renal function in diabetic patients with and without albuminuria. Diabetes. 1994;43:649-55.
8. Bermejo S, Pascual J, Soler MJ. The large spectrum of renal disease in diabetic patients. Clin Kidney J. 2017;10:255-6.
9. Jastaniah SM, Alsayed NA, Awad IR, et al. Evaluation of renal disorders in type 2 diabetic patients using ultrsonography. Open J Med Imaging. 2013;03:165-70.

62 CHAPTER Clinical Approach to Diagnose Diabetic Cardiomyopathy

Anil Kumar Virmani

INTRODUCTION

Diabetic cardiomyopathy has been defined as the presence of abnormal myocardial structure and performance, in a patient with diabetes in absence of other causes like coronary artery disease, hypertension, dyslipidemia, valvular disease, etc. (ACC/AHA/ESC and EASD-2013). It is a diagnosis of exclusion.[1]

It was first described in 1972, on autopsy findings of four diabetic patients with heart failure by Rubler et al.[2]

Insulin resistance in heart muscle leading to compensatory hyperinsulinemia and hyperglycemia are intrinsically responsible for the earliest abnormalities in the relaxation of the left ventricle (LV) leading to early diastolic dysfunction.

Oxidative stress, inflammation, defective immune modulation and activation of the RAAS system leads to structural abnormalities like interstitial fibrosis of myocardial tissues leading to cardiac stiffness and impaired left ventricular filling.

Diabetic cardiomyopathy has a wide clinical spectrum, ranging from early subtle relaxation abnormalities of the left ventricle due to stiffness leading to early diastolic dysfunction and heart failure with preserved ejection fraction (HFpEF), and later in the advanced stages to heart failure with reduced ejection fraction (HFrEF). The challenge is in the early diagnosis with appropriate interventional treatment.

PREVALENCE

The exact prevalence of diabetic cardiomyopathy is not known, as the initial presentation is often as heart failure.

In T1DM, there is an increased risk of heart failure by 30% for every 1% increase in HbA1c, independent of other risk factors.[3] Early diastolic function is seen in children and adolescents with T1DM, with a lower ratio of early (E') to late (A') peak diastolic velocities measurements , on echocardiographic Doppler imaging.[4]

On the other hand, in T2DM, there is an increase in heart failure by 8% for every 1% rise in HbA1c, independent of other risk factors.[5]

Every 1% reduction in HbA1c was associated with reduction in risk for heart failure, myocardial infarction and mortality by 16%, 14%, and 21% respectively.[6]

CARDIAC STRUCTURAL CHANGES

In early stages, metabolic disturbances like hyper-insulinemia, impaired insulin signaling, impaired glucose uptake, increased myocardial nonesterified fatty acid (NEFA) uptake and mitochondrial dysfunction promote cardiac remodeling and fibrotic diastolic dysfunction with increased LV wall stiffness. Furthermore, impaired cardiomyocyte autophagy and increased apoptosis, oxidative stress, maladaptive responses and inappropriate RAAS activation lead to interstitial fibrosis and cardiac stiffness.[7]

In the later stages, cardiac structural changes become more pronounced with collagen accumulation, interstitial fibrosis, increased cross-linking of connective tissue, microvascular disease and cardiomyocyte necrosis, leading to both diastolic and systolic dysfunction, and ultimately heart failure with reduced ejection fraction.[8]

PATHOPHYSIOLOGY

Insulin resistance associated with impaired insulin signaling, leads to hyperinsulinemia along with hyperglycemia. This leads to increased production of advanced Glycation end products (AGE's) and RAAS activation. Associated cardiac lipotoxicity (Steatosis due to increased uptake of NEFA by cardiomyocytes), leads to coronary endothelial dysfunction and dysregulation of exosomes.

These processes ultimately lead to oxidative stress, mitochondrial dysfunction, endothelial reticulum stress and impaired calcium homeostasis. There occurs a subcellular low grade inflammation leading chronically to cardiac hypertrophy, fibrosis and apoptosis with subsequent cardiac stiffness, diastolic and systolic dysfunction, and heart failure.

The heart is metabolically flexible and consumes the highest amount of adenosine triphosphate (ATP) (almost about 6 kg of ATP or about 20 times its weight per day) in the body. Changes in the substrate and energy metabolism lead to the heart becoming metabolically inflexible, with a shift away from utilization of glucose primarily, to reliance on fatty acids for source of energy, thus consuming almost 30% more oxygen than a nondiabetic heart to generate similar levels of ATP.

Moreover, the cardiomyocyte in diabetes has decreased SERCA2a (sarcoplasmic/endoplasmic reticulum calcium ATPase 2a) activity, thus decreasing transport of calcium ions during cardiac relaxation and leading to impaired relaxation.

There is also a marked downregulation of the novel cardioprotective microRNAs in the diabetic heart.[9] Both circulating and cardiac miR-19b-3p and miR-181b-5p levels have shown to be associated with cardiac dysfunction in mice fed with high fat during the development of diabetic cardiomyopathy and could serve as useful biomarkers to detect early asymptomatic diabetic cardiomyopathy.[10]

CLINICAL DIAGNOSIS

Since cardiac remodeling occurs in various phases, it may remain asymptomatic early in the course of diabetic cardiomyopathy. However, vague symptoms of easy fatigability or breathlessness or mild pedal edema may give some clue.

Since, the pathology starts at the subcellular level, the earliest clinical manifestation will be concentric left ventricular hypertrophy, which can be picked up by a thorough clinical examination, ECG, or echocardiography. There is a direct correlation between the presence of diabetes and the left ventricular mass, which is independent of the body mass or presence of hypertension.[11]

As the duration of diabetes increases, interstitial and perivascular fibrosis along with hypertrophy of left ventricle leads to impaired filling due to diastolic stiffness. Echocardiographic Doppler imaging can detect theses subtle changes by measurement of various cardiac parameters. This diastolic dysfunction is very common and will be asymptomatic in the early stages with preserved ejection fraction.

The natural course of diabetic cardiomyopathy is to develop systolic dysfunction in the later stages with heart failure and reduced ejection fraction in a small percentage of patients.[12]

Patients with diabetes-associated fibrosis may also present with atrial fibrillation or other arrhythmias.[13]

The clinical diagnosis of diabetic cardiomyopathy is very challenging in the early stages, due to the absence of specific morphological changes, biochemical markers or specific clinical manifestations. It is primarily based on exclusion of other risk factors and a high index of suspicion, along with the judicious use of echocardiographic Doppler imaging (both transmitral and tissue Doppler), magnetic resonance imaging (MRI) and positron emission tomography (PET) imaging to characterize cardiac morphology and function at the earliest.

The ratio between early passive transmitral inflow velocity (E) and velocity of the medial mitral annulus (e') is a substitute for invasively measured left ventricular filling pressure and a reliable prognostic marker for diabetic patients, and correlate with the development of heart failure and mortality.[14]

SCREENING FOR HIGH RISK PATIENTS

In the absence of traditional risk factors, symptoms of fatigue or breathlessness, or presence of pedal edema, should prompt for further investigations. A detailed clinical history and a thorough physical examination is essential, along with a high index of suspicion.

Recommended tests are:

- Resting ECG, at initial visit and annually thereafter
- Measurement of albuminuria and e-GFR
- Echocardiography, especially with Doppler imaging to detect the earliest abnormalities of impaired LV filling and stiffness.
- In suspected early heart failure, NT-pro BNP with levels >125 pg/mL would indicate the presence of heart failure (European Society of Cardiology).

THERAPEUTIC STRATEGIES

- Lifestyle modification with appropriate diet and physical activity
- Good glycemic control with use of novel cardiorenal-protective proven glucose-lowering therapies,

especially SGLT2 inhibitors or GLP-1RA (especially liraglutide or dulaglutide)

- Treatment of heart failure is independent of the presence of diabetes and should be as per the current guidelines and include ACEi/ARBs, beta-blockers, MRAs (mineral receptor antagonists), ARNIs (angiotensin receptor neprilysin inhibitors), and judicious use of diuretics. Cardiac resynchronization therapy should be considered in patients with sinus rhythm and wide QRS complex (≥130 ms)
- Potential targets for future:
  - *Gene therapy*: Modulating gene expression in vivo for therapeutic purposes, basically to attenuate mitochondrial dysfunction.[15]
  - *Modulation of oxidative stress*: Supplementation of coenzyme Q10
  - *miRNA and Inc-based treatment*: Multi-target therapy to regulate crucial pathways involved in the pathogenesis of diabetic cardiomyopathy.

CONCLUSION

Diabetes confers a higher risk of cardiovascular disease and heart failure, especially in women, probably because of sex hormones, neurohormonal diversity and gender-specific activation of molecular pathways involved in cardiac metabolism and remodeling.

Diabetic cardiomyopathy is a diagnosis of exclusion, independent of other comorbidities with cardiac structural and functional abnormalities which need to be further characterized for their specificity.

Clinicians need to have a high index of suspicion.

Lifestyle modification (balanced calorie intake, physical exercise), use of cardiorenal protective antidiabetic agents, statins, and guideline directed use of agents for heart failure are the current therapeutic strategies.

Besides achieving a good glycemic control, targeted therapeutic strategies are needed for this specific population.

Early detection with the help of novel biomarkers like miRNAs will enhance therapeutic efficacy.

REFERENCES

1. Yancy CW, Jessup M, Bozkurt B, et al. 2013 ACCF/AHA guideline for the management of heart failure: a report of the American College of Cardiology Foundation/American Heart Association Task Force on Practice Guidelines. J Am Coll Cardiol. 2013;62:e147-e239.
2. Rubler S, Dlugash J, Yuceoglu YZ, et al. New type of cardiomyopathy associated with diabetic glomerulosclerosis. Am J Cardiol. 1972;30: 595-602.
3. Lind M, Bounias I, Olsson M, et al. Glycaemic control and incidence of heart failure in 20,985 patients with type 1 diabetes: an observational study. Lancet. 2011;378:140-6.
4. Brunvand L, Fugelseth D, Stensaeth KH, et al. Early reduced myocardial diastolic function in children and adolescents with type 1 diabetes mellitus a population-based study. BMC Cardiovasc Disord. 2016;16:103.
5. Iribarren C, Karter AJ, Go AS, et al. Glycemic control and heart failure among adult patients with diabetes. Circulation. 2001;103:2668-73.
6. Stratton IM, Adler AI, Neil HA, et al. Association of glycaemia with macrovascular and microvascular complications of type 2 diabetes (UKPDS 35): prospective observational study. BMJ. 2000;321:405-12.
7. Adeghate E, Singh J. Structural changes in the myocardium during diabetes-induced cardiomyopathy. Heart Fail Rev. 2014;19: 15-23.
8. Mytas DZ, Stougiannos PN, ZairisMN, et al. Diabetic myocardial disease: pathophysiology, early diagnosis and therapeutic options. J Diabetes Complications. 2009;23:273-82.
9. Mishra PK, Ying W, Nandi SS, et al, Diabetic Cardiomyopathy: An Immunometabolic Perspective. Front Endocrinol (Lausanne). 2017;8:72.
10. Copier CU, Leon L, Fernandez M, et al. Circulating miR-19b and miR-181b are potential biomarkers for diabetic cardiomyopathy. Sci Rep. 2017;7: 13514.
11. Eguchi K, Boden-Albala B, Jin Z, et al. Association between diabetes mellitus and left ventricular hypertrophy in a multiethnic population. Am J Cardiol. 2008;101:1787-91.
12. Palomer X, Pizarro-Delgado J, Vazquez-Carrera M. Emerging actors in diabetic cardiomyopathy: heartbreaker biomarkers or therapeutic targets? Trends Pharmacol Sci. 2018;39:452-67.
13. Russo I, Frangogiannis NG. Diabetes-associated cardiac fibrosis: cellular effectors, molecular mechanisms and therapeutic opportunities. J Mol Cell Cardiol. 2016;90:84-93.
14. Levelt E, Gulsin G, Neubauer S, et al. Mechanisms in endocrinology: diabetic cardiomyopathy: pathophysiology and potential metabolic interventions state of the art review. Eur J Endocrinol. 2018;178; R127-39.
15. Shepherd DL, Hathaway QA, Nichols CE, et al. Mitochondrial proteome disruption in the diabetic heart through targeted epigenetic regulation at the mitochondrial heat shock protein 70 (mtHsp70) nuclear locus. J Mol Cell Cardiol. 2018;119:104-15.

63 CHAPTER Peculiar Infection in Diabetes

Puneet Saxena, Aradhana Sharma, Suresh Kumar Yadav, SS Dariya

INTRODUCTION

Diabetes mellitus (DM) is a clinical syndrome caused by deficiency of insulin secretion or action. It is considered to be one of the largest emerging threats to health in 21st century. Besides the classical complications of the disease, infectious diseases are more frequent and even more serious in patients with diabetes mellitus, which potentially increases the morbidity and mortality. The increase in frequency of infections in patients with diabetes may be because of the hyperglycemic environment, which favors immune dysfunctions such as the neutrophil function damage, depression of the antioxidant system and humoral immunity, as well as micro and macroangiopathies, neuropathy, gastrointestinal and urinary dysmotility, decline in the antibacterial activity of urine, and number of medical interventions. All organs and systems are affected by the infection. Some problems, such as malignant external otitis (MEO), foot infections, gangrenous cholecystitis, and rhinocerebral mucormycosis, are seen mostly in people with diabetes. This article aims to review the current knowledge on peculiar infection in diabetes mellitus.

DIABETES MELLITUS AND INFECTIONS: PHYSIOPATHOLOGY (FIG. 1)

Infections Strongly Associated with Diabetes: Peculiar Infection in Diabetes

- Rhinocerebral mucormycosis
- Malignant otitis externa
- Emphysematous cholecystitis
- Emphysematous pyelonephritis (EPN)
- Emphysematous cystitis
- Necrotizing fasciitis
- Fournier's gangrene.

Infections possibly related to diabetes but not peculiar are urinary tract infection (bacteriuria, pyelonephritis and renal papillary necrosis, renal abscess, perinephric abscess), fungal infections (oral and vulvovaginal candidiasis, fungal urinary tract infections),[1] *Staphylococcus aureus* infections, tuberculosis, H1N1, influenza, etc.

Rhinocerebral Mucormycosis

The disease is usually defined by hyphae growing in and around the blood vessels and may be potentially life-threatening among people with diabetes or severely immunocompromised individuals. It is an aggressive fulminant invasive fungal infection that can occur in patients with diverse precipitating factors such as uncontrolled diabetes. Mucormycosis is a fungal infection caused by fungi in the order Mucorales (class Zygomycetes).[2-4] *Rhizopus* is the most common genus that is associated with infections in human, followed by Mucor and Cunninghamella.[5]

This infection occurs in nearly 50% cases among patients with DM because of the greater accessibility of glucose, reduced serum inhibitory activity against the *Rhizopus* in lower pH, and enhanced expression of certain host receptors, which is followed by invasion and damage to human epithelial cells caused by *Rhizopus*.[6] In contrast to normal human serum, the serum of patients with diabetes with ketoacidosis does not inhibit the growth of *Rhizopus oryzae*. Acidosis disrupts the ability of transferrin to bind iron, a deficiency results release of free iron into

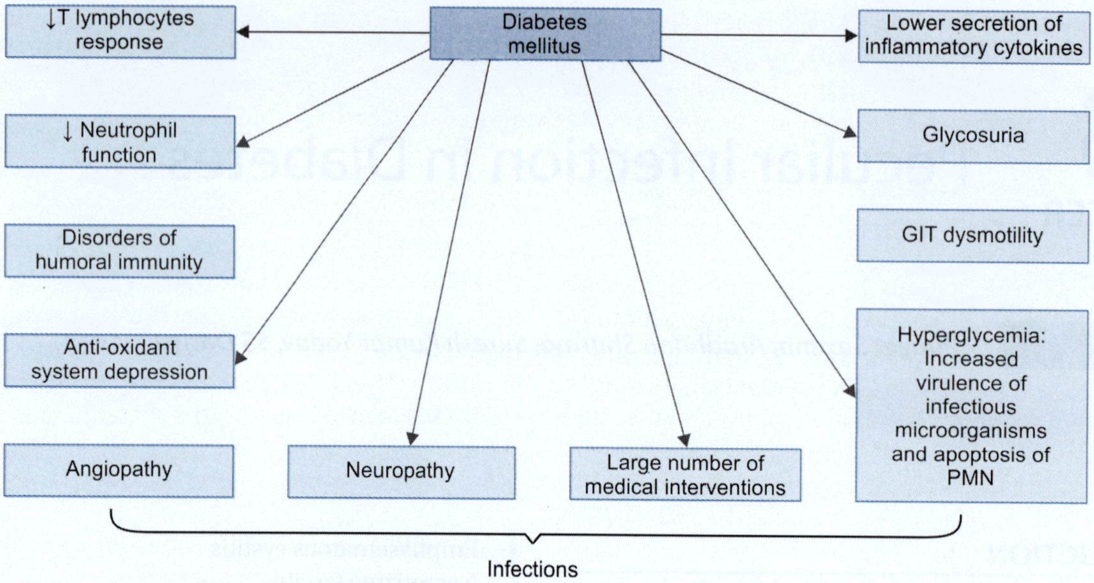

(GIT: gastrointestinal tract; PMN: polymorphonuclear leukocyte)

Figure 1 Diabetes mellitus—infection pathophysiology.

the serum perhaps to an interference in the host defenses against *Rhizopus*, an iron requiring organism.

Mucormycosis may present as a rhinocerebral, pulmonary, cutaneous, gastrointestinal, or disseminated. Rhinocerebral mucormycosis typicaly present with ketoacidosis.

The Rhinocerebral mucormycosis can be acute and chronic.[5,7,8] It is characterized by classical triad of paranasal sinusitis, ophthalmoplegia, and unilateral proptosis.[8,9] A characteristic sign is facial or eye pain as well as necrotic wound of the palate of the nasal mucosa, also necrotic black eschar can occur in the nasal cornets.[5,9] Invasion of brain results in meningoencephalitis or abscess formation with deterioration of neurological function. Aggressive surgical management is mandatory with concomitantly underlying metabolic disorder must be corrected. Amphotericin B remains the standard antifungal therapy and must be used in conjugation with surgery.

The remaining form of mucormycosis does not have a predilection for a specific host, although the pulmonary disease may have a distinctive presentation in patients with diabetes.

Malignant External Otitis

In 1838, Toulmouche was possibly the first physician who reported a case of MEO case. In 1959, Meltzer documented a case of pseudomonal osteomyelitis of the temporal bone. Malignant external otitis is an infection that impacts the temporal bone and the external auditory canal. Necrotizing external otitis is another name for malignant otitis externa. *Pseudomonas aeruginosa* is usually the causative organism and frequently manifests in elderly diabetic patients.[9,10] The infection starts as an external otitis, which advances into the osteomyelitis of temporal bone and adjoining areas.[9,11] Through the Santorini fissures and the osseocartilaginous junction, disease spread outside the external auditory canal.

Bacteria such as *P. aeruginosa* and *S. aureus* often cause malignant otitis externa. Most patients are elderly and 75–90% of people have diabetes who develop malignant otitis externa.

Malignant otitis externa is an aggressive infection rather than a malignancy if it is not treated malignant otitis externa can be life-threatening. Excruciating pain, otorrhea, and hearing loss are the characteristics.[11] But skull base osteomyelitis and cranial nerve involvement may occur. The best diagnostic method is the magnetic resonance imaging.[9] Monotherapy with antipseudomonal cephalosporin ceftazidime for 4–6 week have favorable response in most of patients.

Emphysematous Cholecystitis

It is characterized by perforation of the gallbladder, early gangrene, and increased mortality. Elder males, specifically those with diabetes, are in particular susceptible to the clostridial cholecystitis (emphysematous cholecystitis).

A rare variant of acute cholecystitis is emphysematous cholecystitis, which is caused due to gallbladder wall ischemia and infection with the gas-producing organism such as *Bacteroides fragilis* and *Clostridium perfringens*. It is caused due to acalculous cystic duct obstruction with inflammation and edema that result in cystic artery occlusion with colonization by gas-forming organism. The emphysematous cholecystitis is more frequent in males with DM.[6] The clinical presentation is same as in that of noncomplicated cholecystitis like right upper quadrant abdominal pain, vomiting, and fever.[11] Crackles can be felt on abdominal palpation, which shows worse prognosis.[11] The diagnosis is made by gas inside the gallbladder, demonstrated in radiograph or computerized tomography scan.[6] Cholecystectomy performed as soon as the diagnosis is established with anaerobes as well as both gram-negative and gram-positive organism.

Emphysematous Pyelonephritis

Emphysematous pyelonephritis is a rare, life-threatening acute suppurative infection of the kidney that is characterized by production of gas in and around the kidney. Gas can occur in the calices, collecting system or bladder, but if it is limited to these sites, it distinct from true EPN and carry different prognosis.[12] It is most commonly observed in DM women.[9]

Emphysematous pyelonephritis is characterized by necrosis and gas in the renal parenchyma and in the perinephric tissues. *Escherichia coli* and Enterobacter aerogenes are the most frequent pathogens, followed by *Klebsiella* sp., *Proteus* sp., *Candida*, and *Streptococcus* sp.[6,11] but typically anaerobes are not found. Initially most common clinical presentation is fever, chills, mass and flank pain, nausea, and vomiting.[13] Crackles in the flank or thigh are less frequent.[6,9] Gas in the urinary tract in abdominal computerized tomography allows the identification.[6,9,11] Antibiotics directed at the offending agent with diabetes management imperative but the role of surgery is much less well defined in EPN.

Emphysematous Cystitis

Emphysematous cystitis affects DM persons more frequently than nondiabetics. Also women are more affected than men. It is characterized by the presence of gas in the bladder cavity due to infection by bacteria that produce carbon dioxide. The most common pathogen is *E. coli*, followed by *Enterobacter, Proteus, Klebsiella*, and *Candida*.[6] Standard diagnostic method is computerized tomography.

Necrotizing Fasciitis

It is characterized by fast and progressive deep seated infection of the fascia and subcutaneous tissue, causing fulminant local tissue destruction, microvascular thrombosis, and systemic signs of toxicity. Mortality occurs in approximately 40% of the cases.[11,14-16] Necrotizing fasciitis spreads initially along facial planes progress to muscle, subcutaneous tissues and skin. It is comparatively not common and occurs in people with diabetes and other immunocompromised individuals; it is life-threatening condition. The usual sites are limbs, abdominal wall, perineum and groin.[15,16] Fever and intense local pain are the initial symptoms, followed by areas of skin necrosis with small ulcers draining a colorless fluid and having unpleasant smell.[6,9] Air in the soft tissues can be detected by radiograph.[6] In DM, fasciitis is typically polymicrobial, with one anaerobic and many aerobic microorganisms.[9] Necrotizing fasciitis is divided into two types. Type I fasciitis is caused due to combination of an anaerobic microorganism along with one or more facultative aerobic microorganisms. Group A streptococcus with/without the involvement of staphylococci causes type II fasciitis.[16,17] Necrotizing fasciitis carries a high mortality and is rapidly fatal hence high index of suspicion prompt diagnosis and aggressive treatment are necessary. The cornerstone of management is prompt surgical exploration and debridement of all the involved tissue with antibiotics coverage.

Fournier's Gangrene

It is a specific form of necrotizing fasciitis involving the perineum, scrotum and penis. This is associated with a high mortality (20–30%) and cause of mortality is sepsis and multiorgan failure. Up to 70% of the patients with this infection have DM.[6,18,19]

Fournier gangrene is a fasciitis that affects the perineal, genital, and perianal region. The most common etiologic agents includes *Klebsiella* sp., *E. coli*, *Peptostreptococcus*, and *Proteus* sp. from gastrointestinal tract (30–50%); genitourinary tract (20–40%); and cutaneous injury (20%).[19,20] The etiology may also be polymicrobial, comprising Bacteroides, *Clostridium*, and aerobic or anaerobic streptococci.[6,20]

CONCLUSION

Infectious diseases are found to be more prevalent among peoples with DM due to many factors such as hyperglycemic environment enhancing the virulence of some pathogens, decrease in chemotaxis and phagocytic activity, reduced production of interleukins in response to infection, glycosuria, immobilization of polymorphonuclear leukocytes, and gastrointestinal and urinary dysmotility. Some of the infections, such as rhinocerebral mucormycosis, gangrenous cholecystitis, and MEO, almost always have an effect on persons with diabetes only. Besides being potentially more serious, infectious diseases in DM may lead to metabolic complications like hypoglycemia, ketoacidosis, and coma. Hence strong suspicion and early treatment is needed to prevent or decrease morbidity and mortality.

REFERENCES

1. Stapleton A. Urinary tract infections in patients with diabetes. Am J Med. 2002;113:80S-4S.
2. James WD, Berger TG, Elston DM, et al. Andrews' Diseases of the Skin: Clinical Dermatology. Philadelphia: Saunders Elsevier;2006.
3. Rinaldi MG. Zygomycosis. Infect Dis Clin North Am. 1989;3(1):19-41.
4. Lee FY, Mossad SB, Adal KA. Pulmonary mucormycosis: the last 30 years. Arch Intern Med. 1999;159(12):1301-9.
5. Severo CB, Guazzelli LS, Severo LC. Zigomicose. J Bras Pneumol. 2010;36:134-41.
6. Calvet HM, Yoshikawa TT. Infections in diabetes. Infect Dis Clin North Am. 2001;15:407-20.
7. Artal R, Agreda B, Serrano E, et al. Rhinocerebral mucormycosis: report on eight cases. Acta Otorrinolaringol Esp. 2010;61:301-5.
8. Giuliani A, Mettimano M, Viviani D, et al. An uncommon case of systemic mucormycosis associated with spinal cord infarction in a recently diagnosed diabetic. Int J Immunopathol Pharmacol. 2010;23:355-8.
9. Rocha J, Baggio H, Cunha C, et al. Aspectos relevantes da interface entre diabetes mellitus e infecção. Arq Bras Endocrinol Metab. 2002;46:221-9.
10. Carfrae MJ, Kesser BW. Malignant otitis externa. Otolaryngol Clin North Am. 2008;41:537-49.
11. Nirmal J, Caputo GM, Weitekamp MR, et al. Infections in patients with diabetes mellitus. N Engl J Med. 1999;341:1906-12.
12. Pontin AR, Barnes RD. Current management of emphysematous pyelonephritis. Nat Rev Urol. 2009;6:272-9.
13. Hokkam EN. Assessment of risk factors in diabetic foot ulceration and atheir impact on the outcome of the disease. Prim Care Diab. 2009;3:219-24.
14. Zhang WJ, Cai XY, Yang C, et al. Cervical necrotizing fasciitis due to methicillin-resistant Staphylococcus aureus: a case report. Int J Oral Maxillofac Surg. 2010;39:83-4.
15. Oguz H, Demirci M, Arslan N, et al. Necrotizing fasciitis of the head and neck: Report of two cases and literature review. Ear Nose Throat J. 2010;89:E7-10.
16. Shaikh N, Ummunissa F, Hanssen Y, et al. Hospital epidemiology of emergent cervical necrotizing fasciitis. J Emerg Trauma Shock. 2010;3:123-5.
17. Shimizu T, Tokuda Y. Necrotizing fasciitis. Intern Med J. 2010;49:1051-7.
18. Chen SL, Jackson SL, Boyko EJ. Diabetes mellitus and urinary tract infection: epidemiology, pathogenesis and proposed studies in animal models. J Urol. 2009;182:S51-6.
19. Tran HA, Hart AM. Fournier's gangrene. Intern Med J. 2006;36:200-1.
20. Montoya Chinchilla R, Izquierdo Morejon E, Nicolae Pietricâ B, et al. [Fournier's gangrene. Descriptive analysis of 20 cases and literature review]. Actas Urol Esp. 2009;33:873-80.

64 CHAPTER Urinary Tract Infection and Dental Infection: Often Neglected—How to Prevent?

Asha N Shah

INTRODUCTION

Urinary tract infection (UTI) may be asymptomatic (subclinical) or symptomatic (disease). It encompasses many clinical entities like asymptomatic bacteriuria, cystitis, prostatitis, and pyelonephritis. Except among neonates and elderly, UTI occurs far more commonly in females. As many as 50–80% of women in general population acquires at least one UTI during their lifetime. Diabetic patients have the tendency for increased risk of infections and of UTIs in particular which are usually more severe, and also carry worse outcomes as they are frequently caused by resistant pathogens.[1]

The diabetic population is highly heterogeneous, and the risk of UTI and its complications may vary widely depending on age, gender, type of diabetes, duration, and severity of diabetes. Serious complications of UTI, such as emphysematous cystitis/pyelonephritis, xanthogranulomatous pyelonephritis (XGP), renal/perirenal abscess, and renal papillary necrosis are all seen more frequently in type 2 diabetes compared to the general population. Improved outcomes of all these entities could also be achieved by early diagnosis, assessment of predisposing factors, proper diagnosis, and prompt correct management. All type of infections like community-acquired UTI, healthcare-associated UTI, catheter-associated UTI, or postrenal transplant and recurrent UTI are more common in diabetic patients. Diabetics are more prone to have resistant pathogens as the cause of their UTI. The increased risk of UTI in diabetic patients and the increasing incidence of type 2 diabetes mellitus in the world in recent years, may pose a substantial burden on medical costs.[2] Over and above that the high rates of antibiotic prescription, including broad-spectrum antibiotics, for UTI. In these patients may further induce the development of antibiotic-resistant urinary pathogens.

Why hospital acquired urinary tract infection (UTI) is often neglected?

There is less morbidity due to hospital-acquired UTI compared to that seen in surgical site infections, pneumonia, and bacteremia. Death directly attributable to hospital-acquired UTI is also uncommon. Treatment is generally straightforward. The estimated costs of hospital-acquired UTI are markedly lower than those for the other major healthcare-associated infections. In addition, the healthcare professionals probably perceive an indwelling urethral catheter as less dangerous as and of less concern than an endotracheal tube, surgical incision, or indwelling vascular.

INCIDENCE OF URINARY TRACT INFECTION IN DIABETES

All varieties of UTI are more common in patients having type 2 diabetes. As per report of a Danish study patients with diabetes mellitus were 3 times more likely to be hospitalized with pyelonephritis, as compared to subjects without diabetes.[1] An observational study of all the patients with type 2 diabetes in the United Kingdom found that the incidence rate of UTI was 46.9 per 1,000 person-years among diabetic patients compared to 29.9 for patients without diabetes.[3] Women with recently diagnosed diabetes (within 6 months) had increased risk of UTI compared to previously diagnosed women. A cohort study of over 6,000 patients enrolled in ten clinical trials found an incidence rate of 91.5 per 1,000 person-years in women and 28 per 1,000 person-years in men. Increase in incidence of UTI was observed at all age groups in women.[4] American study based on data of 89,790 patients who were matched pairs from 2014 found that a UTI diagnosis was more common in men and women with diabetes than in those without diabetes (9.4% vs 5.7%, respectively).[5]

PREVALENCE OF URINARY TRACT INFECTION, BY GENDER AND AGE GROUP[2]

It is known that cases of UTI are more in all age groups in female patients and also increase with age.

RISK FACTORS FOR URINARY TRACT INFECTION IN DIABETES

- History of previous UTI and recent or frequent sexual activity increase UTI risk
- Bladder dysfunction and residual urine
- Inadequate fluid intake
- Support for an effect of glycosuria or poor diabetic control, in UTI risk among persons with diabetes, HbA1c levels, and specific diabetic complications is weak
- Urinary tract anatomical defects
- Kidney stones may obstruct the flow of urine and sets the stage for an infection.
- An enlarged prostate
- Menopause
- Pregnancy
- Females using a diaphragm for birth control
- Maternal history of UTI
- New sexual partner
- Use of urinary catheter for long time
- Having surgery on the urinary tract system
- Urinary or fecal incontinence
- Because of diabetic cystopathy vesicourethral reflux results leading to recurrent UTIs. Over and above that, some degree of cystocele, rectocele, and cystourethrocele is present in 30% women with diabetes.

ASYMPTOMATIC BACTERIURIA

Asymptomatic bacteriuria (ASB or ABU) is defined as growth of the same uropathogen ($\geq 10^5$ cfu/mL) in two consecutive urine samples. Women with diabetes have an increased prevalence of ASB in comparison to women without diabetes. A meta-analysis of 22 studies, published in 2011, found a point prevalence of 12.2% of ASB among diabetic patients versus 4.5% in healthy control subjects, etc., asymptomatic bacteriuria.[6]

Increased prevalence of ASB in diabetic patients has been reported in numerous studies with percentage ranging from 8% to 26%. A recent prospective study of indoor patients at an Indian hospital found that prevalence rate of ASB was 30% among diabetic patients ASB is more common in women, due to a short urethra which is in proximity to the, moist, warm vulval, and perianal areas and these areas are more commonly colonized with enteric bacteria. ASB increases with age and is also associated with urinary tract abnormalities or foreign bodies (urethral catheters, stents, etc.). Risk factors for ASB for all women with DM are: age, duration of DM, retinopathy, macroalbuminuria, a lower BMI and a symptomatic UTI in the previous year.

URINARY TRACT INFECTION IN DIABETIC MAN

- Risk of acute bacterial prostatitis
- Prostatic abscess
- Progression to chronic prostatitis
- Lack of circumcision
- An infection following prostatic manipulations, such as transrectal prostate biopsy, is increased in patients with diabetes mellitus.

PATHOGENESIS OF URINARY TRACT INFECTION IN DIABETES

- High renal parenchymal glucose levels create a favorable environment for the growth and multiplication of microorganisms and they adhere to the uroepithelium.
- Impairments in the immune system, including humoral, cellular, and innate immunity.
- Lower urinary interleukin-6 and -8 levels.
- Autonomic neuropathy leading to bladder dysfunction occurs in 26–85% women and leads to dysfunctional voiding and urinary retention, decreasing physical bacterial clearance through micturition, thereby facilitating bacterial growth.
- Hyperglycemia causes dysfunction of neutrophils by increasing intracellular calcium levels and thereby interfering with actin and, so also interferes with, diapedesis and phagocytosis.
- Only dapagliflozin was associated with a slight increase in UTI (4.8% vs 3.7%) but no difference with canagliflozin.[7]
- Emphysematous complications in the kidney or the bladder are likely to be due to the presence of

organisms that rapidly ferment glucose and produce carbon dioxide. Impaired tissue perfusion in diabetes leads to impairment in transport of metabolic end products which may also be a contributing factor.

- The pathogenesis of XGP which is seen in diabetic patients is still not very well-known. It is a chronic granulomatous process and It is associated with Proteus or *Escherichia coli* infection. Proposed etiologies of XGP include chronic renal obstruction and infection, lymphatic obstruction, alterations in lipid metabolism and renal ischemia. In XGP kidney tissue is destroyed and replaced by yellow hard xanthogranulomatous material and treatment is nephrectomy.

Pathogens

The most common pathogens are *Escherichia coli*, other Enterobacteriaceae such as *Klebsiella spp.*, *Proteus spp.*, *Enterobacter spp.*, and Enterococci-resistant pathogens like extended-spectrum β-lactamase-positive Enterobacteriaceae, fluoroquinolone-resistant uropathogens, carbapenem-resistant Enterobacteriaceae, and vancomycin-resistant Enterococci,[8] fungal infections.

Prevention

- Control of blood sugar and hypertension
- Avoidance of risk factors when possible
- Plenty of fluids
- Avoidance of alcohol
- Personal hygiene
- Voiding when there is urge
- The use of cranberry as prophylaxis for UTI is a conditional recommendation (level C evidence).
- Cranberry in juice or tablet form and its effect has been studied by many randomized controlled trials (RCTs)[9]
  - The mechanism of action is supposed to be related to the ability of the proanthocyanidins present in cranberries which may prevent bacteria from adhering to the epithelium of urinary tract.
- As per American urological association guidelines, the use of vaginal estrogen treatment to decrease future UTI risk in peri- and postmenopausal women with recurrent UTIs is a moderate
- Recommendation (level B evidence).
- Routine screening for ASB is not recommended in diabetics
- The strong recommendation is that clinicians should not treat ASB as it may lead to development of infections with Clostridium deficiency, and leads antibiotic resistance, except in few conditions like:
  - Pregnancy
  - Before urological intervention
  - Renal transplant patient
- Immunotherapy with Solco-Urovac, which is a vaccine active against *Escherichia coli, Klebsiella, Proteus, Streptococcus faecalis* organisms may be useful for treatment of UTI
- More RCTs are needed to know the duration of treatment in diabetics with UTI.
- The prevention of hospital-acquired UTI in diabetes
- Urethral catheter should be inserted only when indicated, and it should be removed at the earliest.
- Insert catheter under all aseptic precautions and meatal care
- Maintain a closed drainage system. Before collecting urine specimens by aspirating with a sterile needle from the bag sample port, cleaning the port with 70% isopropyl alcohol should be done and let it dry thoroughly.
- Keep the collection bag at a lower level to bladder so as to prevent backflow of urine.
- Empty the urine collection bag regularly.
- Development of biofilm on the indwelling urinary catheter is the primary cause of catheter-associated UTI.
- Development of catheter materials that do not support biofilm formation could, theoretically, eliminate most bacteriuria and, one assumes, symptomatic infection.

Prevention of Recurrent Urinary Tract Infection

- Prophylactic strategies like continuous, postcoital, or patient initiated therapy.

DIABETES AND DENTAL INFECTIONS

Risk factors for dental infections in diabetes are:[10]

- Diabetics may have xerostomia.
- Normally saliva protects teeth, so they are at a higher risk of cavities.
- More prone to Gingivitis (early gum disease) and Periodontitis (advanced gum disease)
- May have impaired taste sensations.
- Susceptible to infections inside mouth and delayed wound healing
- Children with diabetes may have earlier eruption of teeth
- Diabetics are more prone to different types of dental abscesses like

- Periapical abscess: Collection of pus at the tip of the root.
- Gingival abscess: Localized pus collection involves only gum tissue.
- Periodontal abscess: Pus collection involving bone adjacent to the tooth.
- Pericoronal abscess: Localized abscess of the gum tissue surrounding the crown of tooth (often may be associated with lower wisdom tooth).
- Combined endodontic or peridontal abscess.

Pathophysiological Relationship between Diabetes and Dental Disease

The relationship between diabetes and dental disease has been described in Figure 1.

Prevention of Dental Infections

- Regular dental checkups are important. Treating gum disease can help controlling blood sugar in patients with diabetes as per research studies and also may decrease the progression of the disease. Good oral hygiene is extremely important and deep cleanings by professionals will help greatly.
- Control blood sugar
- Healthy diet
- Avoid smoking
- Regular brushing twice/day with cleaning between teeth (Table 1).

CONCLUSION

Urinary tract infection is common and painful illness which is very common in females and in people with diabetes. As macrovascular and microvascular complications of diabetes occupy major share of concern, infections associated with it take a backseat. More awareness of asymptomatic bacteriuria[11] and its management is needed along with awareness and management of risk factors and preventive measures for UTI. Similarly importance of dental infections and ways of prevention will help physicians take care of their diabetic patients in a better way.

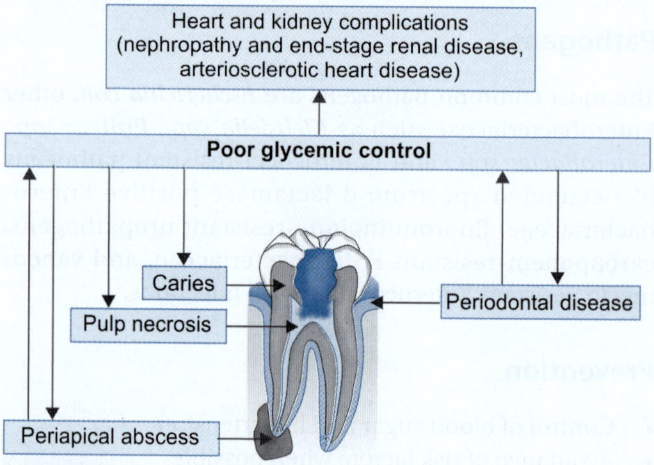

Figure 1 Relationship between diabetes and urinary tract infection (UTI).

TABLE 1: Pathophysiology of relationship between UTI and diabetes.

Oral pathology related to DM	Pathogenesis	Treatment and Prevention
Periodontal disease	Accumulation of AGEs in periodontal tissues, decreased periodontal regenerative capacity, and defective immune regulation	Assessment of risk of disease progression periodic reviews, dietary advice, and periodontal therapy
Dry mouth	Reduced salivary flow as a result of polyuria and dehydration	Proper control diabetes and dental hygiene
Root caries	As a result of gingival resorption and decreased salivary flow	Use of fluoridated pastes, restorative treatments. The optimal glycemic control prevents progression
Oral Candidiasis	Because salivary dysfunction, hyperglycemia and impaired immune system	Antifungal nystatin or miconazole treatment. Good glycemic control and prevention
Pulp necrosis and periodontal abscess	Ischemic tissue damage related pulp own vascular damage from diabetes	Endodontic treatment and control of diabetes
Delayed wound healing and increased incidence of infections following surgery	Caused by vascular dysfunction and decreased immune on diabetes	Preventive administration of antibiotics and good glycemic control

(AGEs: advanced glycation end-products; DM: diabetes mellitus)

REFERENCES

1. Nitzan O, Elias M, Chazan B, et al. Urinary tract infections in patients with type 2 diabetes mellitus: review of prevalence, diagnosis, and management. Diabetes Metab Syndr Obes. 2015;8:129-36.
2. Yu S, Fu AZ, Qiu Y, et al. Disease burden of urinary tract infections among type 2 diabetes mellitus patients in the U.S. J Diabetes Complications. 2014;28(5):621-6.
3. Hirji I, Guo Z, Andersson SW, et al. Incidence of urinary tract infection among patients with type 2 diabetes in the UK General Practice Research Database (GPRD). J Diabetes Complications. 2012;26(6):513-6.
4. Hammar N, Farahmand B, Gran M, et al. Incidence of urinary tract infection in patients with type 2 diabetes. Experience from adverse event reporting in clinical trials. Pharmacoepidemiol Drug Saf. 2010;19(12):1287-92.
5. Fu AZ, Iglay K, Qiu Y, et al. Risk characterization for urinary tract infections in subjects with newly diagnosed type 2 diabetes. J Diabetes Complications. 2014;28(6):805-10.
6. Renko M, Tapanainen P, Tossavainen P, et al. Meta-analysis of the significance of asymptomatic bacteriuria in diabetes. Diabetes Care. 2011;34(1):230-5.
7. Ptaszynska A, Johnsson KM, Parikh SJ, et al. Safety profile of dapagliflozin for type 2 diabetes: pooled analysis of clinical studies for overall safety and rare events. Drug Saf. 2014;37(10):815-29.
8. Wu YH, Chen PL, Hung YP, et al. Risk factors and clinical impact of levofloxacin or cefazolin nonsusceptibility or ESBL production among uropathogens in adults with community-onset urinary tract infections. J Microbiol Immunol Infect. 2014;47(3):197-203.
9. Chambers BK, Camire ME. Can cranberry supplementation benefit adults with type 2 diabetes? Diabetes Care. 2003;26(9):2695-6.
10. Shah BR, Hux JE. Quantifying the risk of infectious diseases for people with diabetes. Diabetes Care. 2003;26(2):510-3.
11. Nicolle LE. Asymptomatic bacteriuria. Curr Opin Infect Dis. 2014;27(1): 90-6.

65 CHAPTER Role of Immunization in Preventing Infections in Diabetes Mellitus

A Muruganathan, D Suresh Kumar, Rohit Vashisht

INTRODUCTION

Diabetics (both type 1 and type 2) are at higher risk for common vaccine-preventable diseases like pneumonia, influenza and hepatitis B.[1] Even if the sugars are well managed, it is harder for the immune system to fight against these infections, hence diabetics are at higher risk for serious complications from an illness compared to people without diabetes. Some illnesses, like influenza, can raise the blood glucose to dangerously high levels. People with diabetes have higher rates of hepatitis B than the rest of the population due to blood glucose monitoring procedures. Immunization protects against these diseases.

COMMON VACCINES FOR PEOPLE WITH DIABETES

Influenza Vaccine

Complications from the flu, such as sinus and ear infections, pneumonia and bronchitis can lead to hospitalization or sometimes death for diabetics. People with diabetes are *six times* more likely to be hospitalized during an influenza epidemic than those without diabetes.[2]

American Diabetes Association (ADA) **2019 Standards of Medical Care in Diabetes** recommends influenza vaccine annually for all diabetic patients more than or equal to 6 months of age.

Centers for Disease Control and Prevention (CDC)/Advisory Committee on Immunization Practices (ACIP) **2019–20** also recommends influenza vaccine to above age group in diabetics. Inactivated trivalent or quadrivalent influenza vaccines are recommended to use. The Live attenuated (LAIV 4) is contraindicated in immunocompromised population; however diabetes has not been mentioned in that list. Hence, it can be used on case to case basis.

In Indian setting also, we should recommend the influenza vaccine to all the diabetics more than or equal to 6 months of age.

Pneumococcal Vaccine

People with diabetes are almost three times at higher risk of death due to pneumonia-related complications.[3] The **ADA 2019** Standards of Medical Care in Diabetes and the **CDC-2018** have recommended that all diabetics with 2 years of age and older below 65 years should receive one dose of 23 valent pneumococcal polysaccharide vaccine (PPSV 23). After 65 years, 13 valent pneumococcal conjugate vaccine (PCV 13) to be given and followed by PPSV 23 after 1 year.

ACIP 2019 also recommends 1 dose of PPSV 23 at age 2 years through 64 years in the diabetic population. It recommends to administer PCV 13 doses needed to complete series to children through age 71 months.

In Indian setting also, we should recommend PPSV 23 to all diabetics between 2 years and 65 years of age. Persons more than 65 years should receive PCV 13 followed by PPSV 23 after 1 year.

Hepatitis B Vaccine

Patients with diabetes are at a 2.1 times increased risk of infection by the hepatitis B vaccine (HBV) than nondiabe-

TABLE 1: Recommended vaccines for diabetic patients.

Vaccine	Frequency and route	Comments
Inactivated influenza vaccine	Annually, intramuscular (IM)	Either trivalent/quadrivalent
Live attenuated vaccine	Annually, intranasal	Caution needed in poorly controlled diabetic
23 valent pneumococcal polysaccharide vaccine (PPV)	One dose between 19 years and 64 years, IM	Booster after the age of 65 years, if vaccinate 5 years before
13 valent pneumococcal conjugate vaccine	Above 65 years, IM	Other immunosuppressing conditions, advised before 65 years age
Hepatitis B	3 doses, IM	0, 1, and 6 months
Tdap	1 dose of Tdap, IM	Then every 10 years Td
Zoster vaccine	1 dose above 60 years, SC	If recombinant vaccine 2 doses above the age of 50 years with 4 weeks gap

tics. The relative risk (RR) of HBV infection was 43% higher amongst those diagnosed with diabetes than amongst those not diagnosed [RR 1.43, 95% confidence interval (CI) 1.26–1.63]. These results suggest that the risk of HBV infection is higher amongst individuals diagnosed with diabetes mellitus. CDC recommends the HBV for any unvaccinated adults under the age of 60 years. It consists of three doses of vaccine administered intramuscularly at 0, 1, and 6 months.[4]

As per latest ACIP, it also recommends Heplisav-B® (HepB-CpG) as an option for adults age 18 years or greater for vaccination against HBV. HepB-CpG is given as a two-dose series separated by 1 month (compared to the standard 3-dose vaccine at months 0, 1 and 6), which may result in better compliance.

In Indian setting also, routine HBV vaccine (e.g. Engerix) is to be offered to all diabetics under the age of 60 years with three-dose schedule of 0, 1 and 6 months.

Herpes Zoster Vaccine

Approximately 13% of cases of herpes zoster infection occur in patients with T2DM.[5]

CDC-2018 recommends this vaccine for people age 50 years and older. Shingrix® (RZV), the recombinant adjuvanted herpes zoster vaccine, is administered intramuscularly in two doses given 2–6 months apart. RZV is the preferred shingles vaccine due to its higher efficacy and longer duration of protection. **In Indian setting,** Shingerix (RZV) is a good option for all diabetics 50 years and older.

Tetanus, Diphtheria, and Pertussis Vaccine

It is administered to protect against tetanus, diphtheria and pertussis. **CDC 2018** recommends all adults get the tetanus, diphtheria, and pertussis (Tdap) vaccine once, and a Td vaccine booster dose every 10 years. Similar recommendations can be applicable to the Indian set up. In summary, following vaccines are recommended for diabetic population (Table 1).

CONCLUSION

Infections in diabetic host increases not only the morbidity but also mortality. Unfortunately most of the common infections are preventable with vaccinations. All diabetic care providers and patients should be sensitized about the vaccinations and simple check lists should be included in the case records to improve the adherence to above practices.

REFERENCES

1. Shah BR, Hux JE. Quantifying the risk of infectious diseases for people with diabetes. Diabetes Care. 2003;26:510-32.
2. Smith SA, Poland GA. Use of influenza and pneumococcal vaccines in people with diabetes. Diabetes Care. 2000;23:95-108.
3. Akbar DH. Bacterial pneumonia: comparison between diabetics and non-diabetics. Acta Diabetol. 2001;38:77-82.
4. Spradling PR, Byrd KK, Xing J, et al. Centers for Disease Control and Prevention (CDC). Use of hepatitis B vaccination for adults with diabetes mellitus: recommendations of the Advisory Committee on Immunization Practices (ACIP). MMWR Morb Mortal Wkly Rep. 2011;60:1709-11.
5. Suaya JA et al. Incidence of herpes zoster and persistent post zoster pain in adults with or without diabetes in the United States. Open forum Infect Dis. 2014;1(2):ofu049.

66 CHAPTER Congenital and Acquired Lipodystrophies

Rohit Kapoor, Rishabh Kapoor, Shivam Kapoor

INTRODUCTION

Lipodystrophies, also termed lipodystrophic syndromes, are a heterogeneous group of rare disorders characterized by either complete or partial loss of adipose tissue (lipoatrophy). The loss of body fat in many patients is developed due to underlying genetic defects and it can also be developed due to various acquired conditions.[1]

Depending on the extent of loss of body fat, lipodystrophies can be classified as generalized (affect nearly the entire body), partial (only certain body part) or localized (small areas under the skin).[2] The genetic lipodystrophies include autosomal-recessive or autosomal-dominant disorders while acquired lipodystrophies include autoimmune mechanisms or drug-induced lipodystrophy [like highly active antiretroviral therapy (HAART)-induces partial lipodystrophy in human immunodeficiency virus (HIV)-infected patients or insulin and other injected drugs results in localized lipodystrophy].[1,2] Table 1 summarizes the major subtypes of lipodystrophies.

Lipodystrophies appeared in the medical pieces of literature for more than 100 years. Approximately 125 years ago, the first type of lipodystrophy reported was acquired partial lipodystrophy (APL),[3] followed by the acquired generalized lipodystrophy (AGL) variety.[4] The phenotype of the first genetic variety, congenital generalized lipodystrophy (CGL), was reported only 56 years ago while HAART-induces partial lipodystrophy in HIV-infected patients was recognized only about two decades ago.[5,6] The most prevalent subtype of lipodystrophies is the localized lipodystrophies and lipodystrophy in HIV-infected patients. Comparatively, the other genetic and acquired lipodystrophies are rare types.[1]

The severity and extent of body fat loss also decide the predisposition of the patients to metabolic disorders associated with insulin resistance, including early onset of diabetes mellitus, hypertriglyceridemia, and hepatic steatosis. Localized lipodystrophies do not predispose to metabolic complications because the loss of fat is trivial; however, other generalized and partial lipodystrophies are associated with variable predisposition to metabolic complications, while localized lipodystrophies do not predispose to metabolic complications.[1,2] In some patients, these metabolic disorders can further lead to complications such as diabetic nephropathy and retinopathy, acute pancreatitis, hepatic cirrhosis, premature cardiovascular disease, etc.[2] Apart from these complications, other common clinical outcomes of lipodystrophies include polycystic ovarian syndrome (PCOS), severe insulin resistance caused acanthosis

TABLE 1: Major subtypes of lipodystrophies.

	Genetic lipodystrophies	Acquired lipodystrophies
Generalized	Congenital generalized lipodystrophy	Acquired generalized lipodystrophy
Partial	Familial partial lipodystrophy	Acquired partial lipodystrophy HAART-induced partial lipodystrophy in HIV patients
Localized		Acquired localized lipodystrophy

(HAART: highly active antiretroviral therapy; HIV: human immunodeficiency virus)

TABLE 2: Subtypes of genetic lipodystrophies.[1,2,7,10,11]

Subtypes	Gene	Prevalence
Congenital generalized lipodystrophy (CGL)		
CGL type 1	AGPAT2	Most common subtype
CGL type 2	BSCL2	Second most common subtype
CGL type 3	CAV1	Only one patient reported
CGL type 4	PTRF	About 20 patients reported
Familial partial lipodystrophy (FPL)		
FPL type 1 Kobberling-type	Unknown	Rare
FPL Type 2 (Dunnigan-type)	LMNA	Most common subtype; more than 500 patients reported
FPL type 3	PPARγ	Second most common subtype; about 30–50 patients reported
FPL type 4	PLIN1	Reported in three families
FPL type 5	CIDEC	One patient reported
FPL type 6	LIPE	Six patients reported
FPL type 7	ADRA2A	Reported in one family

(AGPAT2: 1-acylglycerol-3-phosphate O-acyltransferase 2; BSCL2: berardinelli-Seip congenital lipodystrophy 2; CAV1: caveolin 1; PTRF: polymerase I and transcript release factor; CIDEC: cell death-inducing DFFA-like effector c; LIPE: hormone-sensitive lipase; LMNA: lamin A/C; PLIN1: perilipin 1; PPARγ: peroxisome proliferator-activated receptor-gamma)

nigricans, extreme hypertriglyceridemia caused eruptive xanthomas etc.[1,2,7] Regardless of the etiology, serum levels of adipocytokines, leptin, and adiponectin, are extremely low in patients with generalized lipodystrophy.[8,9]

The present article discusses the major types of lipodystrophies with respect to their molecular basis and key clinical features, along with the current therapy and feature perspectives.

GENETIC LIPODYSTROPHIES

With the advancement in the characterization of the phenotypes of various types of genetic lipodystrophies and the understanding of molecular mechanisms has increased, revealing of these syndromes.[1] There are two major types of genetic lipodystrophies, CGL and familial partial lipodystrophy (FPL) (Table 2).

Congenital generalized lipodystrophy is autosomal-recessive syndrome which is further divided into four subtypes. CGL type 1 is associated with 1-acylglycerol-3-phosphate O-acyltransferase 2 (AGPAT2) gene. This type is the most common subtype of CGL. AGPAT enzymes have an important role in the biosynthesis of triglycerides and phospholipids in various organs. Adipose tissue highly expresses AGPAT isoform 2. CGL type 2 involves Berardinelli-seip congenital lipodystrophy 2 (BSCL2) genes and is the second most common subtype. BSCL2 encode for seipin, which plays an important role in the fusion of small lipid droplets in adipocytes and in adipocyte differentiation. CGL type 3 is associated with caveolin 1 (CAV1) gene. Caveolin 1 is an integral part of caveolae which translocate fatty acids and other lipids to lipid droplets. Only one patient of this type is reported. Polymerase I and transcript release factor (PTRF), also known as cavin-1, is involved in the biogenesis of caveolae and regulates expression of caveolins 1 and 3. PTFR gene mutation is responsible for type 4 CGL. About 20 patients are reported with this type.[2,10,11] Clinical features of each of these types of CGL is summarized in Table 3.

The second major type of genetic lipodystrophies is FPL which is mainly categorized under seven subtypes. FPL type 1 (Köbberling-type) is a rare subtype with unknown pathological mechanism. FPL2 (Dunnigan-type) is the most common subtype of FPL, which is associated with lamin A/C (LMNA) gene. LMNA codes nuclear lamina proteins, lamin A and C. Mutation of lamins disrupts interaction between nuclear lamina and chromatin resulting in apoptosis which may be followed by premature adipocyte death. Followed by FPL2, FPL3 is the second most common subtype involving peroxisome proliferator-activated receptor gamma (PPARγ) gene. PPARγ plays a major role in regulation of adiposity

TABLE 3: Clinical features in congenital generalized lipodystrophy (CGL) subtypes.[1,10,11]

Subtypes	Clinical features
CGL type 1	Near-total fat loss, preserved mechanical fat, severe insulin resistance, metabolic abnormalities, cystic lesions in long bones.
CGL type 2	Severe near-total fat loss, almost no mechanical fat, severe insulin resistance, metabolic abnormalities, and occasionally cystic lesions in long bones, may be associated with delayed mental development and cardiomyopathy
CGL type 3	Near-total fat loss, preserved bone marrow fat, severe insulin resistance, metabolic abnormalities, delayed growth, short stature, hypocalcemia, vitamin D resistance, and osteopenia
CGL type 4	Near-total fat loss, partially preserved bone marrow fat, myopathy with elevated CK levels, percussion-induced muscle mounding, scoliosis, atlantoaxial instability, pyloric stenosis, gastrointestinal dysmotility, cardiac arrhythmias (catecholaminergic polymorphic ventricular tachycardia, atrial fibrillation, prolonged QT), and sudden death

TABLE 4: Clinical features in familial partial lipodystrophy (FPL) subtypes.[1,10,11]

Subtypes	Clinical features
FPL type 1	Fat loss mainly limited to the extremities, truncal obesity, palpable "ledge" between lipodystrophic and non-lipodystrophic areas, severe insulin resistance and metabolic abnormalities
FPL type 2	Fat loss dominantly affects limbs, increased muscularity, excess fat in the face and neck, labial pseudo-hypertrophy, increased mons pubis fat, severe insulin resistance, and metabolic abnormalities
FPL type 3	Milder fat loss mostly affects the distal limbs, no accumulation of adipose tissue in the face and neck, severe insulin resistance and metabolic abnormalities
FPL type 4	Fat loss in lower limbs and femorogluteal depot, severe insulin resistance, and metabolic abnormalities
FPL type 5	Partial lipodystrophy, acanthosis nigricans, severe insulin resistance, metabolic abnormalities, and diabetic ketoacidosis
FPL type 6	Late-onset partial fat loss affecting the lower limbs, multiple lipomatosis, and progressive distal symmetric myopathy.
FPL type 7	FPL phenotype, increased muscularity, needs to be confirmed in further pedigrees.

differentiation. Perilipin 1 (PLIN1) gene is involved in FPL type 4. Perilipin coats lipid droplet and it is required for optimal lipid incorporation and release from droplet. Cell death-inducing DFFA-like effector c (CIDEC) is expressed in lipid droplets. Pathogenic variants of CIDEC gene may result in loss of ability of lipid droplets to store fat and defects in adipocyte differentiation and cause FPL type 5. Hormone-sensitive lipase (LIPE) gene is involved in the pathogenesis of FPL6. LIPE encodes hormone-sensitive lipase, involved in lipolysis regulation. FPL type 7 involved (ADRA2A) gene, activation of which inhibits cAMP production and reduces lipolysis.[2,10,11] Clinical features of FPL are summarized in Table 4.

ACQUIRED LIPODYSTROPHIES

Despite recognition for more than 100 years, understanding underlying mechanisms of acquired lipodystrophies have been slow.[1] Acquired lipodystrophies are more common than the genetic lipodystrophies. Each acquired lipodystrophy expresses unique clinical features and underlying pathogenic mechanism (Table 5).

MANAGEMENT OF LIPODYSTROPHIES

Treatment of lipodystrophies is challenging. Currently, there is no specific treatment available for lipodystrophy. Although lipodystrophy is not cured, morbidity and mortality are improved through early intervention. The management of lipodystrophy is focused on the metabolic abnormalities to prevent complications and cosmetic appearance.

Diet and exercise are an integral part of the treatment plan.[2] A well-balanced diet with macronutrient composed of about 50–60% carbohydrates, 20–30% fat, and about 10–20% protein is suitable for most patients. In infants and children, overfeeding should be avoided, as this can accelerate hepatic steatosis and worsen diabetes and hyperlipidemia, while for adults, energy-restricted diets are more appropriate. Energy-restricted diets are not appropriate in children with growth and developmental needs as they may otherwise develop deficiencies. Patients should be encouraged to be physically active.

If not contraindicated, exercise can help improve metabolic parameters. For patients predisposed to

TABLE 5: Types, subtypes, molecular basis, and clinical features of acquired lipodystrophies.[1]

Types	Subtypes	Molecular basis	Clinical features
Acquired generalized lipodystrophy	• Autoimmune • Panniculitis associated • Idiopathic	Panniculitis preceding loss of subcutaneous fat and association of autoimmune diseases suggests immune-mediated loss of adipose tissue. Other mechanisms may also be involved	Generalized loss of fat associated with tender subcutaneous nodules, autoimmune, or other diseases
Acquired partial lipodystrophy	• Autoimmune • MPGN associated • Idiopathic	Low serum complement 3 levels and presence of autoantibody, complement 3 nephritic factor, in most of the patients suggests autoimmune-mediated loss of adipose tissue.	Loss of subcutaneous fat from the face, neck, upper limbs, and trunk, sparing lower abdomen and lower limbs.
Lipodystrophy in HIV-infected patients	• PI-induced • NRTI-induced	PI may inhibit ZMPSTE24 and/or cause dysregulation of transcription factors involved in adipogenesis. NRTI may inhibit mitochondrial polymerase and cause mitochondrial toxicity	Loss of subcutaneous fat from the face and extremities and excess fat deposition in the neck and abdomen
Localized lipodystrophy	• Drug-induced • Panniculitis-induced • Pressure-induced • Centrifugal • Idiopathic	Multiple mechanisms, including local drug-induced, immune-mediated, or pressure-induced atrophy of adipose tissue. Other unknown mechanisms may also be involved	Loss of subcutaneous fat from small areas of body.

(MPGN: membranoproliferative glomerulonephritis)

TABLE 6: Approval and indications of metreleptin therapy.[9]

Type of lipodystrophy	Indications	Approval status
Generalized lipodystrophy (both CGL and AGL)	First-line drug treatment (after diet/exercise intervention) for metabolic and endocrine abnormalities May prevent comorbidities and metabolic complications in young children	*United States:* Approved as adjunct to diet for treatment of metabolic complications *Japan:* Approved *Europe:* Available through compassionate care programs
Partial lipodystrophy (both FPLD and APL)	May be considered for patients with hypoleptinemia (leptin < 4 ng/mL) who have severe metabolic abnormalities, such as HbA1c > 8% and/or triglycerides > 500 mg/dL	*United States:* Not approved *Japan:* Approved as an adjunct to diet *Europe:* Through compassionate care programs

(AGL: acquired generalized lipodystrophy; APL: acquired partial lipodystrophy; CGL: congenital generalized lipodystrophy; FPLD: familial partial lipodystrophy)

cardiomyopathy, a cardiac evaluation before engaging in an exercise program is necessary.[2]

Lifestyle intervention is great strategies to reduce hypertriglyceridemia. In patients who have not reached lipid-lowering goals after these interventions, lipid-lowering drugs can be used.[2] Insulin resistance and diabetes mellitus are treated with conventional therapies.[2] The treatment goals in patients with lipodystrophy are similar to patients with diabetes without lipodystrophy. Uncontrolled hypertension in patients with lipodystrophy can be treated with angiotensin-converting enzyme inhibitors or angiotensin receptor blockers. Currently, no specific treatments are found effective in hepatic steatosis or steatohepatitis associated with lipodystrophy.

Low serum leptin levels are characteristics of generalized lipodystrophies. This led to the development of recombinant human leptin (metreleptin) as a treatment option (Table 6). Clinical evaluation has shown that metreleptin therapy can improve metabolic abnormalities in patients with generalized lipodystrophy, where leptin therapy ameliorates hypertriglyceridemia, insulin resistance and diabetes, nonalcoholic fatty liver disease, and reproductive abnormalities.[9] Metreleptin is administered as a daily subcutaneous injection with dose adjustments at an interval of every 3–6 months based on metabolic parameters and weight change. Approval of metreleptin for different types of lipodystrophy varies by country.

Lipodystrophy can often lead to psychological distress and even physical discomfort in some cases. In such cases, patients should be directed to appropriate mental health providers. Although supporting data is not available, plastic surgery may provide benefit in some patients. Surgical transfer/removal of fat and cosmetic transplant surgeries can be done to improve the esthetic look in some patients.

CONCLUSION

Congenital and acquired lipodystrophies are heterogeneous disorders characterized by loss of subcutaneous fat and metabolic abnormalities and are accompanied by comorbidities. The most common metabolic complications include severe insulin resistance, hypertriglyceridemia, and ectopic fat deposition, especially hepatic steatosis (Box 1). Genetic mutations involved in lipodystrophies have been identified, which has improved disease classification and provided valuable information on the basic physiologic mechanisms. With this development in the knowledge, the therapy for lipodystrophy syndromes is likely to improve.

BOX 1 Metabolic complications of lipodystrophy.[9]

Glucose metabolism:
- Insulin resistance
- Diabetes
- Acanthosis nigricans

Reproductive:
- Polycystic ovary syndrome (PCOS)
- Abnormal gonadotropin secretion

Lipid metabolism:
- High triglycerides
  - Eruptive xanthomata
  - Pancreatitis
- Nonalcoholic fatty liver disease (NAFLD)
  - Steatosis →
  - Nonalcoholic steatohepatitis (NASH) →
  - Cirrhosis

REFERENCES

1. Garg A. Clinical review#: Lipodystrophies: genetic and acquired body fat disorders. J Clinl Endocrinol Metab. 2011;96(11):3313-25.
2. Hussain I, Garg A. Lipodystrophy syndromes. Endocrinol Metab Clin North Am. 2016;45(4):783-97.
3. Enzi G, Busetto L, Sergi G, Pigozzo S. Non-AIDS Lipodystrophy Syndrome. In: Mantovani G, Anker SD, Inui A, Morley JE, Fanelli FR, Scevola D, Schuster MW, Yeh SS (Eds). Cachexia and Wasting: A Modern Approach. Milano: Springer; 2006.
4. Ziegler LH. Lipodystrophies: report of seven cases. Brain. 1928;51(2): 147-67.
5. Berardinelli W. An undiagnosed endocrinometabolic syndrome: report of 2 cases. J Clin Endocrinol Metab. 1954;14(2):193-204.
6. Carr A, Samaras K, Burton S, et al. A syndrome of peripheral lipodystrophy, hyperlipidaemia and insulin resistance in patients receiving HIV protease inhibitors. Aids. 1998;12(7):F51-8.
7. Garg A. Acquired and inherited lipodystrophies. N Engl J Med. 2004;350(12):1220-34.
8. Haque WA, Shimomura I, Matsuzawa Y, et al. Serum adiponectin and leptin levels in patients with lipodystrophies. J Clin Endocrinol Metabol. 2002;87(5):2395-8.
9. Brown RJ, Gorden P. Leptin therapy in patients with lipodystrophy and syndromic insulin resistance. In: Dagogo-Jack S (Ed). Leptin: Regulation and Clinical Applications. New York: Springer International Publishing; 2015. pp. 225-36.
10. Lightbourne M, Brown RJ. Genetics of lipodystrophy. Endocrinol Metab Clin. 2017;46(2):539-54.
11. Ozen S, Akinci B, Oral EA. Current Diagnosis and Treatment, and Clinical Challenges in the Management of Lipodystrophy Syndromes in Children and Youth. J Clin Res Pediatr Endocrinol. 2019. doi: 10.4274/jcrpe.galenos.2019.2019.0124. [Epub ahead of print].

67 CHAPTER

Rheumatological Manifestations of Diabetes Mellitus

Bharat Panigrahy, Jayanta Kumar Panda

INTRODUCTION

Diabetes mellitus (DM) is a major public health problem worldwide. The global burden of diabetes is about 425 million, of which 82 million are living in Southeast Asia. Diabetes population in India is about 72 million with a prevalence of 8.8% International Diabetes Federation (IDF). Patients with diabetes may develop several musculoskeletal syndromes or symptoms, many of which are associated with the severity and duration of the disease. In contrast to microvascular and macrovascular complications of diabetes which are widely discussed musculoskeletal complications are discussed sparingly and neglected. Poor glycemic control is associated with increased prevalence of rheumatologic manifestations.[1] These complications cause significant disability and negatively affect the quality of life (QoL).

PREVALENCE

Prevalence of rheumatologic complications in diabetes vary from 30% to 35%, depending on study population and definitions used for the problem.[2] Most of the studies assess individual components. The prevalence depends on various factors like age, gender, BMI, diabetes type, duration and control of diabetes, and ethnicity. In one study from South India the prevalence of rheumatic-musculoskeletal manifestations in diabetes in 310 cases and controls was 42.58%; (95% confidence interval (CI): 37.08–48.08) and 31.61%; (95% CI: 26.43–36.79), respectively (Table 1).[2]

PATHOGENESIS

Pathogenesis of the musculoskeletal complications is not clear. Accumulation of advanced glycation end-products (AGEs) and their cross-linking of collagen is thought to be the cause of these complications. Diabetes duration and severity both influence the glycosylation of collagen.[3]

TABLE 1: Prevalence of musculoskeletal disorders in patients with or without diabetes.

Musculoskeletal disorder	With diabetes	Without diabetes
Adhesive capsulitis (frozen shoulder)[5-8]	11–30%	2–10%
Limited joint mobility[9-11]	8–50%	0–26%
Dupuytren's contracture[12-15]	20–63%	13%
Carpal tunnel syndrome[16,17]	11–16%	125/100000*
Flexor tenosynovitis[18]	11%	

*Incidence estimate over 5 years.

Rheumatological complications in diabetes are classified as:

- *Syndromes of limited joint mobility*:
    - Frozen shoulder (adhesive capsulitis)
    - Carpal tunnel syndrome (CTS)
    - Dupuytren contracture (DC)
    - Stiff hand syndrome (diabetic cheiroarthropathy)
    - Flexor tenosynovitis (trigger finger)
- *Muscle disorders*:
    - Diabetic muscle infarction
    - Diabetic amyotrophy
- *Joint disorders*:
    - Charcot joint
    - Osteoarthritis
    - Rheumatoid arthritis
    - Gouty arthritis
- *Skeletal disorders*:
    - Osteoporosis
    - Diffuse idiopathic skeletal hyperostosis (DISH)

Frozen Shoulder (Adhesive Capsulitis)

Frozen shoulder is defined as "a condition of uncertain etiology characterized by significant restriction of both active and passive shoulder motion that occurs in the absence of a known intrinsic shoulder disorder".

Incidence is 10–30% in diabetes in comparison to 2–5% in nondiabetics. More seen in females with a peak age of 50 years.[4]

It progresses in three phases:

1. Initial painful phase with severe disabling pain, which worsens at night, and continues for 3–6 months.
2. Intermediate phase of stiffness with severe restriction of both active as well as passive motion lasts for 6–10 months.
3. Recovery phase lasts from 6–24 months with gradual improvement of range of motion.[5]

The abduction and external movements are mostly affected. Frozen shoulder is a clinical diagnosis. A plain X-ray may be done to exclude glenohumeral osteoarthritis (Figs. 1A to F).

The treatment includes nonsteroidal anti-inflammatory drugs (NSAIDs), physiotherapy, intra-articular corticosteroid and intra-articular dilatation.[6]

Stiff Hand Syndrome (Diabetic Cheiroarthropathy)

It is found in 10–50% of both type 1 and type 2 diabetes compares to 4–20% among individuals without DM.[7]

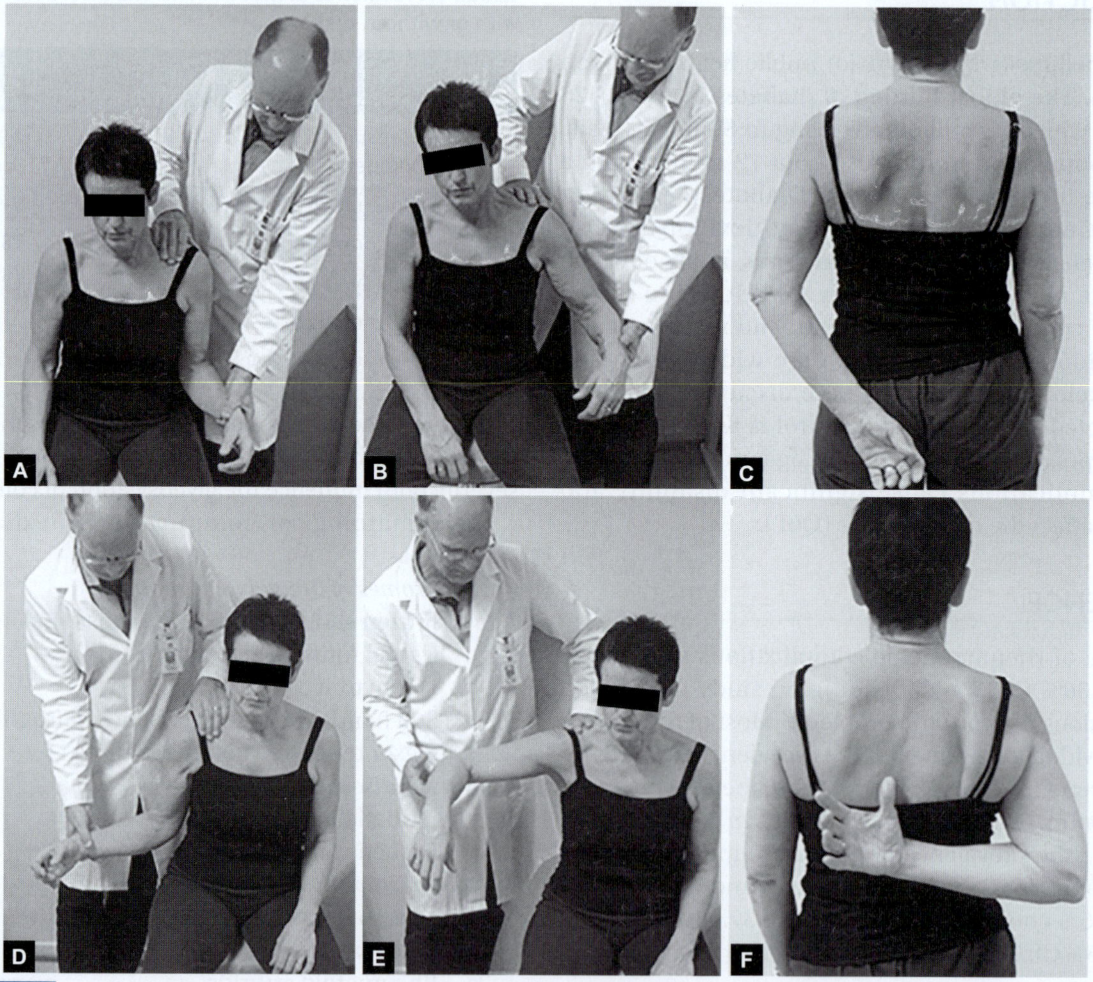

Figures 1A to F Frozen shoulder: Restrictions in motion. The photographs above show common motion restrictions that are found with frozen shoulder. Note how the affected left shoulder is limited in external rotation (A) abduction (B) internal rotation (C) compared with the unaffected shoulder (photographs D, E, and F). Photographs A, B, D, and E depict passive glenohumeral motion while the scapula is stabilized.

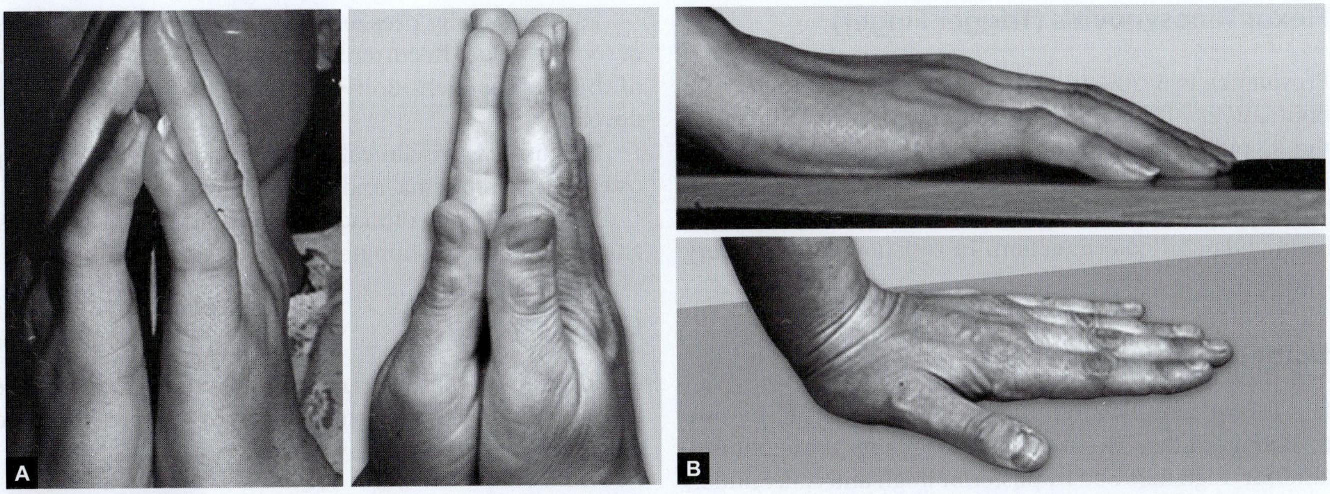

Figures 2A and B Contractures in the metacarpophalangeal joints in diabetes mellitus: (A) Prayer sign and (B) Table top test.

Characterized painless limitations of mobility of the small joints of hands. Examination shows tight, thick, waxy skin of dorsum of fingers and contractures moistly affecting the proximal phalanges and metacarpophalangeal joints (Figs. 2A and B).

Diagnosis by:

- *Prayer sign*: Inability to flatten both the hands as in a prayer.
- *Table top test*: To assess the ability to flatten the palm against the surface of a table.

Treatment: No definite treatment is available. Good glycemic control, smoking cessation, physiotherapy with passive palmar stretching, and occupational therapy may improve function.

Carpal Tunnel Syndrome

It is a painful disorder caused by the compression of the median nerve in the carpal tunnel. Incidence is 15–20% in diabetes versus 1–5% in nondiabetes. Typically the paresthesia occurs in the palm and fingers in the median nerve distribution, being worsened at night. Certain tests may help in diagnosis.

Shaking sign: Disappearance of the symptoms after vigorous flapping of the hands.

Tinel test: Tapping over the compressed nerve at the wrist reproduces pain and paresthesia (Fig. 3).

Phalen maneuver: Fully flexed hands are pressed with each other at the dorsum for 30 seconds reproduce the symptoms.

Nerve conduction velocity can help in diagnosing CTS.

Treatment consists of conservative therapy and surgical. Splinting, glucocorticoid injections, and oral glucocorticoids are useful for symptom relief of CTS, but surgery is the treatment of choice for patients with evidence of ongoing nerve damage.[8]

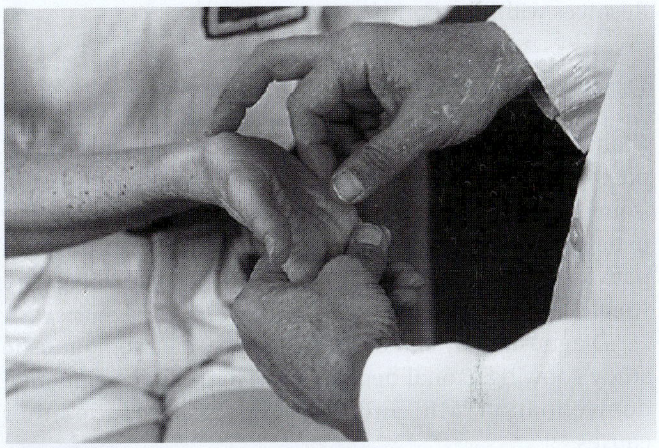

Figure 3 The Tinel test for median nerve injury at the carpal tunnel.

Dupuytren Contracture

It is characterized by progressive fibrosis of palmar fascia causing a contracture in flexion of the fingers. Incidence is 20–60% higher than people without diabetes.[9] While DC affects the 4th and 5th fingers in nondiabetics, the 3rd and 4th fingers are affected in diabetics and frequently bilateral.

Treatment consists of good glycemic control, physiotherapy, local steroid, and in nonresponsive cases surgery.

Flexor Tenosynovitis (Trigger Finger)

Prevalence is 5–30% in DM in contrast to 2% in general population.[10] It is caused by inflammation and fibrosis at the A1 pulley of the flexor tendon causing finger blocking in flexion.

Diagnosis is clinical. Treatment consists of NSAIDs and local glucocorticoid injection. In resistant cases surgery helps.

Diabetic Muscle Infarction

It is a rare complication of diabetes. Thought to be due to vasculopathy. The most common site of affection is anterior thigh followed by posterior thigh and calf. Sudden acute pain and swelling is the presenting feature. MRI is mostly diagnostic.

Treatment is with analgesics, rest and low dose aspirin. Resolves within a month in most cases.[11]

Diabetic Amyotrophy

Diabetic amyotrophy, also known as "diabetic lumbosacral plexopathy" is thought to be due to immune-mediated ischemic injury from a nonsystemic microvasculitis.[12] The usual presentation is acute, asymmetric, focal onset of pain followed by weakness involving the proximal leg, and weight loss.

Diagnosis is by clinical presentation, electrodiagnostic study showing axonal degeneration more than segmental demyelination, MRI and CT imaging to exclude other causes.

Treatment consists of immunosuppressants and symptomatic therapy. Some observational studies found IV methylprednisolone and cyclophosphamide to be effective,[13] however a 2017 systematic review found no published randomized controlled trials evaluating immunotherapy for diabetic amyotrophy. Symptomatic management includes narcotic analgesics, amitriptyline, pregabalin, and duloxetine. Physical and occupational therapy, patient education, and reassurance are a necessity.

Charcot Joint (Charcot's Arthropathy)

Commonly affects the foot. It occurs due to a combination of mechanical and vascular factors secondary to diabetic neuropathy. Lack of proprioception leads to microtrauma, looseness of ligaments, and joint instability.[14] An initial phase of resorption followed by a stage of repair and hypertrophy occurs.

Patient usually presents with erythema and swelling of foot or ankle. Recurrent such attacks leads to collapse of the plantar arch. Bony prominences and ulcers may develop.

Diagnosis is by clinical features and imaging showing osteolysis, osteopenia, and joint subluxation.

Treatment is by offloading with plaster, foot orthoses, and use of bisphosphonates.

Osteoarthritis

Obesity and osteoarthritis relationship is well known.[4] The increased incidence of osteoarthritis in diabetes is due to obesity or diabetes itself is not clear.

Rheumatoid Arthritis

Occurrence of T1DM is 2.8% among first-degree relatives of rheumatoid arthritis patients suggests some common genetic markers and familial clustering.[15]

Gouty Arthritis

Prevalence of gout is around 20% in diabetes whereas it is 2% in nondiabetics.[7] In patients with gout, co-occurrence of diabetes and metabolic syndrome is much higher than in healthy individuals.[16]

Osteoporosis

Diabetes itself and the treatment consequences increase the risk of osteoporosis. Women with T1DM do have higher frequency of hip fracture than nondiabetics.[17] For a given FRAX score, the risk of fracture may be higher in diabetes patients compared with those without diabetes.

Diffuse Idiopathic Skeletal Hyperostosis

Diffuse idiopathic skeletal hyperostosis is an idiopathic, noninflammatory condition characterized by diffuse calcific ossification of predominantly anterior longitudinal ligament of spine and entheses. Insulin and IGF-1 are thought to be responsible for this ossification process.[18]

Often asymptomatic, but may be associated with pain, stiffness and restricted range of motion of spine. Thoracic spine is affected in majority cases. Dysphagia, respiratory distress and compressive myelopathy are rare complications.

Diagnosis is mostly by imaging. Utsinger 1985 revised diagnostic criteria: DISH may be diagnosed by symmetrical peripheral enthesopathy and continuous ossification of anterolateral aspect of the two or more contiguous vertebral bodies.

Treatment is mostly symptomatic; physical therapy, exercise, and symptomatic pain management.

CONCLUSION

Diabetes mellitus is associated with a number of rheumatologic disorders due to long duration of diabetes and poor glycemic control. Early detection and proper treatment can decrease morbidity, mortality, and improve quality of life.

REFERENCES

1. Silverstein JH, Gordon G, Pollock BH, et al. Long-term glycemic control influences the onset of limited joint mobility in type 1 diabetes. J Pediatr. 1998;132(6):944-7.
2. Agrawal RP, Gothwal S, Tantia P, et al. Prevalence of Rheumatological Manifestations in Diabetic Population from North-West India. J Assoc Physicians India. 2014;62(9):788-92.
3. Huang SW, Wang WT, Chou LC, et al. Diabetes mellitus increases the risk of rotator cuff tear repair surgery: a population-based cohort study. J Diabetes Complications. 2016;30(8):1473-7.
4. Huang YP, Fann CY, Chiu YH, et.al. Association of diabetes mellitus with the risk of developing adhesive capsulitis of the shoulder: a longitudinal population-based follow-up study. Arthritis Care Res (Hoboken). 2013;65(7):1197-202.
5. Reeves B. The natural history of the frozen shoulder syndrome. Scand J Rheumatol. 1975;4(4):193-6.
6. Favejee MM, Huisstede BM, Koes BW. Frozen shoulder: the effectiveness of conservative and surgical interventions—systematic review. Br J Sports Med. 2011;45(1):49-56.
7. Smith L, Burnet S, McNeil J. Musculoskeletal manifestations of diabetes mellitus. Br J Sports Med. 2003;37:30-5.
8. Marshall S, Tardif G, Ashworth N. Local corticosteroid injection for carpal tunnel syndrome. Cochrane Database Syst Rev. 2007;(2):CD001554.
9. Crispin JC, Alcocer-Varela J. Rheumatologic manifestations of diabetes mellitus. Am J Med. 2003;114(9):753-7.
10. Cagliero E, Apruzzese W, Perlmutter GS, et al. Musculoskeletal disorders of the hand and shoulder in patients with diabetes mellitus. Am J Med. 2002;112(6):487-90.
11. Arkkila PE, Gautier JF. Musculoskeletal disorders in diabetes mellitus: an update. Best Pract Res Clin Rheumatol. 2003;17:945-70.
12. Kawamura N, Dyck PJ, Schmeichel AM, et al. Inflammatory mediators in diabetic and non-diabetic lumbosacral radiculoplexus neuropathy. Acta Neuropathol. 2008;115(2):231-9.
13. Kilfoyle D, Kelkar P, Parry GJ. Pulsed methylprednisolone is a safe and effective treatment for diabetic amyotrophy. J Clin Neuromuscul Dis. 2003;4(4):168-70.
14. Nielson DL, Armstrong DG. The natural history of Charcot's neuroarthropathy. Clin Podiatr Med Surg. 2008;25(1):53-62, vi.
15. Kuo CF, Grainge MJ, Valdes AM, et al. Familial aggregation of rheumatoid arthritis and co-aggregation of autoimmune diseases in affected families: a nationwide population-based study. Rheumatology (Oxford). 2017;56(6):928-33.
16. Choi HK, Ford ES. Prevalence of the metabolic syndrome in individuals with hyperuricemia. Am J Med. 2007;120(5):442-7.
17. Forsén L, Meyer HE, Midthjell K, et al. Diabetes mellitus and the incidence of hip fracture: results from the Nord-Trøndelag Health Survey. Diabetologia. 1999;42(8):920-5.
18. Denko CW, Boja B, Moskowitz RW. Growth promoting peptides in osteoarthritis and diffuse idiopathic skeletal hyperostosis—insulin, insulin-like growth factor-I, growth hormone. J Rheumatol. 1994;21(9):1725-30.

68 CHAPTER Achievement and Future Plans of IWGDF Consensus on Diabetic Foot

Ashish Sewaram Dengra

INTRODUCTION

The International Working Group on the Diabetic Foot (IWGDF) was founded in the year of 1996. The IWGDF published the first-ever International Consensus on the Diabetic Foot and Practical Guidelines on the Management and Prevention of the Diabetic Foot in the year 1999.

In International Working Group on the Diabetic Foot (IWGDF) Practical Guidelines we describe the basic principles of prevention and management of diabetic foot disease. The Practical Guidelines are based on the IWGDF Guidelines 2019, consisting of evidence-based guideline on:

- Prevention of foot ulcers in persons with diabetes[1]
- Offloading foot ulcers in persons with diabetes[2]
- Diagnosis, prognosis and management of peripheral artery disease in patients with a foot ulcer and diabetes[3]
- Diagnosis and treatment of foot infection in persons with diabetes[4]
- Interventions to enhance healing of foot ulcers in persons with diabetes[5]
- Classification of diabetic foot ulcers[6]

For implementing the International Consensus, the IWGDF had recruited national foot champions to become the members of the IWGDF. Every four years, working groups of experts in the specialized fields were asked to revise and renew the consensus chapters based upon up-to-date published evidence or consensus standards.[7] The implementation group of IWGDF is known as D-Foot International.[8] The objective of D-Foot International is to prevent and decrease the number of amputations from diabetes globally. Implementing the "International Consensus on the Management and Prevention of the Diabetic Foot" guidelines—training healthcare professionals on how to manage diabetic foot problems effectively and prevent amputations; giving healthcare professionals strategies to implement, develop, and sustain foot services; guiding healthcare professionals on how to train and support their colleagues; and promoting the recognition of diabetic foot specialists—has been focused upon. Headquarters of D-Foot International is in Antwerpen, Belgium.

PROGRAMS

Step-by-Step

A foot care project called "Step-by-Step, improving diabetic foot care in the developing world" has been initiated by the International Diabetes Federation (IDF) Consultative Section and IWGDF, together with the Diabetic Foot Society of India (DFSI) and the Muhimbili University College of Health Sciences, Dar-es-Salaam, Tanzania (MUCHS). India, Bangladesh, Sri Lanka, and Tanzania were the participating countries. Teams, consisting of a doctor and a nurse or paramedic, were invited for attending a basic and an advanced course. The objective was to develop educational skills and the management of diabetic foot problems. For teaching and conducting the practical sessions, an experienced national and international faculty was responsible.[3] The first courses were initiated in the autumn of 2004.

The goals and objectives of Step-by-Step program are mentioned herein:

- To create more awareness of diabetic foot problems in India and Tanzania (and possibly other developing countries)

- To offer sustainable training of healthcare professionals for managing diabetic foot
- To facilitate the information cascade from healthcare professionals who have undergone training to other healthcare professionals and hence exporting expertise
- To decrease the risk of lower limb complications in people with diabetes
- To empower people with diabetes to better care for their feet, earlier detection of problems and seek help timely when problems occur.

The Step-by-Step program (SbS) is a 2-year project, where teams, which include a doctor and a nurse or paramedic, are invited to attend a basic and an advanced course. Collecting the data is mandatory during the 2 years. The aim is to improve educational skills and manage diabetic foot problems. A cascade effect and sustainability in the region/country has been created by doing so. An experienced national and international faculty is accountable for teaching and the practical sessions. All participants received medical equipment and educational materials. Successful pilot programs and studies were held in India and Tanzania in 2004 and 2005.[3]

For India, physicians from remote places were invited along with their paramedics (to build up a concept of the team approach). They were offered a basic and an advanced course after 1 year. From 600 applications, 100 teams were selected—94 pairs from India, three from Bangladesh, two from Sri Lanka, and one from Nepal. A basic course of 2.5 days in four metros of India in 2004 and an advanced course in 2005 in India, again of 2.5 days were offered to the selected participants.

The principles of basic foot care, including nail cutting and callus removal education courses were taught. The practical management guidelines were also taught, such as how to:

- Record a history
- Perform a physical examination
- Screen for neuropathy and ischemia
- Classify and stage the foot.

Having identified feet at risk, delegates were trained how to organize appropriate foot care and education and take appropriate action on time in cases of ulceration or advanced foot problems, and in case of patients in trouble, when and where to refer, taking local circumstances into account.

Education and training was also focused on teaching others. Participants are expected to educate people with diabetes along with cascading their acquired knowledge and skills to colleagues in their regions. A spin-off effect is created by the teaching colleagues and can hence help for perpetuating and sustaining the achievements of the project. An explicit focus on audiovisual materials and pictures with little supporting text was of key importance since many languages and dialects exist in the developing world and levels of literacy are low.

Expected impacts of the project:[3]

- Implementation of regular screening programs
- Patient education
- Management of basic foot lesions
- Reduction of amputations
- Cascading effect
- Sustainability
- Extending the project to other parts of the developing world.

Train-the-Foot-Trainer

At the end of 2010, the Step-by-Step Development and Research Group (SSDRG) of the IWGFD started the idea of developing a Train-the-Foot-Trainer (TtFT) program, by setting up a Step-by-Step project, which aimed to reach more regions in a shorter period and to respond in a competent way to the demands. As a result, in Brasilia, Brazil (5–8 December 2012), the first Train-the-Foot-Trainer course was held. This was the first of a series intended to be executed in various regions around the world.[2]

The TtFT course consists of four major parts. The first part deals with general considerations such as history, background, and overview of the significant success of the SbS projects to decrease the number of amputations throughout the world, and aspects of attitude and motivation. The second part consists of content and procedures—how to install the basic course of the SbS program in one's own country. Implementing the advanced course of the SbS program is dealt by the third part. The fourth part deals with effectively implementing the SbS program, creating sustainability, proceeding with data collection, regional networking, and publicity and creating further awareness. Moreover, special information on funding of these programs was provided.

Training of Certified Diabetic Foot Care Assistants

The IDF DFP/IWGDF offers proposals for foot care training courses for educating certified Diabetic Foot Care Assistants (DFCAss). This was started considering the need for diabetic foot education to be available in every country. Podiatry does not exist in several countries. In such countries, interested health professionals should be presented a standardized form of diabetic foot care education to put into their healthcare setting as an adjunct to their professional responsibilities. The requirement of affordable and practical diabetic foot care education below the level of podiatry must be recognized by designing suitable programs to improve care in the absence of podiatry. To address local diabetic foot care issues, successful courses are already in practice in a few countries. The aim of DFCAss courses offered by the IWGDF working group on Diabetic Foot Care Education (DFCE) is not to detract from courses that are already in place. Its goal is to offer a standardized international course to countries who have no podiatry services. These countries can apply to undertake these courses instead of setting up their own individual courses. This education program was launched in September 2008.[2]

GUIDELINES

The international, multidisciplinary, evidence-based guidance documents is produced by the IWGDF to enlighten health professionals all over the world on the prevention and management of diabetic foot disease. The IWGDF published the first-ever International Consensus on the Diabetic Foot and Practical Guidelines on the Management and Prevention of the Diabetic Foot in 1999. This publication has been translated into 26 languages, and more than 80,000 copies have been distributed worldwide. In order to implement the International Consensus, the IWGDF recruited national foot champions as its members. As of now, the organization is represented by 188 members from 170 countries.[1]

The basic principles of prevention and management of diabetic foot disease has been described by the IWGDF Guidelines. These guidelines are based on the systematic reviews of the literature. Guidelines involve the formulation of clinical questions and key outcome measures "that clinicians would care about" when treating patients with diabetic foot problems. These questions were reviewed by clinicians from all over the world and a systematic review of the complete scientific literature was subsequently performed. Once this had been achieved, recommendations were graded to establish how useful they might be.[4]

The new 2019 guidelines consist of 87 evidence-based practice recommendations and 44 future research priorities across 8 chapters and 194 pages. The guidelines include the following subjects:

- Prevention of foot ulcers in persons with diabetes
- Offloading foot ulcers in persons with diabetes
- Diagnosis, prognosis, and management of peripheral artery disease in patients with a foot ulcer and diabetes
- Diagnosis and treatment of foot infection in persons with diabetes
- Interventions to enhance healing of foot ulcers in persons with diabetes
- Classification of diabetic foot ulcers.

INTERNATIONAL SYMPOSIUM ON THE DIABETIC FOOT

In 1991, the quadrennial International Symposium on the Diabetic Foot (ISDF) is the showcase meeting of IWGDF first took place in Noordwijkerhout (The Netherlands). However, it now takes place in the Hague. The symposium is held once every 4 years. It is said to be the largest and most prestigious meeting dedicated to lower extremity problems in people with diabetes. Delegates from many specialties and the leading experts in various fields, both from all over the world can be successfully brought together through this symposium. The most recent symposium was held in May 2019.[5]

CONCLUSION

Studies around the world have shown that setting up an interdisciplinary foot care team and implementing prevention and management of diabetic foot disease according to the principles outlined in this guideline, is associated with a decrease in the frequency of diabetes related lower-extremity amputations. If it is not possible to create a full team from the outset, aim to build one step-by-step, introducing the various disciplines as possible. This team must first and foremost act with mutual respect and understanding, work in both primary and secondary care settings, and have at least one member available for consultation or patient assessment at all times.

REFERENCES

1. Bus SA, Lavery LA, Monteiro-Soares M, et al. On behalf of the International Working Group on the Diabetic Foot (IWGDF). IWGDF guideline on the prevention of foot ulcers in persons with diabetes. Diabetes Metab. Res. Rev. 2019; in press.
2. Bus SA, Armstrong DG, Gooday C, et al. On behalf of the the International Working Group on the Diabetic Foot (IWGDF). IWGDF Guideline on offloading foot ulcers in persons with diabetes. Diabetes Metab. Res. Rev. 2019; in press.

3. Hinchliffe RJ, Forsythe R, Apelqvist J, et al. IWGDF Guideline on diagnosis, prognosis and management of peripheral artery disease in patients with a foot ulcer and diabetes. Diabetes Metab. Res. Rev. 2019; in press.
4. Lipsky BA, Senneville, Abbas Z, et al. IWGDF Guideline on the diagnosis and treatment of foot infection in persons with diabetes. Diabetes Metab. Res. Rev. 2019; in press.
5. Rayman G, Vas P, Dhatariya K, et al. IWGDF Guideline on interventions to enhance healing of foot ulcers in persons with diabetes. Diabetes Metab. Res. Rev. 2019; in press.
6. Monteiro-Soares M, Russell D, Boyko EJ, et al. IWGDF Guidelines on the classification of diabetic foot ulcers. Diabetes Metab. Res. Rev. 2019; in press.
7. International working group on the diabetic foot-implementation. (2019). Who we are. [online]. Available fromhttp://www.d-foot.org/d-foot/ who—we are/?direct=843[Last accessed September, 2019].
8. International working group on diabetic foot. (2019) Diabetic foot internationall [online]. Available from http://www.d-foot.org/dfootinternational/diabetic-foot-international/. [Last accessed September, 2019].
9. Bakker k, Abbas ZG, Pendsey S, STEP, improving diabetic foot care in the developing world . practical diabetes international. 2006:23(8):365-9.
10. nternation working group on diabetic foot. (2019). IWGDF Guidlines [online]. Available from https://iwgdfguidelines.org/guidelines.
11. Symposium profile—diabetes foot [internet]. Diabtes foot 2019 [cited 14 september 2019]. Available from: https://diabetic foot.nl/about/ symposium-profole. [Last accssed September, 2019].

9 SECTION Diabetes and Co-Morbidities

69 CHAPTER Residual Cardiovascular Risk in Statin Era: Should We Focus on Non-high-density Lipoprotein Cholesterol?

Vitull K Gupta, Meghna Gupta, Varun Gupta

INTRODUCTION

Cardiovascular diseases (CVDs) are increasingly being recognized as an important global public health problem in both developed and developing countries leading to increased morbidity and mortality and high healthcare costs.[1] Rapid epidemiological transition in India associated with aging, increasing urbanization, population growth, and economic prosperity has led to risk factor transition[2] dramatically transforming disease characteristics to noncommunicable diseases (NCDs) from infectious, undernutritional, and maternal and childhood diseases.[3] Traditional CVD risk factors along with adverse lifestyles, greater tobacco use, unhealthy nutritional habits, and increasing sedentary lifestyle have added to increasing prevalence of NCDs especially CVDs.[4]

CARDIOVASCULAR RISK FACTORS

Cardiovascular risk factors are discussed as conventional and emerging risk factors.

Traditional or Conventional Risk Factors

Traditional risk factors for CVDs can be divided into two main categories:

1. *Modifiable risk factors*: Hypertension, dyslipidemia, tobacco use, diabetes, obesity, physical inactivity, and unhealthy diet. Other modifiable risk factors include: low socioeconomic status, alcohol use, mental ill health, psychological stress, use of certain medicines, and left ventricular hypertrophy.
2. *Nonmodifiable risk factors*: Advancing age, heredity or family history, gender and ethnicity, or race.

Emerging Risk Factors[5]

Emerging risk factors are the risk factors recently recognized to have independent risk predictive of potential directly associated with increased CVD risk but still their independent role is not fully defined in comparison to the conventional risk factors.

Emerging risk factors for atherosclerotic CVD:

- *Lipid-related biomarkers*:
  - High-density lipoprotein cholesterol
  - Triglycerides
  - Lipoprotein(a)
  - Apolipoprotein A1 and B
  - Lipoprotein-associated phospholipase A2
- *Inflammatory biomarkers*:
  - C-reactive protein
  - Interleukin (IL)-1, IL-6, and IL-18
  - Tumor necrosis factor-α
  - Matrix metalloproteinase-9
  - Soluble CD40 ligand
  - Vascular and cellular adhesion molecule
  - Leukocyte count.
- *Biomarkers of hemostasis and thrombosis*:
  - Fibrinogen
  - Coagulation factors II, V, and VIII
  - von Willebrand factor antigen
  - Tissue plasminogen activator (t-PA)\
  - Plasminogen activator inhibitor-1
  - D-dimer.
- *Cardiac-related biomarkers*:
  - High-sensitivity troponin
  - B-type natriuretic peptide.
- *Kidney-related biomarkers*:
  - Creatinine

- Microalbuminuria
- Cystatin C
- Calcium phosphate/fibroblast growth factor 23
- Uric acid.

• *Other factors*:

- Homocysteine
- Vitamin D
- Metabolism related [e.g. hemoglobin A1c (HbA1c)]
- Platelet-related factors (e.g. platelet volume)
- Endothelial dysfunction (e.g. nitric oxide)
- Environmental exposures (e.g. air pollution, radiation)
- Other noninvasive measures of vascular disease (e.g. carotid plaque).

What is Residual Risk?[6]

The residual risk is the risk that remains after the natural or inherent risks that have been decreased or reduced by risk controls measures or treatment.

Residual risk can be measured by applying subjective judgment or mathematical method. The mathematical method to calculate residual risk is:

Residual risk = Inherent risk – Impact of risk controls.

RESIDUAL CARDIOVASCULAR RISK IN STATIN ERA

Solid evidence exists to define the association between plasma low-density lipoprotein cholesterol (LDL-C) levels and risks of congenital heart defect (CHD) along with beneficial effects of lipid-lowering therapy of statins so that all the guidelines recommend statins for primary and secondary prevention of coronary artery disease (CAD). A number of large randomized controlled trials (RCTs) like the Scandinavian Simvastatin Survival Study (4S), the Long-term Intervention with Pravastatin in Ischemic Disease (LIPID) study, and the Justification for the Use of Statins in Prevention: An Intervention Trial Evaluating Rosuvastatin (JUPITER) study have shown reduction of CAD with statin therapy.[7] Evidence shows that in spite of statin therapy and achieving the optimal LDL-C targets, still risk of CAD is persisting that is known as the residual risk.[8] Several trials like 4S trial, the Cholesterol and Recurrent Events (CARE) trials, and the Heart Protection Study (HPS) showed persistence of CHD event rates in patients treated with statins observing decreased level of LDL-C.[7] A large meta-analysis of 14 randomized trials showed decreased risk of major events by 23% for each 1 mmol/L LDL-C lowering with statin treatment but the residual risk of major adverse cardiac events (MACE) remained high with 14% of patients reporting CV events in statin group and 18% in placebo group.[9] Atorvastatin 80 mg daily in the Treating to New Targets (TNTs) trial reported 22% relative risk reduction of MACE in comparison with atorvastatin 10 mg daily, still CV events were experienced by one in 11 patients during 5 years follow-up. More CVD risk reduction was observed in high-intensity statin treatment as compared to moderate-intensity statin treatment, but residual risk was 22.4% even when LDL-C levels were not increased in the Pravastatin or Atorvastatin Evaluation and Infarction Therapy-Thrombolysis In Myocardial Infarction 22 (PROVE IT-TIMI22) trial. A residual risk reduction of 12% was observed in similar conditions in the Incremental Decrease in Endpoints through Aggressive Lipid Lowering (IDEAL) trials.[7,10] In another trial, lipid-lowering therapy was able to significantly decrease rate of MACE, but residual risk of 32.7% persisted.[11] Evidence suggested that with statin therapy, more residual CV events occur than could be prevented and the residual risk remained elevated even when LDL-C levels were aggressively reduced in clinical trials. It is now well-documented that the present lipid-lowering treatment especially statins targeting to reduce LDL-C levels are not sufficient to prevent all CV events and the residual risk remains elevated in clinical trials aggressively reducing LDL-C levels.[12,13] Presence of residual risk in spite of aggressive lowering of LDL-C with statins has resulted in an increased focus on elevated triglycerides (TGs), low levels of HDL-C, and non-high-density lipoprotein cholesterol (non-HDL-C) levels.[14]

Should We Focus on Non-high-density Lipoprotein Cholesterol?

With current guidelines, non-HDL-C has received less importance as compared to LDL-C so much so that non-HDL-C remains a co-primary therapeutic target with LDL-C, but non-HDL-C quantifies all atherogenic apolipoprotein B (ApoB)-containing lipoproteins [LDL, very low-density lipoprotein (VLDL), intermediate-density lipoprotein (IDL), chylomicrons (CMs), and their TG-rich lipoprotein remnants] accounting for the atherogenic risk, so non-HDL-C is being well-recognized as a significant CHD risk factor.[7] Non-HDL-C is not affected by fasting state and is estimated by subtracting HDL-C from total cholesterol (TC). Atherogenic dyslipidemia (AC) is a typical phenotype of insulin resistance and metabolic syndrome characterized by high TG, HDL-C, and small, dense LDL particles. In Indians, the CVD risk increases with increased levels of non-HDL-C[15] and Indians generally have increased level of non-HDL-C because of high TGs and low-HDL-C. Evidence suggests that more so in diabetics, non-HDL-C predicts CV mortality more strongly than LDL-C. It has been observed that non-HDL-C shows predictive accuracy in both elevated TG (>400 mg/dL) and relatively low TG (<200 mg/dL), whereas LDL-C does not show its predictive value in elevated TG levels (>400 mg/dL).[16] A study conducted in 75 patients with angiographically proven CHD demonstrated close association of non-HDL-C with severity of CHD. Non-HDL-C levels were lowest in single vessel disease and highest in triple vessel disease.[17] A meta-analysis in 2011 including 233,455 subjects in 12 observational studies demonstrated prevention of 300,000 more events by non-HDL-C strategy as compared to a LDL strategy over a 10-year period.[18] Another large meta-analysis of 25 trials including 131,134 patients in 2012 showed that non-HDL-C was better in predicting CVD than ApoB.[19] Meta-analysis including eight trials done in 2012 studied 62,154 patients treated with statins showed that even if LDL-C is controlled, increased risk of future CV events was associated with uncontrolled non-HDL-C.[20] A prospective cohort study, the Second Manifestations of Arterial Disease (SMART) study conducted in 2016 included clinically manifest arterial disease patients showed that the relationship of LDL-C and non-HDL-C with CV events was same among all types of arterial diseases.[21]

Results of the Lipid Research Clinics Program Follow-up Study conducted with a follow-up period of over 19-year in 2001 with an aim to explore the usefulness of non-HDL-C in predicting CHD mortality showed that the baseline levels of non-HDL-C was a strong and significant predictor of CHD deaths as compared to LDL-C level which was shown as somewhat weaker predictor in both males and females.[22] The Health Professionals Follow-up Study compared non-HDL-C and LDL-C as predictors of CHD and showed that for non-HDL-C after adjusting the matching factors, the CHD relative risk in the highest quintile versus the lowest quintile was 2.76 [95% confidence interval (CI), 1.66–4.58] and for LDL-C was 1.81 (95% CI, 1.12–2.93). After mutually adjusting non-HDL-C and LDL-C, it was found that only non-HDL-C predicted the risk of CHD, leading to conclusion that non-HDL-C could be a better and strong predictor of CHD risk as compared to LDL-C.[23] The Framingham Heart Study showed that after multivariate adjustment on the basis of the joint distributions of LDL-C and non-HDL-C, no association of risk of CHD was found between LDL-C within non-HDL-C level, but a strong, graded, and positive association of risk of CHD was found between non-HDL-C within the LDL-C levels.[24] The European Prospective Investigation into Cancer and Nutrition (EPIC)-Norfolk prospective population study in 2013 showed that for LDL-C, the multivariable-adjusted hazard ratio (HR) of future CHD was 1.22 (95% CI, 1.17–1.27) and 1.67 (95% CI, 1.47–1.91) for non-HDL-C. Similarly, for LDL-C, the multivariable-adjusted HR of future CHD was 1.26 (95% CI, 1.20–1.31) and 1.87 (95% CI, 1.62–2.15) for non-HDL-C in the highest quartile.[25] A retrospective study in 2017 explored in 868 post-acute myocardial infarction (AMI) patients the predictability of attaining non-HDL-C goal and long-term MACE as compared to attaining LDL-C target with a mean follow-up of 2.6 years and concluded that future MACE following AMI was better predicted by non-HDL-C.[26]

Several epidemiological studies have shown strong association of non-HDL-C with CHD risk than LDL-C.[22] Post hoc analyses have shown that after lipid-lowering therapy, residual risk is better quantified by non-HDL-C levels than LDL-C because CV outcome is closely associated with on-treatment level of non-HDL-C than levels of LDL-C.[27] Role of non-HDL-C goals for primary prevention of CHD was studied in a large cohort analysis in statin-treated type 2 diabetes mellitus patients and found that in these statin-treated patients after adjustment, the risk of CHD was lower with decreased levels of non-HDL-C ($P < 0.001$). Findings of 13 studies involving 156,381 subjects supported the use of non-HDL-C treatment goals for CHD primary prevention in diabetic patients and suggested that non-HDL-C was a better predictor of future MACE than LDL-C. Existing evidence suggests a positive relationship between non-HDL-C lowering and reduction of CV risk and is superior to LDL-C in its ability to predict MACE. Non-HDL-C is a more comprehensive measure of atherogenic dyslipidemia than LDL-C.[7]

Do Guidelines Support Non-high-density Lipoprotein Cholesterol?[28]

Several important guidelines have stressed non-HDL-C as an important primary target for risk reduction in patients with CHD, but it still remains controversial as to which out of non-HDL-C or LDL-C is the better marker to access the atherogenic coronary risk. Non-HDL-C over LDL-C is preferred as a treatment goal by the Joint British Societies. The 2014 National Institute for Health and Care Excellence (NICE) guidelines states that at least one lipid sample to estimate full lipid profile including TC, HDL-C, non-HDL-C, and TG should be done before starting lipid modification therapy for the primary prevention of atherosclerotic cardiovascular disease (ASCVD) and fasting estimation is not needed. Greater weight age is given to non-HDL-C as compared to LDL-C by the American National Lipid Association (NLA) guidelines. Non HDL-C along with LDL-C as a target is also recommended by the International Atherosclerosis Society (IAS). If insulin resistance is suspected, the American Association of Clinical Endocrinologists (AACE) 2017 guidelines suggest evaluation of non-HDL-C. Since Indians have high incidence of metabolic syndrome, diabetes and obesity are characterized by atherogenic dyslipidemia that is high TG, low HDL-C, and higher small dense LDL particles, so non-HDL-C becomes an important target for therapy in Indians.[16]

RECOMMENDED LEVELS OF NON-HIGH-DENSITY LIPOPROTEIN CHOLESTEROL GOALS[7]

Non-HDL-C has been suggested to be an important risk factor for CHD, but recommended levels of non-HDL-C still remain ambiguous. Currently, 30 mg/dL higher levels of non-HDL-C to the corresponding LDL-C levels is recommended, that is, if non-HDL-C is 100 mg/dL than corresponding LDL-C level will be 70 mg/dL. But large-scale prospective studies are needed to determine the validity of these levels in CHD patients.

CONCLUSION

Significant residual CV risk remains despite aggressive lipid-lowering therapy. Growing evidence has led to increased focus on non-HDL-C lowering and reduction of CV risk. Non-HDL-C is superior measure of atherogenic particles as compared to LDL-C and has better ability to predict CVD risk. Evidence suggests that non-HDL-C deserves more attention and recommendation to achieving non-HDL-C goals in patients at increased CV risk. Superiority of non-HDL-C in CV risk prediction and benefit of non-HDL-C lowering has been shown as compared to LDL-C. So, for residual CV risk reduction in statin era, we should focus on non-HDL-C especially for guiding CV prevention strategies. The recommended levels of non-HDL-C still remain ambiguous and large-scale prospective studies are needed to determine the optimum non-HDL-C levels for residual risk reduction.

REFERENCES

1. GBD 2013 Mortality and Causes of Death Collaborators. Global, regional, and national age-sex specific all-cause and cause-specific mortality for 240 causes of death, 1990-2013: a systematic analysis for the Global Burden of Disease Study 2013. Lancet. 2015;385:117-71.
2. Gupta R, Gupta KD. Coronary heart disease in low socioeconomic status subjects in India: an evolving epidemic. Indian Heart J. 2009;61:358-67.
3. Institute for Health Metrics and Evaluation. (2010). GBD Profile: India. [online] Available from http://www.healthdata.org/sites/default/files/files/country_profiles/GBD/ihme_gbd_country_report_india.pdf. [Last accessed October, 2019].
4. Gupta R, Guptha S, Sharma KK, et al. Regional variations in cardiovascular risk factors in India: India heart watch. World J Cardiol. 2012;4:112-20.
5. Hackman DG, Anand SS. Emerging risk factors for atherosclerotic vascular disease: A critical review of the evidence. JAMA. 2003;290:932-40.
6. Monahan G. Enterprise Risk Management: A Methodology for Achieving Strategic Objectives. United States: John Wiley & Sons; 2008.
7. Xin Su, Yi Kong, Peng D. Evidence for changing lipid management strategy to focus on non-high density lipoprotein cholesterol. Lipids Health Dis. 2019;18:134.
8. Lawler PR, Akinkuolie AO, Chu AY, et al. Atherogenic Lipoprotein Determinants of Cardiovascular Disease and Residual Risk Among Individuals With Low Low-Density Lipoprotein Cholesterol. J Am Heart Assoc. 2017;6:e005549.
9. Baigent C, Keech A, Kearney PM, et al. Efficacy and safety of cholesterol-lowering treatment: prospective meta-analysis of data from 90,056 participants in 14 randomised trials of statins. Lancet. 2005;366:1267-78.
10. Wilson SR, Sabatine MS, Wiviott SD, et al. Assessment of adiponectin and the risk of recurrent cardiovascular events in patients presenting with an acute coronary syndrome: observations from the Pravastatin Or atorVastatin Evaluation and Infection Trial-Thrombolysis in Myocardial Infarction 22(PROVE IT-TIMI 22). Am Heart J. 2011;161:1147-55.e1.
11. Bohula EA, Wiviott SD, Giugliano RP, et al. Prevention of Stroke with the Addition of Ezetimibe to Statin Therapy in Patients With Acute Coronary Syndrome in IMPROVE-IT (Improved Reduction of Outcomes: Vytorin Efficacy International Trial). Circulation. 2017;136:2440-50.
12. Cannon CP, Braunwald E, McCabe CH, et al. Intensive versus moderate lipid lowering with statins after acute coronary syndromes. N Engl J Med. 2004;350:1495-504.
13. Mehra S, Movahed H, Movahed A. Emerging therapies for residual risk. Rev Cardiovasc Med. 2012;13:e24-31.
14. Alagona P. Beyond LDL cholesterol: the role of elevated triglycerides and low HDL cholesterol in residual CVD risk remaining after statin therapy. Am J Manag Care. 2009;15:S65-73.
15. Joshi P, Islam S, Pais P, et al. Risk factors for early myocardial infarction in South Asians compared with individuals in other countries. JAMA. 2007;297:286-94.
16. Iyengar SS, Puri R, Narasingan SN, et al. Lipid Association of India expert consensus statement on management of dyslipidemia in Indians. Part 1. J Assoc Physicians India. 2016;64:S7-52.
17. Aggarwal J, Reddy S, Nagtilak S, et al. Non-high density lipoprotein cholesterol-risk predictor for coronary heart disease in Indian population. Int J Adv Res. 2014;2:810-7.

18. Sniderman AD, Williams K, Contois JH, et al. A meta-analysis of low-density lipoprotein cholesterol, non-high-density lipoprotein cholesterol, and apolipoprotein B as markers of cardiovascular risk. Circ Cardiovasc Qual Outcomes. 2011;4:337-45.
19. Robinson JG, Wang S, Jacobson TA. Meta-analysis of comparison of effectiveness of lowering apolipoprotein B versus low-density lipoprotein cholesterol and non high-density lipoprotein cholesterol for cardiovascular risk reduction in randomized trials. Am J Cardiol. 2012;110:1468-76.
20. Boekholdt SM, Arsenault BJ, Mora S, et al. Association of LDL cholesterol, non-HDL cholesterol, and apolipoprotein B levels with risk of cardiovascular events among patients treated with statins: a meta-analysis. JAMA. 2012;307:1302-9.
21. van den Berg MJ, van der Graaf Y, de Borst GJ, et al. Low-density lipoprotein cholesterol, non-high-density lipoprotein cholesterol, triglycerides, and apolipoprotein b and cardiovascular risk in patients with manifest arterial disease. Am J Cardiol. 2016;118:804-10.
22. Cui Y, Blumenthal RS, Flaws JA, et al. Non-high-density lipoprotein cholesterol level as a predictor of cardiovascular disease mortality. Arch Intern Med. 2001;161:1413-9.
23. Pischon T, Girman CJ, Sacks FM, et al. Non-high-density lipoprotein cholesterol and apolipoprotein B in the prediction of coronary heart disease in men. Circulation. 2005;112:3375-83.
24. Mora S, Ridker PM. Justification for the use of statins in primary prevention: an intervention trial evaluating rosuvastatin (JUPITER) - can C-reactive protein be used to target statin therapy in primary prevention? Am J Cardiol. 2006;97:33-41.
25. Sondermeijer BM, Rana JS, Arsenault BJ, et al. Non-HDL cholesterol vs. apo B for risk of coronary heart disease in healthy individuals: the EPIC-Norfolk prospective population study. Eur J Clin Investig. 2013;43:1009-15.
26. Wongcharoen W, Sutthiwutthichai S, Gunaparn S, et al. Is non-HDL-cholesterol a better predictor of long-term outcome in patients after acute myocardial infarction compared to LDL-cholesterol?: A retrospective study. BMC Cardiovasc Disord. 2017;17:10.
27. Kastelein JJ, van der Steeg WA, Holme I, et al. Lipids, apolipoproteins, and their ratios in relation to cardiovascular events with statin treatment. Circulation. 2008;117:3002-9.
28. Dalal JJ, Mohan JC, Dasbiswas A, et al. Cholesterol Management in Indians: Should We Treat the Targets or Treat the Risk? J Clin Diagn Res. 2018;12:OE01-5.

70 CHAPTER Triglyceride and CV Risk: Emerging Link in Diabetes

Dheeraj Kapoor, Ranjana Bhatt

INTRODUCTION

Type 2 diabetes mellitus (T2DM) is a metabolic disorder with chronic hyperglycemia resulting in disability and macrovascular or microvascular complications that can lead to impairment in quality of life and increased mortality. As per a number of recent updates, cardiovascular diseases in diabetic population contribute to be a major cause of morbidity and it is the reason behind 70–75% of mortality in this set of population. Rising trend of cardiovascular diseases and the associated morbidity is more commonly seen in present times and has become a common cause of global mortality and disability round the world with a projected estimate of around 17.7 million deaths attributed to the cardiovascular diseases as per World Health Organization (WHO) in 2015.[1] Hence preventive measures for all the possible risk factors causing cardiovascular diseases are of utmost priority.[2] Similar alarming rising trend of diabetes is seen in the present times at global level. T2DM has a significant patient burden and is a very well-known and a significant risk factor for various cardiovascular outcomes like coronary heart disease, stroke, and peripheral arterial disease with 2–4 times increased risk than the nondiabetic counter population.[3] Cardiovascular outcomes in diabetes are responsible for approximately 60% of the associated mortality.[4,5]

EPIDEMIOLOGY

India carries a burden of around 72 million diabetic patients and this figure is expected to double to 134 million by 2025. Most of these individuals from the diabetic group also suffer from dyslipidemia. Among diabetics, this impairment in blood lipid profile is seen commonly as a mixed profile with various combinations like higher levels of small dense low-density lipoprotein (LDL) particles, elevated levels of triglycerides, and low high-density lipoprotein (HDL) cholesterol levels. This particular pattern of dyslipidemia in view of its potential to cause progression of atherosclerosis is also known as an atherogenic diabetic dyslipidemia (ADD). Ratio of dyslipidemia among the Indian diabetic population is seen as affecting 85.5% of males and 97.2% of the females.[6] It has also been seen and published that higher triglyceride levels are an important and independent risk factor in terms of possible cardiovascular risk in future. Indian population is at risk of metabolic disorders like diabetes and dyslipidemia due to following factors:[7]

- Lack of physical activity
- Poor diet—intake of carbohydrate enriched food and fat with less omega-3 PUFA triggers hypertriglyceridemia
- Overweight and obesity—excessive accumulation of visceral and abdominal fat disproportionate to the BMI
- Genetics—abnormality in lipoprotein lipase (LPL), apoC3 (causing lipoprotein lipase inhibition), and apoE3 (formation of VLDL) genes causing dyslipidemia and various HLA variants and genes predisposing for maturity-onset diabetes of the young (MODY) and T2DM
- Metabolic syndrome
- Alcohol intake
- Females with polycystic ovarian syndrome have high triglyceride levels[8]
- Use of oral contraceptives or estrogen therapy causes dyslipidemia with increased triglycerides[9]
- Maternal hypertriglyceridemia is also seen during gestational diabetes mellitus.

PATHOGENESIS

Triglycerides in plasma come both from de novo synthesis as well as from diet.[10] While passage through the digestive tract, the fat from the diet undergoes lipolysis, dissolution into micelles, and hydrolysis by the pancreatic lipase enzyme followed by the uptake of the free fatty acid (FFA) molecules thus produced in the small intestine.[11] These FFA molecules on entering the enterocyte get converted into the triglyceride moiety by the enzyme acyl-CoA:diacylglycerol acyltransferase 2 (DGAT2)[10] and most of these triglyceride particles get packed in apoB48-containing lipoprotein particles (chylomicrons) by the microsomal triglyceride transfer protein (MTTP) and thereby gets secreted into the lymphatic system, draining in the systemic circulation finally, thus bypassing the liver; however some amount of triglycerides can get stored in form of lipid droplets.[12] After its secretion, these triglyceride particles undergo lipolysis via the enzyme known as lipoprotein lipase which is usually present in the capillary beds of skeletal muscle and adipose tissue. Another particle called as ApoC-II is an important cofactor for this process. Fatty acid molecules thus produced are taken up at the level of skeletal muscle as an energy source and by the adipose tissue as a storage moiety. Cardiac myocytes derive 60% of their energy expenditure from fatty acids mobilized by the lipoprotein lipase enzyme.[13] The remaining particles like apoB-48 carrying the chylomicron residue and the apoB-100 particle carrying the very low-density lipoprotein (VLDL) residues after various modulations are taken up by the hepatocytes through the LDL-receptor situated on the plasma membrane.[14] Hypertriglyceridemia is a frequently seen phenomenon in patients with metabolic syndrome or diabetes mellitus or as a familial combined hyperlipidemia moiety.[15] The primary basis of all of the above phenotypes is the same that is insulin resistance.[16] Insulin has an important position in regulation and homeostasis of lipids. Hence in a background of insulin resistance there is defective maneuvering of lipid particles in the organs sensitive to insulin which are mainly adipose tissue, skeletal muscle, and liver. In the postprandial state, insulin stimulates the lipoprotein lipase enzyme in adipocytes followed by a shift to cause FFA uptake and storage as lipid droplets in adipose tissue. While in a fasting state where insulin levels fall, compensatory high glucagon levels act by upregulation of the hormone-sensitive lipase enzyme via inhibition of cAMP-associated and PKA-dependent phosphorylation, by ultimately providing the FFA moiety which is secreted and taken up at the level of peripheral tissues.[17] In the state of adipose tissue insulin resistance there is an increased supply of FFA in the hepatocytes which results in synthesis and secretion of abnormal VLDL particles. These FFA particles are recognized as significant ligands for various nuclear receptors in metabolism of lipids. Hence impaired signaling in case of resistance to insulin will lead to accumulation of abnormal lipoprotein and ultimately hypertriglyceridemia. It is seen that triglyceride particles are involved in the process of atherogenesis.[18] There is a combined effect and interaction between diabetes with its associated factors and dyslipidemia in stimulation and progression of atherosclerosis. High triglyceride levels along with esterified FFA levels, diacylglycerol, and various serine/threonine kinases worsen diabetes by hampering the beta cell function and enhancing peripheral insulin resistance. Decline in function of beta cell predisposes to hyperglycemia which further increases risk of cardiovascular diseases. Insulin resistance results in proinflammatory state along with impaired coagulation profile. Triglyceride levels are also believed to cause alteration in size of LDL particles in an inverse manner such as elevated triglycerides would produce small and dense LDL particles (Fig. 1).[19]

Various cardiovascular studies have shown supporting evidence that these small dense LDL particles are strongly atherogenic than the larger LDL moiety.[20,21] Various other mechanisms also play a role in accelerating atherogenesis. Triglyceride particles also upregulate activation of various cytokines, coagulation factors along with collection of leukocyte adhesion molecules, disproportionate vasodilation, and impair fibrinolysis in this process. Various published longitudinal or cross-sectional studies that have been done till now suggest that high triglyceride level can be a strong predictor for cardiovascular disease risk. Like a hypertriglyceridemic waist which was characterized by marked triglyceride levels plus high circumference of waist was correlated with risk of cardiovascular disease arteriographically.[22]

CONCLUSION

Hence it is of utmost importance that diabetic dyslipidemia is a significant and independent factor involved in the process of an accelerated macrovascular disease among the diabetic population. Various primary mechanisms involved in pathogenesis of dyslipidemia in diabetic patients mainly include postprandial lipemia, increased plasma VLDL levels, and increased production of small dense LDL particles indirectly via triglyceride influx. These abnormal lipid particles then further stimulate a

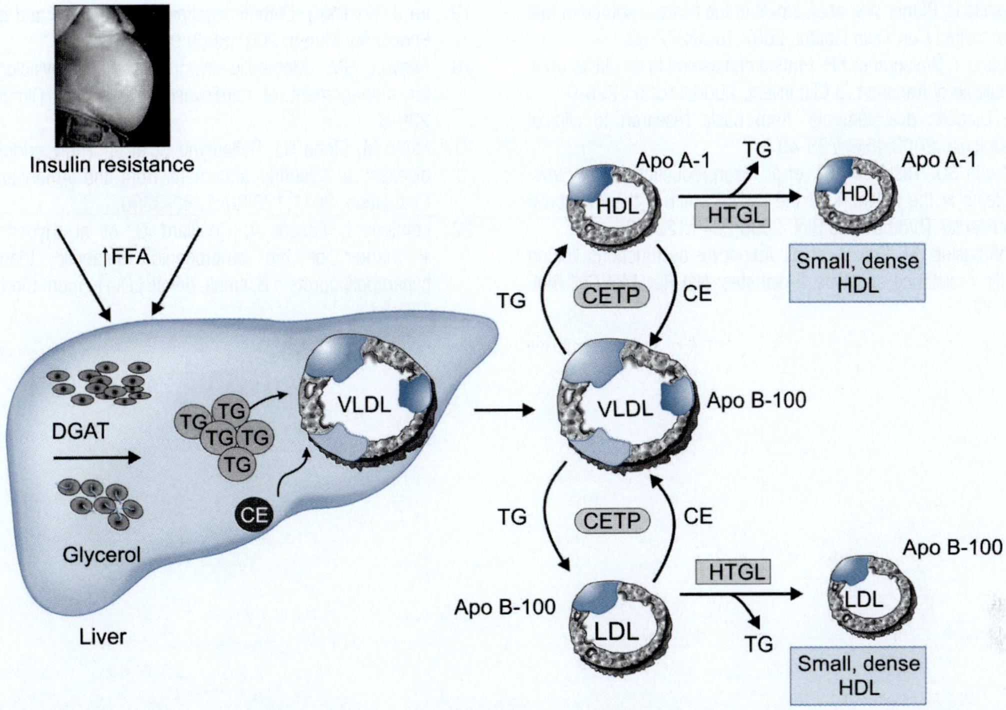

(CETP: cholesteryl ester transfer protein; CE: cholesteryl ester; DGAT: diacylglycerol acyltransferase; FFA: free fatty acid; HDL: high-density lipoprotein; HTGL: hepatic triglyceride lipase; LDL: low-density lipoprotein; TG: triglyceride)

Figure 1 Pathogenesis of diabetic dyslipidemia.

proinflammatory state causing cardiovascular morbidity and mortality. Thus high triglyceride levels and low HDL levels in Indian population have a predisposition to develop cardiovascular diseases. So management of these abovementioned abnormalities in lipid metabolism has an equal and important potential in reducing occurrence of cardiovascular events and burden. This leads to the formulation that management of triglycerides and small dense LDL particles will provide a window period for all diabetic patients and will allow these patients to lead a longer and a healthier life.

REFERENCES

1. WHO. World Health Statistics 2017: Monitoring health for the SDGs. Geneva: WHO; 2017.
2. De Backer G, Ambrosioni E, Borch-Johnsen K, et al. European guidelines on cardiovascular disease prevention in clinical practice: third joint task force of European and other societies on cardiovascular disease prevention in clinical practice (constituted by representatives of eight societies and by invited experts). Eur J Cardiovasc Prev Rehabil. 2003;10(4):S1-10.
3. Emerging Risk Factors Collaboration; Sarwar N, Gao P, Seshasai SR, et al. Diabetes mellitus, fasting blood glucose concentration, and risk of vascular disease: a collaborative meta-analysis of 102 prospective studies. Lancet. 2010;375(9733):2215-22.
4. Moss SE, Klein R, Klein BE. Cause-specific mortality in a population-based study of diabetes. Am J Public Health. 1991;81(9):1158-62.
5. Laakso M. Hyperglycemia and cardiovascular disease in type 2 diabetes. Diabetes. 1999;48(5):937-42.
6. Parikh RM, Joshi SR, Menon PS, et al. Prevalence and pattern of diabetic dyslipidemia in Indian type 2 diabetic patients. Diabetes Metab Syndr. 2010;4(1):10-2.
7. American Association of Physicians of Indian Origin. (2002). Clinical Implications: Dyslipidemia in the Asian Indian Population. Unique aspects and implications for treatment. 20th Annual Convention of the American Association of Physicians of Indian Origin. [Online]. Available from https://cadiresearch.org/wp-content/themes/twentyeleven/pdf/AAPI-monograph.pdf [Last accessed September, 2019].
8. Talbott E, Guzick D, Clerici A, et al. Coronary heart disease risk factors in women with polycystic ovary syndrome. Arterioscler Thromb Vasc Biol. 1995;15(7):821-6.
9. Greenlund KJ, Webber LS, Srinivasan S, et al. Associations of oral contraceptive use with serum lipids and lipoproteins in young women: the Bogalusa Heart Study. Ann Epidemiol. 1997;7(8):561-7.
10. Yen CL, Stone SJ, Koliwad S, et al. Thematic Review Series: Glycerolipids. DGAT enzymes and triacylglycerol biosynthesis. J Lipid Res. 2008;49(11):2283-301.
11. Mu H, Hoy CE. The digestion of dietary triacylglycerols. Prog Lipid Res. 2004;43(2):105-33.
12. Williams KJ. Molecular processes that handle - and mishandle - dietary lipids. J Clin Invest. 2008;118(10):3247-59.
13. Twickler T, Dallinga-Thie GM, Chapman MJ, et al. Remnant lipoproteins and atherosclerosis. Curr Atheroscler Rep. 2005;7:140-7.

14. Park TS, Yamashita H, Blaner WS, et al. Lipids in the heart: a source of fuel and a source of toxins. Curr Opin Lipidol. 2007;18(3):277-82.
15. Mahley RW, Huang Y, Weisgraber KH. Putting cholesterol in its place: apoE and reverse cholesterol transport. J Clin Invest. 2006;116(5):1226-9.
16. Taskinen MR. Diabetic dyslipidaemia: from basic research to clinical practice. Diabetologia. 2003;46(6):733-49.
17. Adiels M, Olofsson SO, Taskinen MR, et al. Overproduction of very low-density lipoproteins is the hallmark of the dyslipidemia in the metabolic syndrome. Arterioscler Thromb Vasc Biol. 2008;28(7):1225-36.
18. Guilherme A, Virbasius JV, Puri V, et al. Adipocyte dysfunctions linking obesity to insulin resistance and type 2 diabetes. Nat Rev Mol Cell Biol. 2008;9(5):367-77.
19. Ira J. Goldberg, Diabetic dyslipidemia: Causes and consequences. J Clin Endocrinol Metab. 2001;86(3):965-71.
20. Reaven GM. Metabolic syndrome. Pathophysiology and implications for management of cardiovascular disease. Circulation. 2002;106(3):286-8.
21. Miller M, Stone NJ, Ballantyne C, et al. Triglycerides and cardiovascular disease: a scientific statement from the American Heart Association. Circulation. 2011;123(20):2292-3330.
22. Lemieux I, Pascot A, Couillard C, et al. Hypertriglyceridemic waist: a marker of the atherogenic metabolic triad (hyperinsulinemia; hyperapolipoprotein B; small, dense LDL) in men. Circulation. 2000;102(2):179-84.

71 CHAPTER Screening for Silent CVD in Diabetics: What is the Best Approach?

S Arulrhaj, Aarathy Kannan, Gurunadha Rao, Ankita Bajpai

INTRODUCTION

The patients who have type 2 diabetes mellitus (T2DM) may have apparently asymptomatic cardiovascular (CV) damage,[1,2] along with the ischemic episodes that remain undetected at a reported prevalence of one in three diabetic patients in comparison to one in five patients without diabetes.[3] Thus, development of CV sequelae can occur much earlier than detected; the disease is only identified when there is presence of more pronounced symptoms.[2,4]

As reported by Shah et al. (2015), the risk of stroke, peripheral artery disease (PAD), and coronary heart disease (CHD) is increased by two-to fourfold by diabetes. In diabetes, the leading cause of mortality are the macrovascular events. Over the past two decades, there is an increase in the burden of cardiovascular disease (CVD) that is attributable to diabetes. Insulin resistance is the underlying factor for all the features of metabolic syndrome and is considered crucial in the pathophysiology of vascular damage.

INCIDENCE

In the Framingham cohort, it was reported that the incidence of CVD in diabetic men as well as women was twice and three times as compared to nondiabetic men as well as women, respectively. It was reported in a 25-year follow-up of middle-aged men and women that the mortality among men with diabetes and without previous CHD was comparable to that of men with CHD and without diabetes (54.0 vs. 50.5 deaths per 1,000 person-years). In women with diabetes only, the risk of death was considerably higher than in women with CHD only (46.7 vs. 29.2 deaths per 1,000 person-years) (Flowchart 1).

CLINICAL PRESENTATION (FLOWCHART 2)

Cardiac

In patients with type 1 diabetes mellitus (T1DM) and T2DM, hypertension is very common. Prevalence rate of hypertension in T1DM is 30% and in T2DM is 60%. The development of diabetic nephropathy (DN) is closely associated with hypertension in diabetic patients.

Diabetes mellitus appears to contribute directly to the development of diabetic cardiomyopathy (CMP). Annual mortality rates up to 20%.

Myocardial Infarction

Patients with DM are in a prothrombotic and procoagulant state, which may account for the higher rates of MI. The prevalence of diabetes in patients with CAD is up to 40% in many countries.

Silent CAD is far more prevalent in patients with DM (10–20%) than those without DM (1–4%). Diabetic neuropathy is one factor that may explain the increased incidence of silent ischemia in patients with DM.

Heart Failure

Risk for heart failure increases 2.4-fold in men and 5-fold in women in comparison with those without diabetes mellitus. Microvascular disease, characterized by arterial

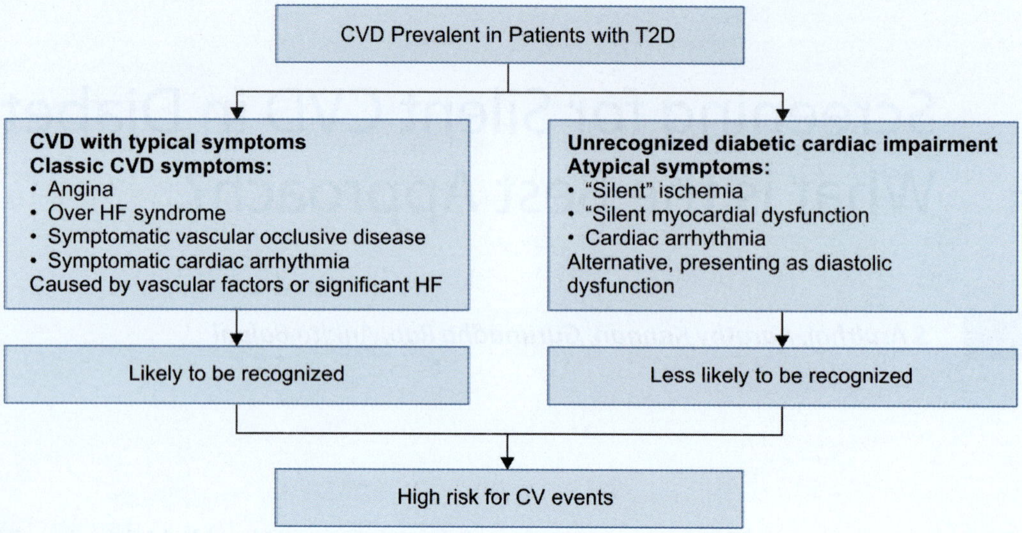

(CVD: cardiovascular disease; HF: heart failure; T2D type 2 diabetes mellitus)

Flowchart 1 Prevalence of cardiovascular disease in type 2 diabetes patient.

(*Source*: Schernthaner G, Lotan C, Baltadzhieva-Trendafilova E, et al. Unrecognised cardiovascular disease in type 2 diabetes: is it time to act earlier? Cardiovasc Diabetol. 2018;17:145.)

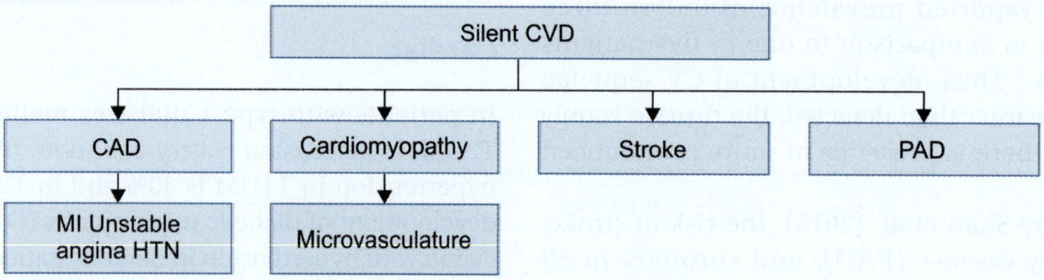

(CVD: cardiovascular disease; CAD: coronary artery disease; HTN: hypertension; PAD: peripheral artery disease; MI: myocardial infarction)

Flowchart 2 Clinical presentation of cardiovascular disease.

thickening and fibrosis, as well as endothelial and vasomotor dysfunction, can increase the risk of heart failure in diabetes mellitus.

Vascular

Cerebrovascular Disease

Diabetes is a major risk factor for development of carotid atherosclerosis and stroke, both ischemic and hemorrhagic. Data from the Emerging Risk Factors Collaboration found that diabetes was associated with a 2.27-fold increase in the risk of ischemic stroke and a 1.56-fold increase in the risk of hemorrhagic stroke. Diabetes is actually considered an established risk factor for cognitive impairment, dementia, and Alzheimer disease.

Peripheral Artery Disease

Diabetes is also associated with a twofold increase in the risk of lower limb ischemia, and an estimated 21% of patients have signs of PAD. The ankle-brachial index (ABI) is the most widely and validated tool to diagnose PAD and normally ranges from 0.9 to 1.3. An ABI lower than 0.9 is commonly used to diagnose PAD, both symptomatic and asymptomatic.

Cardiovascular Autonomic Neuropathy

Common among patients with DM and is correlated with an increased 5-year mortality rate from CVD. Up to 34% of the patients with type 2 diabetes (T2D) may be affected by diabetic cardiac autonomic neuropathy (CAN).

It can cause abnormalities in heart rate control as well as vascular dynamics, which can lead to asymptomatic ischemia, exercise intolerance, painless myocardial infarction, and orthostatic hypotension. In patients with T2D, CAN has been reported to be associated with increase in prevalence of left ventricular diastolic dysfunction (LVDD), arrhythmia, and sudden death. The LVDD can progress to heart failure with preserved ejection fraction (HFpEF), with increase in morbidity as well as mortality. There is an increase in incidence of CAN with age and inadequate glycemic control; this places patients having DM at increased risk of developing CVD and CAN.

The development as well as progression of CAN is possibly associated with dysregulation of the autonomic nervous system with enhanced sympathetic activity and increased inflammatory markers. Coronary artery disease (CAD) is a leading cause of morbidity and mortality in patients with diabetes. Therefore, for prevention as well as early and successful treatment of coronary events, proper screening and diagnosis of CAD is important.

APPROACH TO SILENT CVD IN T2DM (TABLE 1)

Silent Coronary Artery Disease

Among all the CVD complications of DM, CAD plays the major role in mortality and morbidity. Hence the diagnosis of silent CAD is the need of the hour. For prevention as well as early and successful treatment of coronary events, proper screening and diagnosis of CAD is important.

TABLE 1: Tools with advantages and disadvantages to approach silent cardiovascular disease in type 2 diabetes mellitus.

Tool	Advantages	Disadvantages
Questionnaires	• Can be carried out by a variety of people with limited affect to its validity and reliability • Results can be quickly and easily quantified • Can be analysed more 'scientifically' and objectively than other forms of research • Can be used to compare and contrast data and to measure change	• Patients may provide the answers that they think are expected • Lacks validity • It is difficult to assess how much thought a patient has given to each question • The interpretation of each question may differ
Digital data gathering (e.g. wearable personal health tracker)	• Provide continuous, objective, remote monitoring • Patients can monitor and self-manage behaviors • A significant volume of data can be captured • Data collected may promote beneficial lifestyle changes	• Accuracy may be affected by factors such as individual gait characteristics, body morphology, and where and how a device is worn on the body • Patients may place greater faith in the accuracy of the device than is warranted • Sensitive data may be captured with resultant privacy issues
Stress test or 6-minute walking test	• Practical and simple requiring no specialized equipment • Evaluates the global and integrated responses of all the systems involved during exercise • Useful for measuring the response to medical interventions • Findings are reproducible	• Additional cardiopulmonary exercise testing may be required • Adherence to strict protocols is required to ensure validity of data collected
Biomarkers (B-type natriuretic peptide (BNP) or N-terminal pro BNP)	• Free from recall bias • Can provide sensitive and specific early detection of disease	• Usually require a sample of body fluid to be taken • Inter-individual variability may be a concern • Specialized laboratory analysis may be required • Reproducibility could be a concern • May not be cost-effective

Type 2 diabetes mellitus is considered a "coronary artery disease" equivalent.[5] CAD is often asymptomatic in diabetic patients, and up to 60% of myocardial infarctions may be clinically silent and detected only by systematic electrocardiogram (ECG) screening.[5] Silent myocardial ischemia (SMI) has been reported to be associated with significant coronary stenosis on angiography in 35–70% of patients. Nonspecific or atypical symptoms, such as dyspnea, giddiness, abdominal pain, and confusion were reported by 32% to 42% of diabetic patients with SMI compared with 6–15% of nondiabetic patients.[6]

According to ICMR-INDIAB (The Indian Council of Medical Research–India Diabetes) study, 62.4 million people have diabetes in India. It is expected to increase to 101 million by 2030. The prevalence of SMI is 10–20% in diabetic patients compared to 1–4% in nondiabetic patients. 12.5 million diabetic patients have asymptomatic CAD.[7]

The Detection of Ischemia in Asymptomatic Diabetics (DIAD) study (Young et al. 2009) is the only randomized trial to investigate the clinical value of CAD screening in asymptomatic diabetic patients.[8]

Definition

Silent myocardial ischemia defined as objective evidence of myocardial ischemia in the absence of chest discomfort or other anginal equivalents.[9] This objective evidence includes ST-segment shifts (usually depression), reversible regional wall motion abnormalities, and perfusion defects on scintigraphic studies.[10]

Classification

Silent myocardial ischemia is divided into three categories:[11]

1. *Type I*: Least common form, occurs in completely asymptomatic patients with CAD in the absence of anginal symptoms.
2. *Type II*: It occurs in patients with documented previous MI.
3. *Type III*: Most common form and occurs in patients with chronic stable angina, unstable angina and vasospastic angina.

Mechanisms of SMI

Diabetic patients often present with less severe chest pain than nondiabetic patients and that their presenting symptoms of cardiac events are frequently unrelated to chest pain.[12]

Silent ischemia results from variable combinations of decreased sensitivity to painful stimuli and coronary microvascular dysfunction.[13] The association between diabetes and both silent ischemia and "painless infarctions" has been attributed to autonomic neuropathy.[14]

The data from the Framingham study confirmed that truly silent myocardial infarction, as documented by biennial ECGs, occurs in ≈12% of patients and is more common in diabetic patients. These clinical findings are supported by autopsy data from patients without a clinical history of myocardial infarction, showing that myocardial scar is more likely to be present in diabetics than nondiabetics.[15] Histological changes in intracardiac sympathetic and parasympathetic afferent fibers are often cited as a potential mechanism for the diminished, altered, or absent sensation of chest pain experienced by diabetic patients with acute myocardial infarction (AMI).[16]

As compared to the overall population, CAD is usually detected at more advanced stages of the disease in the patients with diabetes. It is because in diabetic subjects, there is faster and earlier development of arteriosclerotic process; the patient stays asymptomatic for CAD for a long duration.[17] In DM, the atherosclerotic plaques are generally characterized by their large volumes as well as lipid cores. This cause large remodeling rates among the affected vascular segment and have thin fibrous caps with intense inflammatory process, which renders them more vulnerable to rupture and may induce an acute coronary event.[17] In patients with diabetes, there is a more diffuse, extensive, and severe coronary artery involvement. These are the factors that are associated with worse prognosis.[17]

Another area of investigation suggests that silent ischemia may be due to cerebral cortical dysfunction, rather than peripheral nerve dysfunction. Frontal cortical activation appears to be necessary to experience cardiac pain, and some evidence indicates that in patients with silent ischemia, afferent pain impulses from the heart are subject to abnormal neural processing.[18]

Whom to Screen

Screening for asymptomatic CAD among diabetics is recommended especially among those who have diabetes for more than 5 years or have additional risk factors like hypertension, smoking, dyslipidemia, family history of CAD, and micro- or macrovascular complications of diabetes.

European Association for the Study of Diabetes (EASD) suggests to perform the screening also in asymptomatic patients at particular high risk such as those with evidence of target organ damage. These include patients with PAD, high coronary artery calcium (CAC) score, low ABI, increased carotid intima-media thickness, microalbuminuria, chronic kidney disease, photocoagulated retinopathy, autonomic neuropathy, and erectile dysfunction.

The American Diabetes Association (ADA) consensus statement on CAD recommends screening in the following cases:
- Typical or atypical chest pain
- Abnormal electrocardiogram (ECG) suggestive of ischemia or infarction
- Peripheral or carotid arterial occlusive disease
- 35 years with sedentary lifestyle in a patient who plans a vigorous exercise program.
- Two or more risk factors in addition to diabetes, such as dyslipidemia, hypertension, tobacco use, family history for premature CAD, or micro- or macroalbuminuria

When to Screen

Flowchart 3 shows when to screen for ischemic heart disease in diabetic patients.

Available Modalities in the Diagnosis of SMI

Objective evidence of SMI in diabetics may be obtained through several ways, and its prevalence depends significantly on the method of screening and what test result is considered diagnostic for CHD. The available screening tests can be divided into mechanical, pharmacological, and nuclear.

Exercise ECG

Treadmill exercise ECG should be considered as initial screening test in asymptomatic population of diabetics. It is diagnostic tool for the diagnosis and risk stratification of CHD whose diagnostic and prognostic value has been studied extensively.

Myocardial ischemia is indirectly detected by the exercise ECG. Myocardial ischemia is the result of a mismatch among myocardial oxygen delivery (i.e. coronary blood flow) and myocardial oxygen demand (i.e. myocardial work).

The graded exercise tests are broadly used clinically for evaluating the ability of a person to safely tolerate increase in physical activity. Whereas, ECG, hemodynamic, as well as symptomatic responses are used for monitoring the development of electrical instability, myocardial ischemia, as well as other abnormalities related to exertion.

Silent myocardial ischemia has been defined as exercise-induced ST depression of >1 mm in the absence of CAD symptoms. Patients with a resting ECG suggestive of ischemia or infarction should undergo stress testing. Furthermore, asymptomatic patients with diabetes and two or more CV risk factors should also undergo stress testing.

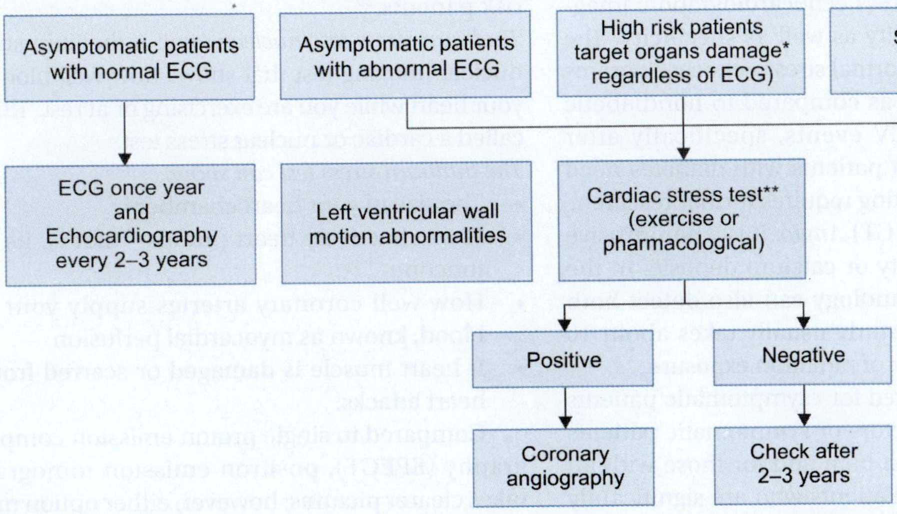

*Target organ damage includes peripheral artery disease, high coronary artery calcium (CAC) score, low ankle-brachial index (ABI), increased carotid intima-media thickness, proteinuria, chronic kidney disease, laser-treated retinopathy, autonomic neuropathy, and erectile dysfunction.

**Cardiac stress tests include ECG exercise tolerance test, pharmacological myocardial perfusion imaging, or pharmacological stress echocardiography.

Flowchart 3 Diagnostic flowchart for ischemic heart disease in diabetic patients.

(*Source*: 2016 Italian Standard of Care in Diabetes.)

Non-ST-segment variables:

- Duke Treadmill Exercise Score: Assess exercise capacity which is predictor of CV mortality.
- Heart rate recovery (HRR) after exercise and chronotropic response (percentage of heart rate reserve used): Diabetic patients have a higher incidence of autonomic dysfunction--prolonged HRR after exercise predicts mortality in the general population.

The low risk group by treadmill exercise ECG should not be routinely advised for coronary angiogram. The medium risk group should be advised for further investigation by coronary angiogram only in the presence of additional risk factors for CAD. The high risk group should strongly be recommended for coronary angiogram and considered for revascularization therapy where indicated.

ECHO: Echocardiogram can identify the majority of patients likely to have significant ischemia during their daily activities and remains the most important screening test for significant CAD. The presence of resting RWMA might represent underlying myocardial damage due to infarction, hibernation or stunning secondary to atherosclerotic CAD or nonischemic insult to myocardium. Echo is the only independent 2-D echo predictor of high risk CAD. Elderly diabetic patients unable to exercise with low EF and RWMA appeared to be of highest risk of severe CAD.

Stress Echo: Stress testing with imaging is well recognized to provide greater diagnostic accuracy than exercise ECG testing in the general clinical population. Dobutamine and dipyridamole can be used as stressors. As compared to exercise ECG testing, the stress echocardiographic imaging gives improved sensitivity as well as specificity. The patients with diabetes and normal stress echocardiograms seem to have a higher risk as compared to nondiabetic patients for subsequent CV events, specifically after 2 years. The hypothesis that patients with diabetes need more frequent follow-up testing requires further research.

Computed tomography (CT) *Angio*: It is a noninvasive imaging test to evaluate fatty or calcium deposits in the coronary arteries. This technology can also detect both soft and hard plaque. The study usually takes about 10 minutes, and there is the risk of radiation exposure.

This test can be considered for asymptomatic patients who have significant risk factors or symptomatic patients with typical or atypical chest pain and for those with an equivocal stress test result. Patients who are significantly overweight or who have an abnormal rhythm, such as atrial fibrillation, are not good candidates for this study because imaging quality may be compromised. A functional study is recommended if the study reveals a >50% lesion or a CAC score >1,000.

Computed tomography coronary angiography has a high accuracy for detecting CAC score, degree, and extent of SMI compared with invasive coronary angiography.

Cardiac fat (Echo and CTA): Cardiac fat [including epicardial adipose tissue (EAT) and pericardial adipose tissue (PAT) fat] is an imaging biomarker of CAD due to its intimate relation to the myocardium and coronary arteries. EAT thickness was measured as the echo-free space above the free wall of the right ventricle to the epicardium at end-systole in the parasternal long axis view perpendicular to the aortic annulus. PAT thickness was measured as the hypoechoic space in front of EAT and on the external pericardium. EAT and PAT were combined to obtain CAT.[19]

Magnetic resonance imaging (MRI): Cardiovascular magnetic resonance (CMR) imaging data are sparse but evolving rapidly. These studies can provide information regarding coronary stenosis and flow, evaluation of myocardial perfusion and metabolism, wall motion during stress, and evidence of infarction. The absence of ionizing radiation in CMR is an attractive feature because all imaging studies except echocardiography require exposure to ionizing radiation. Myocardial perfusion imaging helps to identify whether anatomical stenosis causes myocardial dysfunction and to assess the risk stratification and prognosis of SMI. Myocardial perfusion imaging, which provides evidence of ischemia by directly measuring the "total ischemic burden", is clearly the method of choice in low- and intermediate-risk patients.[20]

Thallium stress test/nuclear scan: A thallium stress test is a nuclear imaging test that shows how well blood flows into your heart while you are exercising or at rest. This test is also called a cardiac or nuclear stress test.

The thallium stress test can show:

- The size of your heart chambers
- How effectively heart pumps—that is, its ventricular function
- How well coronary arteries supply your heart with blood, known as myocardial perfusion
- If heart muscle is damaged or scarred from previous heart attacks.

Compared to single proton emission computed tomography (SPECT), positron emission tomography (PET) takes clearer pictures; however, either option may be used.

Nuclear heart scans have few risks like small amount of and in rare instances, some people have a treatable allergic reaction to the tracer. If there is CHD, patient may have chest pain during the stress test that can be relieved with medication.

Cardiac catheterization—angiogram: Coronary angiography is considered the gold standard for identifying obstructive lesions. It is reserved for patients who have evidence of ischemia on a stress test or for further assessment of the coronary anatomy in patients with a negative stress test who continue to have symptoms (suspected false negative results).

Percutaneous coronary intervention (PCI): There are two reasons to perform coronary revascularization—to improve survival and to improve symptoms. Patients with stable CAD and silent ischemia who are treated with PCI guided by fractional flow reserve (FFR) had a lower composite rate of death or myocardial infarction at 5 years than those who were treated with medical therapy alone (Table 2).

TABLE 2: Screening methods for detecting asymptomatic coronary artery ischemia in patients with diabetes.

Screening methods	Detection of prevalent coronary heart disease	Comments
Functional tests		
Resting electrocardiogram (ECG)	• Low sensitivity and specificity	• Widely available, very low cost
Exercise ECG	• Moderate sensitivity (45–61%) and specificity (70–90%)	• Relatively low cost, widely available • Many patients unable to exercise • Some have uninterpretable baseline ECGs
Radionuclide single proton emission computed tomography (SPECT)	• Good sensitivity(80–90%)and specificity (75–90%) • The most widely used test to assess silent myocardial ischemia	• Moderate to high cost • Widely available • High negative predictive value(95%) • Image quality affected by body habitus and large breasts • Screening of asymptomatic patients not prognostically useful unless high-risk patients are selected
Myocardial perfusion imaging (MPI) with positron emission tomography (PET)	• High sensitivity for myocardial viability studies • Accurate global and regional measurements of myocardial perfusion, blood flow, and function at stress and rest in a single study	• Better image quality because of higher spatial resolution, less scattered, and fewer attenuation artifacts • Lower radiation exposure than SPECT • Costly, not universally available
• *Stress echocardiography Exercise stress echo* • *Pharmacologic stress echo (dobutamine, adenosine, and dipyridamole)*	• The sensitivity and specificity are satisfactory (80–85%) • Able to assess left ventricular function and valvular abnormalities	• Low cost, widely available • Operator dependent • Difficulty in interpreting the images in obese persons
Anatomic (imaging) techniques		
Coronary artery calcium score (CAC)	• CAC more prevalent in people with diabetes than nondiabetes • Closely associated with total coronary artery atherosclerotic plaque burden • Predicts incident ischemia, CHD morbidity and mortality	• Moderate to high cost • No differentiation between obstructive and nonobstructive CHD • Up to 25% of patients have minimal or no CAC at the time of screening
Multidetector-row computed tomography (MRCT) angiography	• High sensitivity (83–99%) and specificity (93–98%)	• Good sensitivity, specificity, and negative predictive value. • High radiation doses • High cost
Magnetic resonance imaging (MRI)	• Good sensitivity (83–90%) and specificity (72–84%) • Delayed gadolinium hyperenhancement linked to increased risk of major cardiovascular events • Not adequately investigated	• Able to assess myocardial structure and function and characterize ischemic, inflammatory and various types of cardiomyopathies • High cost

Silent Stroke Screening

Magnetic resonance angiography (MRA)

A specific type of MRI examination that allows to look specifically at the arteries, without seeing all the overlying tissues. It may or may not require the injection of a contrast material, depending on the specific vessels being scanned. The contrast material used for MRA is less likely to cause an allergic reaction than the contrast material used for CT.

Magnetic resonance venography (MRV)

A specific type of MRI that examines the veins without the overlying tissues being visible. Typically, this examination will require an injection of a contrast material to enhance the visibility of the veins.

Carotid artery screening

In individuals without signs or symptoms of carotid artery disease ultrasound (US) imaging of the carotid arteries can be performed, like:

- *Carotid duplex ultrasound*: It uses A combination of conventional and Doppler ultrasound is used in carotid duplex ultrasound for—
  - Evaluating the blood flow in carotid arteries
  - Measuring the speed of the blood flow
  - Estimating the diameter of a blood vessel as well as degree of obstruction, if present.
- *Carotid intima media thickness (IMT) ultrasound*: In this technique, the ultrasound pictures of the carotid arteries are used for measuring the thickness of the two innermost layers of the carotid artery walls (i.e. the intima and media) and for identifying the plaque buildup. An abnormal arterial wall thickening can indicate the development of CVD.

Transcranial Doppler (TCD): It is aptly known as the "doctor's stethoscope of the brain". It is a noninvasive ultrasound method, which is utilized for assessing the blood circulation in brain. Inaudible sound waves (which cannot be heard) are transmitted through the tissues of the skull during TCD. Such sound waves reflect off the blood cells that are moving within the blood vessels; this enables the radiologist to interpret their speed as well as direction. The TCD ultrasound images are useful in the diagnosis of a variety of conditions that affect blood flow to the brain as well as within the brain.

Silent PAD Screening

Ankle-brachial index

The test compares the blood pressure at your ankle with the blood pressure at your arm. A low ABI number can indicate narrowing or blockage of the arteries in your legs. You may have ABI testing before and immediately after walking on a treadmill. An exercise ABI test can assess the severity of the narrowed arteries during walking. The device uses sound waves to produce images and allows your pulse to be heard in your ankle arteries after the cuff is deflated.

Arterial Doppler

Doppler ultrasound is a painless way to detect blood flowing through a small artery. It uses sound waves and a type of sonar detection system to make noise when blood flow is detected. For arterial studies of the legs (called segmental Doppler pressures), Doppler ultrasound is used in place of the stethoscope that doctors usually use when taking blood pressures.

MARKERS OF SILENT CVD

1. *Erectile dysfunction* is red flag for silent early CVD - Because vascular disturbance of the penile endothelium leads to ED, the possibility arises that ED may be an early indicator for systemic endothelial dysfunction and subsequent CVD.
2. *Micro- or macroproteinuria*: Proteinuria has also been associated with increased risk of atherosclerotic events affecting the peripheral vasculature. Patients with proteinuria have been shown to have increased risk of incident stroke.
3. *Retinal artery narrowing*: Microvascular dysfunction leads to atherosclerosis by inducing endothelial dysfunction of the large vessels. There is a correlation between retinal arteriolar narrowing and decreased myocardial blood flow and perfusion reserve.[21]
4. The presence of plaque and thickness of intima and medial layers in carotid arteries, measured as *carotid intima media thickness*, is considered a marker for CAD. The test is performed with high-frequency B-mode ultrasonography. It is simple and reproducible, widely available, well-validated, and does not expose patients to ionizing radiation.
5. Emerging data on circulating markers such as *high-sensitivity C-reactive protein and high-sensitivity troponin T (hsTroponin T)* report on aspects of atherosclerosis pathogenesis distinct from traditional risk factors and may ultimately improve the utility of risk engines in nominating candidates for further testing.
6. Patients with T2DM and *microalbuminuria* were more likely to have SMI. Microalbuminuria is now recognized as a marker of endothelial dysfunction. Endothelial dysfunction is considered to be one of

the most important pathophysiological precursors to the development of CVD. Thus the presence of microalbuminuria can be an important clue to identify asymptomatic diabetic patients with underlying CVD.

7. *Copeptin* is released very early during the onset of an SMI. Copeptin is released much earlier than troponin, given that copeptin is actively released from the hypothalamus. It has been shown that the combination of a negative result of troponin together with a negative result of copeptin can rule out AMI at emergency department presentation with a negative predictive value ranging from 95% to 100% (Flowchart 4).[22]

SUMMARY FOR EVALUATING SILENT CVD IN DM

Evaluation of silent CVD in DM is shown in Flowchart 5.

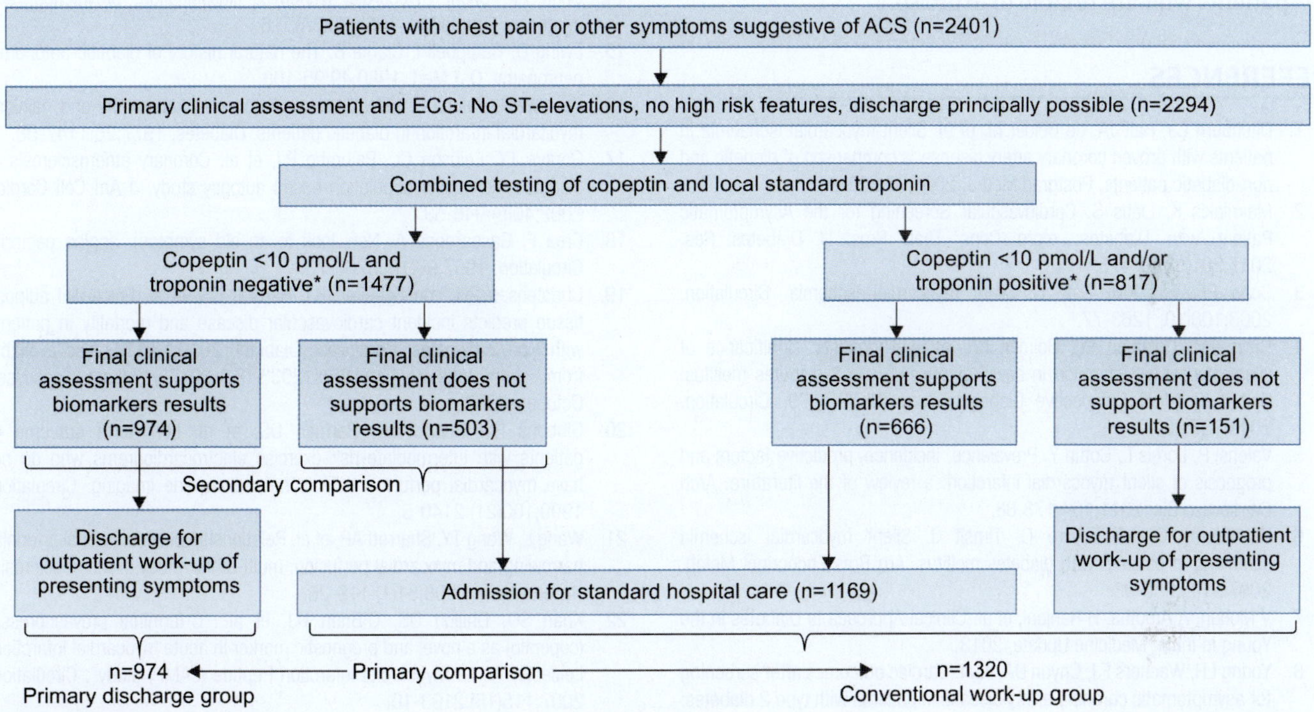

(ACS: acute coronary syndrome)

Flowchart 4 Early rule-out strategy and guidance of primary early discharge vs. general hospital admission (conventional workup).

(*Source*: Giannitsis E, Clifford P, Slagman A, et al. Multicenter cross-sectional observational registry to monitor the safety of early discharge after rule-out of acute myocardial infarction by copeptin and troponin: the Pro-Core registry. BMJ Open. 2019;9:e028311.)

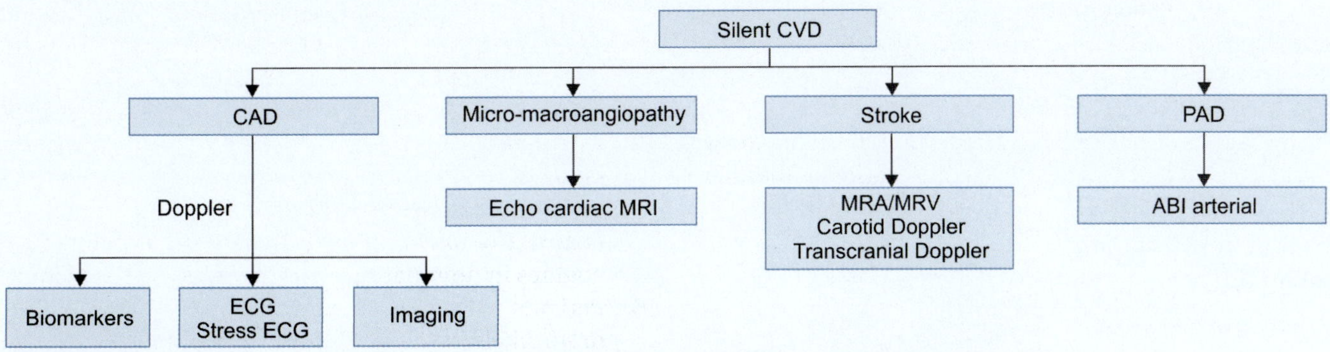

(CVD: cardiovascular disease; CAD: coronary artery disease; PAD: peripheral artery disease; ABI: ankle-brachial index)

Flowchart 5 Evaluation of silent cardiovascular disease.

CONCLUSION

- The most appropriate test to establish a diagnosis of CAD is treadmill exercise ECG.
- Coronary artery calcium scoring has evolved as a broadly accessible, consistent, and reproducible means of evaluating risk for major CV outcomes, particularly when planning primary prevention interventions like aspirin and statins.
- Stress echo and stress thallium can be reserved for patients who are unable to exercise.

REFERENCES

1. Ditchburn CJ, Hall JA, de Belder M, et al. Silent myocardial ischaemia in patients with proved coronary artery disease: a comparison of diabetic and non-diabetic patients. Postgrad Med J. 2001;77:395-8.
2. Makrilakis K, Liatis S. Cardiovascular Screening for the Asymptomatic Patient with Diabetes: more Cons Than Pros. J Diabetes Res. 2017;2017:8927473.
3. Cohn PF, Fox KM, Daly C. Silent myocardial ischemia. Circulation. 2003;108(10):1263-77.
4. Davis TM, Coleman RL, Holman RR, et al. Prognostic significance of silent myocardial infarction in newly diagnosed type 2 diabetes mellitus: United Kingdom Prospective Diabetes Study (UKPDS) 79. Circulation. 2013;127:980-7.
5. Valensi P, Lorgis L, Cottin Y. Prevalence, incidence, predictive factors and prognosis of silent myocardial infarction: a review of the literature. Arch Cardiovasc Dis. 2011;104:178-88.
6. Barthelemy O, Lê Feuvre C, Timsit J. Silent myocardial ischemia screening in patients with diabetes mellitus. Arq Bras Endocrinol Metab. 2007;51(2):285-93.
7. V Mohan, A Amutha, H Ranjani, et al. Clinical Approach to Diabetes in the Young in India. Medicine Update; 2013.
8. Young LH, Wackers FJ, Chyun DA, et al. Cardiac outcomes after screening for asymptomatic coronary artery disease in patients with type 2 diabetes: the DIAD study: a randomized controlled trial. JAMA. 2009;301:1547-55.
9. Hollenberg NK. Controversies in cardiovascular care: Silent myocardial Ischemia. Complicat Card Patient. 1987;1:24-30.
10. Hollenberg NK. Controversies in cardiovascular care: silent myocardial ischemia. Complicat Card Patient. 1987 Spring; 1(2):24-30.
11. Cohn PF. Silent myocardial ischemia: Classification, prevalence, and prognosis. Am J Med. 1985;79:2-6.
12. Soler NG, Bennett MA, Pentecost BL, et al. Myocardial infarction in diabetics. Q J Med. 1975;44:125-32.
13. Maseri A. Ischemic Heart Disease: A Rational Basis for Clinical Practice and Clinical Research. New York: Churchill Livingstone; 1995.
14. Cohn PF. Silent myocardial ischemia: classification, prevalence, and prognosis. Am J Med. 1985;79(3A):2-6.
15. Ewing D, Campbell I, Clarke B. The natural history of diabetic autonomic neuropathy. Q J Med. 1980;49:95-108.
16. Faerman I, Faccio E, Milei J, et al. Autonomic neuropathy and painless myocardial infarction in diabetic patients. Diabetes. 1977;26:1147-58.
17. Goraya TY, Leibson CL, Palumbo PJ, et al. Coronary atherosclerosis in diabetes mellitus: a population-based autopsy study. J Am Coll Cardiol. 2002;40(5):946-53.
18. Crea F, Gaspardone A. New look to an old symptom: angina pectoris. Circulation. 1997;96(10):3766-73.
19. Christensen RH, von Scholten BJ, Hansen CS, et al. Epicardial adipose tissue predicts incident cardiovascular disease and mortality in patients with type 2 diabetes. Cardiovasc Diabetol. 2019;18:114. Also available from https://doi.org/10.1186/s12933-019-0917-y [Last accessed October, 2019].
20. Gibbons RJ, Hodge DO, Berman DS, et al. Long-term outcome of patients with intermediate-risk exercise electrocardiograms who do not have myocardial perfusion defects on radionuclide imaging. Circulation. 1999;100(21):2140-5.
21. Wang L, Wong TY, Sharrett AR, et al. Relationship between retinal arteriolar narrowing and myocardial perfusion: multi-ethnic study of atherosclerosis. Hypertension. 2008;51(1):119-26.
22. Khan SQ, Dhillon OS, O'Brien RJ, et al. "C-terminal provasopressin (copeptin) as a novel and prognostic marker in acute myocardial infarction: Leicester Acute Myocardial Infarction Peptide (LAMP) study". Circulation. 2007;115(16):2103-10.

72 CHAPTER Cardiovascular Risk Stratification in Diabetes: Options and Approach

Sanjiv Shah, Usha Ayyagari

INTRODUCTION

Cardiovascular disease (CVD) is the major cause of morbidity and mortality in patients with diabetes. It is often silent, more advanced, frequently at younger age in India, and associated with less favorable prognosis (more so in post-menopausal women).[1] Clinical trials have shown the benefit of early intervention and management, which needs early diagnosis through systematic screening and primary prevention in all at risk individuals.[2]

Diabetes has long been considered as a cardiovascular (CV) risk equivalent which could be challenged in low risk younger individuals with a shorter duration of diabetes mellitus (DM) and no preexisting CVD/risk factors. But, patients with hyperglycemia, hypertension, and hyperlipidemia run a very high risk for CVD. Therefore, current guidelines recommend management based on multimodal risk stratification.[2]

RISK FACTORS FOR CARDIOVASCULAR DISEASE

Traditional risk factors for CVD include age, body mass index (BMI), gender, hypertension, dyslipidemia, smoking, and family history of CVD at a younger age. Current guidelines recommend stratifying risk using multiple modalities including nephropathy, retinopathy, and biomarkers to recognize individuals at highest risk who would benefit from either early or aggressive therapy.[2]

Age and Gender

The continuum of increasing CVD with age represents the strongest, nonmodifiable risk factor. However, it is difficult to define an exact age at which risk changes. For a threshold of >20% in 10 years of myocardial infarction (MI), stroke, and death from any cause as a composite outcome, transition from a low- to high-risk category happens at an age of 48 years and 54 years in men and women, respectively. Women have lower incidence of MI but higher mortality post-MI and in heart failure (HF).[3]

Hypertension

As a strong, continuous risk factor for CVD and stroke, hypertension should be treated to 130/80 target in all diabetics. The strongest risk predictor for CVD in the Framingham study was diastolic BP (DBP) at ≤50 years of age, all measures of BP at age 50–59 years, and pulse pressure in those ≥60 years in age. Each 10 mm Hg reduction in systolic BP (SBP) significantly lowered the risk for many outcomes such as mortality by 13%, cardiovascular event (CVE) by 11%, CVD by 12%, and stroke by 27%.[4]

Hypercholesterolemia

Low-density lipoprotein cholesterol (LDL-C) is one of the most important modifiable CV risk factors. Prior to the extensive use of statins, MRFIT study showed an increased risk of CV mortality in men with higher cholesterol. Cholesterol Treatment Trialists' (CTT) Collaborators meta-analysis showed that for every 1 mmol/L (38.7 mg) reduction in LDL-C (up to 50 mg/dL), there is a significant reduction in AMI, a 21% relative risk reduction in CVE, and a 9% relative risk reduction in all-cause mortality.[5]

Smoking

Smoking is the most important reversible risk factor for CV morbidity and mortality. Smokers have a 54% higher risk of CVEs, 52% higher risk of MI, 44% higher risk of stroke, and 48% higher risk of total CV mortality. The risk is proportional to pack year history and improves with smoking cessation.[6]

Family History

The risk of CVD for an individual with DM increases with the number of first-degree relatives with CVD, especially those with premature CVD: one first-degree relative with CVD confers a 50% increased CVD risk, and two relatives confer a 75% increased risk.[2]

Body Mass Index

Higher BMI is associated with both DM and CVD. The Dallas Heart Study showed significant heterogeneity in the phenotype associated with increased CV risk even when adjusted for BMI. Visceral adipose tissue (VAT) showed a step-wise increase in association with CVD with an approximate doubling in CV risk from the lowest VAT quartile to the highest.[7]

Nonalcoholic Fatty Liver Disease, Obstructive Sleep Apnea, and Cardiovascular Risk

The coexistence of nonalcoholic fatty liver disease (NAFLD) with type 2 diabetes mellitus (T2DM) is independently associated with an increased CV risk over and above other coexisting risk factors. In the Valpolicella Heart Diabetes Study, among 2103 type 2 DM participants, with an unadjusted prevalence of NAFLD of 69.5% who were followed up for 6.5 years, 384 participants subsequently developed CVD events.[8] Severe obstructive sleep apnea (OSA) with apnea-hypopnea index >30/h is strongly associated with increased CV mortality.

Glomerular Filtration Rate, Albuminuria, and Cardiovascular Risk

Microalbuminuria, the earliest sign of kidney-vascular disease is strongly associated with CVD and also with other traditional risk factors for CVD. It is associated with worse CVD outcomes and all-cause mortality. An estimated glomerular filtration rate (eGFR) < 75 mL/min/1.73 m^2 is independently associated with increased CV mortality and the combination of lowered eGFR with raised ACR is additive.[9]

Hypoglycemia and Cardiovascular Risk

Epidemiological as well as longitudinal studies have shown severe hypoglycemia (SH) as an independent risk factor for CV and all-cause mortality. In the Hong Kong Diabetes Registry, individuals with SH had a threefold higher mortality. In a prospective observational study of 1,260 adult T2DM patients with median follow-up of 10.4 years, SH was associated with 2.64-fold increased risk of all-cause mortality.[10]

Erectile Dysfunction, Autonomic Neuropathy, and Cardiovascular Risk

Erectile dysfunction, marker of vascular disease in uncontrolled diabetes is associated with higher mortality and higher risk of CVD and stroke, independent of traditional risk factors, in a meta-analysis.[9] The American Diabetes Association (ADA) recommends exercise stress testing in both symptomatic and asymptomatic patients with autonomic neuropathy who have higher CV risk.[11]

CARDIOVASCULAR RISK STRATIFICATION

Risk stratification is a step further in the direction of precision medicine to improve physician intervention. Using data from lifestyle, clinical history, and laboratory tests on a risk calculator apps (smart phone) will provide 10 year-risk stratification.

Risk Calculators

The reduction in CVD over the past decade was likely driven by higher awareness, detection and treatment of risk factors (probably using statistical risk models). The development of all statistical risk models has allowed the probability of future CVEs to be calculated based on multiple risk factors, however, its application in different ethnic population is questionable.[12] These risk equations are not validated in diabetic population and they either underestimate or overestimate cardiovascular risk.[13] Such risk calculators should at least prompt physician to treat high-risk patients more intensively and it is proven that documentation of CV risk prediction score on medical records was associated with more intensive antihypertensive and hypolipidemic treatment.[14] Out of multitude of risk scores developed, only 12 models have been specifically developed for use in the diabetic population in a systematic review on the subject.[15] The majority of these predicted 5-year risk of CVD, using predictor's age, sex, smoking, duration of diabetes, and HbA1c.

High Cardiovascular Risk in Diabetes

Patients at very high risk of developing CVD with one or more risk factors like age above 60 years, albuminuria, reduced eGFR, SBP > 180 mm Hg or DBP > 110 mm Hg, familial hypercholesterolemia should not undergo risk calculation.[16]

ASSESSMENT OF ASYMPTOMATIC OR SUBCLINICAL CARDIOVASCULAR DISEASE

Diabetes patients at high risk should routinely be managed with maximum medical therapy and routine screening for SC CVD has not proven to add value in these patients. Although coronary artery calcium (CAC) score showed some initial promise for independent risk prediction, this was not borne out in a subsequent RCT in patients with normal electrocardiogram (ECG). Furthermore, in patients who are initially screened with a risk factor-based approach, subsequent CAC did not identify those who have silent ischemia. Patients identified to have higher coronary disease burden on CAC and other tests may go on to develop more CVEs.

Studies have demonstrated that a significant percentage of patients with diabetes who have no symptoms of CAD have abnormal stress tests, either by stress ECG, stress echocardiogram or stress nuclear perfusion imaging. Carotid intima-media thickness (CIMT) and carotid plaque, and ankle-brachial index (ABI) show promise for assessing subclinical-CVD, but none have proven outcome measures and ADA guidelines does not recommended for routine clinical risk assessment.[2]

Undiagnosed Heart Failure in Patients with Diabetes

In an epidemiological investigation of 581 diabetics over age 60 years, 25.8% had LV dysfunction and 25.1% had diastolic dysfunction. Previously unknown HF was diagnosed in 161 patients (27.7%), 28(4.8%) with reduced ejection fraction, and 133(22.9%) with preserved ejection fraction. To diagnose early, HF prediction scoring is recommended, especially in the elderly and in women.[17]

Heart Failure Risk Score

The Get With The Guidelines-Heart Failure (GWTG-HF) risk score, ADMIRE-HF risk score and 6-minute walking tests can diagnose HF early. Independent predictors of HF are: age, renal dysfunction, diuretic use, HbA1c, duration of diabetes, LDL-C, microalbuminuria, heart rate, RBBB/LBBB, previous MI and pioglitazone treatment.[18] TIMI risk score (TRS 2°P) was developed from 16,488 type 2 diabetes patients with CV disease in SAVOR-TIMI 53, and tested in diabetes cohort from REACH registry. TRS 2°P used nine predictor variables: (1) age ≥ 75 years, (2) diabetes, (3) hypertension, (4) current smoking, (5) prior stroke, (6) prior CABG, (7) history of HF, (8) renal dysfunction (eGFR < 60), and (9) peripheral arterial disease. Powerful risk gradient for the composite of CV death, MI, and ischemic stroke was observed, with 2-year event rates of 19.8% in the highest-risk versus 0.9% in the lowest-risk groups.[19]

BIOMARKERS

Various biomarkers hsCRP, ApoB, hsTnT, NT-proBNP, galectin-3, copeptin are currently under investigation for their potential predictive value for CVE. In a subgroup analysis of the SAVOR-TIMI 35 study evaluating multiple biomarkers including hsCRP, hsTnT, and NT-proBNP, inclusion of these markers in the risk model improved the predictive value for MACE. In an 8-year observational study of 27,939 presumed healthy American women followed up for incident MI, ischemic stroke, coronary revascularization or death from cardiovascular causes, hsCRP was independently correlated with incidence of CVE, even after adjustment for multiple confounding factors. However, unlike in nondiabetics, the predictive value of biomarkers for CVD in diabetics is less certain and requires further evaluation.[2]

CONCLUSION

Type 2 diabetes is a heterogeneous disorder with variable CV risk, higher risk in patients with metabolic syndrome. Exact calculation of risk helps physician to decide appropriate diagnostic test and the right intensity of treatment. Patients with high risk should be offered counseling to improve compliance with intensified treatment. Treating CV risk with SGLT2-i or GLP1-RA is well established. Prevention of CVD still should be top priority while treating diabetes.

REFERENCES

1. International Diabetes Federation. IDF Diabetes Atlas, 8th edition. Brussels, Belgium: International Diabetes Federation; 2017.
2. Arnett DK, Blumenthal RS, Albert MA, et al. 2019 ACC/AHA guideline on the primary prevention of cardiovascular disease: a report of the American College of Cardiology/American Heart Association Task Force on Clinical Practice Guidelines. Circulation. 2019;140:e596-e646.
3. Bertoluci MC, Rocha VZ. Cardiovascular risk assessment in patients with diabetes. Diabetol Metab Syndr. 2017;9:25.
4. Emdin CA, Rahimi K, Neal B, et al. Blood pressure lowering in type 2 diabetes: a systematic review and meta-analysis. JAMA. 2015;313:603-15.
5. Cholesterol Treatment Trialists' (CTT) Collaborators, Kearney PM, Blackwell L, et al. Efficacy of cholesterol-lowering therapy in 18,686 people with diabetes in 14 randomised trials of statins: a meta-analysis. Lancet. 2008;371:117-25.
6. Qin R, Chen T, Lou Q, et al. Excess risk of mortality and cardiovascular events associated with smoking among patients with diabetes: meta-analysis of observational prospective studies. Int J Cardiol. 2013;167:342-50.
7. Neeland IJ, Turer AT, Ayers CR, et al. Body fat distribution and incident cardiovascular disease in obese adults. J Am Coll Cardiol. 2015;65:2150-1.
8. Targher G, Bertolini L, Rodella S, et al. Nonalcoholic fatty liver disease is independently associated with an increased incidence of cardiovascular events in type 2 diabetic patients. Diabetes Care. 2007;30:2119-21.
9. Chronic Kidney Disease Prognosis Consortium, Matsushita K, van der Velde M, et al. Association of estimated glomerular filtration rate and albuminuria with all-cause and cardiovascular mortality in general population cohorts: a collaborative meta-analysis. Lancet. 2010;375:2073-81.
10. Cha SA, Yun JS, Lim TS, et al. Severe hypoglycemia and cardiovascular or all-cause mortality in patients with type 2 diabetes. Diabetes Metab J. 2016;40:202-10.
11. Dong JY, Zhang YH, Qin LQ. Erectile dysfunction and risk of cardiovascular disease. J Am Coll Cardiol. 2011;58:1378-85.
12. Kengne AP, Patel A, Colagiuri S, et al. The Framingham and UK Prospective Diabetes Study (UKPDS) risk equations do not reliably estimate the probability of cardiovascular events in a large ethnically diverse sample of patients with diabetes: the Action in Diabetes and Vascular Disease: Preterax and Diamicron-MR Controlled Evaluation (ADVANCE) Study. Diabetologia. 2010;53:821-31.
13. Simmons RK, Coleman RL, Price HC, et al. Performance of the UK Prospective Diabetes Study Risk Engine and the Framingham Risk Equations in Estimating Cardiovascular Disease in the EPIC-Norfolk Cohort. Diabetes Care. 2008;32:708-13.
14. Hall LM, Jung RT, Leese GP. Controlled trial of effect of documented cardiovascular risk scores on prescribing. BMJ. 2003;326:251-2.
15. van Dieren S, Beulens JW, Kengne AP, et al. Prediction models for the risk of cardiovascular disease in patients with type 2 diabetes: a systematic review. Heart. 2012;98:360-9.
16. National Stroke Foundation. National Vascular Disease Prevention Alliance. Guidelines for the management of absolute cardiovascular disease risk. Australia: National Stroke Foundation; 2012.
17. Boonman-de Winter LJ, Rutten FH, Cramer MJM, et al. High prevalence of previously unknown heart failure and left ventricular dysfunction in patients with type 2 diabetes. Diabetologia. 2012;55:2154-62.
18. Bergmark BA, Bhatt DL, Braunwald E, et al. Risk Assessment in Patients With Diabetes With the TIMI Risk Score for Atherothrombotic Disease. Diabetes Care. 2017;41:577-85.
19. Pfister R, Cairns R, Erdmann E, et al. A clinical risk score for heart failure in patients with type 2 diabetes and macrovascular disease: an analysis of the PROactive study. Int J Cardiol. 2013;162:112-6.

73 CHAPTER It is Time to Declare Victory over Heart Failure in Diabetes

Raj Kumar Lalwani

INTRODUCTION

The title is suggestive of an inherent euphoria which deserves to be appreciated in the following three areas, related to heart failure (HF) management in diabetes:

1. *Understanding HF in diabetes and how big is the problem?*
2. *What therapeutic solutions we have and what are the limitations and unmet needs?*
3. *What is the cause of this newfound excitement, prompting clinicians to think of declaring victory over HF?*

UNDERSTANDING HEART FAILURE IN DIABETES

Diabetes profoundly affects every component of cardiovascular (CV) system, the pipes (arteries—through atherothrombosis), the pump (causing HF), and damages the filters (diabetic renal disease). These cardiorenal complications of diabetes are the major cause of huge morbidity, mortality, and economic burden.[1] Conceptually, comorbidities such as type 2 diabetes mellitus (DM), obesity or chronic kidney disease (CKD), all are highly prevalent in HF populations, and actually are driving forces of HF, especially of HF with preserved ejection fraction (HFpEF), a phenotype which is prevalent as almost half of HF cases and for which we do not have any approved therapy at all.

Epidemiology

In patients with DM, the prevalence of HF is four times, which is, between 10% and 22%, as compared to the general population. Conversely, HF is also an independent risk factor for the development of diabetes, shown in a follow up where 29% of HF patients without diabetes developed DM, compared to 18% in matched control subjects without HF. Nearly 25% HF patients have coexisting diabetes and this number goes up to 40% in patients hospitalized for acute decompensated HF.[2]

It must be noted that when both are present, long-term prognosis and survival are determined largely by HF rather than diabetes, making HF a therapeutic priority.

For people over the age of 65 years, HF has been a major health problem and is a leading cause for hospitalization. Diabetes is a risk factor for congestive HF, and was documented in Framingham Heart Study over 20 years ago. Framingham study recorded risk of HF as two times higher in men and five times higher in women with diabetes.[3] In patients aged ≤65 years, it was 4-fold more in males and 8-fold in females with diabetes, as compared to nondiabetics. Kaiser Permanente data showed that diabetes doubled HF with each decade of age.[3]

In ALLHAT trial, patients with diabetes had a nearly 2-fold risk for HF hospitalization or death, even when adjusted for other risk factors [relative risk (RR) = 1.95]. The UKPDS showed links of HF risk with HbA1c levels.

Identifiable risk factors for developing diabetic cardiomyopathy are increased HbA1c, high body mass index, advanced age, use of insulin, proteinuria, the coexistence of coronary artery disease (CAD) and/or peripheral target organ diseases such as retinopathy and nephropathy.[4]

Diabetic Cardiomyopathy

Clinically, diabetic cardiomyopathy diagnosis requires a history of longstanding, poorly controlled type 2 DM, and exclusion of significant CAD, hypertensive cardiomyopathy, valvular and/or congenital heart disease and of familial, viral, toxic/drug related or infiltrative cardiomyopathy. Traditionally, it was seen as a dilated heart with reduced ejection fraction or HFrEF occurring in diabetic patients having nephropathy and/or retinopathy.[5] Lately, few authors labeled restrictive, HFpEF or diastolic HF as early phenotype of diabetic cardiomyopathy. Occurring more commonly in obese women with poor glycemic control. The debate on whether HFpEF at all is an entity, is more or less resolved with majority of clinicians agreeing to >50% of ejection fraction as preserved and <40% as reduced ejection fraction.[5]

Pathobiology and Pathophysiology

Cardiomyopathies can be either *primary*, with cardiac function impaired due to a defect in the heart muscle itself, or *secondary*, where cardiac performance is impaired because of other systemic conditions.

Any cardiomyopathy leading to HF, can be either as *diastolic dysfunction* and failure, with preserved ejection fraction, or *systolic heart failure, with reduced ejection fraction,* or a combination of both.

Diabetes is peculiar; it can lead to HF by both mechanisms. Impairing and augmenting all the classical CV risk factors (e.g. accelerating the appearance and progression of CAD, hypertension, and also by a direct suppressive and deleterious effect on the heart muscle directly).

Diabetic cardiomyopathy, therefore, is defined as:

- Dilatation and hypertrophy of the left ventricle
- With the concomitant appearance of diastolic and/or systolic dysfunction
- Without the coexistence of ischemic or hypertensive or valvular heart disease syndromes.

Myocardial fibrosis and hypertrophy are the most frequently reported changes and are well documented. Defective cellular calcium transport has been shown in many studies,[6] while defective myocardial contractile proteins and an increased collagen deposition also add to dysfunction, resulting in anatomic and physiological changes in the myocardium (Table 1).

Increased collagen synthesis and defective matrix synthesis are documented.[7]

*Myocyte defects as m*icroscopic anomalies in myocardial cells of diabetic animals like: (1) loss of microfibrils, (2) loss of cell-to-cell adhesions and connection in the intermediate disks, and (3) increased lipid accumulation in the cytoplasm with loss of the endoplasmic reticulum. Concentric left ventricular hypertrophy and remodeling are seen with DM, are independent of other confounders like age, obesity and hypertension.

Mechanisms of Heart Failure in Diabetes Mellitus

What initiates or triggers can be different in patients, but direct myocardial injury (e.g. in myocardial ischemia or cardiomyopathy), volume overload (e.g. in aortic valve insufficiency), and pressure overload (e.g. in arterial hypertension) all add up to the process.

Diabetes accelerates atherosclerosis in epicardial coronary arteries, and impairs the structural and functional integrity of smaller vessels, causing variable but increased ischemic burden which may not be fully visible in coronary arteries.

TABLE 1: Evaluation of heart failure; AHS/ACC-stages of heart failure.

Evaluation of heart failure AHS/ACC-stages of heart failure			
Stage A	**Stage B**		**Stages C and D**
Rick factors	Cellular pathophysiology	Ventricular remodeling	Ventricular dysfunction
Aging Hypertension Smoking Dyslipidemia Diabetes Obesity Toxins Genes	→ Hypertrophy infarction Accelerated apoptosis fibrosis	LVH Dilatation Both	→ Systolic Diastolic Both
	Structural heart disease no symptoms		Symptomatic heart failure

(LVH: left ventricular hypertrophy; AHS/ACC: American Heart Association/American College of Cardiology)

Diabetic cardiomyopathy aggravates BP, adds to afterload and pressure overload, and coexisting renal failure may further add to the preload through salt and water retention.[8]

Molecular Mechanisms

Hyperglycemia induces advanced glycation end products (AGEs) and reactive oxygen species (ROS) or free radicals. Soluble AGEs, produced locally or arriving with circulation when get connected to receptor for advanced glycation end products (RAGEs), trigger NADPH oxidase and then production of peroxide, thereby generating more ROS. These can cause more damage to cell organelles and its DNA as well through numerous inflammatory cytokines.[9]

Myocardial energy substrate anomalies:

Human heart mainly consumes free fatty acids (FFA; almost 70%) and glucose (almost 30%). This can interchange readily through "Randle cycle", by which high circulating glucose can decrease FFA consumption and vice versa.

- Myocytes uptake more of glucose and FFA HF, but both are reduced in mitochondria. Metabolic intermediates, accumulating in the cytoplasm, add to maladaptive signals.
- Peroxisome proliferator activated receptor-alpha (PPAR-α) gets activated by FFA, which are used as substrate.

Insulin resistance disallows use of glucose by heart, adding up energetic inefficiency to heart muscle. This creates a situation where more O_2 is now needed for each ATP produced, a process called "mitochondrial uncoupling".

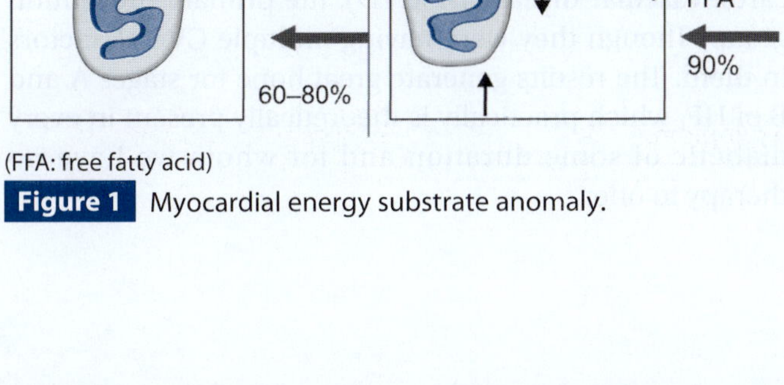

(FFA: free fatty acid)

Figure 1 Myocardial energy substrate anomaly.

In HF, sympathetic activation promotes lipolysis and release of FFA from adipose tissue into the plasma. This adds to left ventricular diastolic dysfunction.

Ketone bodies like BHOB when available, (energy depletion/starvation) get their enzyme pathways activated in HF. Furthermore, ketone bodies by inducing FFA uptake into adipocytes, decrease FFA in plasma, facilitating Glucose use by myocytes[10] (Fig. 1).

Therefore, mechanisms of HF in diabetic patients involve reduced contractility, metabolic disturbances, accumulation of AGE, myocardial fibrosis, small vessel disease, impaired calcium homeostasis, autonomic neuropathy and insulin resistance (Flowchart 1) all adding up and propagating each other in a cascade, perpetuated by Hyperglycemia. (Flowchart 1).

TREATMENT AND UNMET NEEDS IN HEART FAILURE WITH DIABETES

Patients with DM may not have symptoms of HF but often have subclinical abnormalities of cardiac structure and function as pointed earlier, corresponding to ACC/AHA Stage A and Stage B HF. These include left ventricular systolic dysfunction, increased left ventricular mass, increased wall thickness, enlarged left atrium with diastolic dysfunction, and an increased extracellular fluid fraction in total fluid volume. Each of these abnormalities is linked with increased risk of symptomatic HF and death.[11] There are no approved treatments for this category of diastolic HF or HFpEF.

Guidelines with approved treatment plans are only available for HFrEF, which include the following validated treatment options:[12]

The MICRO-HOPE with ramipril and EUROPA trial with perindopril reported an impressive decline in the rates of HF hospitalizations. In ATLAS trial, lisinopril in high doses was shown to be effective and well tolerated.

Angiotensin receptor blockers (ARBs) like valsartan and candesartan have proved their value in Val-HeFT and CHARM (candesartan), while LIFE and the RENAAL studies showed that losartan significantly brought down the incidence of first hospitalization for HF.

Aldosterone antagonists: Mineralocorticoid receptor antagonist (MRA) eplerenone was tested with placebo in patients with left ventricular systolic dysfunction, symptoms of HF following an acute myocardial infarction, RALES and EPHESUS were both encouraging regular serum potassium monitoring as advised with all renin-angiotensin-aldosterone system (RAAS) blocking

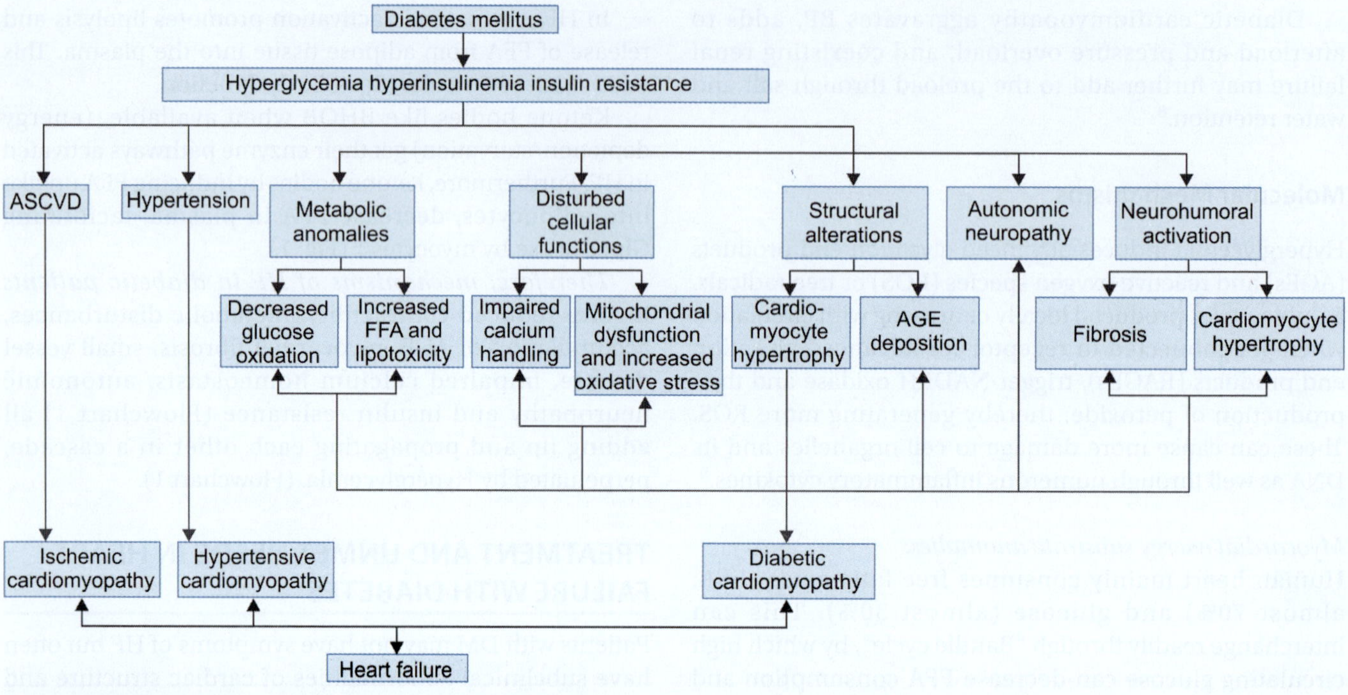

(ASCVD: atherosclerotic cardiovascular disease; FFA: free fatty acids)

Flowchart 1 Mechanism of heart failure in diabetic patients.

therapies, and to keep the serum potassium below 5 mmol/L.

Beta-blockers: COPERNICUS, MERIT-HF and CIBIS II trials brought carvedilol, metoprolol and bisoprolol as standard therapies for HF including those for diabetics.

Diuretics: Work well in congested states. Potassium, intravascular volume depletion and aggravation of renal failure, etc. are big concerns.

Ivabradine: It significantly reduced CV deaths and HF hospitalizations in the SHIFT trial, in patients with HF in sinus rhythm and with heart rates over 70 bpm. The trial had 30% of patients as diabetics type 2. The benefits were similar for patients with and without diabetes.[13]

PARADIGM-HF has demonstrated impressive benefits with the angiotensin receptor-neprilysin inhibitor (ARNI) therapy and sacubitril/valsartan (Sac/Val) in patients with and without DM.

Implantable cardioverter-defibrillator, cardiac resynchronization therapy, etc. are beyond the scope of this chapter.

All these therapies have no place in HFpEF or prevention of HF in diabetics who are prone to develop HF and are having subclinical HF. Simplified algorithm is given in (Flowchart 2).

WHAT HAS CAUSED THE PRESENT EXCITEMENT?

Now, we have sodium-glucose cotransporter-2 (SGLT2) inhibitors. This class of glucose-lowering drugs have shown substantial CV benefits, especially towards HF and renal disease in respective CVOT trials.[14,15] DECLARE–TIMI 58 compared dapagliflozin 10 mg daily to placebo[16] and showed substantial reduction of composite primary outcome of CV deaths and hospitalization from HF, with gross and significant reduction in new onset of HF even in those patients who did not have HF or any evidence of a CV disease at the time of entry into the trial. This has given an all-new exciting perspective to clinicians. Because as many as 60% of 17,160 enrolled patients in this trial were not having any atherosclerotic cardiovascular disease (ASCVD), the primary prevention group. Though they were having multiple CV risk factors in them. The results generate great hope for stages A and B of HF, which practically is theoretically present in every diabetic of some duration and for whom we have no therapy to offer.

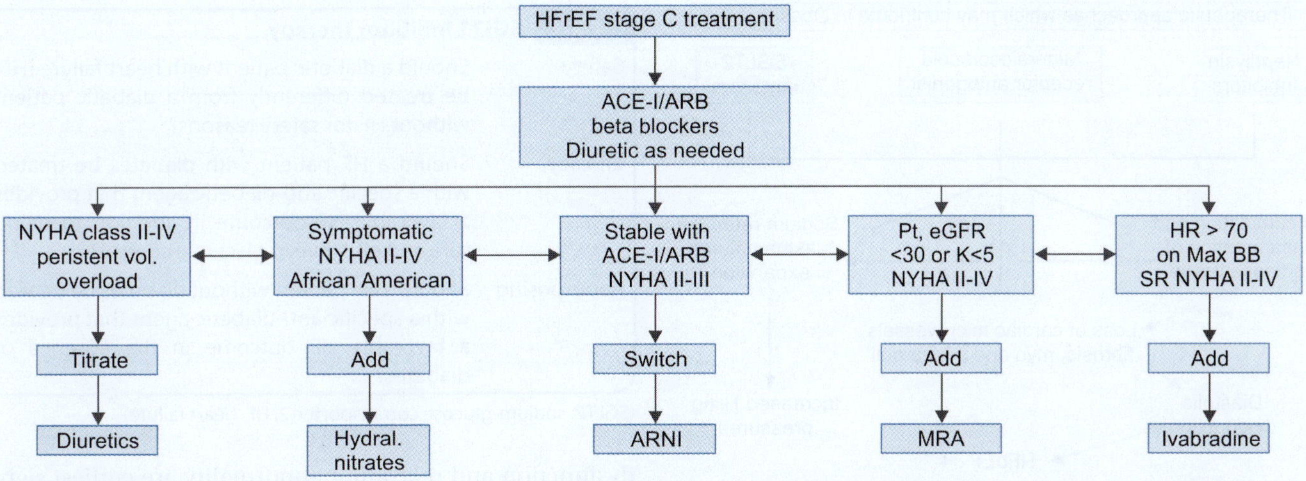

(HFrEF: heart failure with reduced ejection fraction; ACE: angiotensin-converting enzyme; ARB: angiotensin receptor blocker; NYHA: New York Heart Association; eGFR: estimated glomerular filtration rate; HR: heart rate; SR: sinus rhythm; ARNI: Angiotensin receptor-neprilysin inhibitor; MRA: mineralocorticoid receptor antagonist)

Flowchart 2 HFrEF treatment algorithm.

Another exciting point from DECLARE–TIMI 58 is that they considered a composite endpoint of HF hospitalizations and CV deaths as co-primary outcome, along with major adverse cardiovascular events (MACE), which traditionally has always been used to measure CV outcomes of any new drug. MACE and HF are related to two differing pathobiological processes, unrelated to each other.

Dapagliflozin did reduce CV death and HF, but not MACE in both patient groups of so-called primary and secondary prevention.

A meta-analysis of the three SGLT2 inhibitor-analyzed CV outcome trials,[15] revealed that specifically in those with established ASCVD, SGLT2 inhibitor drugs did significantly reduce MACE, hospitalizations due to heart failure (HHF), and progression of kidney disease in all its forms and stages. Interestingly MACE benefits were modest, while HF, HHF, and renal benefits were profound with all three drugs of the class, that too to the extents of 30–40%. And these benefits were seen across the participants irrespective of H/O HF, renal disease or presence of ASCVD at the baseline.[16]

Osmotic diuresis, natriuresis, changes in myocardial substrate utilization, alterations in myocardial sodium-hydrogen exchange, reduction in left ventricular mass, blood pressure/afterload reduction, glomerular afferent arteriolar constriction (with resultant drop in intraglomerular pressure), etc. have been explained by authors of many papers trying to explain mechanisms involved. But most intriguingly, all the HF benefits appear to be unrelated to the level of glycemic controls, and also are not explainable by traditional risk factors.

DECLARE–TIMI 58 trial, therefore convincingly changes the way we should think of choosing antihyperglycemic therapies in type 2 diabetes, even for those who have no ASCVD.

In contrast, GLP1RA have shown reductions in ischemic events, but these are mostly confined to patients with ASCVD.[17] Therefore, dapagliflozin reducing HF-related hospitalizations with benefits on progressive renal deterioration in primary prevention population, announces a new era and a new day for type 2 diabetes.

For a change, now we have a drug class improving HF and HF deaths in patients, which can be considered for an earlier use, in vast majority and, where HF or renal defects are not yet evident.

A detailed cost analysis in terms of cost of pill versus cost of disease prevention, etc. should settle the issue in favor of SGLT2 inhibitors because benefits are huge. SGLT2 inhibitors are also being tested as HF drugs or renoprotective drugs in patients with and without diabetes.[18]

Obesity-related HF brought into focus another conceptual breakthrough for non-coronary myocardial affliction, adding more to prevention of diabetic HFpEF. Bariatric surgery and weight loss show reductions in HF; this has prompted using SGLT2 inhibitors as add-on therapy, and trials are ongoing[19] (Flowchart 3).

Very recently DAPA HF results were declared, in 4,744 adults in 20 countries who had HFrEF (left ventricular EF

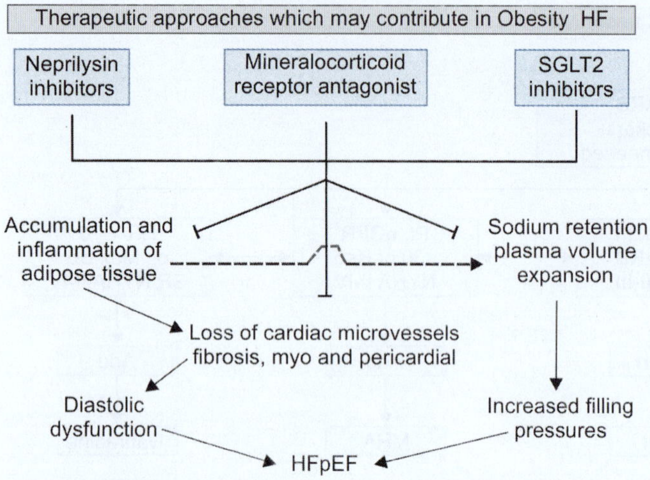

(HF: heart failure; SGLT2: sodium-glucose cotransporter-2; HFpEF: heart failure with preserved ejection fraction)

Flowchart 3 Therapeutic approaches which may contribute to obesity heart failure.

<40%). At baseline, of which 45% had type 2 diabetes and 55% patients had raised N-terminal pro-B-type natriuretic peptide and an estimated glomerular filtration rate of 30 mL/min/1.732 or higher. Once-daily dapagliflozin 10 mg compared with matching placebo, reduced risk for worsening HF and CV death, when added to standard therapy in patients with HFrEF, regardless of diabetes status. Benefits persisted in all subgroup analyses and were consistently seen in all receiving dapagliflozin, irrespective of even Sac/Val therapy, which was in the background as standard care in substantial number of HF cases in the trial.

At the press conference, McMurray said:[20]

- Type 2 diabetes-associated cardiac failure and renal disease appear to benefit from SGLT2 Inhibition: SGLT2 inhibitors provide marked benefits to reduce HF and progressive renal decline by promoting sodium loss, reducing volume, and modulating other pathways of neurohumoral activation and cellular metabolism.
- Renin-angiotensin-aldosterone system (RAAS): Individuals with ASCVD, HF, and CKD, as well as those with multiple risk factors, appear to benefit from SGLT2 inhibitor therapy (Box 1).[21]

BOX 1	**SGLT2 inhibitor therapy.**
Safety	Should a diabetic patient with heart failure (HF) be treated differently from a diabetic patient without HF for safety reasons?
Efficacy	Should a HF patient with diabetes be treated with a specific anti-diabetic agent that provides a favorable HF outcome in addition to being safe and effective in glycemic control?
Repurposing	Should a HF patient without diabetes be treated with a specific anti-diabetic agent that provides a favorable HF outcome in the absence of diabetes?

(SGLT2: sodium-glucose cotransporter-2; HF: heart failure)

CONCLUSION

Heart failure in diabetics remains largely undiagnosed, though appears early in subclinical form. Diastolic dysfunction and relaxation abnormality are earliest signs, but remain asymptomatic and undetected.

HF is serious, lethal, and high-cost comorbidity, grossly reducing quality of life and life expectancy. Despite good BP control and CAD management, the overall prevention and control of HF remains incomplete. Lack of agreement on detection criteria and treatment of subclinical HF frustrated prevention strategies for HF and related CV mortality.

The advances in diabetes and CV therapeutics, which actually came as pleasant unexpected outcome in trials with SGLT2 inhibitors, has opened up an absolutely new exciting era, which may cause significant improvements in the prognosis of patients with diabetes and HF, that too right from the subclinical stages. We can see a huge scope for well-powered, well-designed, prospective, randomized controlled trials to look into the mortality and morbidity benefits comparing various HF treatment modalities in subjects with SGLT2 inhibitors and who knows SGLT2 inhibitor therapies may become Gold Standard for HF soon. For now, however, IT IS TIME WE CAN DECLARE an important victory on HF in type 2 diabetes.[21]

REFERENCES

1. Verma S, Juni P, Mazer CD. Pump, pipes, and filter: Do SGLT2 inhibitors cover it all? Lancet. 2019;393(10166):3-5.
2. Greenberg BH, Abraham WT, Albert NM, et al. Influence of diabetes on characteristics and outcomes in patients hospitalized with heart failure: a report from the Organized Program to Initiate Lifesaving treatment in Hospitalized Patients with Heart Failure (OPTIMIZE-HF). Am Heart J. 2007;154(2):277.e1-8.
3. Nichols GA, Hillier TA, Erbey JR, et al. Congestive heart failure in type 2 diabetes: Prevalence, incidence, and risk factors. Diabetes Care. 2001;24(9):1614-9.
4. Vermes E, Ducharme A, Bourassa MG, et al. Enalapril reduces the incidence of diabetes in patients with chronic heart failure: Insight from the Studies Of Left Ventricular Dysfunction (SOLVD). Circulation. 2003;107(9):1291-6.

5. Seferovic PM, Paulus WJ. Clinical diabetic cardiomyopathy: a two-faced disease with restrictive and dilated phenotypes. Eur Heart J. 2015;36(27):1718-1727, 1727a-c.
6. Regan TJ, Wu CF, Yeh CK, et al. Myocardial composition and function in diabetes. The effects of chronic insulin use. Circ Res. 1981;49(6):1268-77.
7. Ban CR, Twigg SM, Franjic B, et al. Serum MMP-7 is increased in diabetic renal disease and diabetic diastolic dysfunction. Diabetes Res Clin Pract. 2010;87(3):335-41.
8. Voulgari C, Papadogiannis D, Tentolouris N. Diabetic cardiomyopathy: from the pathophysiology of the cardiac myocytes to current diagnosis and management strategies. Vasc Health Risk Manag. 2010;6:883-903.
9. Ernande L, Rietzschel ER, Bergerot C, et al. Impaired myocardial radial function in asymptomatic patients with type 2diabetes mellitus: a speckle-tracking imaging study. J Am Soc Echocardiogr. 2010;23(12):1266-72.
10. Maack C, Lehrke M, Backs J, et al. Heart failure and diabetes: metabolic alterations and therapeutic interventions: a state-of-the-art review from the Translational Research Committee of the Heart Failure Association-European Society of Cardiology. Heart J. 2018;39(48):4243-54.
11. Dunlay SM, Givertz MM, Aguillar D, et al. Type 2 Diabetes Mellitus and Heart Failure: A Scientific Statement From the American Heart Association and the Heart Failure Society of America: This statement does not represent an update of the 2017 ACC/AHA/HFSA heart failure guideline update. Circulation. 2019;140(7):e294-324.
12. Shekelle PG, Rich MW, Morton SC, et al. Efficacy of angiotensin-converting enzyme inhibitors and beta-blockers in the management of left ventricular systolic dysfunction according to race, gender, and diabetic status: A meta-analysis of major clinical trials. J Am Coll Cardiol. 2003;41(9):1529-38.
13. Wlodarczyk JH, Keogh A, Smith K, et al. CHART: Congestive cardiac failure in hospitals, an Australian review of treatment. Heart Lung Circ. 2003;12(2):94-102.
14. Fichett DH, Udell JA, Inzucci SE, et al. Heart failure outcomes in clinical trials of glucose-lowering agents in patients with diabetes. Eur J Heart Fail. 2017;19(1):43-53.
15. Zelniker TA, Wiviott SD, Raz I, et al. SGLT2 inhibitors for primary and secondary prevention of cardiovascular and renal outcomes in type 2 diabetes: a systematic review and meta-analysis of cardiovascular outcome trials. Lancet. 2018;393(10166):P31-9.
16. Wiviott SD, Raz I, Bonaca MP, et al. Dapagliflozin and cardiovascular outcomes in type 2 diabetes. N Engl J Med. 2019;380(4):347-57.
17. Marso SP, Daniels GH, Brown-Frandsen K, et al. Liraglutide and cardiovascular outcomes in type 2 diabetes. N Engl J Med. 2016; 375(4):311-22.
18. Butler J, Hamo CE, Filippatos G, et al. The potential role and rationale for treatment of heart failure with sodium-glucose co-transporter 2 inhibitors. Eur J Heart Fail. 2017;19(11):1390-1400.
19. Packer M, Kitzman DW. Obesity-Related Heart Failure With a Preserved Ejection Fraction: The Mechanistic Rationale for Combining Inhibitors of Aldosterone, Neprilysin, and Sodium-Glucose Cotransporter-2. JACC Heart Fail. 2018;6(8):633-9.
20. McMurray J. DAPA HF-The Dapagliflozin And Prevention Of Adverse-outcomes In Heart Failure Trial (Press release). Paris, France: European Society of Cardiology Congress; 2019.
21. Verma S, McMurray JJV. SGLT2 inhibitors and mechanisms of cardiovascular benefit: a state-of-the-art review. Diabetologia. 2018;61 (10):2108-17.

74 CHAPTER Secondary Diabetes

SS Dariya, Puneet Saxena, Aradhana Sharma, Suresh Kumar Yadav, Rishika Goyal, Deepak Chadha

INTRODUCTION

Secondary diabetes can be defined as a diabetic condition that develops after the destruction of the beta-cells in the pancreatic islets and/or the induction of insulin resistance by an acquired disease (e.g. endocrinopathies) or others.[1]

Secondary diabetes accounts for 1–2% of all cases of diabetes with net reported prevalence of 1.8%; however, concrete data is not available in Asians as prevalence could be more.[2]

Etiologic classification of diabetes: According to the classification system developed by the Expert Committee on the Diagnosis and Classification of Diabetes Mellitus, diabetes is classified into four broad categories:

1. Type 1 diabetes
2. Type 2 diabetes
3. Gestational diabetes
4. Other specific types of diabetes.

Secondary diabetes is now redefined as "*other specific type of diabetes*".

CAUSES OF SECONDARY DIABETES

- Diseases of the exocrine pancreas
  - Cystic fibrosis
  - Pancreatitis
  - Hemochromatosis
  - Neoplasm
  - Fibrocalculous pancreatopathy
- Endocrinopathies
  - Acromegaly
  - Cushing's syndrome
  - Pheochromocytoma
  - Glucagonoma
  - Primary hyperaldosteronism
  - Hyperthyroidism
- Drug-induced diabetes mellitus
- Viruses and diabetes mellitus
- Genetic syndromes associated with diabetes mellitus
- Genetic defects in insulin action
- Genetic defects of beta-cell function

PANCREATIC DIABETES/TYPE 3C DIABETES

Pancreatic or pancreatogenic diabetes is a form of secondary diabetes where pancreatic disease with exocrine deficiency leads to endocrine dysfunction resulting in defective glucose homeostasis. Clinical features of pancreatic diabetes are different from type 1 diabetes mellitus (T1DM) and type 2 diabetes mellitus (T2DM), thus it is now considered as a separate entity.

Etiology of Pancreatic Diabetes

- Acute pancreatitis
- Chronic pancreatitis
- Relapsing pancreatitis
- Alcohol
- Gallstone
- Hypertriglyceridemia
- Congenital anomalies of pancreatic duct system—pancreatic divisum
- Ectopic pancreas
- Annular pancreas
- Autoimmune pancreatitis
- Hereditary pancreatitis
- Genetic pancreatitis
- Drug-causing pancreatitis

- Trauma
- Hemochromatosis

Pathophysiology

Pathophysiology of pancreatic diabetes has been shown in Flowchart 1.

Clinical Features

Clinical manifestations—when compared to T1DM and T2DM have been shown in Table 1.

There is no insulin resistance in pancreatic diabetes. Hormonal and metabolic changes in pancreatic diabetes compared to T1DM and T2DM have been shown in Table 2.

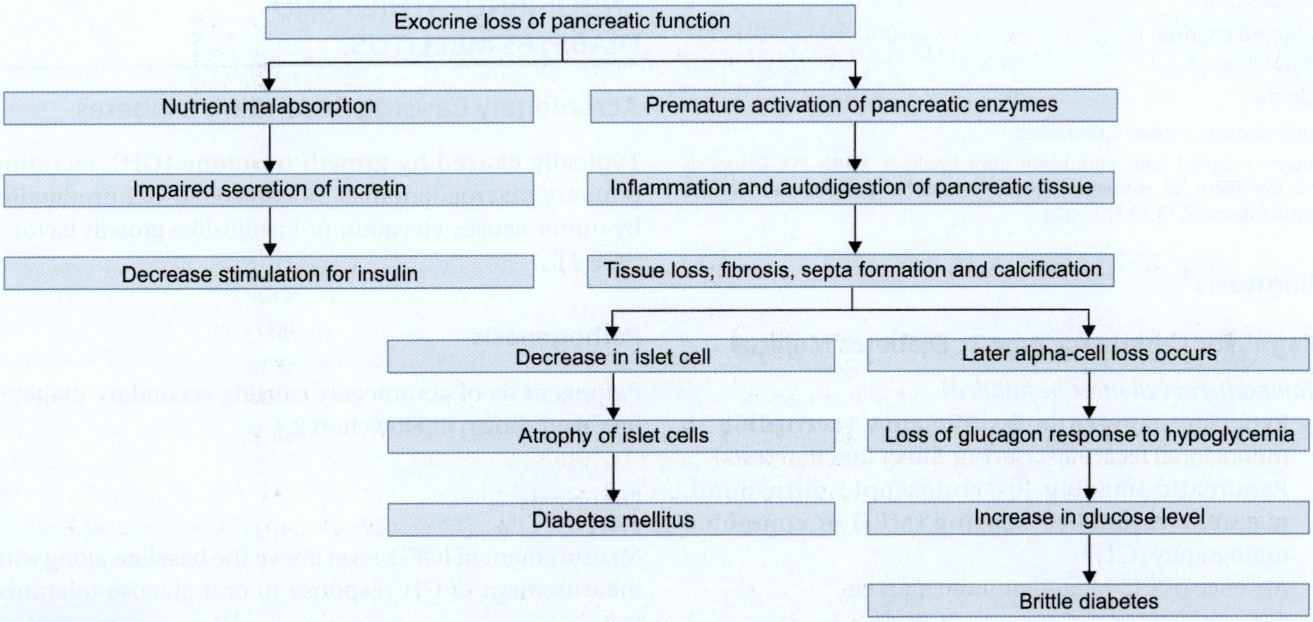

Flowchart 1 Pathophysiology of pancreatic diabetes.

TABLE 1: Clinical features of type 1, type 2 and type 3c diabetes mellitus.[2]

	T1DM	T2DM	T3cDM		
Associated with	Autoimmunity	Obesity	Chronic pancreatitis	Cystic fibrosis	Pancreatic resection
Median age of onset	2nd decade of life	6th decade of life	5th decade of life	3rd decade of life	within 5 years of surgery
Pancreatic insufficiency	No	No	Yes	Yes	Yes
Pain abdomen	No	No	Yes	Yes	No
Hepatic insulin sensitivity	Normal or decreased	Decreased	Normal or decreased	?	Normal or decreased
Peripheral insulin sensitivity	Normal or decreased	Decreased	Normal	?	Normal
Diabetic ketoacidosis	Yes	No	No	No	No
Hypoglycemia risk	Increased	Normal or increased	Normal or increased	Normal or increased	Normal or increased
Pancreatic polypeptide response	Normal or decreased	Decreased or absent	Decreased or absent	Absent	Absent

(*Source:* Adapted with permission from Gudipaty L, Rickels MR. Pancreatogenic (type 3c) diabetes. Pancreapedia: Exocrine Pancreas Knowledge Base; 2015.)

TABLE 2: Hormonal and metabolic derangements in pancreatic diabetes compared to type 1 and type 2 diabetes.[3]

	Pancreatic diabetes	Type-1 DM	Type-2 DM
Insulin secretion	↓↓	↓↓↓	↓
Insulin sensitivity	0	↓	↓↓
Glucagon secretion	↓↓	↑/↓	↑/↓
Plasma amino acids	↑↑	↑/0	↑/0
Ketosis prone	↑↑	↑↑↑	↑
Glucose counter regulation	↓	0/↓	0/↓
Lipids	0	↑	↑↑

↑, increased; 0, normal; ↓,decreased

(*Source:* Adapted with permission from Ewald N, Hardt PD. Diagnosis and treatment of diabetes mellitus in chronic pancreatitis. World J Gastroenterol. 2013;19:7276-81.)

Diagnosis[4]

Diagnostic Criteria for Type 3c Diabetes Mellitus

Major criteria (all must be fulfilled):

- Exocrine pancreatic insufficiency (according to monoclonal fecal elastase-1 or direct function tests)
- Pancreatic imaging [by endoscopic ultrasound, magnetic resonance imaging (MRI) or computed tomography (CT)]
- Absence of T1DM autoimmune markers.

Minor criteria:

- Impaired beta-cell function [as measured by homeostasis model assessment of β-cell function (HOMA-β), C-peptide/glucose ratio]
- Absence of insulin resistance [measured by HOMA of insulin resistance (IR)]
- Impaired incretin [e.g. gastric inhibitory polypeptide (GIP)] or pancreatic polypeptide secretion
- Low serum levels of lipid soluble vitamins (A, D, E, and K) (Ewald and Bretz et al.).

Management

- Control of hyperglycemia (HbA1c < 7%): Insulin therapy, drugs enhancing insulin secretion or insulin sensitizers have a little role to play.
- Care of exocrine deficiency—supplementation with enzymes like lipase and fat-soluble vitamins.
- Lifestyle modifications:
    - Cessation of smoking
    - Abstinence from alcohol
    - Low-fat diet.

Surgical Treatment

- Fibrocalculous pancreatic diabetes (FCPD)—Peustow's operation
- Large stone—extracorporeal lithotripsy (ECLT)
- Pancreatic cancer—total pancreatectomy with islet autotransplantation (TPIAT).

ENDOCRINOPATHIES AND DIABETES MELLITUS

Acromegaly Causing Secondary Diabetes

Typically caused by growth hormone (GH)-secreting pituitary macroadenomas, uncontrolled GH production by tumor causes elevation of insulin-like growth factor-1 (IGF-1).

Pathogenesis

Pathogenesis of acromegaly causing secondary diabetes has been shown in Flowchart 2.

Diagnosis

Measurement of IGF-1 level above the baseline along with measurement of GH response to oral glucose tolerance test.

Treatment

It is mainly surgical especially transsphenoidal surgery supported by medical management including GH receptor antagonists like *pegvisomant* and somatostatin receptor analogs like *octreotide* that may cause hyperglycemia.

Radiotherapy including external beam radiotherapy along with stereotactic surgery with gamma knife is also indicated.

Cushing's Syndrome

It is defined as hypercortisolism either due to autonomous hypersecretion or due to adrenocorticotropic hormone (ACTH) stimulation. Diabetes observed in 30–65% of Cushing's disease patients.

Mechanism[5]

Cortisol induces diabetes by following underlying mechanisms (Fig. 1):

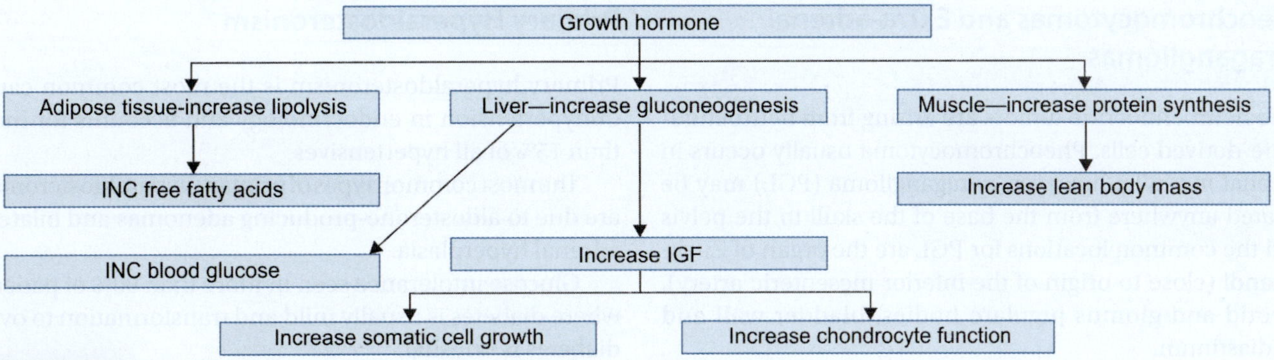

Flowchart 2 Pathogenesis of acromegaly causing secondary diabetes.

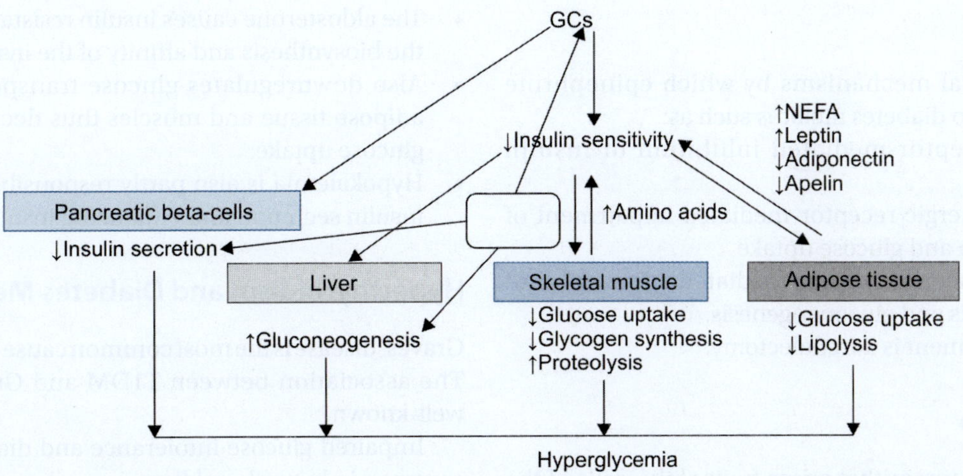

Figure 1 Diabetes induced by cortisol.

- Visceral obesity
- Increased hepatic glucose output
- Increased insulin resistance
- Impaired beta-cell function.

Treatment

Broadly divided into two categories:

1. Acute setting (preoperative setting)
2. Chronic setting (diabetes prevails due to incomplete control of hypercortisolemia following surgery or radiotherapy).

In preoperative settings:

- Cortisol-lowering agents to be used like metyrapone, ketoconazole or in rare occasion by mitotane.
- Metformin alone or its combination with insulin to be used to achieve glycemic control
- *Transsphenoidal resection of the pituitary tumor* is the treatment of choice in case of ACTH-dependent Cushing's disease
- *Surgical adrenalectomy* is the treatment of choice in case of adrenal-related Cushing's syndrome

In chronic setting:

- Glycemic control can be achieved by oral antidiabetic agents alone or in combination with insulin. Among all oral hypoglycemic agents (OHAs), metformin is first choice as it acts by improving the insulin resistance.
- Other agents like sulfonylureas and peroxisome proliferator-activated receptor-gamma (PPAR-γ) agonists are also effective. Rosiglitazone is a PPAR-γ agonist also found effective in lowering corticosterone levels by suppressing ACTH secretion in Cushing's syndrome.

Pheochromocytomas and Extra-adrenal Paragangliomas

Rare neuroendocrine tumors are arising from neuroendocrine-derived cells. Pheochromocytoma usually occurs in adrenal medulla; however, paraganglioma (PGL) may be located anywhere from the base of the skull to the pelvis and the common locations for PGL are the organ of Zuckerkandl (close to origin of the inferior mesenteric artery), carotid and glomus jugulare bodies, bladder wall and mediastinum.

Diabetes is seen in almost 25–75% of patients with pheochromocytoma.

Mechanism[6-9]

There are several mechanisms by which epinephrine excess can lead to diabetes mellitus such as:

- Alpha-2 receptor-mediated inhibition of insulin release
- Beta-2 adrenergic receptor-mediated impairment of insulin action and glucose uptake
- Beta-2 adrenergic receptor-mediated stimulation of glycogenolysis and gluconeogenesis.

Surgical management is adrenalectomy.

Glucagonoma

Neuroendocrine tumor that arises from alpha-cells of the pancreas.

These tumors are located in the tail of pancreas and are usually encapsulated, glucagonoma is a slow growing tumor; therefore, the average delay in diagnosis is approximately 3 years and nearly half of them present with metastasis at the time of diagnosis.

Glucagonoma is characterized by "4Ds": (1) diabetes, (2) dermatitis (rash), (3) deep vein thrombosis (DVT), and (4) depression.

The association of diabetes with glucagonoma ranges variably between 25% and 95% and the underlying mechanism behind its causation is glucagon stimulation of hepatic gluconeogenesis.

Diagnosis

- High fasting glucagon level in the absence of other causes of hyperglucagonemia.
- Localization of pancreatic mass on imaging modalities.
- Other neuroendocrine tumors associated with diabetes are VIPomas and somatostatinomas.

Primary Hyperaldosteronism

Primary hyperaldosteronism is the most common cause of hypertension in endocrinology and accounts for more than 15% of all hypertensives.

The most common types of primary hyperaldosteronism are due to aldosterone-producing adenomas and bilateral adrenal hyperplasia.

Glucose intolerance seen in more than 60% of patients where diabetes is usually mild and transformation to overt diabetes is unusual.

Mechanism

- The aldosterone causes insulin resistance by inhibiting the biosynthesis and affinity of the insulin receptor.
- Also downregulates glucose transporter (GLUT) in adipose tissue and muscles thus decreases the tissue glucose uptake.
- Hypokalemia is also partly responsible for decreasing insulin secretion and enhancing insulin resistance.

Hyperthyroidism and Diabetes Mellitus

Graves' disease is the most common cause of thyrotoxicosis. The association between T1DM and Graves' disease is well-known.

Impaired glucose intolerance and diabetes mellitus is common in hyperthyroidism.

Mechanism

Hyperthyroidism can cause diabete by several mechanisms such as:

- Increased intestinal hexose absorption
- Impair insulin action
- Decreased half-life of insulin due to increased degradation and excess release of inactive insulin precursors
- Increased hepatic glucose output due to increased hepatocyte GLUT-2 expressions, increased fatty acid production and gluconeogenesis
- Increased levels of GH, catecholamine and glucagon can also contribute to glucose intolerance in hyperthyroidism.

The thionamides (NeoMercazole and propylthiouracil) are the primary drugs used to treat Graves' hyperthyroidism.

NeoMercazole is preferred because of its longer duration of action and thus can be administered once daily.

TABLE 3: Drug-induced diabetes.

Drugs that cause diabetes by interfering with insulin-synthesis and secretion:	
Phenytoin	L-asparaginase
Pentamidine	Tacrolimus
B-blockers	Didanosine
Diazoxide	Opiates
Calcium channel blockers	
Drugs that cause diabetes by interfering insulin action:	
Glucocorticoids	β-adrenoreceptor agonist
Megasterol acetate	Clonazepine, olanzapine (antipsychotics)
Oral contraceptives	SSRI
Growth hormone	Protease inhibitors
Drugs that cause diabetes by interfering with insulin secretion and insulin action:	
Thiazide diuretics	Cyclosporine
Diazoxide	Atypical antipsychotic
Drugs that cause diabetes independent of insulin:	
Nicotinic acid	
Statin	
Aspirin	
Total parental nutrition	

DRUG-INDUCED DIABETES

The exact mechanism by which drugs causing disturbances in glucose intolerance remains uncertain; however, the diabetogenic mechanism can be classified into four broad categories (Table 3):

1. Impairment of insulin synthesis and secretion
2. Impairment of insulin action
3. Impairment of both insulin secretion and insulin action
4. Independent of insulin action.

VIRUSES AND DIABETES MELLITUS

There are several mechanisms by which viral infections can lead to diabetes (Table 4):[10]

- Direct cytopathic effect and death of beta-cells
- Immune-mediated destruction of beta-cells (molecular mimicry is one mechanism that entitles a cross-reactive immunity against epitopes that are shared between viral structure and beta-cell antigens.)
- Bystander activation of unrelated T cells which leads to production of inflammatory mediators and beta-cell destruction.

GENETIC SYNDROMES ASSOCIATED WITH DIABETES MELLITUS

Genetic syndrome associated with diabetes accounts for less than 1% of the total diabetes mellitus.

There are four categorizations of syndromes associated with diabetes:

1. Chromosomal disorders linked up with diabetes like—Down's/Turner's/Klinefelter's syndrome
2. Genetic syndromes associated with metabolic syndromes include—Laurence-Moon-Biedl syndrome, Bardet-Biedl syndrome and Prader-Willi Syndrome
3. Hereditary neuromuscular disorders such as Huntington's chorea, Friedreich ataxia (FRDA) and diabetes insipidus, diabetes mellitus, optic atrophy, deafness (DIDMOAD)
4. Several mitochondrial disorders like Kearns-Sayre syndrome, Leber's hereditary optic neuropathy (LHON), myoclonic epilepsy with ragged-red fibers (MERRF) and mitochondrial myopathy, encephalopathy, lactic acidosis and stroke-like episodes (MELAS) syndrome.

GENETIC DEFECTS IN INSULIN ACTION

Insulin resistance defined as a state in which a more than normal amount of insulin is actually required to generate a quantitatively normal response.

Examples of some of the acquired conditions causing insulin resistance are obesity, polycystic ovarian disease, T2DM and metabolic syndrome while inherited syndromes are also present that are characterized by a scenario of insulin resistance are mainly arising due to mutations affecting either the insulin receptors or post-receptor cascade pathway.

The most common conditions are:

- Type 1 insulin resistance
- Leprechaunism
- Rabson-Mendenhall syndrome.

The clinical spectrums that are shared between these above-mentioned syndromes are hyperinsulinemia, disturbances in glucose homeostasis, ovarian hyperandrogenism and acanthosis nigricans.

Lipodystrophy Syndromes

These disorders characterized by selective loss of adipose tissue and are clinically manifested by dyslipidemia, insulin resistance, diabetes mellitus, hepatic steatosis and acanthosis nigricans.

TABLE 4: Viruses and diabetes mellitus.

	Species	Genetic factor	Effects
RNA virus			
Coxsackie B	Human, mice, nonhuman primates	ND	Associated with induction of inlet autoantibodies, cytolytic destruction of β-cells Virus isolated pancreas of diabetes animal
Enterovirus	Mice	Yes	Virus-induced β-cell lysis Molecular mimicry Virus-induced bystander damage
Encephalomyocarditis	Mice	Yes	*High dose*: virus-induced β-cell lysis *Low dose*: infection of β-cells, activation of macrophage and destruction of β-cells
Toga virus	Human	Yes	Associated with development islet cell autoantibodies
Rubella virus	Human/Hamsters	ND	T-cell cross-reactivity between rubella antigens and GAD infection of β-cell without cytolytic effects
Paramyxovirus family (Mumps virus)	Human	ND	Induction of islet autoantibodies Infection of β-cells without cytolytic effect Increased expression of HLA class I and II on β-cells
Rota virus	Mice	Yes	Infection of β-cells Molecular mimicry
Reovirus	Human	ND	Infection of β-cells
DNA viruses			
Parvovirus	Human/Rat	ND	Associated with induction of autoimmune disease Virus associated macrophage—breakdown of tolerance Th-1 type immune response is enhanced
Cytomegalovirus	Human/Rat	ND	Associated with induction of islets autoantibodies Infection of β-cells but without cytolytic effects T-cells cross reactivity between HCMB and GAD-65
Epstein-Barr virus	Human		Induction of autoimmunity mediated by recognition of epitope by HLA-DQ8
Varicella Zoster	Human		Indirect evidence of association
Kilham rat virus	Rats	ND	No β-cell infection. Autoimmune mediated development of diabetes

GENETIC DEFECTS OF BETA-CELL FUNCTION

The most common forms of diabetes T1DM and T2DM are polygenic in nature, meaning the risk of developing these disorders is related to multiple genes. However, additional and rare forms of diabetes, termed *monogenic*, result from mutations in a single gene.

Neonatal diabetes (ND) and maturity-onset diabetes of the young (MODY) are the two main forms of monogenic diabetes (Table 5).

Neonatal Diabetes

Neonatal diabetes is a monogenic form of diabetes that occurs in the first 6 months of life.

Symptoms of ND mimic those of T1DM.

Maturity-Onset Diabetes of the Young

Hallmark features are:

- Usually occurs during adolescence or early adulthood

TABLE 5: Monogenic forms of diabetes.

Forms associated with insulin resistance
Mutations in the insulin receptor gene
Type A insulin resistance
Leprechaunism
Rabson-Mendenhall syndrome
Lipoatrophic diabetes
Mutations in the PPARγ gene
Form associated with defective insulin secretion
Mutations in insulin or proinsulin genes
Mitochondrial gene mutations
Maturity-onset diabetes of the young (MODY)
HNF-4α (MODY 1)
Glucokinase (MODY 2)
HNF-1α (MODY 3)
IPF 1 (MODY 4)
HNF-1β (MODY 5)
NeuroD1/Beta 2 (MODY 6)

- Strong family history of diabetes (typically 2–3 generations affected)
- MODY patients often are asymptomatic or demonstrate only mild hyperglycemia. They are generally not overweight.
- Hyperglycemia worsens with age and develops in frank diabetes—slow progression.

CONCLUSION

A relatively very minor of population subset belongs to the category of secondary diabetes as comparison to type 1 and type 2 forms.[11] Treatment of causative agent may cure diabetes in these patients thereby forming secondary diabetes as the only diabetes of its kind that is *reversible*; therefore, it is imperative on the part of treating physicians to be cautious for such causative factors as early recognition and treatment of underlying causation can remold the final outcome easily.

REFERENCES

1. Podolsky S, Viswanathan M (Eds). Secondary Diabetes: The Spectrum of Diabetic Syndromes. New York: Raven Press; 1980.
2. Ganda OP. Diabetologist. Joslin Diabetes Center, Boston, MA, United States.
3. Gudipaty L, Rickels MR. Pancreatogenic (type 3c) diabetes. Pancreapedia: Exocrine Pancreas Knowledge Base; 2015.
4. Ewald N, Hardt PD. Diagnosis and treatment of diabetes mellitus in chronic pancreatitis. World J Gastroenterol. 2013;19:7276-81.
5. Ewald N, Bretzel RG. Diabetes mellitus secondary to pancreatic diseases (type 3c)—are we neglecting an important disease? Eur J Intern Med. 2013;24:203-6. PMID: 23375619.
6. Page R, Boolell M, Kalfas A, et al. Insulin secretion, insulin sensitivity and glucose-mediated glucose disposal in Cushing's disease: a minimal model analysis. Clin Endocrinol (Oxf). 1991;35(6):509-17.
7. La Batide-Alanore A, Chatellier G, Plouin PF. Diabetes as a marker of pheochromocytoma in hypertensive patients. J Hypertens. 2003;21(9):1703-7.
8. Hamaji M. Pancreatic alpha- and beta-cell function in pheochromocytoma. J Clin Endocrinol Metab. 1979;49(3):322-5.
9. Saccà L, Vigorito C, Cicala M, et al. Role of gluconeogenesis in epinephrine-stimulated hepatic glucose production in humans. Am J Physiol. 1983;245(3):E294-302.
10. Turnbull DM, Johnston DG, Alberti KG, et al. Hormonal and metabolic studies in a patient with pheochromocytoma. J Clin Endocrinol Metab. 1980;51(4):930-3.
11. Genuth S, Alberti KG, Bennett P, et al. Follow-up report on the diagnosis of diabetes mellitus. Diabetes Care. 2003;26(11):3160-7.

75 CHAPTER Optical Coherence Tomography: Useful Tool for Retinal Problems

Kiran Shah

INTRODUCTION

Every diabetic is a potential candidate for diabetic retinopathy (DR). Diabetic macular edema (DME) is the thickening of the central retina or macula, is responsible for a significant degree of visual loss in diabetic patients.[1] The International Diabetes Federation (IDF) estimates that among all people with diabetes, 11% have DME[2] and that percentage increases to 29% among people who have lived with diabetes for 20 years or more.[3] Optical coherence tomography (OCT) was first introduced in 1991.[4] OCT is a noninvasive imaging modality which uses low-coherence interferometry to produce quick, precise, reproducible high-definition cross-sectional images of retina up to 10 micron resolution.[5] Conventional practice of assessing the macula for its thickness, involving slit-lamp biomicroscopy, fundus photography, and fluorescein angiography, is less sensitive to subtle changes and is only qualitative. OCT provides anatomical extent of macular edema such as extent of thickening and retinal layers involved. Thus, OCT plays vital role in the diagnosis, management, and follow-up of DME.[6]

OPTICAL COHERENCE TOMOGRAPHY INTERPRETATION

The OCT has greatly enhanced our ability to understand the complex nature of DME. It provides us with quantitative and qualitative analysis on how to interpret DME.

Quantitative Analysis

It refers to measuring the thickness of the retina. This is a standard report from Zeiss Cirrus HD OCT Device (Fig. 1). The report provides lot of information (Table 1):

Qualitative Analysis

It refers to interpreting scan to see, if there is a disease and to understand what this disease might be.

This analysis aims to serve as guide to OCT features of common retinal conditions such as:[7]

- *Disorders of vitreomacular interface:* These include vitreomacular adhesion, vitreomacular traction (Fig. 2) and macular hole (Fig. 3).
- *Choroidal neovascular (CNV) membrane* (Fig. 4): Further classified based on OCT features as: type 1 well-defined hyper-reflective tissue between the retinal pigment epithelium (RPE) or Bruch's membrane, type 2 CNV above RPE[8,9] and type 3 sub-RPE CNV with intraretinal hyper-reflective foci along with subretinal neovascularization and intraretinal cystoid changes.[10,11]
- *Macular edema*: It based on OCT that takes into account five simple parameters like retinal thickness, extension of retinal thickening, macular volume, retinal morphology, and vitreoretinal relationship, DME can be classified as (a) Sponge-like retinal swelling (Fig. 5), (b) Cystoid macular edema (Fig. 6), (c) Sponge-like retinal swelling + CME or serous foveal detachment (Fig. 7), and (d) Combination of all types.
- *Clinically significant macular edema (CSME):* CSME was originally defined by the early treatment diabetic retinopathy study (ETDRS) in terms of retinal thickening as detected by stereo retinal photography or clinical examination with stereo biomicroscopy. Criteria for diagnosis of CSME: (a) Thickening of the retina at or within 500 μm of the center of the macula. (b) Hard exudates at or within 500 μm of the center of the macula, if associated with thickening of adjacent retina.[12] (c) Any zone (s) of retinal thickening

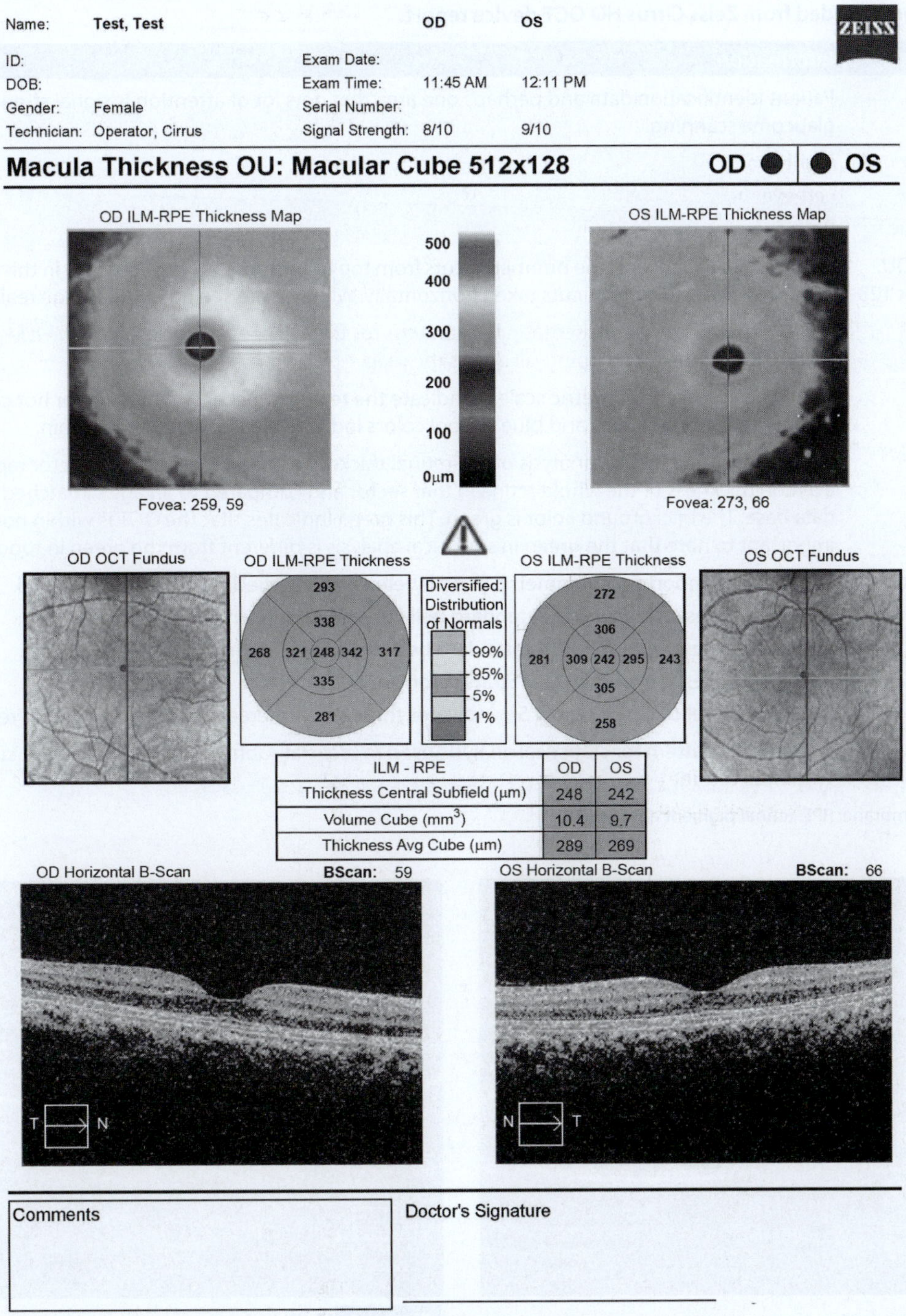

Figure 1 Standard report from Zeiss Cirrus HD OCT device. ***(For color version see color plate No. 4)***

1 disk area or larger, any part of which is within 1 disk diameter of the center of the macula (Fig. 8).

- *Conditions causing serous detachment at macula*: Central serous chorioretinopathy (Fig. 9) and age-related macular degeneration (Fig. 10).
- Retinal pigment epithelial detachments (Fig. 11).

LIMITATIONS OF OPTICAL COHERENCE TOMOGRAPHY

Optical coherence tomography does not show accuracy:

- In presence of media opacities like cataract, vitreous hemorrhage, asteroids, etc.

TABLE 1: Information provided from Zeiss Cirrus HD OCT device report.

Device	Information
Topmost Section	Patient identification data and perhaps one area that gets lot of attention is signal strength especially in glaucoma scanning.
OD—Oculus dexter OS—Oculus sinister OU—Oculus uterque	Right eye Left eye Both eyes
Macular thickness OU: Macular Cube 512 × 128	The number 512 means: the number of cuts from top to bottom running vertically in this plane. The number 128 means: the number of cuts taken horizontally. What we are seeing in this image really is one single cut.
OD and OS ILM-RPE Thickness Map	This is a topographic representation that measures the thickness of retina from the ILM all the way to the RPE, at almost thousand points all across the map.
Colorimetric scale	The device uses a colorimetric scale to indicate the relative thickness where red or hot colors indicate areas where retina is thick and blue or cool colors indicate areas where retina is thin.
OD and OS ILM-RPE Thickness	This represents statistical analysis of the retinal thickness. The number in each sector represents the average thickness of the whole retina in that sector and compared to an age – matched normative data base. The background color is green. This green indicates that the OCT is within normal limits. It is important to note that the green in statistical analysis is different from the green in topographic map.
Diversified distribution of normals	This is a very important colorimetric band labeled as diversified distribution of normal. Retinal thickness within 5–95% standard bell curve: Within Normal Limits Retinal Thickness within 95–99% standard bell curve: Bit Thicker Retina. Retinal Thickness beyond 99% or Straw color: Very Thick Retina. Similarly the yellow color below 5% indicates thin retina whereas red means very thin retina.
ILM–RPE	Calorimetric pattern for statistical analysis used for central subfield Thickness, volume cube and average Thickness of cube.

(ILM: inner limiting membrane; RPE: retinal pigment epithelium)

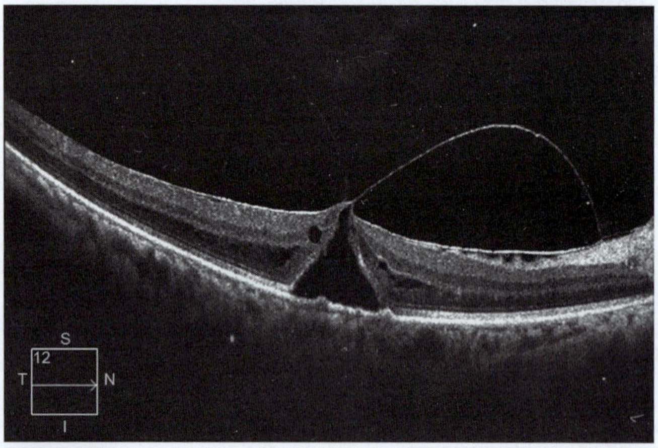

Figure 2 Vitreomacular traction.

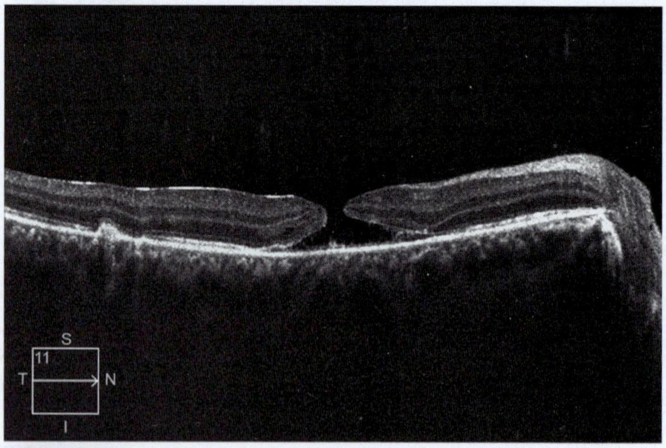

Figure 3 Full thickness macular hole.

- In noncooperative patients.
- Needs minimal pupil diameter > 3 mm

It does not provide information on functional and dynamic changes like vascular permeability, difference between afferent arteries and efferent veins, and velocity of blood flow.

TECHNOLOGICAL ADVANCES IN OPTICAL COHERENCE TOMOGRAPHY

The hallmark of DR is vascular changes involving different retinal layers. OCT angiography (OCTA) provides data on vascular, morphological, and distributional features

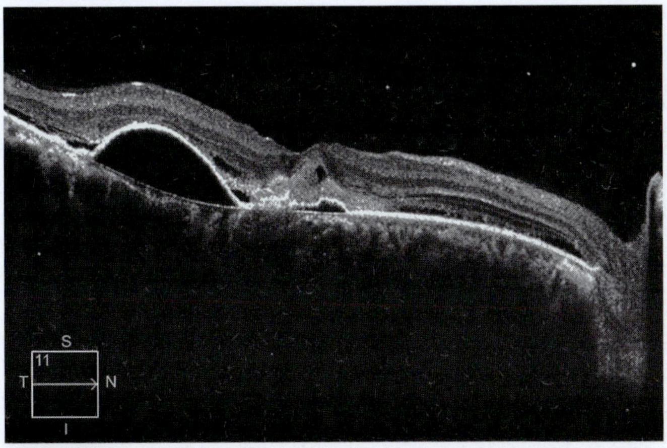

Figure 4 Choroidal neovascular membrane.

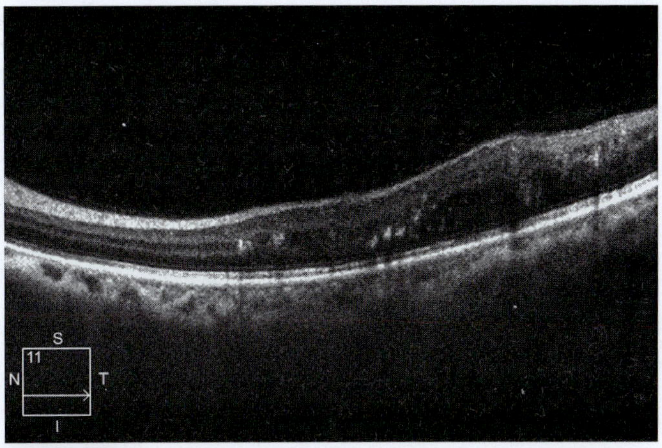

Figure 5 Sponge-like retinal swelling with hard exudates.

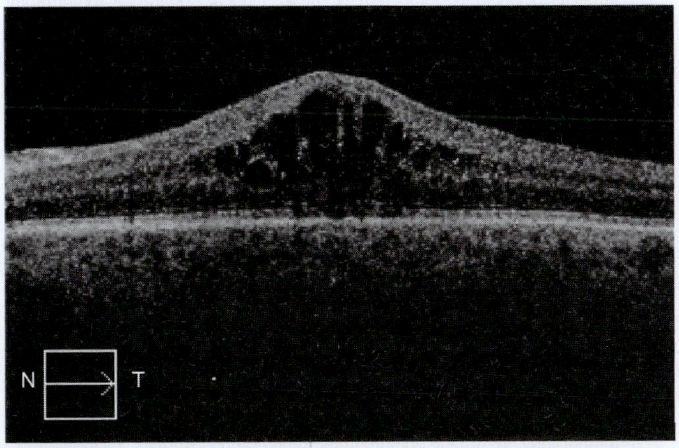

Figure 6 Cystoid macular edema. ***(For color version see color plate No. 5)***

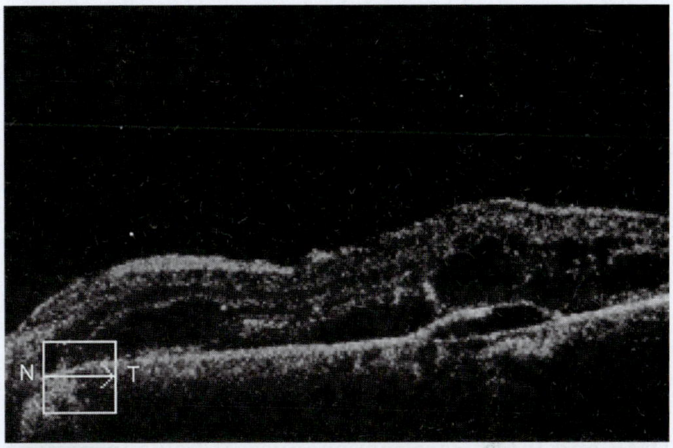

Figure 7 Sponge-like retinal swelling + CME/serous foveal detachment. ***(For color version see color plate No. 5)***

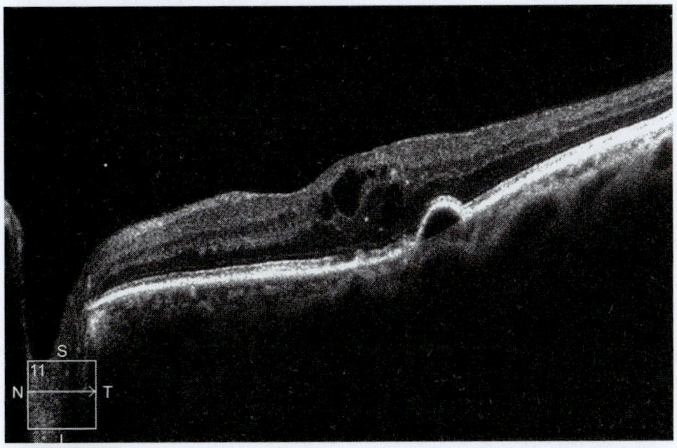

Figure 8 Clinically significant macular edema with hard exudates and pigment epithelial detachment.

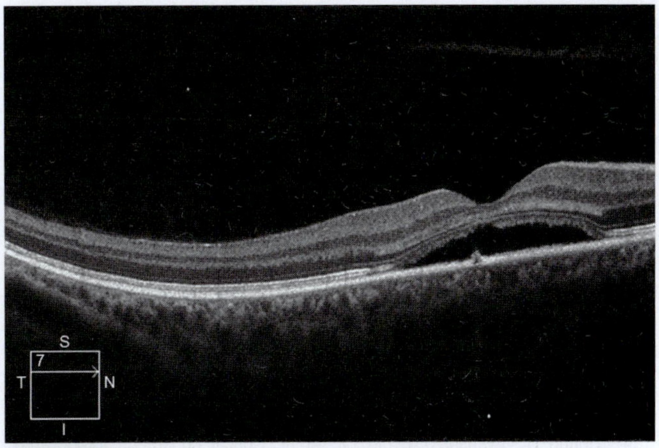

Figure 9 Central serous chorioretinopathy.

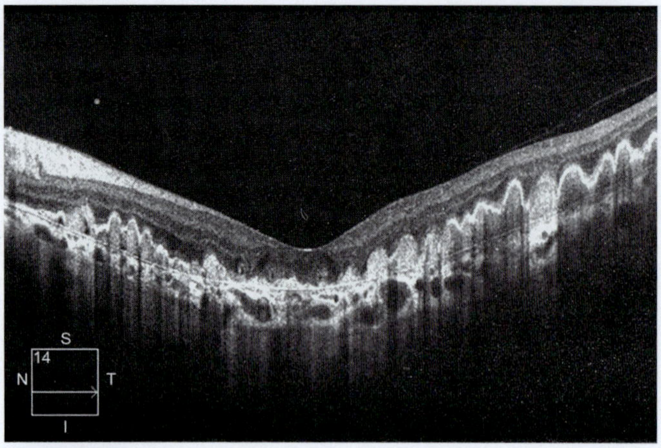

Figure 10 Age-related macular degeneration.

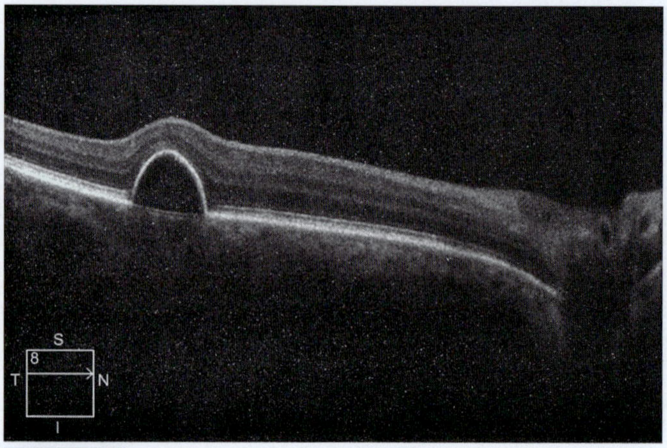

Figure 11 Pigment epithelial detachment.

in different retinal layers. It is also superior to fluorescein angiography to visualize foveal avascular zone as the dye leakage does not cover it. OCTA elucidates central and parafoveal microvasculature.[13]

Advantages of OCTA:

- Identifies DR before it is clinically detectable.
- Visualizes morphological changes in DR.[14]
- Identifies vascular changes in choriocapillaries in DR.[15]
- Quantitative assessment of vascular changes in DR.[16,17]

CONCLUSION

Optical coherence tomography defines the anatomy of DME and the intraretinal changes. It helps in patient selection especially those who can benefit from treatment, selection of treatment indicated, guide its implementation, and allow monitoring of treatment response. The American Diabetes Association promotes the adoption of OCT to assess retinal thickness and intraretinal pathology to identify clinically silent microvascular lesions.[18]

REFERENCES

1. Klein R, Klein BE, Moss SE, et al. The Wisconsin epidemiologic study of diabetic retinopathy. XV. The long-term incidence of macular edema. Ophthalmology. 1995;102:7-16.
2. International Diabetes Federation (Europe). Diabetes and blindness due to DME. Brussels, Belgium: International Diabetes Federation. [online] Available from www.idf.org/sites/default/files/IDF%2520Toolkit_Backgrounder_FINAL.pdf.
3. Klein R, Klein BE, Moss SE. The Wisconsin epidemiologic study of diabetic retinopathy. IV. Diabetic macular edema. Ophthalmology. 1984;91:1464-74.
4. Huang D, Swanson EA, Lin CP, et al. Optical coherence tomography. Science. 1991;254:1178-81.
5. Virgili G, Menchini F, Casazza G, et al. Optical coherence tomography (OCT) for detection of macular edema in patients with diabetic retinopathy. Cochrane Database Syst Rev. 2015;1:CD008081.
6. Browning DJ, Fraser CM, Propst BW. The variation in optical coherence tomography-measured macular thickness in diabetic eyes without clinical macular edema. Am J Opthalmol. 2008;145:889-93.
7. Bhende M, Shetty S, Parthasarthy MK, et al. Optical coherence tomography: A guide to interpretation of common macular diseases. Indian J Opthalmol. 2018;66:20-35.
8. Gass JD. Biomicroscopic and histopathologic considerations regarding the feasibility of surgical excision of subfoveal neovascular membranes. Am J Ophthalmol. 1994;118:285-98.
9. Regatieri CV, Branchini L, Duker JS. The role of spectral-domain OCT in the diagnosis and management of neovascular age-related macular degeneration. Ophthalmic Surg Lasers Imaging. 2011;42 Suppl:S56-66.
10. Lim EH, Han JI, Kim CG, et al. Characteristic findings of optical coherence tomography in retinal angiomatous proliferation. Korean J Ophthalmol. 2013;27:351-60.
11. Freund KB, Ho IV, Barbazetto IA, et al. Type 3 neovascularization: The expanded spectrum of retinal angiomatous proliferation. Retina. 2008;28:201-11.
12. Photocoagulation for diabetic macular edema. Early Treatment Diabetic Retinopathy Study report number 1. Early Treatment Diabetic Retinopathy Study research group. Arch Ophthalmol. 1985;103:1796-806.
13. Soares M, Neves C, Marques IP, et al. Comparison of diabetic retinopathy classification using fluorescein angiography and optical coherence tomography angiography. Br J Opthalmol. 2017;101:62-8.
14. Matsunaga DR, Yi JJ, De Koo LO, et al. Opitcal coherence tomography angiography of diabetic retinopathy in human subjects. Opthalmic Surg Lasers Imaging Retina. 2015;46:796-805.
15. Melancia D, Vicente A, Cunha JP, et al. Diabetic choroidopathy: A review of current literature. Graefes Arch Clin Exp Opthalmol. 2016;254:1453-61.
16. Park JJ, Soetikno BT, Fawzi AA. Characterization of middle capillary plexus using optical coherence tomography angiography in healthy and diabetic eyes. Retina. 2016;36:2039-50.
17. Bhanushali D, Anegondi N, Gadde SG, et al. Linking retinal microvasculature features with severity of diabetic retinopathy using optical coherence tomography angiography. Invest Opthalmol Vis Sci. 2016;57:OCT519-25.
18. Solomon SD, Chew E, Duh EJ, et al. Diabetic retinopathy: A position statement by American Diabetes Association. Diabetes Care. 2017;40:412-8.

10 SECTION Diabetes and Women

76 CHAPTER Diagnosis of Gestational Diabetes Mellitus—Indian Context

Shalini Jaggi, Rajeev Chawla

INTRODUCTION

The epidemic of diabetes and obesity gripping the world today has resulted in a proportionate increase in the number of cases of gestational diabetes mellitus (GDM) globally, more so in the high-risk ethnic populations. India is no different with about 4 million women having GDM in India alone.[1] The region-wise prevalence varies from 3.8% to 21% in different parts of the country, with a higher incidence in urban population.[2,3] GDM is associated with not only adverse pregnancy outcomes, but also predisposes both the mother and her baby to developing diabetes and metabolic disorders including obesity later in life. An early diagnosis and screening strategy go a long way in detecting GDM early and providing an effective management strategy to reduce its implications. Hence, GDM provides a golden window of opportunity for intervention benefiting not only the pregnant woman but also her baby. There have been various different recommendations for screening and diagnosis as well as management of GDM which vary from region to region with no global single set of guidelines to follow. In this chapter, we will focus on putting facts in the Indian context and focus on the India specific recommendations for the screening and diagnosis of GDM.

What is gestational diabetes mellitus and why is it important?

Gestational diabetes mellitus is defined as "glucose intolerance of any degree with the onset or first recognition during pregnancy" which may or may not resolve after delivery; women with known diabetes, who have an hemoglobin A1c (HbA1c) ≥ 6.5% in the first trimester, type 1 diabetes, and monogenic diabetes can sometimes present in pregnancy are said to have overt diabetes and have to be differentiated from true GDM.[4,5]

Gestational diabetes mellitus is associated with an increase in maternal as well as fetal morbidity and mortality (Box 1).[6,7] Not only does it increase the risk of development of type 2 diabetes in the mother, but also makes the baby more prone to develop obesity as well

BOX 1 Hyperglycemia-related maternal and fetal complications.[7]

Maternal complications:
- Miscarriages in early pregnancy
- Higher incidence of infections
- Preeclampsia
- Preterm labor
- Birth trauma
- Assisted delivery and cesarean sections
- Hypoglycemia
- Acute metabolic complications such as diabetic ketoacidosis (DKA)
- Worsening of preexisting microvascular complications.

Fetal complications:
- Congenital malformations particularly cardiac and neural tube defects but sacral agenesis is the most pathognomonic
- Higher incidence of stillbirths
- Polyhydramnios
- Macrosomia
- Shoulder dystocia
- Prolonged labor
- Birth trauma and Erb's palsy
- Neonatal asphyxia
- Neonatal hypoglycemia.

as glucose intolerance in the future, thus affecting two generations. Hence, an early diagnosis and adequate management of GDM provides us with a golden window of opportunity for intervention which has beneficial effects both on the present pregnancy and the future risk for both mother and baby.

PATHOPHYSIOLOGY OF GESTATIONAL DIABETES MELLITUS

Pregnancy involves a major alteration in the mother's hormonal milieu, characterized by an increase in estrogen, progesterone, prolactin, cortisol, human chorionic gonadotropin (hCG), prolactin as well as placental hormones. These hormones alter the maternal insulin resistance to enable adequate supply of nutrients to the fetoplacental unit for growth. These metabolic changes promote adipose tissue deposition in early pregnancy, followed by increasing insulin resistance and facilitated lipolysis in late pregnancy.

The hallmark of late second and third trimesters is increasing insulin resistance, caused by alterations in adipocytokines such as lower levels of adiponectin, and increase in leptin, tumor necrosis factor-α (TNF-α), interleukin-6, and resistin, etc. as well as marked increase in counterregulatory hormones .These include human placental lactogen (30-fold rise), human placental growth hormone (6–8-fold rise), prolactin (7–10-fold rise), and cortisol. As a consequence, insulin-mediated glucose disposal is reduced by almost 50% and there is a compensatory 200–250% increase in insulin secretion in late pregnancy.[8,9]

The increased insulin resistance and diabetogenic stress due to placental hormone surge in the second half of pregnancy places a huge demand for compensatory increase in insulin secretion. If this demand for massive increase in insulin secretion is not adequately fulfilled, it leads to dysglycemia and a clinical presentation of GDM.

RISK FACTORS FOR DEVELOPMENT OF GESTATIONAL DIABETES MELLITUS

- Obesity [body mass index (BMI) ≥ 30 kg/m^2]
- Family history of diabetes (first-degree relative with diabetes)
- Bad obstetric history
- Previous macrosomic baby weighing ≥4.5 kg
- Previous history of GDM
- Elderly primigravida
- Hydramnios
- Multiparity or twin gestation
- Previous or current pregnancy-induced hypertension (PIH)
- *High-risk ethnicity*: South Asian, Black Caribbean, and Middle Eastern.

DIAGNOSIS OF GESTATIONAL DIABETES MELLITUS

The screening strategy for GDM has been controversial and has been changed from time to time. Many international diabetes associations and organizations recommend screening only the high-risk pregnancies for GDM, but universal screening is recommended for all high-risk ethnicities such as Asian Indians, Hispanics, Pacific islanders, and Afro-Americans, etc. All Indian pregnant women, being part of the high-risk ethnic group, need to be screened for diabetes at their first antenatal visit itself. Those found to be normal should be screened again at 24–28 weeks for GDM.

Current American Diabetes Association 2019 Recommendations[10]

As per the American Diabetes Association (ADA), diagnosis of GDM can be made by either one-step or a two-step screening approach as shown here (Table 1):

- "One-step" method with 2-hour 75 g oral glucose tolerance test (OGTT) [International Association of Diabetes and Pregnancy Study Groups (IADPSG) consensus]
- "Two-step" approach with a 1-hour 50 g (nonfasting) screen followed by a 3-hour 100 g OGTT for those who screen positive, i.e. 1 hour ≥ 140 mg/dL [National Institutes of Health (NIH) consensus].

Different diagnostic criteria will identify different magnitudes of maternal hyperglycemia and maternal/fetal risk.

INDIAN SCENARIO

Who to screen and when to screen?

Indian women are at an 11 times greater risk of developing GDM than Caucasians, making universal screening mandatory for all pregnant Indian women. A joint Diabetes in Pregnancy Study Group of India-Federation of Obstetric and Gynecological Societies of India (DIPSI-FOGSI) study demonstrated that GDM is diagnosed in about one-third of women in the first trimester itself contrary to the usual

TABLE 1: Current screening and diagnosis of GDM as per the ADA.

"One-step" (IADPSG consensus)			
Perform a 75-g OGTT, with plasma glucose measurement fasting and at 1 and 2 h, at 24–28 weeks of gestation in women not previously diagnosed with overt diabetes			
The OGTT should be performed in the morning after an overnight fast of at least 8 h			
The diagnosis of GDM is made when any of the following plasma glucose values are exceeded:			
• Fasting: ≥92 mg/dL (5.1 mmol/L)			
• 1 h: ≥180 mg/dL (10.0 mmol/L)			
• 2 h: ≥153 mg/dL (8.5 mmol/L)			
"Two-step" (NIH consensus)			
• Perform a 50-g GLT, (nonfasting), with plasma glucose measurement at 1 h (Step 1), at 24–28 weeks of gestation in women not previously diagnosed with overt diabetes			
• If the plasma glucose level measured 1 h after the load is ≥140 mg/dL* (7.8 mmol/L), proceed to 100-g OGTT (Step 2). The 100-g OGTT should be performed when the patient is fasting			
• The diagnosis of GDM is made when at least two of the following four plasma glucose levels (measured fasting, 1 h, 2 h, 3 h after the OGTT) are meat or exceeded:			
	Carpenter/Coustan	or	NDDG
• Fasting	95 mg/dL (5.3 mmol/L)		105 mg/dL (5.8 mmol/L)
• 1 h	180 mg/dL (10.0 mmol/L)		190 mg/dL (10.6 mmol/L)
• 2 h	155 mg/dL (8.6 mmol/L)		165 mg/dL (9.2 mmol/L)
• 3 h	140 mg/dL (7.8 mmol/L)		145 mg/dL (8.0 mmol/L)

*The American College of Obstetricians and Gynecologists (ACOG) recommends a lower threshold of 135 mg/dL (7.5 mmol/L) in high-risk ethnic minorities with higher prevalence of GDM; some experts also recommend 130 mg/dL (7.2 mmol/L).

(ADA: American Diabetes Association; GDM: gestational diabetes mellitus; GLT: glucose load test; IADPSG: International Association of Diabetes and Pregnancy Study Groups; NDDG: National Diabetes Data Group; NIH: National Institutes of Health; OGTT: oral glucose tolerance test)

(*Source*: American Diabetes Association. 14. Management of Diabetes in Pregnancy: Standards of Medical Care in Diabetes-2019. Diabetes Care. 2019;42(Suppl 1):S165-72.)

occurrence in the 2nd to 3rd trimesters, and more than a 25% of these women have a history of fetal loss in their previous pregnancies.[11] This makes it important for Indian women to be screened early in pregnancy rather than later as mandated globally. Besides ethnicity, advancing age and increasing BMI are predominant risk factors predisposing to GDM in Indian women, and the incidence is much more in urban women than rural women in India. A diagnosis of GDM not only has a psychosocial impact on the pregnant woman and her family, but its implications make it necessary to screen early and manage it timely to reduce maternofetal complications and improve pregnancy outcomes. The DIPSI mandates screening at first point of contact in the antenatal screening to pick up any case of early GDM as well as any pregestational diabetes for timely diagnosis and management of any degree of hyperglycemia in pregnancy.

Hence, in all Indian pregnant women:

- *Universal screening for GDM is recommended preferably at first visit to the antenatal clinic.*
- *If she tests negative in early pregnancy, a repeat testing must be done at 24–28 weeks again to rule out development of GDM at this time.*

How to screen?

As recommended by the ADA earlier, either of the two strategies may be followed to screen for GDM. Due to ease and convenience, the one-step strategy of a fasting 75-g OGTT with 1 hour and 2-hour postglucose testing is followed in many parts of the globe. The American College of Obstetricians and Gynecologists (ACOG), however, recommends the two-step strategy requiring first a 50-g glucose load test (GLT), and then proceeding for a 100 g OGTT in women with a 1-hour postglucose (PG) load reading of 130 mg/dL, 135 mg/dL, or 140 mg/dL. However, in contrast to the ADA, the ACOG recommends any one positive value in the GTT as a diagnosis of GDM and recommends management as per the GDM pathway.

However, India has its own limitations and a huge urban-rural divide besides a socioeconomic as well as literacy divide. In rural settings, even basic healthcare infrastructure is still a challenge. Furthermore, asking a pregnant woman to come fasting the next day for a OGTT has the inherent risk of losing them to follow-up as they may not turn up as needed due to a plethora of reasons. Keeping in mind all the different challenges, there has been a need for an easy and economical single-step screening strategy that can help in picking up potential GDM cases early so that proper treatment can be given at the right time to prevent all the complications associated with GDM.

A prospective study performed in India established that a 2-hour PG ≥ 140 mg/dL with 75 g oral glucose administered to pregnant women in the fasting or nonfasting state can diagnose GDM irrespective of the last meal timing.[12] A normal woman without any dysglycemia would have a brisk and sufficient insulin response after a meal/glucose enough to maintain euglycemia. On the other hand, in a woman with GDM who has impaired insulin secretion, her glycemic levels would increase with a meal, and when challenged with glucose the glycemic excursion would be further exaggerated. Thus, the cut-off value of 2-hour plasma glucose above 140 mg/dL, which is considered impaired in nonpregnant adults, was proposed as the single-step cut-off value for diagnosing GDM in pregnant women. Even the National Institute for Health and Care Excellence (NICE) guidelines recommend 2-hour PG > 140 mg/dL as diagnostic criteria for GDM based on the study performed in multiethnic population of UK.[13]

The DIPSI in 2006 proposed this "single-step strategy" (Box 2).[14] of screening all pregnant women coming to antenatal care (ANC) clinic irrespective of their fasting/nonfasting state which has eventually been endorsed by the International Diabetes Federation (IDF), the International Federation of Gynecology and Obstetrics (FIGO) Society, and the World Health Organization (WHO) and has been approved by the Ministry of Health, Government of India.

BOX 2 DIPSI-GDM screening protocol.[14]

- In the antenatal clinic, a pregnant woman after undergoing preliminary clinical examination has to be given a *75-g oral glucose* dissolved in about 300 mL of water over 5–10 minutes *without regard to the time of the last meal.*
- *GDM is diagnosed if 2-hour plasma glucose is ≥140 mg/dL.*
- The first testing should be done during the first trimester as almost one-third of GDM-positive women are detected during this period or first antenatal contact as early as possible in pregnancy.
- If found negative at this time, the second screening test is to be performed again around 24–28th weeks.

(DIPSI: Diabetes in Pregnancy Study Group of India; GDM: gestational diabetes mellitus)

PROTOCOL FOR INVESTIGATION

The first screening procedure should be done during the first trimester itself as almost one-third of GDM-positive women are detected during this period or at the first antenatal contact as early as possible in pregnancy. The second testing should be done during 24–28 weeks of pregnancy. If the first test is negative, it is important to ensure second test as many pregnant women develop glucose intolerance during this period (24–28 weeks). If it could not be done during this time, then it can be done any time after 24 weeks of pregnancy with at least a month's gap between the two tests.

The test is to be conducted for all pregnant women even if she comes late in pregnancy for ANC clinic at the time of first contact. For women who present beyond 28 weeks of pregnancy, only one test is done at the first point of contact.

A few studies comparing the DIPSI criteria with the IADPSG 75-g OGTT have pointed out a few limitations of the DIPSI criteria as it tends to miss out on cases of fasting dysglycemia which are also seen in quite a few cases of hyperglycemia in pregnancy.[15,16] Hence, although the single-step or the two-step OGTT remains the standardized recommended tests for GDM screening globally as well as in urban India, DIPSI can be used as an effective screening tool in cases where it is not possible to carry out the fasting GTT due to different reasons, especially in primary health centers (PHCs) as well as resource-strapped areas.

CONCLUSION

Early diagnosis and optimum management of GDM is very important not only for preventing adverse maternofetal outcomes in the ongoing pregnancy, but also to institute effective preventive strategies for future risk of developing type 2 diabetes in the mother as well as her offspring. Although the one-step or two-step strategies recommended by the ADA are followed globally and even in urban India, they may be challenging to implement in a resource-strapped rural setting with poor healthcare infrastructure or poor patient compliance. In such settings, the single-step DIPSI screening strategy can be an effective step to diagnose GDM early in pregnant women and start an effective management plan to optimize outcomes and minimize complications.

REFERENCES

1. International Diabetes Federation (IDF). (2017). Gestational diabetes. [online] Available from https://www.idf.org/our-activities/care-prevention/gdm#targetText=Approximately%20half%20of%20women%20with,over%20the%20age%20of%2045. [Last accessed October, 2019].
2. American Diabetes Association. Diagnosis and Classification of Diabetes Mellitus. Diabetes Care. 2010;33(Suppl 1):S62-9.
3. Barbour LA. Diabetes and pregnancy. In: McDermott MT (Ed). Endocrine Secrets, 6th edition. Philadelphia: Elsevier Saunders; 2013. p. 45.
4. Seshiah V, Balaji V, Balaji MS, et al. Prevalence of gestational diabetes mellitus in South India (Tamil Nadu)—a community based study. J Assoc Physicians India. 2008;56:329-33.
5. Seshiah V, Balaji V, Balaji MS, et al. Pregnancy and diabetes scenario around the world: India. Int J Gynaecol Obstet. 2009;104 Suppl 1:S35-8.
6. Macintosh MC, Fleming KM, Bailey JA, et al. Perinatal mortality and congenital anomalies in babies of women with type 1 and type 2 diabetes in England, Wales, and Northern Ireland: population based study. BMJ. 2006;333(7560):177.
7. Lambert K, Germain S. Pre-existing type 1 and type 2 diabetes in pregnancy. Obstet Gynaecol Reprod Med. 2010;20(10):353-8.
8. Barbour LA, McCurdy CE, Hernandez TL, et al. Cellular mechanisms for insulin resistance in normal pregnancy and gestational diabetes. Diabetes Care. 2007;30 Suppl 2:S112-9.
9. Catalano PM, Huston L, Amini SB, et al. Longitudinal changes in glucose metabolism during pregnancy in obese women with normal glucose tolerance and gestational diabetes mellitus. Am J Obstet Gynecol. 1999;180(4):903-16.
10. Management of diabetes in pregnancy: standards of medical care in diabetes-2019. Diabetes Care. 2019;42(Suppl 1):S165-72.
11. Maternal Health Division. Ministry of Health & Family Welfare, Government of India. [online] www.mohfw.gov.in and www.nhm.gov.in. [Last accessed October, 2019].
12. Anjalkshi C, Balaji V, Balaji MS, et al. A single step procedure to diagnose gestational diabetes mellitus. Acta Diabetol. 2009;46(2):52-4.
13. National Institute for Health and Care Excellence (NICE). (2015). Diabetes in pregnancy: management from preconception to the postnatal period. [online] Available from https://www.nice.org.uk/guidance/ng3. [Last accessed October, 2019].
14. Seshiah V, Das AK, Balaji V, et al. Gestational diabetes mellitus—guidelines. J Assoc Physicians India. 2006;54:622-8.
15. Mohan V, Mahalakshmi MM, Bhavadharini B, et al. Comparison of screening for gestational diabetes mellitus by oral glucose tolerance tests done in the non-fasting (random) and fasting states. Acta Diabetol. 2014;51(6):1007-13.
16. Vij P, Jha S, Gupta SK, et al. Comparison of DIPSI and IADPSG criteria for diagnosis of GDM: a study in a north Indian tertiary care center. Int J Diabetes Dev Ctries. 2015;35(3):285-8.

CHAPTER 77 Medical Nutrition Therapy and Oral Therapy in Gestational Diabetes Mellitus

Purvi Chawla

INTRODUCTION

Pregnancy-driven complications like hypertensive disorders, gestational diabetes mellitus (GDM) and many others may arise from imbalanced, maternal nourishment, underlying inflammation and impaired glucose tolerance. While reporting a direct and continuous relationship between maternal hyperglycemia and perinatal complications, the Hyperglycemia and Adverse Pregnancy Outcomes Study clearly demonstrated that even mild hyperglycemia could have a negative impact on outcomes; necessitating meticulous management of the same to reduce perinatal morbidity and mortality.[1] Thus, we review the management of GDM using nutritional intervention and other medical measures in this chapter.

MEDICAL NUTRITION THERAPY (MNT)

Advances in nutritional sciences have made it possible for MNT, a customized nutritional plan drawn up by a qualified and experienced dietitian along with the patient, as the mainstay of managing GDM. Thus, MNT in GDM aims to provide optimal nutrition and calories for the developing fetus and mother without distorting diet preferences, maintaining maternal euglycemia, promoting appropriate gestational weight gain (GWG), imparting good nutritional patterns to the family "gatekeeper" and encouraging nutritional choices that prevent recurrence of GDM or onset of type 2 diabetes mellitus (T2DM). It also aims to ensure nutritional intervention for optimal fetal development and proper fetal programming.[2]

Due to inadequate evidence from non-extensive studies, there is a dearth of harmonious consensus statements globally recommending a specific caloric intake for women with GDM. The food plan from dietary reference intakes recommends at least 175 g of carbohydrate, 71 g of proteins and 28 g of fiber for every woman with GDM.[3] Not just the quantity of carbohydrates, but the type of carbohydrate is also important while prescribing MNT.

A systematic review[4] critically appraising MNT guidelines for GDM concluded that it requires enhanced dietitian-patient involvement, facilitators and monitoring tools for translating recommendations into practice. It suggested that future guidance documents should be high-quality based on evidence, clarity, pragmatism and individualization to support clinicians in improving outcomes for patients with GDM. Among 1,200 guidelines, only 21 fulfilled the criteria for the review. The majority (n = 13) of the guidelines provided evidence on GDM management with nutrition recommendations; some (n = 7) focused on MNT for diabetes with additional pointers for GDM. Most guidelines (at least 15) were written under the auspices of medical/professional/scientific organizations while few (n = 6) were drawn up under the auspices of governmental organizations. Different guidelines fared differently in terms of scope and purpose, stakeholder involvement, scientific vigor, clarity and applicability with most (n = 12) scoring above average (>50%) and a few (n = 7) scoring more than 90%.

The American College of Obstetricians and Gynaecologists (ACOG),[5] American Diabetes Association,[6] Academy of Nutrition and Dietetics,[7] Diabetes UK,[8] International Diabetes Federation (IDF)[9] and many other international societies have recommended MNT in pre-GDM, GDM, defined MNT and have recommend individualizing plans in a culture-sensitive manner with nutritional education.

The Ministry of Health and Family Welfare (New Delhi, India)[10] endorses an additional 350 kcal/day over the adult requirement during the second and third trimesters of pregnancy. As per the Indian Centre of Medical Research (ICMR) guidelines, an average weight gain of 10–12 kg is recommended using the following equations for calculating adult energy requirement:

Energy requirement (kcal/day) = BMR (basal metabolic rate) × PAL (physical activity level)

BMR (kcal/day) for adult females (18–30 years) = 14 × BW (kg) + 471

BMR (kcal/day) for adult females (30–60 years) = 8.3 × BW (kg) + 788,

where, BW is the body weight.

A simple calculation for the total energy requirement during pregnancy based on the level of physical activity is given in Table 1.

Table 2 describes the energy requirement during pregnancy based on the body mass index (BMI) level. Thus, moderate energy restriction of 30% of the estimated energy needs in obese women with GDM is associated with decreased complications, improved glycemia without causing ketonemia or decreased maternal weight gain.

In terms of the macronutrient distribution,[10] 50–60% of energy intake should be from complex carbohydrates (whole-grain cereals, whole pulses, vegetables and fruits) rather than simple carbohydrates, 10–20% from proteins; 20–30% from fats with saturated fat (coconut oil, ghee, palm oil, organ meat, full fat cream, red meat) content <10% of the total fat intake and regular fiber intake. A low-fat diet should be considered in obese women with GDM. It is also recommended that the carbohydrate-containing foods are spread over three small meals and 2–3 snacks per day with an aim to include 2–3 carbohydrate servings per meal and 1–2 carbohydrate servings per snack, by encouraging carbohydrate counting. Breakfast should include 1–2 carbohydrate servings and one protein-rich serving. The total protein intake should be increased by 23 g/day and distributed as three daily servings.

TABLE 1: Total energy requirement during pregnancy (based on physical activity level).

Level of activity	Energy requirement during pregnancy	Total energy requirement (kcal/d)
Sedentary work	1900 + 350	2250
Moderate work	2230 + 350	2580
Heavy work	2850 + 350	3200

TABLE 2: Energy requirement during pregnancy (based on the BMI).

Weight category	BMI (kg/m²)	Total energy requirement (kcal/day)
Underweight	<18.5	Energy requirement as per level of activity + 500 kcal/day
Normal weight	18.5–22.9	Energy requirement as per level of activity
Overweight	23–24.9	Energy requirement as per level of activity
Obese	>25	Energy requirement as per level of activity–500 kcal/day

(BMI: body mass index)

The ACOG and the Endocrine Society endorse low fat diets in GDM. In terms of other scientific evidence, meta-analyses[11] of 18 randomized controlled trials demonstrated an improvement in perinatal outcomes with dietary interventions as opposed to routine care in patients of GDM; underscoring the significance of MNT in GDM as the first line of treatment and also the need to develop the optimal guidance for MNT.

Restricting carbohydrates or increasing complex carbohydrates in the diet were studied and it was found that a higher complex carbohydrate/lower fat diet as compared to a low-carbohydrate/higher fat one, improved insulin resistance in the mother and adiposity in the infant.[12] A diet with consistent low glycemic index food items also resulted in lowered maternal insulin resistance, lower insulin doses and risk of macrosomia.[13]

Another trial found that dietary patterns with vegetables, fruits, fiber, fish, legumes, whole-wheat cereals and vegetable oil were associated with improvement in insulin sensitivity and inflammation. Among other trials evaluating potential benefits of dietary interventions in reducing the risk of GDM, the "Low-GI Diet in Pregnancy" study in 62 pregnant women randomized to receive either a diet low in glycemic index or a diet with high fiber and moderate-to-high glycemic index foods, found no difference in GDM incidence and fetal birth weight. No significant differences were found in the incidence of GDM in 100 pregnant women although there was significant less GWG with an intervention involving focused dietary counseling, encouraging exercise and advice regarding appropriate weight gain.

Studies that examined the effect of Dietary Approaches to Stop Hypertension (DASH) or Mediterranean (MED)[14] diets in approximately 460 women with or without GDM, found a negative relation with fasting blood glucose, glycated hemoglobin (HbA1c) or serum triglycerides with lower adherence. Patients with the greatest adherence to the MED and DASH diets respectively had an 80% and 71% lower risk for GDM ($p_{trend} = 0.006$) after adjusting for potential confounding factors.

Following this retrospective analysis, the St. Carlos GDM prevention[15] trial evaluated the MedDiet, reinforced with daily consumption of extra virgin olive oil (EVOO) (40 mL/day) and 25–30 g of nuts (pistachios), as an intervention-based diet in preventing GDM, cardiovascular disease (CVD) and T2DM, especially at 24–28 gestational weeks in approximately 1,000 pregnant women with less than 12 gestational weeks and normal glucose tolerance (NGT). Besides basic dietary and walking recommendations given to both the arms, the intervention arm received a unique 1-h group guidance session and EVOO and pistachios whereas the control arm received instructions to restrict dietary fat including EVOO and nuts. Overall, GDM rate was significantly reduced to 13.9% in the intervention arm as compared to the control arm (RR 0.81 (0.73–0.93), p<0.001); lower GWG (10.88 ± 6.46 vs 12.30 ± 5.42 kg, p = 0.013) in diabetic women; lower excessive weight gain in (RR 0.91 (0.86-0.96; p<0.001)) in GDM patients without significant increase of insufficient weight gain and lower rates of large/small for gestational age born babies in the intervention arm than in the control arm. In conclusion, dietary intervention like MedDiet earlier on during pregnancy reduced the incidence of GDM and prevented adverse maternal-fetal outcomes, demonstrating its effective use as the first-line therapy for GDM. The key attributes of this diet were polyunsaturated and monounsaturated fatty acids, high-quality vegetable protein, fiber, minerals, tocopherols, phytosterols and phenolic compounds in nuts that improved glycemia and the underlying inflammation.

A secondary analysis of the St. Carlos GDM Prevention study[16] was also conducted to compare the HbA1c levels at 36–38 gestational weeks in women with GDM as compared to those with NGT. Of the total 874 women included in the final analysis, 177 women were diagnosed with GDM while 697 had NGT. The MedDiet with daily EVOO of ≥40 mL and 25–30 g of pistachios continued throughout pregnancy. Although a significantly higher HbA1c level was observed in women with GDM (5.1% ± 0.3%) as compared to those with NGT (4.9% ± 0.3%, p = 0.001) at 24–28 gestational weeks. The levels were comparable at 36–38 gestational weeks with a similar trend observed in fasting serum insulin and homeostatic model assessment insulin resistance (HOMA-IR). A total of 26.6% of women with GDM required insulin therapy for glycemic management; higher rates of insufficient weight gain (39.5% vs. 22.0%, p = 0.001), small for gestational age (6.8% vs. 2.6%, p = 0.009) and neonatal intensive care unit admission (5.6% vs. 1.7%, p = 0.006) in women with GDM versus NGT. However, rates of macrosomia, large for gestational age, pregnancy-induced hypertensive disorders, prematurity and cesarean sections were comparable with women with NGT. A positive reinforcement of the intervention and higher adherence after the diagnosis of GDM was observed with lower weight gain in the intervention arm. Thus, universal and early (end of first trimester) nutritional intervention using the MedDiet reduced the incidence of GDM and other adverse outcomes while providing long-term benefits to the mother and offspring and translated observations to results.

Besides, the focus on macronutrients, guidelines also recommend supplementation with vitamins D and B12 during pregnancy, especially in vegetarians; abstinence from alcohol consumption and smoking, limiting non-nutritive sweeteners[7] and coffee consumption to not more than 300 mg/day and deciding a postpartum diet plan with the patient of GDM.

PHYSICAL ACTIVITY AND SELF-MONITORING OF BLOOD GLUCOSE

The keys to managing glycemic targets during pregnancy also include physical activity and exercise as medically advised, in the absence of complications and maintenance of a regular schedule of self-monitoring of blood glucose as decided between the treating physician and the patient, using home blood glucose meters. Enhanced physical activity and self-monitoring of blood glucose have been associated with improved HbA1c and perinatal outcomes.

ORAL THERAPY

Despite MNT, when blood sugars are not at target (fasting <95 mg/dL and post-meals < 120 mg/dL), medical management of GDM is recommended. In the US, India and many countries, insulin is the first drug of choice for the medical management of GDM.[3,10] The Indian guidelines suggest that metformin (500 mg of metformin twice daily up to a total dose of 2000 mg/day)[10] may be considered after 20 weeks of gestation for GDM whereas insulin may be started at any time during pregnancy. Although there was lower risk of neonatal hypoglycemia and lower weight gain in the mother taking metformin as opposed to insulin as reported in literature,[17,18] it was associated with premature delivery as metformin does cross the placenta and gets concentrated in the umbilical cord. The MiG TOFU (the Metformin in Gestational Diabetes: The Offspring Follow-Up), one of the largest studies conducted with metformin in pregnancy tracked up to 7–9 year old offspring exposed to metformin therapy for GDM and found that they were larger than those exposed to insulin.[19] Results of two large trials evaluating metformin use continued in pregnancy following polycystic ovarian syndrome, also demonstrated higher BMI and increased obesity in the offspring exposed to metformin at the 4-year follow-up; thus, clearly necessitating the need for long-term outcomes study in the offspring exposed to these drugs.[19] A systematic review and meta-analyses[20] of 28 randomized, controlled studies including 3976 participants from GDM-affected pregnancies either treated with metformin or insulin across various continents found that neonates born to metformin-treated mothers were significantly smaller than those treated with insulin during pregnancy. However, there was accelerated growth, higher weight and BMI by mid-childhood in those exposed to metformin *in utero* as compared to those treated with insulin. Trends of low-birth weight and post-natal catch-up growth with increased adiposity are potential risk factors for disturbances in long-term cardio-metabolic health; robust studies are required to evaluate the effect of intra-uterine exposure of metformin in the offspring.

Sulfonylureas and acarbose, a type of α-glucosidase inhibitor have also been used in pregnant women with GDM with varying success. Glyburide has been known to cross the placenta, found in high concentrations in the umbilical cord and was associated with neonatal hypoglycemia.[17,18] A systematic review and meta-analyses revealed that it caused more neonatal hypoglycemia and macrosomia as compared to insulin or metformin.[17] In one study, it was comparable with insulin based on the composite outcome of neonatal hypoglycemia, macrosomia and hyperbilirubinemia although long-term safety data for offspring were not available. In two large trials, 46% and 18% of women with GDM on metformin and glyburide, respectively progressed to insulin use.

A small case series of women treated with thrice a day, acarbose found that postprandial hyperglycemia was mitigated and infants were healthy. Another randomized controlled trial in Brazil[20] comparing insulin versus glyburide versus acarbose in 70 patients, reported no significant differences in LGA or cesarean section rates among any of the three treatment groups; however, acarbose had higher gastrointestinal adverse effects. Other classes of oral antidiabetic agents have none or limited data in pregnant women, hence should not be used.

CONCLUSION

Gestational diabetes mellitus provides a window of opportunity to the physician to understand the future metabolic risks in the patient and to intervene adequately in order to prevent adverse perinatal outcomes. When the patient with GDM and a well-qualified and experienced dietitian develop an individualized nutritional plan, i.e. MNT as therapy, it may be used as the first line of management in GDM. Physical activity and self-monitoring of blood glucose at a regular frequency also enhances glycemic control. If glycemic control is not achieved despite great adherence to MNT, insulin may be offered as the first line of medical management to the patient. According to the Indian guidelines, metformin may be used up to a maximum dose of 2 g/day in GDM post 20 gestational weeks although it crosses the placenta. The MiG TOFU study that tracked offspring of mothers exposed to metformin during GDM in pregnancy, found that it was associated with higher BMI and fat percentage at 7–9 years of age. Sulfonylureas and acarbose have been used with limited efficacy and require more robust studies to determine their efficacy and safety long-term on mothers and offspring. Due to inadequate data on the long-term effects of the intra-uterine exposure and trans-placental transfer of metformin and other oral drugs, they are not generally recommended as first-line treatment for GDM. Thus, there is no controversy that well-tailored MNT plans for patients of GDM provide long-term improvement in outcomes but also foster healthy eating in at least two generations—mother and the child.

REFERENCES

1. Metzger BE, Lowe LP, Dyer AR, et al. HAPO Study Cooperative Research Group. Hyperglycemia and adverse pregnancy outcomes. N Engl J Med. 2008;358:1991-2002.
2. Dabelea D, Mayer-Davis EJ, Lamicchane AP, et al. Association of intrauterine exposure to maternal diabetes and obesity with type 2 diabetes in youth: The Search case-control study. Diab Care. 2008;31(7):1422-6.
3. Management of diabetes in pregnancy: Standards of Medical Care in Diabetes—2019. Diab Care. 2019;42(Suppl.1):S165-S172.
4. Tsirou E, Grammatikopoulou MG, Theodoridis X, et al. Guidelines for Medical Nutrition Therapy in Gestational Diabetes Mellitus: Systematic Review and Critical Appraisal. J Acad of Nutr and Diet. 2019:119(8);1320-39.
5. Committee on Practice Bulletins – Obstetrics. ACOG Practice Bulletin No. 190: Gestational diabetes mellitus. Obstet Gynecol. 2018;131(2): e49-e64.
6. Management of diabetes in pregnancy. Standards of Medical Care in Diabetes -2018. Diab Care. 2018;41(Suppl 1):S137-S143.
7. Duarte-Gardea MO, Gonzales-Pacheco DM, Reader DM, et al. Academy of Nutrition and Dietetics gestational diabetes evidence-based nutrition practice guideline. J Acad Nutr Diet. 2018;118(9):1719-42.

8. Evidence-Based Nutrition Guidelines for the Prevention and Management of Diabetes. London: Diabetes UK; 2018.
9. IDF. Pregnancy and Diabetes: Global Guideline. Brussels, Belgium: International Diabetes Federation; 2009.
10. National Guidelines for Diagnosis and Management of Gestational Diabetes Mellitus. New Delhi: Indian Ministry of Health and Family Welfare; 2018.
11. Yamamoto JM, Kellett JE, Balsells M, et al. Gestational diabetes mellitus and diet: a systematic review and meta-analysis of randomized controlled trials examining the impact of modified dietary interventions on maternal glucose control and neonatal birth weight. Diab Care. 2018;41: 1346-61.
12. Hernandez TL. Carbohydrate content in the GDM diet: Two views: View 1: nutrition therapy in gestational diabetes: the case for complex carbohydrates. Diabetes Spectr. 2016;29:82-8.
13. Wei J, Heng W, Gao J. Effects of low glycemic index diets on gestational diabetes mellitus: a meta-analysis of randomized controlled clinical trials. Medicine. 2016;95:e3792.
14. Izadi V, Tehrani H, Haghighatdoost F, et al. Adherence to the DASH and Mediterranean diets is associated with decreased risk for gestational diabetes mellitus. Nutrition. 2016;32:1092-6.
15. Assaf-Balut C, García de la Torre N, Durán A, et al. A Mediterranean diet with additional extra virgin olive oil and pistachios reduces the incidence of gestational diabetes mellitus (GDM): A randomized controlled trial: The St. Carlos GDM prevention study. PLoS One. 2017;12(10):e0185873.
16. Assaf-Balut C, Garcia de la Torre N, Durán A, et al. Medical nutrition therapy for gestational diabetes mellitus based on Mediterranean Diet principles: a subanalysis of the St Carlos GDM Prevention Study. BMJ Open Diab Res Care. 2018;6:e000550.
17. Balsells M, García-Patterson A, Solà I, et al. Glibenclamide, metformin, and insulin for the treatment of gestational diabetes: a systematic review and meta-analysis. BMJ. 2015;350:h102.
18. Jiang Y-F, Chen X-Y, Ding T, et al. Comparative efficacy and safety of OADs in management of GDM: network meta-analysis of randomized controlled trials. J Clin Endocrinol Metab. 2015;100:2071-80.
19. Rowan JA, Rush EC, Plank LD, et al. Metformin in Gestational Diabetes: The Offspring Follow-Up (MiG TOFU): body composition and metabolic outcomes at 7-9 years of age. BMJ Open Diab Res Care. 2018;6:e000456.
20. Tarry-Adkins JL, Aiken CE, Ozanne SE. Neonatal, infant, and childhood growth following metformin versus insulin treatment for gestational diabetes: A systematic review and meta-analysis. PLoS Med. 2019.16(8): e1002848.

78 CHAPTER Is Metabolic Syndrome a Subclinical Cushing's Syndrome? Yes

Sunil Kumar Kota, Abhay Kumar Sahoo

INTRODUCTION

Metabolic syndrome (MetS) consists of a group of disorders including abdominal obesity, hyperglycemia, hypertension and altered lipid parameters like reduced high-density lipoprotein cholesterol (HDL-C) levels, and elevated triglycerides (TG).[1,2] The associated endothelial dysfunction and atherosclerosis increases the risk of diabetes by fivefold and cardiovascular disease (CVD) by twofold after 5–10 years.[3,4]

Subclinical Cushing's syndrome (SCS) refers to adrenocorticotropic hormone-independent subclinical hypercortisolism in absence of clear-cut Cushingoid phenotype and is usually seen in patients harboring adrenal incidentaloma.[5] In SCS, even a very low elevated serum cortisol level may lead to occurrence of metabolic and cardiovascular disorders including obesity, diabetes, hypertension, carotid atherosclerosis, and osteoporosis.[6]

The common characteristics of MetS and SCS suggest common etiology of excessive and prolonged glucocorticoid exposure. Both basal and stimulated cortisol values are higher in patients with MetS.[7] Hyperactivity of the hypothalamic-pituitary-adrenal (HPA) axis gives rise to functional hypercortisolism in MetS. Sometimes there are normal cortisol levels with increased activity at periphery. Chronic stress and/or low birth weight can both be associated with greater HPA axis responsiveness and increased circulating cortisol levels, which contributes to increased visceral fat deposition. Increased hepatic and adipose tissue activity of 11β-hydroxysteroid dehydrogenase type 1 (11β-HSD1) enzyme activity might give rise to several features of MetS. Furthermore, weight loss normalizes cortisol levels, reverses phenotypic abnormalities, and improves insulin resistance.[1,2]

SHARED FEATURES OF METABOLIC SYNDROME AND SUBCLINICAL CUSHING'S SYNDROME

Abdominal Obesity

Both MetS and SCS are characterized by a redistribution of adipose tissue from peripheral to central body regions including the truncal region and visceral depots, giving rise to central obesity.[2] Cortisol appears to play a role in adiposity in MetS with increased urinary free cortisol, being witnessed in patients with MetS.[8] Insulin sensitivity is inversely correlated with cortisol clearance, which is independent of body fat.[9] Glucocorticoids promote proliferation and differentiation of human adipocytes and the receptors are more abundantly present in visceral than in subcutaneous adipose tissue.[10] Additionally, they redistribute adiposity from peripheral to central depots, increase the number and size of fat cells, and stimulate lipolysis giving rise to release of free fatty acids into the circulation.[11] Glucocorticoids stimulate appetite, promote lipoprotein lipase and adipocyte differentiation more strongly in visceral than in subcutaneous adipocytes. The enzyme AMPK is known as the sensor of cellular energy status, in patients with SCS the AMPK activity is 70% lower in visceral adipose tissue giving rise to upregulation of fatty acid synthase (FAS). FAS promotes lipid storage in abdominal visceral tissue. Glucocorticoid mediated insulin resistance also plays a role in abdominal fat deposit.

There is increased responsiveness of the HPA axis to different stimuli including corticotropin-releasing hormone (CRH)-arginine vasopressin and the abdominal adiposity is associated with attenuated negative feedback in the HPA axis with reduced diurnal cortisol variation. The

TABLE 1: Role of cortisol in the pathogenesis of MetS and obesity.

Variables	Features of MetS
Higher fasting cortisol levels	• Central obesity • Waist circumference • TG levels • BP, fasting glucose • Insulin resistance
Increased urinary free cortisol excretion	Central obesity
	High TG and low HDL levels
Increased cortisol response to food intake	Central obesity
Increased cortisol response to low-dose ACTH test	Central obesity
Increased cortisol response to CRH-arginine vasopressin test	Central obesity
Resistance to low oral dexamethasone suppression test	Central obesity
Loss of diurnal cortisol variation	Central obesity

(ACTH: adrenocorticotropic hormone; CRH: Corticotropin-releasing hormone; HDL: high level lipoprotrion; MetS: metabolic syndrome; TG: triglycerides)

various abnormalities of disturbed HPA axis regulation and their correlation with various aspects of MetS are mentioned in Table 1.

In fact MetS is labeled as a Cushing's syndrome of visceral abdominal fat. Cortisol contributes to the pathogenesis of MetS at two different levels. First, there is an activation of the HPA axis, leading to abdominal fat deposit.[12]

Chronic stress, reduced duration of sleep, and low birth weight might give rise to central activation of the HPA axis. Second, there may be defective modulation of cortisol metabolism in abdominal tissues of patients with MetS, due to altered expression of 11β-HSD-1, which converts inactive cortisone to cortisol, the active metabolite.[13]

Hyperglycemia

Subclinical Cushing's syndrome represents an archetype of MetS. Glucocorticoid exposure leads to impaired insulin sensitivity in liver, adipose tissue, and skeletal muscle by its direct effect on insulin signaling pathways, glucose transport, glucose oxidation, and by an indirect effect on lipid metabolism and protein metabolism.[14] In fact increase in urinary free and serum overnight cortisol levels are associated with insulin resistance, assessed by using the homeostasis model assessment.[15] Additionally higher cortisol levels associated with a reduced insulin secretion as well. In subjects with MetS, there is a significant association between serum cortisol levels and fasting glucose concentration, which is due to effects of glucocorticoid on insulin secretion and hepatic gluconeogenesis and insulin secretion.[15]

Hypertension

Association between serum cortisol and systolic and diastolic blood pressure (BP) levels is well documented.[7] Stress might play a role by activating HPA axis and sympathetic nervous system, resulting in higher levels of urinary cortisol and catecholamine metabolites in patients with MetS and hypertension.[16] Reduction in nitric oxide (NO; a vasodilator) production or bioavailability and activation of endothelin system with increased endothelin-1 (ET-1) levels is associated with increased responsiveness to vasoconstrictors with reduced vasodilation in glucocorticoid mediated hypertension.[15] Hyperinsulinemia and insulin resistance induced release of ET-1 leads to renal injury, which can further potentiate hypertension. Again in insulin resistance, there is imbalance between pressor and dilator actions of insulin ultimately favoring a state of vasoconstriction.[17] Obesity, which is found both in MetS and SCS can give rise to hypertension by several mechanisms including increased sodium reabsorption, volume expansion, increased cardiac output and increased sympathetic nervous system, renin-angiotensin-aldosterone system activity mediated rise in systemic vascular resistance. Additionally leptin resistance, increase ET-1 along with decreased NO can also lead to hypertension.[17]

Dyslipidemia

Both MetS and SCS are associated with hypertriglyceridemia and low HDL-C concentration.[2,7] Sometimes, genetic variations in glucocorticoid receptors (GRs) can affect the activity of the HPA axis and metabolism of lipids in MetS (Fig. 1).[15]

Other Shared Features

Uric Acid

Both MetS and SCS are associated with elevation in serum uric acid (SUA) levels,[18] which is a predictor of cardiac and overall mortality in patients having coronary heart disease (CHD) or stroke and is also associated with elevated stroke risk in patients with or without CHD.[15] There is higher SUA

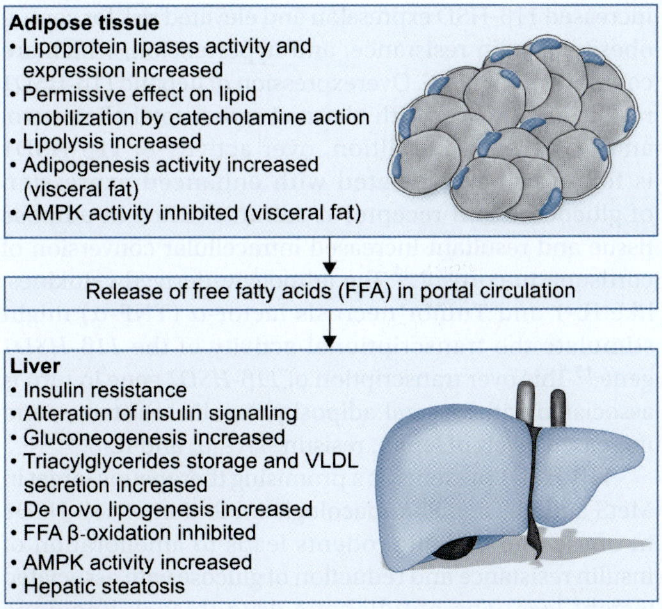

Figure 1 Glucocorticoids' effect on adipose tissue and hepatic fatty acid metabolism.

and urinary uric acid excretion in SCS as a consequence of hypercatabolic state and is correlated with overweight.[18]

Adipokines

Among the several bioactive peptides secreted by adipose tissue, the major components are adiponectin and leptin.[15] Both these proteins enhance insulin sensitivity by fatty acid oxidation. Additionally adiponectin has antidiabetic, antiatherogenic, and anti-inflammatory effects. Insulin resistance mediated leptin resistance and increased leptin. Resistin levels in obesity are associated with low level chronic systemic inflammation and thereby higher CVD risk.[19] Glucocorticoids downregulate adiponectin messenger ribonucleic acid (mRNA) and increase leptin levels in human visceral adipose tissue. In fact adrenalectomy and the resultant normalization of cortisol levels are associated with an increase in adiponectin and reduction in leptin levels.[20]

Endothelial Dysfunction and Hypercoagulability

Endothelial dysfunction is associated with both MetS and SCS, increasing predisposition to CVD.[1,2,4] The associated reduced NO and increased ET-1 concentrations contribute to the progression of atherosclerosis. The higher levels of homocysteine and fibrinogen in SCS and MetS make both the disorders a prothrombotic state, with increased risk of both CVD and venous thrombosis.[15] High cortisol levels are associated with increased activity of factors XII, XI, IX, and VIII, as well as plasminogen and α2-antiplasmin.[21] Additionally, there is increased concentration of von Willebrand factor with elevated thrombin and plasmin generation. There is defective fibrinolytic potential owing to high levels of plasminogen activator inhibitor-1 observed in both MetS and SCS, further contributing to hypercoagulability.

PLAUSIBLE MECHANISMS

Sleep Duration

Sleep deprivation is associated with increased cortisol levels at one hand; while on the other hand there is increased risk of MetS, type 2 diabetes mellitus (T2DM), hypertension, hypertriglyceridemia, and CVD.[22] Reduced sleep is associated with neuroendocrine dysregulation of appetite with reduction of anorexigenic hormone leptin and increase in orexigenic hormone ghrelin.[22] Therefore there is a speculation that shorter sleep duration associated elevated cortisol levels may have a pathogenetic mechanism in the generation of the MetS/SCS phenotype.

The Role of Stress

A variety of stressful situations including chronic work stress, low socioeconomic status, anxiety, and depression may augment neuroendocrine responses. Stress potentiates insulin resistance by activation of HPA axis and sympathetic nervous system leading to excessive cortisol production and intra-abdominal adiposity leading to development of MetS. In MetS, there is higher urinary excretion of cortisol metabolites, metanephrine, and elevated levels of interleukin 6 (IL-6) and C-reactive protein.[15] Chronic activation of HPA axis leads to greater cortisol reactivity and decreased diurnal variability of cortisol levels ultimately leading to central fat distribution.[9] In vitro, cortisol increases lipoprotein lipase levels in adipose tissue, which is a fat-storing enzyme and it is seen particularly in visceral fat.[23] Genetics does play a role in the relationship between stress and central fat, influencing psychological coping with stress and cortisol reactivity and variance in fat distribution.

Low Birth Weight

There is wealth of evidence pointing to association between low birth weight and increased prevalence of adult onset MetS and vascular diseases. There are subtle abnormalities of HPA axis, which may explain linkage between suboptimal fetal growth and adult onset MetS. There is glucocorticoid overproduction in fetal malnutrition, manifested in the form of elevated umbilical cord blood cortisol concentrations, as well as elevated excretion of glucocorticoid metabolites during childhood in low birth weight babies.[24] Indeed both birth and infant weights are inversely associated with the prevalence of impaired glucose tolerance (IGT) and T2DM.[25] This is in tune with experiments on pregnant rats, where it is shown that exposure to stressful stimuli like low-protein diet, nonabortive infections were associated with induction of corticosteroid secretion in adult life.[26]

11β-Hydroxysteroid Dehydrogenase

Overall, relative hypercortisolemia is contributory towards the development of varied features of MetS. However, role of glucocorticoids in pathogenesis of obesity is not clear. In fact circulating cortisol levels in obese subjects are not always elevated and may be lower in some cases than lean subjects.[27] This may possibly due to enhanced metabolic clearance of cortisol, leading to increased urinary excretion of free cortisol and metabolites because obese patients.[15]

As another determinant of cortisol action, the local tissue expression of 11β-HSD plays an important role in the interaction between cortisol and adiposity. 11β-HSD is an enzyme which catalyzes the conversion of the hormonally active C11-hydroxylated glucocorticoids (cortisol and corticosterone) to their inactive C11-keto metabolites (cortisone and 11-dehydrocorticosterone).[28] There are two isoforms of 11β-HSD—11β-HSD1 and 11β-HSD2. 11β-HSD2 is a high-affinity nicotinamide adenine dinucleotide-dependent dehydrogenase enzyme and it helps to protect the mineralocorticoid receptor in renal tubules from excess stimulation by cortisol. It is also found in the salivary glands, colon, and placenta. Mutation in the *11β-HSD2* gene leads to "syndrome of apparent mineralocorticoid excess", which is an inherited form of hypertension, where cortisol acts as a potent mineralocorticoid. On the other hand, 11β-HSD1 predominantly acts as a reductase to convert inactive cortisone to active cortisol. Therefore, 11β-HSD1 helps glucocorticoids to function effectively at target sites including liver and adipose tissue. It is also expressed in gonadal tissue and central nervous system. The 11β-HSD1 is expressed more abundantly in omental fat than subcutaneous fat. In obese subjects, 11β-HSD1 is responsible for higher intra-adipose cortisol levels in obese subjects.[24] In mice, the genetic experiments have documented association between increased 11β-HSD expression and elevated risk for central obesity, insulin resistance, and hypertension, which are components of MetS. Overexpression of hepatic 11β-HSD1 results in fatty liver with elevated serum total cholesterol and TG levels. In addition, over activity of 11β-HSD1 is found to be associated with enhanced expression of glucocorticoid receptor α subunit (GRα) in adipose tissue and resultant increased intracellular conversion of cortisone to cortisol.[29] The adipocyte-derived cytokines, like IL-1 and Tumor necrosis factor-α (TNF-α) might stimulate the transcriptional activity of the *11β-HSD1* gene.[15] This over transcription of *11β-HSD1* gene in turn is associated with visceral adiposity, insulin resistance, and increased levels of leptin, resistin, TNF-α, and IL-6.[30]

11β-HSD1 presents as a promising therapeutic target in MetS and obesity. Pharmacologic inhibition of 11β-HSD1 in obese and diabetic rodents leads to amelioration of insulin resistance and reduction of glucose with associated weight loss. The antidiabetic drug thiazolidinedione [peroxisome proliferator-activated receptor (PPAR)-γ agonists] inhibits the transcriptional activity of adipose tissue 11β-HSD1 leading to decrease in the tissue-specific concentration of glucocorticoids in humans. Other drugs tried to inhibit 11β-HSD1 include PPAR-α agonist (clofibrate), metformin, arylsulfonamidothiazoles, anilinothiazolones, and adamantyl triazoles.[15]

CONCLUSION

As MetS shares many characteristics of SCS, it is hypothesized that the pathogenesis of MetS and associated central obesity involves excessive and prolonged exposure to glucocorticoids. Patients with MetS reveal hyperactivity of the HPA axis leading to functional hypercortisolism. Stress, sleep deprivation, and low birth weight are all implicated in HPA axis activation in MetS. Simultaneously there is over expression of 11β-HSD1 enzyme in adipocytes, more so in central areas leading to increased conversion of cortisone to cortisol and in heightened tissue-specific glucocorticoid activity. Experimental studies with 11 β hydroxy steroid dehydrogenase 1 isoform (11β-HSD1) inhibitors leading to amelioration of components of MetS further point to the role of 11β-HSD1 in the pathogenesis of MetS. This provides a window of opportunity for these novel therapeutic approaches in patients with obesity or MetS.

REFERENCES

1. Obunai K, Jani S, Dangas GD. Cardiovascular morbidity and mortality of the metabolic syndrome. Med Clin North Am. 2007;91:1169-84.
2. Third Report of the National Cholesterol Education Program (NCEP) Expert Panel on Detection, Evaluation, and Treatment of High Blood Cholesterol

in Adults (Adult Treatment Panel III) final report. Circulation. 2002;106: 3143-421.

3. Kolovou GD, Anagnostopoulou KK, Salpea KD. The prevalence of metabolic syndrome in various populations. Am J Med Sci. 2007;333:362-71.
4. Athyros VG, Mikhailidis DP, Papageorgiou AA, et al. Prevalence of atherosclerotic vascular disease among subjects with the metabolic syndrome with or without diabetes mellitus: the METS-GREECE Multicentre Study. Curr Med Res Opin. 2004;20:1691-701.
5. Terzolo M, Pia A, Reimondo G. Subclinical Cushing's syndrome: definition and management. Clin Endocrinol (Oxf). 2012;76:12-8.
6. Anagnostis P, Karagiannis A, Tziomalos K, et al. Adrenal incidentaloma: a diagnostic challenge. Hormones (Athens). 2009;8:163-84.
7. Misra M, Bredella MA, Tsai P, et al. Lower growth hormone and higher cortisol are associated with greater visceral adiposity, intramyocellular lipids, and insulin resistance in overweight girls. Am J Physiol Endocrinol Metab. 2008;295:E385-92.
8. Pasquali R, Cantobelli S, Casimirri F, et al. The hypothalamic-pituitary-adrenal axis in obese women with different patterns of body fat distribution. J Clin Endocrinol Metab. 1993;77:341-6.
9. Holt HB, Wild SH, Postle AD, et al. Cortisol clearance and associations with insulin sensitivity, body fat and fatty liver in middle-aged men. Diabetologia. 2007;50:1024-32.
10. Rebuffe´-Scrive M, Walsh UA, McEwen B, et al. Effect of chronic stress and exogenous glucocorticoids on regional fat distribution and metabolism. Physiol Behav. 1992;52:583-90.
11. Rebuffe´-Scrive M, Krotkiewski M, Elfverson J, et al. Muscle and adipose tissue morphology and metabolism in Cushing's syndrome. J Clin Endocrinol Metab. 1988;67:1122-8.
12. Pasquali R, Vicennati V. The abdominal obesity phenotype and insulin resistance are associated with abnormalities of the hypothalamic-pituitary-adrenal axis in humans. Horm Metab Res. 2000;32:521-5.
13. Rosmond R, Dallman MF, Bjorntorp P. Stress-related cortisol secretion in men: relationships with abdominal obesity and endocrine, metabolic and hemodynamic abnormalities. J Clin Endocrinol Metab. 1998;83:1853-9.
14. Chanson P, Salenave S. Metabolic syndrome in Cushing's syndrome. Neuroendocrinology. 2010;92 Suppl 1:96-101.
15. Anagnostis P, Athyros VG, Tziomalos K, et al. Clinical review: The pathogenetic role of cortisol in the metabolic syndrome: a hypothesis. J Clin Endocrinol Metab. 2009;94(8):2692-701.
16. Brunner EJ, Hemingway H, Walker BR, et al. Adrenocortical, autonomic, and inflammatory causes of the metabolic syndrome: nested case-control study. Circulation. 2002;106:2659-65.
17. Karagiannis A, Mikhailidis DP, Athyros VG, et al. The role of renin-angiotensin system inhibition in the treatment of hypertension in metabolic syndrome: are all the angiotensin receptor blockers equal? Expert Opin Ther Targets. 2007;11:191-205.
18. Faggiano A, Pivonello R, Melis D, et al. Nephrolithiasis in Cushing's disease: prevalence, etiopathogenesis, and modification after disease cure. J Clin Endocrinol Metab. 2003;88:2076-80.
19. Bakhai A. Adipokines-targeting a root cause of cardiometabolic risk. Q J Med. 2008;101:767-76.
20. Ashizawa N, Takagi M, Seto S, et al. Serum adiponectin and leptin in a patient with Cushing's syndrome before and after adrenalectomy. Intern Med. 2007;46:383-5.
21. Patrassi GM, Dal Bo Zanon R, Boscaro M, et al. Further studies on the hypercoagulable state of patients with Cushing's syndrome. Thromb Haemost. 1985;54:518-20.
22. Spiegel K, Leproult R, Van Cauter E. Impact of sleep debt on metabolic and endocrine function. Lancet. 1999;354:1435-9.
23. Rebuffe-Scrive M. Neuroendocrine regulation of adipose tissue: molecular and hormonal mechanisms. Int J Obes. 1991;15 Suppl 2: 83-6.
24. Clark PM, Hindmarsh PC, Sheill AW, et al. Size at birth and adrenocortical function in childhood. Clin Endocrinol (Oxf). 1996;45:721-6.
25. Fall CH, Osmond C, Barker DJ, et al. Fetal and infant growth and cardiovascular risk factors in women. BMJ. 1995;310:428-32.
26. Reul JM, Stec I, Wiegers GJ, et al. Prenatal immune challenge alters the hypothalamic-pituitary-adrenocortical axis in adult rats. J Clin Invest. 1994;93:2600-7.
27. Travison TG, O'Donnell AB, Araujo AB, et al. Cortisol levels and measures of body composition in middle-aged and older men. Clin Endocrinol (Oxf). 2007;67:71-7.
28. Espíndola-Antunes D, Kater CE. Adipose tissue expression of 11β-hydroxysteroid dehydrogenase type 1 in Cushing's syndrome and in obesity. Arq Bras Endocrinol Metab. 2007;51:1397-403.
29. Iwasaki Y, Takayasu S, Nishiyama M, et al. Is the metabolic syndrome an intracellular Cushing state? Effects of multiple humoral factors on the transcriptional activity of the hepatic glucocorticoid-activating enzyme (11β hydroxysteroid dehydrogenase type 1) gene. Mol Cell Endocrinol. 2008;285:10-8.
30. Tomlinson JW, Moore J, Cooper MS, et al. Regulation of expression of 11 β hydroxysteroid dehydrogenase type 1 in adipose tissue: tissue-specific induction by cytokines. Endocrinology. 2001;142:1982-9.

79 CHAPTER Diet is a Magic Pill for Diabetes

Aravinda Jagadeesha

INTRODUCTION

India is the diabetes capital of the world! More than 60 million Indians are diagnosed with diabetes—including, children, young adults, and pregnant women. More often than not, a poor diet, a sedentary lifestyle, and genetics cause diabetes in most people. While not much can be done about the genes you have inherited, changing your diet and lifestyle can help to manage and prevent diabetes.

A healthy eating pattern, regular physical activity, and often pharmacotherapy are key components of diabetes management. For many individuals with diabetes, the most challenging part of the treatment plan is determining what to eat.[1]

The general approach to diabetes in our contemporary times is to start with a "diet". It is a much maligned word, which evokes dread in a lot of common folk. These days, the intellectuals among the population would like to refer to this approach as medical nutrition therapy, abbreviated as MNT, so as to also avoid bringing to the fore even the word "nutrition". This word "nutrition" is also widely bandied about in almost the same context as "diet", which means the much of the negativity of the word "diet" also rubs on to "nutrition" as well. Even though clichéd, "diet", still is important to the management of diabetes, the benefits include—improved metabolic control, weight loss, and reduced risk of vascular disease.[2]

Due to its wide global prevalence, diabetes is keenly studied both academically and clinically. With such level of interest, it is only natural that we are the recipients of huge caches of scientific data on this subject. In recent years, data, from the laboratory and from patient interactions, are pointing toward certain key conclusions—the importance of key nutrients, certain foods, and patterns of diet are necessary for preventing and managing type 2 diabetes.[3] Fats and carbohydrates are crucial but what stands apart is that the quality of the dietary fats and carbohydrates consumed is vital than the amount of these macronutrients ingested. Diets consisting of whole grains, fruits, vegetables, nuts, and legumes; low in refined grains, red or processed meats, and sugar-sweetened beverages along with moderate alcohol intakes are ideal in the case of preventing and managing diabetes. Studies have shown that such diets reduce the risk of diabetes and improve glycemic control. Also, they help to regulate blood lipids in patients with diabetes. In a highly globalized world, dietary patterns from different cultures and geographies can be used to create specialized diets plan tailored for diabetes such as Mediterranean diet, low glycemic index diet, moderately low carbohydrate diet, and vegetarian diets. These plans can be tailored to personal and cultural food preferences as well as for appropriate calorie needs for weight control and for diabetes prevention and management. In developed nations, there has been much progress in the development and implementation of evidence-based nutrition plans, but a concerted worldwide effort along with global policies has been sadly lacking. A more global effort is needed to alleviate global and regional disparities.[4]

Management of diabetes goes hand in hand with dietary and lifestyle modifications. The objectives in managing diabetes are:

- Maintaining normal glucose levels
- Maintaining normal lipid profile and ideal body weight
- Optimal nutrition intake
- Relieving symptoms and minimize chronic degenerative vasculopathies.

Interestingly, a diabetic diet is good for healthy non-diabetic subjects as well, as it meets the daily nutrition intake requirements. These dietary recommendations are evidence based and emphasize more on quality of fat and carbohydrate than quantity alone.[5]

Prediabetes may be understood as impaired fasting glucose (IFG) and impaired glucose tolerance, or clinically diagnosed by having an HbA1c value of 6.0–6.4% (42– 46 mmol/mol). Prediabetes also could entail an independent risk for cardiovascular disease along with the risk of developing type 2 diabetes. Thus, prediabetes risk prevention approaches must also address the prevention of cardiovascular risks along with managing progressive dysglycemia.[6]

Of all the various nutrition-based strategies for managing type 2 diabetes, a personal individualized approach was observed to have the most success. This sort of an approach would consider the cultural influences, nutritional sources, and personal preferences while devising the nutritional plan. Also, along with the earlier considerations, the strategy would also consider bringing in variety in the food as long as they are from the five main food groups. It has been observed that extreme restrictions in diets and exclusion of certain groups of food like dairy and grains may result in weight loss in the short term but may not be a sustainable option on the long term. The best diet should be sustainable, this means that the diet should be able to meet the nutritional intake daily which would help in maintaining an ideal weight, stabilize the blood levels of glucose and other lipids. Dietary consideration should also account for the inclusion of fruits, vegetables, vegetable oils with low content of saturated fat (olive oil), nuts, legumes, unrefined grain (with high fiber content) and fish. Along with these, another key consideration is to limit the intake of highly processed foods.[4]

A short summary of the prevalent dietary approaches is given below.

MEDITERRANEAN DIET PLAN

Mediterranean diet plan may refer to the one that comprises at least two of the following components:[7]

- The diet components have a high monounsaturated to saturated fat ratio
- The diet component consists of low-to-moderate red wine consumption
- The diet component comprises high intake of legumes
- The diet component comprises high intake of grains and cereals
- The diet component comprises high intake of fruits and vegetables
- Low consumption of meat and meat-based products and increased consumption of fish
- The diet component comprises moderate consumption of milk and dairy products.

A Mediterranean kilojoule-reduced diet is known to achieve weight loss and also shows improvement in controlling blood pressure and triglyceride levels. One key benefit of a Mediterranean diet is its suitability for a vegan, vegetarian, or meat-eating palette.[7]

LOW-CARBOHYDRATE DIET PLAN

Based on the quantitative amount of carbohydrates, there are different descriptions in clinical trials, and thus making broad judgments of their effectiveness is rather difficult. Examples could include:

- *Low-carbohydrate ketogenic diet (LCKD)*: <50 g of carbohydrates (10% kilojoules) daily
- *Low-carbohydrate diet (LCD)*: 50–130 g carbohydrates (10–26% of kilojoules) daily
- *Moderate carbohydrate diet (MCD)*: 130–225 g carbohydrates daily (26–45% of kilojoules) daily.

The effects on improved glycemia and weight reduction across this range of diets may be possible due to restrictions in kilojoules. No significant superiority among the various diets was observed in long-term as well as short-term studies.[8,9]

INTERMITTENT OR ALTERNATE DAY FASTING VERSUS CONTINUAL CALORIE RESTRICTION

In the case of the 5:2 diet, despite its popularity, no significant differences in glucose control were observed in a review. In the case of the continual calorie restriction (CCR), more weight loss was observed but both diets produced comparable reductions in visceral fat weight. The review concluded with calls for more research to identify specific benefits in using this approach to manage type 2 diabetes. Interestingly, to avoid hypoglycemia in patients on oral sulfonylureas or insulins, they need to be carefully assessed while fasting.[10]

VERY LOW-ENERGY DIET PLAN

Such an approach may be a useful intervention in adults with a BMI > 30 kg/m^2, or with a BMI > 27 kg/m^2 and T2DM (as per NHMRC guidelines).[11] This sort of an intervention could be effective in achieving weight loss.

LOW-GLYCEMIC INDEX DIET PLAN

This diet plan contains foods with low-glycemic index. Studies in type 2 diabetes case have shown some benefits though the reduction of HbA1c levels (up to 0.5%) was observed to have fewer hypoglycemic events. However, in comparison to other load diets, this dietary approach did not achieve additional weight loss.[12]

ALCOHOL

It is recommended that diabetic patients do not consume alcohol when driving as alcohol and hypoglycemia can have a synergistic effect on cognitive functions. The case against alcohol strengthens as alcohol is known to aggravate existing comorbidities (e.g. liver disease, neuropathy).[13]

LOW-KILOJOULE SWEETENERS

A broad analysis of multiple independent trials pointed to a small amount of weight loss with the use of low-kilojoule sweeteners. In the type 2 diabetes patients, use of such sweeteners could be helpful for weight maintenance. Their ability to assist in prevention of complications in such patients is, however, unsure.[14]

PATIENTS USING INSULIN

Use of ketogenic diets and other low-carbohydrate dietary approaches may cause hypoglycemia in patients with type 2 diabetes. This would complicate the matching of glucose self-monitoring to medical supervision of insulin dose adjustment.[15]

DIET AND HYPOGLYCEMIA[16]

In a situation when the glucose level in blood is <4 mmol/L and patient is symptomatic, awake, and can swallow, the patient is to be managed as per Rule 15 in the following manner:

- 15 g of fast-acting carbohydrate, which is easy to consume, to be provided to the patient [e.g. half a can of regular (non-diet) soft drink, half a glass of fruit juice, 3 teaspoons of sugar or honey, 6–7 jellybeans, and 3 glucose tablets].
- Wait for 15 minutes and recheck the blood glucose levels. If the levels are not rising, suggest eating another quick-acting carbohydrate from the above list.
- In case the patient's next meal is more than 15 minutes away, provide some longer acting carbohydrate (e.g. a sandwich, 1 glass of milk or soy milk, 1 piece of fruit, 2–3 pieces of dried apricots, figs or other dried fruit, 1 tub of natural low-fat yoghurt, 6 small dry biscuits, and cheese).
- Test glucose again during the next 2–4 hours.

DIET AND NEPHROPATHY

A broad statistical evaluation of 13 randomized clinical trials involving 779 patients showed minor evidence that a lowered protein diet assisted with diabetic nephropathy. Using pharmacotherapy and a sodium-restricted diet along with tight control on glycemic and lipid profiles would help to underpin the long-term prevention of this condition in management of hypertension.[17]

CONCLUSION

The model diet for prevention and the management of type 2 diabetes remains an individualized and sustainable dietary approach. This should be able to achieve and maintain an ideal weight range along with addressing major comorbidities such as cardiovascular diseases.

The best way to address weight management is using different dietary approaches to kilojoule restriction [including very low-energy diet (VLED) approaches] that synergistically act with increasing physical activity.

Of the multiple approaches, the diet which has accumulated the most evidence showing cardiovascular risk reduction is the Mediterranean diet. A general protocol of a structured team-based approach will assist the physician in providing a support framework integrating the various dietary principles to support the ever increasing number of identified patients needing dietary advice.

REFERENCES

1. Innucchi E, Bergenstal R, Buse J, et al. Management of hyperglycaemia in type 2 diabetes, 2015: a patient centered approach. Update to a Position Statement of the American Diabetes Association and the European Association for the Study of Diabetes. Diabetes Care. 2015;38(1):140-9.
2. Sawyer L, Gale EA. Diet, Delusion and Diabetes. Diabetologia. 2009;52(1):1-7.
3. Westman EC, Yancy WS, Humphreys M. Dietary treatment of diabetes mellitus in the pre-insulin era (1914–1922). Perspect Biol Med. 2006;49(1):77-83.
4. Portero McLellan KC, Wyne K, Villagomez ET, et al. Therapeutic interventions to reduce the risk of progression from prediabetes to type 2 diabetes mellitus. Ther Clin Risk Manag. 2014;10:173-88.

5. Ramchandran A, Snehalatha C, Vishwanathan V. Dietary management of Diabetes Mellitus in India and South East Asia. In: Defronzo RA, Ferrannini E, Keen H, Zimmet P (Eds). International Textbook of Diabetes Mellitus, 3rd edition. UK: John Wiley & sons Ltd.; 2004.
6. Twigg S, Kamp M, Davis T, et al. Prediabetes: a position statement from the Australian Diabetes Society and Australian Diabetes Educators Association. Med J Aust. 2007;186(9):461-65.
7. Rees K, Hartley L, Flowers N, et al. 'Mediterranean' dietary pattern for the primary prevention of cardiovascular disease. Cochrane Database Syst Rev. 2013;8:CD009825.
8. Santos FL, Esteves SS, Da Costa Pereira A, et al. Systematic review and meta-analysis of clinical trials of the effects of low carbohydrate diets on cardiovascular risk factors. Obes Rev. 2012;13(11):1048-66.
9. Schwingshackl L, Hoffmann G. Long-term effects of low-fat diets either low or high in protein on cardiovascular and metabolic risk factors: a systematic review and meta-analysis. Nutr J. 2013;12:48.
10. Barnosky AR, Hoddy KK, Unterman TG, et al. Intermittent fasting vs daily calorie restriction for type 2 diabetes prevention: a review of human findings. Transl Res. 2014;164(4):302-11.
11. National Health and Medical Research Council. (2013). Clinical practice guidelines for the management of overweight and obesity in adults, adolescents and children in Australia. [online] Available from https://www.nhmrc.gov.au/sites/default/files/documents/reports/clinical%20guidelines/n57-obesity-guidelines-.pdf. [Last accessed October, 2019].
12. Thomas D, Elliot EJ. Low glycaemic index, or low glycaemic load, diets for diabetes mellitus. Cochrane Database Syst Rev. 2009;(1):CD006296.
13. Australian Government Department of Health. Australian guidelines to reduce health risks from drinking alcohol. Canberra: Commonwealth of Australia. [online] Available from www.alcohol.gov.au/internet/alcohol/publishing.nsf/Content/guidelines. [Last accessed October, 2019].
14. Miller PE, Perez V. Low-calorie sweeteners and body weight and composition: a meta-analysis of randomized controlled trials and prospective cohort studies. Am J Clin Nutr. 2014;100(3):765-77.
15. Kelly T, Dyson P. Evidence-based nutrition guidelines for the prevention and management of diabetes. London: Diabetes UK, 2011. [online] Available from www.diabetes.org.uk/documents/reports/nutritional_guidelines 200911.pdf. [Last accessed October, 2019].
16. American Diabetes Association. Lifestyle Management: Standards of Medical Care in Diabetes—2019. Diabetes Care. 2018;42(Supplement 1):S46-S60.
17. Nezu U, Kamiyama H, Kondo Y, et al. Effect of low-protein diet on kidney function in diabetic nephropathy: meta-analysis of randomised controlled trials. BMJ Open. 2013;3:e002934.

80 CHAPTER Reversal of Diabetes: Myth or Reality? A Reality!

Minal Mohit

INTRODUCTION

"Can type 2 diabetes mellitus (T2DM) be treated or reversed? What is the best way of attaining this? Is there any point ahead of which this condition cannot be reversed?"

Every year millions of people around the globe learn that they have T2DM. At the same time millions of people are still missed. Every time the diagnosis is declared to the patient, the common queries that cross the mind of every individual and that every physician is bound to answer are the ones as stated above. So far diabetes has the reputation of being a chronic and irreversible disease. Now, with a better understanding about reversal of the disease, this missed diagnosis or early diagnosis becomes extremely relevant. The time lost is the opportunity lost to revert diabetes. In the World Health Organization (WHO) Global Report 2016, which is on diabetes, a section has been added on reversal on diabetes. It was acknowledged in the report that diabetes can be reversed by calorie restriction and weight loss.[1]

Few terms need to be clarified to know whether the concept of reversal of diabetes is a myth or reality.

Cure

The patient is healed of the disease and the good health has been restored. The risk of recurrence of the disease is small. The term "cure" has not been applied to T2DM, as there does exist the potential for re-occurrence.

Remission

A decrease in or disappearance of signs and symptoms of the disease, so that it does not need pharmacological treatment but it does exist and needs to be taken care of in terms of lifestyle management to maintain the target parameters. A hemoglobin A1c (HbA1c) under the diabetes threshold of 6.5% for an extended period of time without the use of glycemic control medications would qualify for the term remission.[2] Here, metformin is excluded from the glycemic control medications list, as it has indications beyond diabetes. Thus, a patient maintaining HbA1c <6.5% only on metformin can be said to be in the phase of remission.[3,4]

Partial Remission

Here, some, but not all, signs and symptoms of the disease have disappeared. In case of T2DM, the target parameters are not in normal range but below the treatment thresholds. "Partial" remission is when HbA1c <6.5% without glycemic control medications for 1 year.

Complete Remission

Here, all signs and symptoms of the disease disappear, although the disease still persists in the body. In reference to T2DM, the target parameters are within the normal range of the disease free population. "Complete" remission of diabetes is when HbA1c <5.7% without glycemic control medications for 1 year.[5]

Reversal

This means to change drastically or completely the course or effect of the disease, i.e. to initiate recovery or to reverse the disease and restore health. After diagnosis, T2DM has been treated back to below target parameters and is maintained in subclinical state without pharmacological treatment. Diabetes reversal is a term that describes significant improvement in insulin production in the body or effective response of the body to insulin.

Chronic

A disease requiring long term, may be life time, pharmacological management and care.

Conventional Theory

Type 2 diabetes mellitus is a lifelong progressive disorder. The underlying pathophysiology is mainly due to two factors:

1. Insulin resistance, i.e. tissues losing their ability to respond normally to insulin, leading to hyperinsulinemia.
2. Beta cell failure.

The lifelong status of the disease is due to insulin resistance, which remains unchanged over the period of time. Whereas, it is the beta-cell apoptosis, which is the ongoing process that makes the disease progressive. Keeping in mind the above facts, all the patients at diagnosis are informed about lifelong management of the disease, which they need to do as best as possible.[6,7]

Most of the researches so far have always targeted insulin resistance either by drugs or lifestyle management to treat the disease. β-cell dysfunction has proved less amenable to therapy. As already 50% of the function is lost by the time the disease is diagnosed and continue to decline over time irrespective of the treatment interventions by drugs or life style modification (LSM), also irrespective of the glycemic control.

THE TWIN-CYCLE HYPOTHESIS

The hypothesis, which states that the abnormalities of insulin secretion and resistance underlying T2DM has a single, common etiology, i.e. excess accumulation of lipid in the liver and pancreas,[8] gives an unified hypothesis for explaining a common disease. It also provided a common target to knock down for reversing diabetes.

For explaining the potential nutritionally dependent reversal of T2DM, a twin cycle hypothesis was formulated. As per this hypothesis, excess of calories over many years results in accumulation of fat in the liver, and therefore leads to liver insulin resistance. Continuously, liver makes glucose that is only inhibited through insulin action. The liver insulin resistance induced by fat causes a slight increase in the fasting plasma glucose and initiates an increase in production of insulin. As high levels of insulin initiate conversion of carbohydrate to fat in liver, a vicious cycle initiates. The excess liver fat is also expected to result in increased export of fat to the entire body, which can be consumed by many tissues, including pancreatic B cells. Intrapancreatic fat accumulated, thus, causes a decrease in acute insulin production. The drop in insulin production causes postmeal hyperglycemia, which, in turn, would result in higher insulin levels and a greater fat deposition.

AT HEPATIC LEVEL

More than a decade ago, the plasma levels of the liver enzyme alanine aminotransferase (ALT) and triglyceride have been shown to increase steadily over the 18 months prior to T2DM diagnosis.[9]

Overall, the increasing ALT concentrations seen prior to the diagnosis of T2DM[9] tend to indicate increasing accumulation of hepatic fat and gradually resistance to increasing hepatic insulin.

AT PANCREATIC LEVEL

It is an age old concept that fat can impair B-cell function.[10,11] Early studies conducted by Clark et al.[12,13] demonstrated that the ultrastructural intracellular damage in B cells of rodent and insulin-secreting cell lines caused due to fairly reduced levels of saturated fatty acids. Addition of hyperglycemia possibly compound the metabolic insult initiated by fat.[14,15]

People clearly vary in susceptibility to the harmful effects of increased intraorgan accumulation of fat. Importantly, it was predicted by the hypothesis that if the main driver of the twin cycles can be reversed, through negative calorie balance, then T2DM could resolve in some, perhaps many, people.

No correlation exists between indices of insulin secretion and pancreatic fat; this suggests that for such toxic intermediaries, there are individual thresholds of tolerance instead of a simple dose-response relationship within the pancreas.

REVERSAL HYPOTHESIS

Body utilizes its supplies of stored energy, when there is sudden calorie restriction in T2DM patients. This leads to:

- First, the fat that is stored in the liver is used and both the hepatic insulin resistance and the fasting plasma glucose decrease.
- Second, fat content of pancreas reduces and insulin secretion induced by glucose normalizes.

The twin defect of insulin resistance and beta cell failure that underlies the T2DM pathogenesis can be reversed by the acute negative energy balance alone.

Fasting blood glucose and hepatic insulin sensitivity reduce to normal and intrahepatic lipid reduce by 30% in the first 7 days of the decreased energy intake. Beta-cell function increases toward normal and pancreatic fat reduces over the 8 weeks of dietary energy restriction.

In a typical group of people (n = 11) having T2DM, the COUNTERPOINT (counteracting pancreatic inhibition of insulin secretion by triglyceride) study[16] was successful in attaining a 15.3 kg weight loss in the planned 8-week period. The levels of fasting plasma glucose normalized within 7 days of starting sudden negative calorie balance in counterpoint, although metformin was withdrawn on day 1 of the diet. Over the same time course, hepatic insulin sensitivity and liver fat levels also normalized, returning to levels noted in weight-matched nondiabetic control participants (n = 8) within the 7 days. In the study, fat content of pancreas reduced and the first-phase insulin response increased gradually and normalized by 8th week. There was a paradigm shift in findings as it was earlier believed that restoration of normal first-phase insulin secretion cannot be attained among people having T2DM. Therefore, the predictions of the twin-cycle hypothesis had been confirmed.

In counterpoint and subsequent studies, a diet-only approach was followed for achieving the essential 15-kg average weight loss as commencement of exercise programs can induce compensatory eating, and thus limit weight loss.[17-19] However, a very significant component of long-term avoidance of weight regain is a sustained increase in daily physical exercise.[20]

SUCCESS

The steps that can be used to reverse diabetes:
The first step toward reversing diabetes is to prevent the spikes in insulin production. Research shows that this can be done through either or combination of low-carbohydrate diets, very low calorie diets, exercise, and bariatric surgery.

METHODS OF REVERSAL

This is indicated by a significant number of studies that diabetes reversal can be achieved by using bariatric surgery, carbohydrate restriction (LC), and low-calorie diets (LCD).

BARIATRIC SURGERY

For both morbid obesity and the metabolic processes that accompany it, particularly T2DM, bariatric surgery has long been identified as a potential treatment. The efficacy of T2DM reversal depends on the procedure selection; however, there is unilateral improvement in glycemia after operation.[8] It has been reported that bariatric surgery is superior as compared to intensive T2DM medical management. Accordingly, in 2016, the Second Diabetes Surgery Summit (DSS-II) issued recommendations, which were endorsed by 45 medical and scientific societies globally, for using bariatric surgery as a treatment option for T2DM; currently, bariatric surgery is approved by the 2016 recommendations for adults having a body mass index (BMI) >40 kg/m^2 or >35 kg/m^2 along with comorbidities related with obesity.[21] Of interest is the consistent finding present in studies that glycemic improvements take place rapidly, usually within hours to days, and precede loss of weight, which possibly represents the enteroendocrine responses to altered flow of the intestinal contents (i.e. bile acid signaling and alterations in microbiota and their metabolome).[22-28] Laparoscopic and robotic Roux-en-Y gastric bypass (RYGB) or sleeve gastrectomy (SG) are the most commonly performed bariatric surgeries. Surgical treatment is based on the principles of intestinal malabsorption and restriction; however, it is suggested by evidence that there are more complex mechanisms at play. It has been consistently demonstrated that bariatric surgery dramatically and rapidly improves blood glucose levels,[29] while allowing reduced use of oral hypoglycemic medications and insulin that effectively reverses diabetes in nearly 80% of the patients[30] in the short term. Along with the early postoperative improvement in levels of blood glucose and insulin sensitivity, has also been demonstrated that bariatric surgery cause alterations in gastrointestinal (GI) hormone release, comprising leptin, ghrelin, peptide-tyrosine-tyrosine (PYY), glucagon-like peptide 1 (GLP-1), and cholecystokinin (CCK), which can effect feeding behavior through the gut-brain axis along with modulating euglycemia.[31] Moreover, microbial alterations in the human gut have been related to obesity. Surgical changes in GI anatomy have been related with dramatic alterations in the gut microbiota populations with reversion from an "obesogenic" to a lean bacterial population.[22,23,25,28,32,33]

DURABILITY OF THE REVERSAL OF TYPE 2 DIABETES AFTER THE RETURN TO NORMAL EATING

There is a requirement of long-term studies and data for answering this question. However, a general understanding of the concept directs the dictum that reversal is retained as long as the weight regain is prevented. Durability of returning to nondiabetic plasma glucose levels will ensure broader clinical applicability of a nutritional and behavioral approach for attaining long-term isocaloric eating following the acute weight loss.

The COUNTERBALANCE (counteracting β-cell failure by long-term action for normalizing calorie intake) study[34] included rapid weight loss, stepped food reintroduction over 2 weeks, and then 6 months of follow-up by specialists in a research center. In this study, patients were divided into two groups: less than 4 years duration group (n = 15); more than 8 years duration group (n = 14). For inducing weight loss, a liquid diet replacement was used, which was followed by stepped reintroduction of normal foods. Then, supportive follow-up was done emphasizing on the portion size and regular check-ups of body weight. There was no significant weight regain. In contrast, the group lost nearly 14 kg body weight and maintained postweight loss normalization of blood glucose control. The overall remission rate [HbA1c less than 6.5% (48 mmoL/moL) on two occasions, minimum 2 months apart][35] continued to be constant (60% in the short-duration group and 21% in the long-duration group) in the 6-month follow-up.

These findings were extended in the DiRECT trial (Diabetes Remission Clinical Trial),[36,37] that was conducted completely in primary care. DiRECT was much larger as compared to the Counterpoint and Counterbalance studies. There were total 149 subjects in both the intervention group and the control group. Those participants who had T2DM for up to 6 years were included in the study. At 12 months, the mean weight loss in the intervention group was 10 kg (that was analyzed on an intention-to-treat basis). After 12 months, diabetes remission was attained in 46% (n = 68) of 149, and 36% (n = 53) of 149 at 24 months in the intervention group, of all the antidiabetic drugs. In both the DiRECT study and the Counterbalance study, people who had reversed their T2DM following weight loss stayed diabetes free, if they avoided subsequent weight regain.

There are some long-term data available from the Look Ahead study.[38] It reported that mean weight loss was found to be greater in the intensive lifestyle group than the control group receiving standard management by 3.9% after 4 years of follow-up. It was related with 5.3% more participants who underwent remission of the T2DM. In Look Ahead, the focus was on diet as well as on intensive exercise programs from the outset that are not easily sustained, and thus could have resulted in more weight regain. To note, population of The Look Ahead study was different from the direct population in significant ways. In Look Ahead, at the start of the study, nearly a fifth of the patients were on insulin. The median duration of diabetes was longer (5 years in comparison to 3 years in direct). Many participants had diabetes for >10 years. There was a difference in ethnic mix also; nearly 60% were white in Look Ahead, while this figure was approximately 100% in DiRECT. These two trials are therefore not easily comparable. There were many individuals who continued to have BMI more than 30 kg/m^2 after attaining remission of T2DM, the implications of which should be considered. Following acute weight loss, mean BMI was in the Counterbalance study and DiRECT study was 28.6 kg/m^2 and 31.5 kg/m^2, respectively. Therefore, nearly half of the each group remained obese. Therefore, a significant question was if the remaining excess fat might redistribute into the liver and pancreas, when isocaloric eating was resumed. Baseline mean liver fat content in Counterbalance study and DiRECT study was 12.8% and 16.0%, respectively. In Counterbalance study, weight loss was found to be associated with a reduction in liver fat to 2% (low normal) in individuals who reversed their diabetes; this level remained unchanged after 6-month follow up. In the DiRECT Study participants, liver fat content reduced to 3.3% following rapid weight loss and a return to isocaloric eating (5 months), and then to 3.0% at 12 months. It seems that if total body fat burden reduces below an individual threshold, and if this fall is retained, then ectopic fat does not reaccumulate. This finding is in agreement with the personal fat threshold concept[39] that is supported by genetic data relating limited capacity for subcutaneous fat storage with cardiometabolic disease.[40] This suggests BMI to be only a very general guide to a healthy metabolic weight for a person. For pancreatic fat, a parallel pattern of change was noted. Although self-reported observations were open to bias, they suggest that people who lost substantial weight through change in diet remained free of diabetes over many years, if weight regain was avoided.[40,41]

CHALLENGES

Reversal of diabetes, is it a reality? Is it always possible? Or is it the result of some short-term studies? Conducted on a limited population data with selection bias? So there are questions unanswered, there are challenges to overcome. One of the important question: Can T2DM of any duration be reversed?

The Counterpoint study enrolled people having T2DM up to 4 years following diagnosis. However, finding out the effect of a longer duration of diabetes on reversibility was essential. Thus, the subsequent counterbalance study[34] enrolled individual diagnosed with T2DM for 0.5–23 years. By the end of the first week of the study, all 29 participants demonstrated an improvement in fasting plasma glucose.[34] Out of the 15 people, 87% (n = 13) who were diagnosed with diabetes for <4 years attained nondiabetic concentration of fasting plasma glucose (less than 7 mmoL/L). In the subgroup that had been diagnosed for <4 years, the mean fasting plasma glucose after 6 months was 5.8 (se 0.2) mmoL/L. In individuals diagnosed for 8–12 years, it was 6.2 (se 0.7) mmoL/L. For those who were diagnosed for 12 years or more, it was 10.6 (se 1.7) mmoL/L. None of the patients who were diagnosed with diabetes for >11 years returned to nondiabetic fasting plasma glucose concentrations. Probably, the crucial mechanism underlying the conversion to T2DM in susceptible people is loss of the specialized β-cell phenotype (dedifferentiation).[15,42-45] The markers of dedifferentiation are expressed in the beta-cells from pancreas of people having T2DM.[46-48] It is not agreed upon by everyone that dedifferentiation is the only process underlying beta-cell dysfunction in T2DM; however, if this state remains too long in a person, it could lead to irreversible loss of endocrine function. Now, the histological and cell biological processes can be combined with observations during clinical reversal of the disease process.[49] The histological findings of substantially lower number of beta-cell seems likely to associate to the insulin immunostain, such that beta-cells that stopped producing insulin were simply not recognized, and incorrectly considered to be nonviable instead of nonfunctional.

DIFFERENCES BETWEEN PREDIABETES AND POSTDIABETES

Although there are many people achieving and maintaining substantial weight loss return to a state of normal glucose metabolism, other individuals achieve an HbA1c that is nondiabetic (<48 mmoL/moL), but it is not in the normal range. Is this possible that this group re-enter the prediabetes zone? Can such individuals be clubbed with the prediabetes cohort? Or does a different label is required for them?

There was a substantial improvement in individuals in their overall likelihood of long-term good health. Their blood glucose as well as the parallel blood pressure and lipids demonstrate improvements. The Counterbalance study group was supervised for avoiding weight regain during 6-month follow-up. There was a substantial improvement in mean blood pressure and lipids.[34] The 10-year cardiovascular risk, which was assessed by the Q risk score,[50] reduced on average from 23% to 7% in individuals that attained remission in this closely supervised study. In this group, the average age of participants was 55 years. The calculated heart age fell from 71 years to 56 years. In DiRECT, it was reported that in the second year, serious adverse events were substantially lower. This was mainly due to reduced numbers of major vascular events and cancers, although numbers were too small for showing statistical significance in each category.[37] As per the Swedish obese subjects study, weight loss induced by the bariatric surgery brought a 32% reduced risk for macrovascular complications in comparison with the control group in a 15-year follow-up period.[51] When considered together, it was suggested by the findings that major health gains are a result of avoidance of weight gain.

Now, a term is needed for describing people who achieved stable weight with normalized intrapancreatic and intrahepatic fat and reversed their T2DM. Approximately, two-thirds of the individuals in remission in the DiRECT study attained normal fasting plasma glucose and HbA1c. For the third individuals who persisted below the diabetic range but not in the normal range, it would be incorrect to designate these individuals as having prediabetes, because this state is related with cardiovascular risk (associated primarily to the related dyslipidemia). It was proposed that their metabolic condition would be best known as postdiabetes, maintaining the fact that they would remain susceptible to diabetes if weight regain occurs.[52] The return to the previous weight seems to be related uniformly with return of diabetes as evaluated both by informal observation of former study participants, and from the 24-month data of DiRECT.[37] In the DiRECT trial, individuals who were in remission at 12 months but returned to the diabetic state at 24 months regained 7.1 (SD 5.4) kg over this time interval.[37] Those in the postdiabetes state do not have diabetes, and this is significant for insurance purposes; it is also a motivating factor in avoiding weight regain.

It is essential to provide ongoing support for people with postdiabetes as adequate weight regain will enhance the likelihood of diabetes returning.

It is very unlikely that microvascular complications will occur or advance in the postdiabetes state, as noticed after transplantation of pancreas in type 1 diabetes or following bariatric surgery-induced remission of T2DM.[51,53] However, if there is presence of moderately severe retinopathy, then there is a risk of worsening to proliferative retinopathy or treatable maculopathy after the sudden reduction in plasma glucose concentrations.[54,55] Imaging of retina within 4–6 months is needed for people in the postdiabetes state with more than minimal retinopathy.

FUTURE QUESTIONS

Restriction of calories for achieving substantial weight loss and remission of T2DM has been noticed previously[56,57], which raise the question of how the initial advantage provided by a low-calorie liquid diet can be best maintained. It has been emphasized by the recent National Dietary Guidelines that there is a need to provide individualized advice, instead of only one dietary prescription for every individual. Further, high-quality studies are required in primary care for assessing the dietary advice and the nature of the behavioral support that is provided for maintaining remission of T2DM.

Genetic traits appear probably to underlie the variable susceptibility of people to fat-induced beta-cell dedifferentiation, considering the fact that 72% of the people having a BMI >40 kg/m^2 do not have diabetes.[58] These traits possibly operate through both β-cell susceptibility and capacity for safe, subcutaneous storage of fat. There are a large numbers of T2DM people who have a normal BMI (less than 25 kg/m^2); 16% are above 55 years and 10% are in the age range of 16–54 years.[59] To note, all studies on reversing T2DM have enrolled people having a BMI >27 kg/m^2. Thus, it is unknown if people having T2DM as well as normal BMI can also undergo T2DM reversal through calorie restriction-induced weight loss. In this group, it is possible that is an enhanced proportion of individuals who have been not diagnosed correctly and in fact have maturity onset diabetes of the young or slow-onset type 1 diabetes. There could also be unidentified diagnostic categories, though the concept that T2DM itself has more than one cause appears to be unlikely.

The beta-cell factors preventing return to normal plasma glucose control require to be recognized, as weight loss of >15 kg did not reverse T2DM in 5 (14%) out of 36 individuals who were diagnosed with T2DM for up to 6 years in the DiRECT study.[60] Likewise, weight loss of >25 kg following bariatric surgery did not cause remission of diabetes in 13 (39%) out of 33 individuals who were diagnosed as having T2DM for an average of 10 years.[61]

CONCLUSION

A survey was conducted by The James Lind Alliance, in association with Diabetes UK, including people having T2DM to establish their priorities for the research. First research priority was "can T2DM be treated or reversed? What is the best way of achieving this? Is there any point ahead of which the condition cannot be reversed?

Type 2 diabetes is a condition which develops in people consuming more calories than their requirement over a long period of time. There is accumulation of more fat than the individual's body can safely store, which result in excess pancreatic and liver fat and subsequent loss of plasma glucose control. The susceptibility to excess fat appears to differ considerably among individuals. In the early years following onset of diabetes, the removal of excess fat in the pancreas and liver through intensive but achievable weight loss can in several cases result in normalization of hepatic glucose production and possible redifferentiation of beta-cells, and diabetes can be reversed. Now, American Diabetes Association (ADA) identifies remission as an appropriate aim of management.[23] For the benefit of patients, physicians must grasp this paradigm shift in the understanding of T2DM. It has major implications for information that should be given to newly diagnosed patients, who should be aware that they have a potentially reversible condition and not the one that is inevitably progressive.

Established T2DM is now considered to be a reversible condition in the early years. The underlying mechanism includes removal of the excess fat from liver and pancreas in the susceptible people. It was reported by the Diabetes Remission Clinical Trial that nearly half of a primary care population of people having T2DM of <6 years of duration can be returned to nondiabetic blood glucose control that lasts for minimum 12 months. A vital part of our clinical strategy is reframing mass provision of weight loss support for prevention and treatment of T2DM. However, the existing obesogenic environment is a reality in which people must live. A personal account including information about achieving substantial weight loss and maintaining it gives an invaluable insight into the encountered practical problems. This understanding should be assimilated and expressed by all health professionals dealing with weight control.

Effective prevention and long-term reversal of T2DM is possible. This includes the postdiabetes group, and varies significantly from the high cardiovascular risk state of prediabetes. Existing data show long-term stable beta-cell function, which shows that weight regain is prevented. If a person, who has previously demonstrated susceptibility to T2DM, regains their previous weight then recurrence of the condition is certain. It is recommended that the words "reversal" and "remission" be used appropriately with emphasis on the inadequacy of the word "cure".

Bariatric surgery, LC and VLC are evidence-based means of attaining and maintaining remission of T2DM. With increasing duration of T2DM, there is steadily diminishing chance of achieving reversal.

REFERENCES

1. World Health Organization. Global Report on Diabetes. 2016. Available from: https://www.who.int/diabetes/publications/grd-2016/en/. [Last accessed October 2019).
2. Ramos-Levi AM, Cabrerizo L, Matia P, et al. Which criteria should be used to define type 2 diabetes remission after bariatric surgery. BMC Surgery. 2013;13:8.
3. Xiang AH, Trigo E, Martinez M, et al. Impact of gastric banding versus metformin on β-cell function in adults with impaired glucose tolerance or mild type 2 diabetes. Diabetes Care. 2018;41:2544-51.
4. Diabetes Prevention Program Research Group. Long-term effects of metformin on diabetes prevention: Identification of subgroups that benefited most in the diabetes prevention program and diabetes prevention outcomes study. Diabetes Care, 2019;dc181970.
5. Buse JB, Caprio S, Cefalu WT, et al. How do we define cure of diabetes? Diabetes Care. 2009;32:2133-5.
6. Huang CJ, Lin CY, Haataja L, et al. High expression rates of human islet amyloid polypeptide induce endoplasmic reticulum stress mediated β-cell apoptosis, a characteristic of humans with type 2 but not type 1 diabetes. Diabetes. 2007;56:2016-27.
7. Laybutt DR, Preston AM, Akerfeldt MC, et al. Endoplasmic reticulum stress contributes to beta cell apoptosis in type 2 diabetes. Diabetologia. 2007;50:752-63.
8. Steven S, Carey PE, Small PK, et al. Reversal of Type 2 diabetes after bariatric surgery is determined by the degree of achieved weight loss in both short- and long-duration diabetes. Diabet Med. 2015;32: 47-53.
9. Sattar N, McConnachie A, Ford I, et al. Serial metabolic measurements and conversion to type 2 diabetes in the West of Scotland Coronary Prevention Study: specific elevations in alanine aminotransferase and triglycerides suggest hepatic fat accumulation as a potential contributing factor. Diabetes. 2007;56:984-91.
10. McGarry JD. Banting lecture 2001: dysregulation of fatty acid metabolism in the etiology of type 2 diabetes. Diabetes. 2002;51:7-18.
11. Unger RH. Lipotoxicity in the pathogenesis of obesity-dependent NIDDM: genetic and clinical implications. Diabetes. 1995;44:863-70.
12. Pinnick K, Neville M, Clark A, et al. Reversibility of metabolic and morphological changes associated with chronic exposure of pancreatic islet β-cells to fatty acids. J Cell Biochem. 2010;109:683-92.
13. Pinnick KE, Collins SC, Londos C, et al. Pancreatic ectopic fat is characterized by adipocyte infiltration and altered lipid composition. Obesity (Silver Spring). 2008;16:522-30.
14. Poitout V, Amyot J, Semache M, et al. Glucolipotoxicity of the pancreatic beta cell. Biochim Biophys Acta. 2010;1801:289-98.
15. Wang Z, York NW, Nichols CG, et al. Pancreatic β cell dedifferentiation in diabetes and redifferentiation following insulin therapy. Cell Metab. 2014;19:872-82.
16. Lim EL, Hollingsworth KG, Aribisala BS, et al. Reversal of type 2 diabetes: normalisation of beta cell function in association with decreased pancreas and liver triacylglycerol. Diabetologia. 2011;54:2506-14.
17. Finlayson G, Bryant E, Blundell JE, et al. Acute compensatory eating following exercise is associated with implicit hedonic wanting for food. Physiol Behav. 2009;97:62-7.
18. Hopkins M, Blundell JE, King NA. Individual variability in compensatory eating following acute exercise in overweight and obese women. Br J Sports Med. 2014;48:1472-6.
19. King NA, Horner K, Hills AP, et al. Exercise, appetite and weight management: understanding the compensatory responses in eating behaviour and how they contribute to variability in exercise-induced weight loss. Br J Sports Med. 2012;46:315-22.
20. Wing RR, Phelan S. Long-term weight loss maintenance. Am J Clin Nutr. 2005;82(Suppl 1): 222S–5S.
21. Rubino F, Nathan D, Eckel RH, et al. Delegates of the 2nd Diabetes Surgery Summit. Metabolic surgery in the treatment algorithm for type 2 diabetes: A joint statement by International Diabetes Organizations. Diabetes Care. 2016;39:861-77.
22. Anhe FF, Varin TV, Schertzer JD, et al. The Gut Microbiota as a Mediator of Metabolic Benefits after Bariatric Surgery. Can J Diabetes. 2017;41:439-47.
23. Medina DA, Pedreros JP, Turiel D, et al. Distinct patterns in the gut microbiota after surgical or medical therapy in obese patients. Peer J. 2017;5:e3443.
24. Magouliotis DE, Tasiopoulou VS, Sioka E, et al. Impact of bariatric surgery on metabolic and gut microbiota profile: A systematic review and meta-analysis. Obes Surg. 2017;27:1345-57.
25. Murphy R, Tsai P, Jullig M, et al. Differential changes in gut microbiota after gastric bypass and sleeve gastrectomy bariatric surgery vary according to diabetes remission. Obes Surg. 2017;27:917-25.
26. Kaska L, Sledzinski T, Chomiczewska A, et al. Improved glucose metabolism following bariatric surgery is associated with increased circulating bile acid concentrations and remodeling of the gut microbiome. World J Gastroenterol. 2016;22:8698-719.
27. Penney NC, Kinross J, Newton RC, et al. The role of bile acids in reducing the metabolic complications of obesity after bariatric surgery: a systematic review. Int J Obes (Lond). 2015;39:1565-74.
28. Sweeney TE, Morton JM. The human gut microbiome: A review of the effect of obesity and surgically induced weight loss. JAMA Surg. 2013;148:563-9.
29. Rubino F, Gagner M. Potential of surgery for curing type 2 diabetes mellitus. Ann Surg. 2002;236:554-9.
30. Cohen R, Caravatto PP, Correa JL, et al. Glycemic control after stomach-sparing duodenal-jejunal bypass surgery in diabetic patients with low body mass index. Surg Obes Relat Dis. 2012;8:375-80.
31. Federico A, Dallio M, Tolone S, et al. Gastrointestinal hormones, intestinal microbiota and metabolic homeostasis in obese patients: Effect of bariatric surgery. In Vivo. 2016;30:321-30.
32. Peat CM, Kleiman SC, Bulik CM, et al. The intestinal microbiome in bariatric surgery patients. Eur Eat Disord Rev. 2015;23:496-503.
33. Sweeney TE, Morton JM. Metabolicsurgery: Action via hormonal milieu changes, changes in bile acids or gut microbiota? A summary of the literature. Best Pract Res Clin. Gastroenterol. 2014;28:727-40.
34. Steven S, Hollingsworth KG, Al-Mrabeh A, et al. Very low calorie diet and 6 months of weight stability in type 2 diabetes: pathophysiological changes in responders and nonresponders. Diabetes Care. 2016;39:158-65.
35. McCombie L, Leslie W, Taylor R, et al. Beating type 2 diabetes into remission. BMJ. 2017;358:j4030.
36. Lean ME, Leslie WS, Barnes AC, et al. Primary care-led weight management for remission of type 2 diabetes (DiRECT): an open-label, cluster-randomised trial. Lancet. 2017;391:541-51.
37. Lean ME, Leslie W, Barnes AC, et al. Durability of a primary careled weight management intervention for remission of type 2 diabetes: 2-year results of the DiRECT open-label, cluster randomised trial. Lancet Diabetes Endocrinol. 2019;7:344-55.
38. Gregg EW, Chen H, Wagenknecht LE, et al. Association of an intensive lifestyle intervention with remission of type 2 diabetes. JAMA. 2012;308:2489-96.

39. Taylor R, Holman R. Normal weight individuals who develop type 2 diabetes: the personal fat threshold. Clin Sci (Lond). 2015;128: 405-10.
40. Lotta LA, Gulati P, Day FR, et al. Integrative genomic analysis implicates limited peripheral adipose storage capacity in the pathogenesis of human insulin resistance. Nat Genet. 2017;49:17-26.
41. Peters C, Steven S, Taylor R. Reversal of type 2 diabetes by weight loss despite presence of macro- and micro-vascular complications. In: Draznin B (Ed). Diabetes case studies: real problems, practical solutions. Alexandria: American Diabetes Association; 2015. pp. 271-4.
42. Doughty R. Type 2 diabetes and the diet that cured me. The Guardian, May 12, 2013. https://www.theguardian.com/lifeandstyle/2013/may/12/type-2-diabetes-diet-cure. [Last Accessed October, 2019].
43. Brereton MF, Iberl M, Shimomura K, et al. Reversible changes in pancreatic islet structure and function produced by elevated blood glucose. Nat Commun. 2014;5:4639.
44. Spijker HS, Song H, Ellenbroek JH, et al. Loss of β-cell identity occurs in type 2 diabetes and is associated with islet amyloid deposits. Diabetes. 2015;64:2928-38.
45. Talchai C, Xuan S, Lin HV, et al. Pancreatic β cell dedifferentiation as a mechanism of diabetic β cell failure. Cell. 2012;150:1223-34.
46. White MG, Marshall HL, Rigby R, et al. Expression of mesenchymal and α-cell phenotypic markers in islet β-cells in recently diagnosed diabetes. Diabetes Care. 2013;36:3818-20.
47. Cinti F, Bouchi R, Kim-Muller JY, et al. Evidence of β-cell dedifferentiation in human type 2 diabetes. J Clin Endocrinol Metab. 2016;101: 1044-54.
48. Sun J, Ni Q, Xie J, et al. B-Cell dedifferentiation in patients with T2D with adequate glucose control and nondiabetic chronic pancreatitis. J Clin Endocrinol Metab. 2019;104:83-94.
49. White MG, Shaw JAM, Taylor R. Type 2 diabetes: the pathologic basis of reversible β-cell dysfunction. Diabetes Care. 2016;39:2080-88.
50. QRISK. The QRISK2–2017 risk calculator. QRISK, 2017. https://qrisk.org/2017/ [Last Accessed October, 2019].
51. Sjostrom L, Peltonen M, Jacobson P, et al. Association of bariatric surgery with long-term remission of type 2 diabetes and with microvascular and macrovascular complications. JAMA. 2014;311:2297-304.
52. Taylor R, Barnes AC. Can type 2 diabetes be reversed and how can this best be achieved? James Lind Alliance research priority number one. Diabet Med. 2019;36:308-15.
53. Pearce IA, Ilango B, Sells RA, et al. Stabilisation of diabetic retinopathy following simultaneous pancreas and kidney transplant. Br J Ophthalmol. 2000;84:736-40.
54. Arun CS, Pandit R, Taylor R. Long-term progression of retinopathy after initiation of insulin therapy in type 2 diabetes: an observational study. Diabetologia. 2004;47:1380-84.
55. Kroc Collaborative Study Group. Diabetic retinopathy after two years of intensified insulin treatment: follow-up of the Kroc Collaborative Study. JAMA. 1988;260:37-41.
56. Henry RR, Wallace P, Olefsky JM. Effects of weight loss on mechanisms of hyperglycemia in obese non-insulin-dependent diabetes mellitus. Diabetes. 1986;35:990-8.
57. Wing RR, Blair E, Marcus M, et al. Year-long weight loss treatment for obese patients with type II diabetes: does including an intermittent very-low-calorie diet improve outcome? Am J Med. 1994;97:354-62.
58. Gregg EW, Cheng YJ, Narayan KM, et al. The relative contributions of different levels of overweight and obesity to the increased prevalence of diabetes in the United States: 1976–2004. Prev Med. 2007;45:348-52.
59. Public Health England. Adult obesity and type 2 diabetes. July 2014. https://assets.publishing.service.gov.uk/government/uploads/system/uploads/attachment_data/file/338934/Adult_obesity_and_type_2_diabetes_.pdf [Last Accessed October, 2019].
60. Taylor R, Al-Mrabeh A, Zhyzhneuskaya S, et al. Remission of human type 2 diabetes requires decrease in liver and pancreas fat content but is dependent upon capacity for β cell recovery. Cell Metab. 2018;28:547-56.e3.
61. Steven S, Carey PE, Small PK, et al. Reversal of type 2 diabetes after bariatric surgery is determined by the degree of achieved weight loss in both short- and long-duration diabetes. Diabet Med. 2015;32:47-53.

81 CHAPTER What is Next after Metformin: Is Pioglitazone Written Off? Yes

Pratap P Jethwani

INTRODUCTION

Type 2 diabetes is a chronic progressive metabolic disorder characterized by persistent hyperglycemia and it's associated long-term complications resulting in reduced survival along with diminished quality of life.[1] It is increasing globally, particularly in India, requiring particular attention to early diagnosis and effective management to prevent long-term complications.[1] Metformin is endorsed by majority of organizations across the globe as the first-line therapy for management of hyperglycemia in type 2 diabetes unless it is contraindicated. Unfortunately, metformin is not a very powerful and durable antihyperglycemic agent so it may require addition of other agents for glycemic control over a period of time. As per the recent American Diabetes Association (ADA) and European Association for Study of Diabetes (EASD) consensus statement for management of hyperglycemia in diabetes,[2] when metformin monotherapy is not able to reach glycemic targets, one may add any of the available therapies based on various factors like drug efficacy, impact on hypoglycemia risk and body weight, history of atherosclerotic cardiovascular disease or heart failure or renal disease, potential side effects, delivery method (oral versus subcutaneous), cost, and patient preferences. As far as glycemic efficacy is concerned, all agents including thiazolidinediones (TZDs) have almost equivalent A1c lowering effect as an add on to metformin therapy. TZDs (including pioglitazone) have always raised controversies and came under scanner of global drug regulating agencies because of their association with a number of serious side effects. Rosiglitazone was withdrawn from global market because of it's association with an increased risk of cardiovascular events and all-cause mortality (hazard ratio [HR] 1.68 [95% CI 1.27–2.08]) as per a report from the U.S. Food and Drug Administration (FDA).[3] Because of an increased risk of bladder cancer among patients treated with pioglitazone versus placebo in the prospective pioglitazone clinical trial in macrovascular events (PROactive),[4] this drug was banned in 2005 in many countries including India. Pioglitazone is associated with a number of serious adverse events.

BODY WEIGHT GAIN

Many studies of TZDs reported weight gain of ~5 kg over 3–5 years. As per meta-analysis of randomized controlled trials (RCTs) of pioglitazone,[5] it can lead to an increase in body weight by 2.06 kg (WMD: 2.06 kg, 95% CI: 1.11–3.01). Weight gain induced by pioglitazone is not only due to fluid retention but there is also expansion of adipose tissue resulting in an increase in body fat. In a subgroup analysis of The Actos Now (ACT NOW) for the Prevention of Diabetes study, which measured changes in body composition, body weight increased 4.63 ± 0.60 kg in pioglitazone group as compared to 0.98 ± 0.62 kg in placebo group and body fat increased by 4.89 ± 0.42 kg in the pioglitazone group compared to 1.41 ± 0.44 kg in placebo group.[6] This increase in fat is more in legs and trunk as compared to arms and long-term effects of this weight gain are still not studied properly.

FLUID RETENTION AND EDEMA

Glitazones can lead to peripheral edema in 5–10% of patients when used as monotherapy and this may increase to 15–20% when combined with insulin.[7]

As per meta-analysis of RCTs of pioglitazone, there was an increased risk of edema (RR: 2.21, 95% CI: 1.48–3.31) with pioglitazone.[5] Edema results from fluid retention and manifested as the increase in body weight and total body water, small but significant 6–7% increase in plasma volume, and reduction of hematocrit, hemoglobin, and serum albumin concentrations.[7] TZD-induced fluid retention is often resistant to diuretics and is relieved only by drug withdrawal. Exact mechanism for this fluid retention is not known but proposed mechanism is an increase in tubular sodium and water reabsorption in the kidney, but the role of specific nephron segments and sodium carriers involved in this process is less clear.[7]

HEART FAILURE

Heart failure is a common comorbidity of type 2 diabetes with occurrence rates of 8–20% and is associated with a poor outcome requiring special attention in patients with diabetes. In the PROactive trial, pioglitazone use was associated with an increased rate of serious heart failure but without any increase in all-cause mortality.[8] In a retrospective analysis of insurance database by Delea et al.[9] TZD use was associated with an increased risk of heart failure, with an adjusted incidence of heart failure (defined as requiring hospitalization or diagnosed at an outpatient visit) of 8.2% in the TZD group and 5.3% in the control group at 40 months. In the Insulin Resistance Intervention After Stroke (IRIS) study in nondiabetic subjects with insulin resistance, heart failure risk was increased in patients with previous myocardial infarction as compared to those without incident myocardial infarction in both groups (pioglitazone group: 31.4% versus 2.7%; placebo group: 25.7% versus 2.4%; $P <$ 0.0001).[10] However, one should keep in mind that edema, dyspnea, and weight gain in this trial led to more study drug dose reduction with a lower mean dose of pioglitazone versus placebo. With the availability of newer sodium-glucose transporter 2 (SGLT2) inhibitors, which are to be preferred as second-line agents after metformin therapy in people with heart failure or established cardiovascular diseases (CVD), pioglitazone has been pushed to the back bench as far as heart failure in type 2 diabetes in concerned.

PERIPHERAL ARTERIAL DISEASE

In post hoc analyses of PROactive trial, pioglitazone was less effective in decreasing the primary composite and main secondary outcomes in patients with established peripheral arterial disease (PAD) and there was a significant increase in leg revascularization procedures with pioglitazone use.[11]

RENAL DISEASE

Pioglitazone should be used with caution in chronic kidney disease (CKD) stages 4 and 5 because of the risk of water and sodium retention resulting in edema, precipitation of heart failure and anemia.[12]

BONE FRACTURES

ADOPT was the first trial to show increased risk of fractures with rosiglitazone in pre- and postmenopausal women but not in men and the fractures were not at typical osteoporotic sites of spine and hip, but instead at distal parts of the upper and lower extremities.[13] A recent national database cohort study in Scotland showed that risk of hip fracture increased with TZD use in both women and men, risk was cumulative (increased by 18% for each year of TZD exposure), and the 90-day mortality from hip fractures was expectedly high at ~15% with or without TZD. Probable mechanism involves peroxisome proliferator-activated receptor-γ (PPARγ) activation in bony tissue resulting in differentiation of mesenchymal precursor cells to adipocytes rather than osteoblasts, thereby making bones brittle.[14] In the IRIS trial of nondiabetic patients with insulin resistance,[15] pioglitazone was associated with an increased incidence of bone fracture 53% relative increase in risk for any fracture over 5 years and 4.9% absolute risk increment in any fracture with pioglitazone therapy. Also risk for serious fracture was significantly elevated in men in pioglitazone group in this study.[15] Currently, there are no guidelines limiting TZD use because of an increased fracture risk, but it is advisable to monitor bone density in female patients on TZD therapy and to limit TZD use in patients known to have low bone density.[12]

MACULAR EDEMA

Large population-based retrospective cohort study of 103,368 patients with type 2 diabetes and no diabetic macular edema (DME) at baseline, using the Health Improvement Network (THIN) database,[16] has shown that, even after adjustment for a range of confounding variables, TZDs are associated with an increased risk of DME in patients with type 2 diabetes, especially when used in combination with insulin therapy. The risk increased continuously over the 10-year duration of this study. This study advised clinicians to remain vigilant in the clinical screening for DME among those patients taking TZDs.[16]

CANCERS

In 2005, an increased risk of bladder cancer among patients treated with pioglitazone versus placebo was observed in the PROactive trial[4] and this was supported by many subsequent observational studies. Because of this concern of increased risk of bladder cancer, pioglitazone was banned in many countries including Germany, France, and India[5] and the US FDA added a warning against use by patients with active bladder cancer. In a recent meta-analysis of RCTs, an increased risk of bladder cancer was noted in patients treated with pioglitazone versus placebo (OR, 1.84; 95% CI, 0.99–3.42) and in meta-analysis of 20 observational studies (total number of 4,846,088 individuals), the increased risk of bladder cancer was slight but significant among ever-users of pioglitazone versus never-users (OR, 1.13; 95% CI, 1.03–1.25), which appeared to be both time dependent (P = 0.003) as well as dose dependent (P = 0.05), being significantly higher in those with more than 2 years of use or more than 28 grams of cumulative dose of drug.[17] In a biological function, network analysis exploring the direct targets of pioglitazone and genes associated with this drug and then further trying to evaluate the relationships of pioglitazone with prostate cancer and pancreatic cancer by identifying respective genes involved in genesis of this cancers, pioglitazone is likely to be a causal risk factor for prostate cancer and pancreatic cancer suggesting cautious use of this agent.[18]

CONCLUSION

Pioglitazone, although targeting crucial insulin resistance in type 2 diabetes mellitus, is associated with a number of serious adverse events including weight gain, fluid retention, edema, heart failure, bone fracture as well as bladder cancer. In the current era of availability of newer therapies having established cardiovascular benefits in dedicated cardiovascular outcome trials as well as well-established safety, *pioglitazone is no longer to be considered as second-line agent as add on to metformin monotherapy in type 2 diabetes management.*

REFERENCES

1. Joshi SR. Diabetes Care in India. Ann Glob Health. 2015;81(6):830-8.
2. Davies MJ, D'Alessio DA, Fradkin J, et al. Management of Hyperglycemia in Type 2 Diabetes, 2018. A Consensus Report by the American Diabetes Association (ADA) and the European Association for the Study of Diabetes (EASD). Diabetes Care. 2018;41(12):2669-701.
3. Graham DJ, Ouellet-Hellstrom R, MaCurdy TE, et al. Risk of acute myocardial infarction, stroke, heart failure, and death in elderly Medicare patients treated with rosiglitazone or pioglitazone. JAMA. 2010;304:411-8.
4. Lewis JD, Ferrara A, Peng T, et al. Risk of bladder cancer among diabetic patients treated with pioglitazone: interim report of a longitudinal cohort study. Diabetes Care. 2011;34:916-22.
5. Alam F, Islam MA, Mohamed M, et al. Efficacy and safety of pioglitazone monotherapy in type 2 diabetes mellitus: A systemic review and meta-analysis of randomized controlled trials. Sci Rep. 2019;95389.
6. Bray GA, Smith SR, Banerji MA, et al. Effect of pioglitazone on body composition and bone density in subjects with prediabetes in the ACT NOW trial. Diabetes Obes Metab. 2013;15(10):931-7.
7. Bełtowski J, Rachańczyk J, Włodarczyk M. Thiazolidinedione-Induced Fluid Retention: Recent Insights into the Molecular Mechanisms. PPAR Res. 2013;2013:628628.
8. Erdmann E, Charbonnel B, Wilcox RG, et al. Pioglitazone use and heart failure in patients with type 2 diabetes and preexisting cardiovascular disease: Data from PROactive study (PROactive 08). Diabetes Care. 2007;30:2773-8.
9. Delea TE, Edelsberg JS, Hagiwara M, et al. Use of thiazolidinediones and risk of heart failure in people with type 2 diabetes: a retrospective cohort study. Diabetes Care. 2003;26:2983-9.
10. Young LH, Viscoli CM, Schwartz GG, et al. Heart failure after ischemic stroke or transient ischemic attack in insulin-resistant patients without diabetes mellitus treated with pioglitazone. Circulation. 2018;138:1210-20.
11. Betteridge DJ, DeFronzo RA, Chilton RJ. PROactive: time for a critical appraisal. Euro Heart J. 2008;29:969-83.
12. Schernthaner G, Currie CJ, Schernthaner GH. Do We Still Need Pioglitazone for the Treatment of Type 2 Diabetes? A risk-benefit critique in 2013. Diabetes Care. 2013;36(2):s155-61.
13. Kahn SE, Zinman B, Lachin JM, et al. Rosiglitazone-associated fractures in type 2 diabetes: an Analysis from A Diabetes Outcome Progression Trial (ADOPT). Diabetes Care. 2008;31(5):845-51.
14. Colhoun HM, Livingstone SJ, Looker HC, et al. Hospitalised hip fracture risk with rosiglitazone and pioglitazone use compared with other glucose-lowering drugs Diabetologia. 2012;55:2929-37.
15. Viscoli CM, Inzucchi SE, Young LH, et al. Pioglitazone and Risk for Bone Fracture: Safety Data From a Randomized Clinical Trial. J Clin Endocrinol Metab. 2017;102(3):914-22.
16. Idris I, Warren G, Donnelly R. Association between thiazolidinedione treatment and risk of macular edema among patients with type 2 diabetes. Arch Intern Med. 2012;172(13):1005-11.
17. Tang H, Shi W, Fu S, et al. Pioglitazone and bladder cancer risk: a systematic review and meta-analysis. Cancer Medicine. 2018;7(4):1070-80.
18. Wen W, Wu P, Gong J, et al. Association of pioglitazone with increased risk of prostate cancer and pancreatic cancer: A functional network study. Diabetes Ther. 2018;9:2229-43.

82 CHAPTER First Injectable in Type 2 Diabetes: GLP-1 Receptor Agonists

Bhavana Sosale

INTRODUCTION

Glucagon-like peptide 1 receptor agonists (GLP-1RAs) are injectable agents used for the treatment of type 2 diabetes.[1] They are noninsulin injectable formulations in the large armamentarium of therapeutic options. Since early aggressive therapy is now a well-established concept in patient care and injectable drugs are not considered the last resort, GLP-1RAs are a fitting option for management.

Injectable GLP-1RAs include exenatide, liraglutide, dulaglutide, albiglutide, lixisenatide, and semaglutide. Oral semaglutide, a GLP-1RA will not be discussed in this chapter. GLP-1RA may be further classified into short-acting or long-acting agents based on the $T_{1/2}$. Short-acting GLP-1RAs reduce postprandial glucose excursions better than long-acting ones.[2]

The goals of treatment for type 2 diabetes include:

- Achieving normoglycemia
- Minimize hypoglycemia
- Preventing complications and reducing progression of complications.

There are several factors that are taken into consideration while choosing an anti-diabetic agent.[3]

- Ability to address as many pathophysiological defects of type 2 diabetes mellitus (T2DM)
- Evidence in terms of efficacy and safety
- Hypoglycemia risk and effect on body weight
- Cardiovascular safety
- Cost.

Cost being the only limiting factor, GLP-1RAs tick all the other check boxes above. Let us consider each of the factors.

Pathophysiology of Type 2 Diabetes Mellitus

There are several pathophysiological abnormalities that contribute to the development of T2DM. The ominous octet of T2DM is illustrated in Figure 1.[4] During previous decades, management was primarily "beta cell" centric with the use of sulfonylureas and insulin. With the advent of newer therapies and a greater understanding of T2DM, it has come to our understanding that it is important to address as many pathophysiological defects as possible to achieve better glycemic control.

Glucagon-like peptide 1 receptor agonists stimulate glucose-dependent insulin release from the beta cell. They also slow down gastric emptying, reduce appetite, improve satiety and reduce glucagon levels. In animal models, GLP-1RAs have resulted in proliferation and regeneration of beta cells. The mechanism of action of GLP-1RAs is complex and involves multiple systems and pathways. The pathophysiological approach to treatment favors the use of GLP-1RA as they address several defects of T2DM (Fig. 1).[2]

Efficacy and Safety

In head-to-head trials comparing the efficacy and safety of GLP-1RA versus other and injectable therapies, GLP-1RA resulted in HbA1c reduction ranging from 1% to 1.5% across studies. Studies comparing GLP-1RA versus basal insulin indicate that HbA1c reduction is greater with GLP-1RA than insulin in some studies and similar is others (Table 1). A meta-analysis by Wang et al. comparing randomized control trials of GLP-1RA and insulin, showed a greater reduction in HbA1c with GLP-1. In terms of

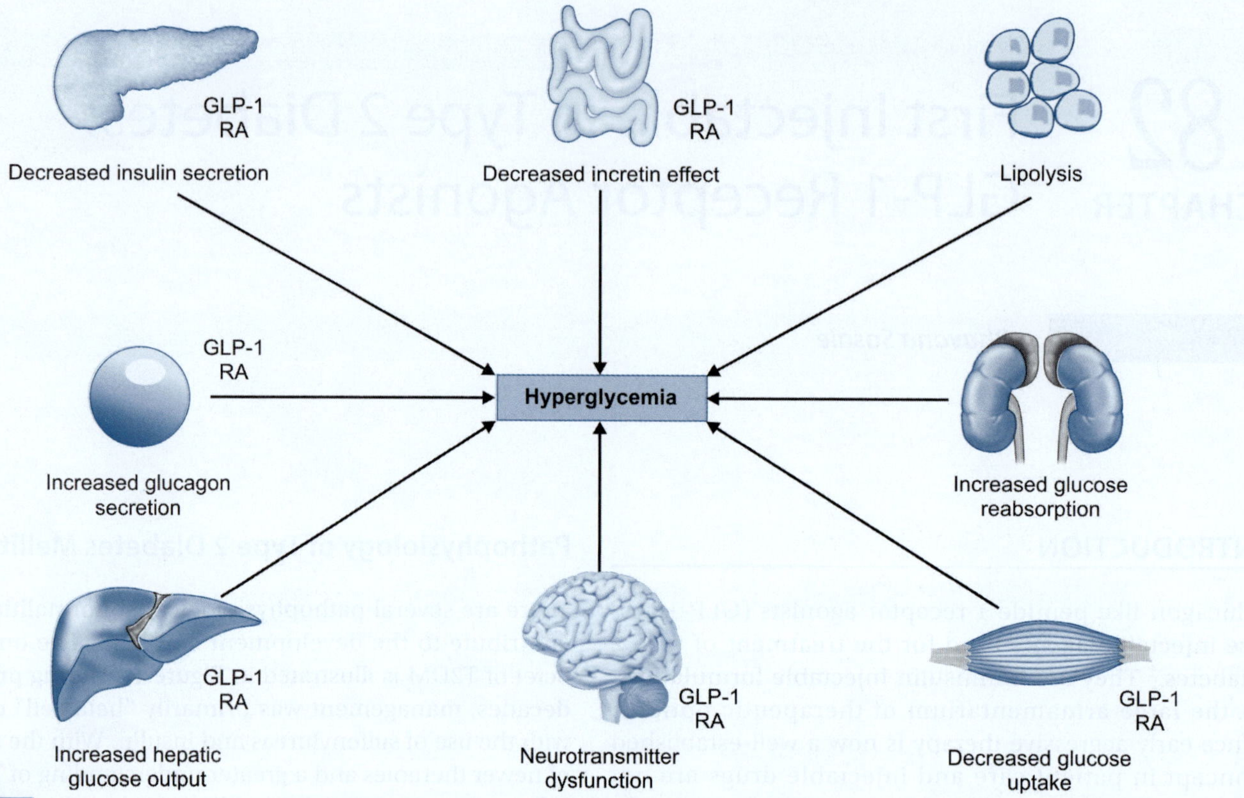

Figure 1 Addressing pathophysiological defects of type 2 diabetes with GLP-1 RA. ***(For color version see color plate No. 6)***

(*Source*: DeFronzo RA. From the triumvirate to the ominous octet: a new paradigm for the treatment of type 2 diabetes mellitus. Diabetes. 2009; 58:773-95.)

TABLE 1: Studies comparing GLP-1RA versus basal insulin.

		HbA1c (%)	Weight (kg)	Hypoglycemia
Wang et al.[5]	Meta-analysis GLP-1RA (exenatide, liraglutide) vs. insulin (glargine, BIAsp)	−0.14% (−0.27 to −0.02)	−4.40 (−5.23 to −3.56)	0.45 (0.27–0.76)
DURATION 3[6]	Exenatide Once weekly vs. glargine	−1.01 vs. −0.81 −0.2 (−0.39 to −0.02)	−2.49 vs. +2.01	3 times higher with glargine
D'Alessio D et al.[7]	Liraglutide vs. glargine	0.15% (0.28 to 0.02)	−3 vs. +2	Reduction in overall hypoglycemic, nocturnal hypoglycemia and severe hypoglycemia

Contd...

Contd...

		HbA1c (%)	Weight (kg)	Hypoglycemia
AWARD 2[8]	Dulaglutide (1.5 mg and 0.75 mg) vs. glargine	1.5 mg −1.08 ± 0.06% 0.75 mg −0.76 ± 0.06% glargine −0.63 ± 0.06%	1.5 mg − 1.87 ± 0.24 0.75 mg −1.33 ± 0.24 glargine + 1.44 ± 0.24	Reduction in overall hypoglycemia and nocturnal hypoglycemia
SUSTAIN 4[9]	Semaglutide (0.5 mg and 1 mg) vs. Glargine	0.5 mg −1·64 (1·54–1·74) 1 mg −1·21 (1·10–1·31) glargine −0·83 (0·73–0·93)	0.5 mg −3.47 (3·00–3·93) 1 mg −5.17 (4·71–5·66) glargine +1.15 (0·70–1·61)	Reduction in hypoglycemia

safety, gastrointestinal (GI) side effects like nausea and vomiting are more frequently observed with GLP-1RA use compared to insulin or sulfonylureas.[2,5] Acute pancreatitis has also been reported with GLP-RA use and hence should not be prescribed in individuals with a history of pancreatitis.

Hypoglycemia Risk and Effect on Body Weight

Minimizing hypoglycemia and avoiding weight gain in addition to control of hyperglycemia are the goals of therapy. GLP-1RAs when compared to other sulfonylureas and insulin have a lower incidence of hypoglycemia. In comparison to other drugs, GLP-1RAs result in a weight loss ranging from 2 kg to 8 kg. In studies comparing GLP-1RA with basal insulin, those on GLP-1RA lost 2.5–4.1 kg and those on basal insulin gained 0.8–2 kg (summarized in Table 1).

Cardiovascular Safety

Results from studies with GLP-1RA and sodium glucose cotransporter uptake 2 inhibitors (SGLT2is) have led to a paradigm shift in management of diabetes. Studies demonstrating a reduction in primary cardiovascular (CV) end points (composite of CV death, nonfatal myocardial infarction, and non-fatal stroke) have translated to an approach centered around cardiovascular and renal disease (in addition to safety, efficacy, and minimizing hypoglycemia and weight gain).[3]

ELIXA and EXSCEL demonstrated the CV safety of lixisenatide and exenatide QW. HARMONY, LEADER, SUSTAIN-6, and REWIND demonstrated the superiority of albiglutide, liraglutide, semaglutide, and dulaglutide over other antihyperglycemic therapy with respected to CV outcomes. Cardiovascular outcome trials (CVOTs) with GLP-1RA are tabulated in Table 2.

The study with albiglutide only included individuals with a preexisting CV disease and thus the results cannot be extrapolated to the primary prevention cohort. Among the drugs which showed CV benefit, heterogeneity (difference in outcomes based on baseline CV disease) was observed with liraglutide. Dulaglutide and semaglutide did not demonstrate heterogeneity. This implies that dulaglutide and semaglutide reduce CV events in both individuals with CV disease and in those with multiple risk factors (MRFs); and that the benefits with liraglutide are only seen in those with established CV disease. While

TABLE 2: Cardiovascular outcome trials with glucagon-like peptide 1 receptor agonist (GLP-1RA).

Name	Study drug	Hazard ratio (95% CI)	Cardiovascular (CV) events	Heterogeneity with respect to baseline CV disease
ELIXA[10]	Lixisenatide	1.02 (0.89–1.17)	CV safe	–
EXSCEL[11]	Exenatide QW	0.91 (0.83–1)	CV safe	No
HARMONY[12]	Albiglutide	0.78 (0.68–0.9)	Reduces CV events	–
LEADER[13]	Liraglutide	0.87 (0.78–0.97)	Reduces CV events	Yes
SUSTAIN-6[14]	Semaglutide	0.74 (0.58–0.95)	Reduces CV events	No
REWIND[15]	Dulaglutide	0.88 (0.79–0.99)	Reduces CV events	No

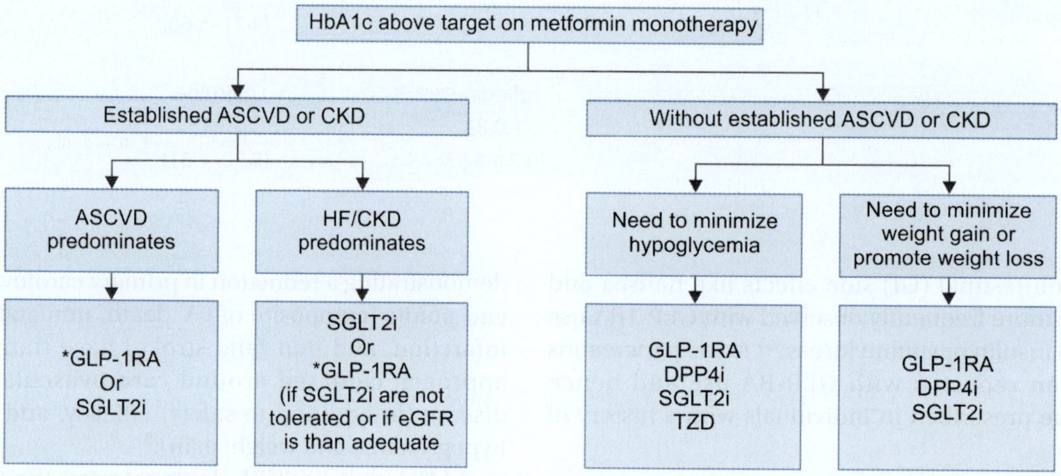

*GLP-1RA that have proven CV benefit

(ASCVD: atherosclerotic cardiovascular disease; CKD: chronic kidney disease; DPP4i : dipeptidyl peptidase 4 inhibitors; eGFR: estimated glomerular filtration rate; GLP-1 RA: glucagon like peptide receptor agonists; HF: heart failure; SGLT2i: sodium glucose co-transporter 2 inhibitors; TZD: thiazolidinediones)

Flowchart 1 ADA/EASD approach to management of uncontrolled type 2 diabetes. ***(For color version see color plate No. 6)***

(*Source*: American Diabetes Association. 9. Pharmacologic Approaches to Glycemic Treatment: Standards of Medical Care in Diabetes-2019. Diabetes Care. 2019;42:S90-102.)

most of the CVOT largely included a population with established CV disease, REWIND included the largest primary prevention cohort (without baseline CV disease). Results of REWIND further reaffirm the benefit of GLP-1RA in individuals with or without CV disease.

Cost

Glucagon-like peptide 1 receptor agonists are expensive compared to other glucose-lowering therapies. Hence, choice of agent usually depends on affordability (in pay out of pocket healthcare systems) and based on availability and insurance reimbursements in the developed countries.

TREATMENT GUIDELINES

The American Diabetes Association/European Association for the Study of Diabetes (ADA/EASD) guidelines (Flowchart 1) recommend a risk-based approach to treatment based on presence of CV disease, kidney disease,

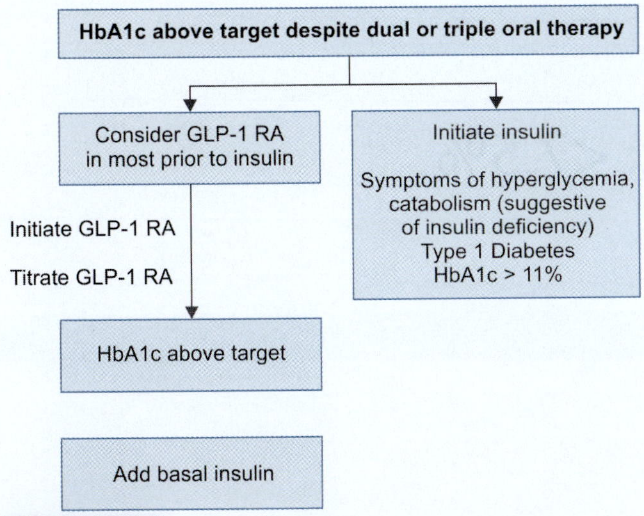

Flowchart 2 Intensification of anti-diabetic drugs with injectable therapies.

(*Source*: American Diabetes Association. 9. Pharmacologic Approaches to Glycemic Treatment: Standards of Medical Care in Diabetes-2019. Diabetes Care. 2019;42:S90-102.)

heart failure, need to minimize hypoglycemia and weight gain, promote weight loss, and lower treatment cost.[3]

In individuals, uncontrolled on dual/triple oral therapy, the addition of a GLP-1RA is recommended. In those with established CV disease and kidney disease, the use of GLP-1RA is recommended based on the evidence from CV outcome trials. Insulin is not recommended as the first injectable owing to the enormous body of evidence with GLP-1RA with efficacy, hypoglycemia risk, weight loss, and CV benefit (Flowchart 2). However, there are some situations where insulin is preferred over GLP-1RA. These include presentation with an acute illness, presence symptoms of hyperglycemia and catabolism (suggestive of insulin deficiency), diabetic ketoacidosis, HbA1c > 11% or in those with type 1 diabetes insulin is the preferred option.[3]

CONCLUSION

When physicians are presented with the task of choosing the first injectable, the choice lies between GLP-1RA and basal insulin. GLP-1RAs score over basal insulin in terms of HbA1c reduction, aiding in weight loss, minimizing hypoglycemia and reducing CV events.

The ADA guidelines also suggest a risk-based approach and recommend the use of GLP-1RA in patients with CV disease and renal disease. Evidence from REWIND (with dulaglutide) demonstrating benefit in a large primary prevention cohort further supports the use of GLP-1RA in all patients with diabetes (with or without CV disease). Cost, a limiting factor in management needs to be considered in addition to science.

REFERENCES

1. Vilsbøll T, Holst JJ. Incretins, insulin secretion and Type 2 diabetes mellitus. Diabetologia. 2004;47:357-66.
2. Rasalam R, Barlow J, Kennedy M, et al. GLP-1 Receptor Agonists for Type 2 Diabetes and Their Role in Primary Care: An Australian Perspective. Diabetes Ther. 2019;10:1205-17.
3. American Diabetes Association. 9. Pharmacologic Approaches to Glycemic Treatment: Standards of Medical Care in Diabetes-2019. Diabetes Care. 2019;42:S90-102.
4. DeFronzo RA. From the triumvirate to the ominous octet: a new paradigm for the treatment of type 2 diabetes mellitus. Diabetes. 2009;58:773-95.
5. Wang Y, Li L, Yang M, et al. Glucagon-like peptide-1 receptor agonists versus insulin in inadequately controlled patients with type 2 diabetes mellitus: a meta-analysis of clinical trials. Diabetes Obes Metab. 2011;13:972-81.
6. Diamant M, Van Gaal L, Stranks S, et al. Once weekly exenatide compared with insulin glargine titrated to target in patients with type 2 diabetes (DURATION-3): an open-label randomised trial. Lancet. 2010;375:2234-43.
7. D'Alessio D, Häring HU, Charbonnel B, et al. Comparison of insulin glargine and liraglutide added to oral agents in patients with poorly controlled type 2 diabetes. Diabetes Obes Metab. 2015;17:170-8.
8. Giorgino F, Benroubi M, Sun JH, et al. Efficacy and Safety of Once-Weekly Dulaglutide Versus Insulin Glargine in Patients with Type 2 Diabetes on Metformin and Glimepiride (AWARD-2). Diabetes Care. 2015;38:2241-9.
9. Aroda VR, Bain SC, Cariou B, et al. Efficacy and safety of once-weekly semaglutide versus once-daily insulin glargine as add-on to metformin (with or without sulfonylureas) in insulin-naive patients with type 2 diabetes (SUSTAIN 4): a randomised, open-label, parallel-group, multicentre, multinational, phase 3a trial. Lancet Diabetes Endocrinol. 2017;5:355-66.
10. Pfeffer MA, Claggett B, Diaz R, et al. Lixisenatide in Patients with Type 2 Diabetes and Acute Coronary Syndrome. N Engl J Med. 2015;373:2247-57.
11. Holman RR, Bethel MA, Mentz RJ, et al. Effects of Once-Weekly Exenatide on Cardiovascular Outcomes in Type 2 Diabetes. N Engl J Med. 2017;377:1228-39.
12. Hernandez AF, Green JB, Janmohamed S, et al. Albiglutide and cardiovascular outcomes in patients with type 2 diabetes and cardiovascular disease (Harmony Outcomes): a double-blind, randomized placebo-controlled trial. Lancet. 2018;392:1519-29.
13. Marso SP, Daniels GH, Brown-Frandsen K, et al. Liraglutide and Cardiovascular Outcomes in Type 2 Diabetes. N Engl J Med. 2016;375:311-22.
14. Marso SP, Bain SC, Consoli A, et al. Semaglutide and Cardiovascular Outcomes in Patients with Type 2 Diabetes. N Engl J Med. 2016;375:1834-44.
15. Gerstein HC, Colhoun HM, Dagenais GR, et al. Dulaglutide and cardiovascular outcomes in type 2 diabetes (REWIND): a double-blind randomised, placebo-controlled trial. Lancet. 2019;394:121-30.

83 CHAPTER Desirable HbA1c: <7.5%

Jugal Kishor Sharma, Amit Gupta

INTRODUCTION

Treatment of type 2 diabetes mellitus (T2DM) is full of complexities and despite all the efforts, many patients develop microvascular and macrovascular complications of diabetes. Cardiovascular (CV) complications remain the leading cause of mortality in patients with diabetes. The UKPDS[1] (United Kingdom Prospective Diabetes Study) has established that intensive glycemic control significantly improves the risk of microvascular complications but the same cannot be said convincingly about the macrovascular complications including myocardial infarction (MI) and stroke. The STENO-2[2] trial has explained that to reduce the risk of macrovascular complications a more pragmatic approach is required, which addresses not only the glycemia but also the dyslipidemia, blood pressure, and smoking. An important debatable and unresolved issue is to determine the safe level of glycemic control as reflected by glycated hemoglobin (HbA1c). Not all the guidelines are on the same page when it comes to define target HbA1c levels in T2DM patients. In 2018, the American College of Physicians (ACP) released its guidance suggesting more relaxed control of diabetes.[3] This has again led to perplexities and confusion among clinicians as well as the patients.

Revised guidelines for T2DM by ACP published in 2018 stated a target HbA1c of 7–8% in most of the patients with diabetes. This guidance is obviously not in line with the guidance of the American Association of Clinical Endocrinologist (AACE)[4] which suggest a target A1c of less than 6.5% (wherever feasible), the American Diabetes Association (ADA)[5] which suggests a target A1c of 7% or less, and NICE (National Institute for Health and Care Excellence) UK[6] which advocates an A1c of 6.5% if achievable without causing hypoglycemia or less than 7% if hypoglycemia is a concern. Similarly, RSSDI (Research Society for the Study of Diabetes in India) also recommends an A1c target of less than 7% in most of the patients with diabetes. The statement of ACP attracted worldwide criticism and did not garner much support; however, it is the responsibility of the scientific mind to critically analyze the two aspects of the same coin (all the guidelines have analyzed the same evidence data and reached different conclusions).

REVIEW OF EVIDENCE

The ACP guidelines evaluated the guidelines of AACE, ADA, NICE, SIGN (Scottish Intercollegiate Guidelines Network),[7] ICSI (Institute of Clinical Systems Improvement),[8] and VA/DoD (Veterans Affairs Department/Department of Defense).[9] The first guidance given by ACP states: "Clinicians should personalize goals for glycemic control in patients with type 2 diabetes on the basis of a discussion of benefits and harms of patients general health and life expectancy, treatment burden, and costs of care." As far as this statement is concerned, there does not seem any difference in opinion and all guidelines recommend patient-centered care where target A1c and drug chosen for therapy is guided by the patient's preference, cost of therapy, life expectancy, comorbid conditions, advanced diabetes complications, risk of hypoglycemia, ability to understand and perform diabetes self-management tasks. All guidelines agree that individualized targets can be higher than those suggested in patients with already advanced diabetes complications with limited life expectancy.

The second guidance statement says: "Clinicians should aim to achieve an HbA_{1c} level between 7% and 8% in most patients with type 2 diabetes." So how does the difference of 0.5–1% in A1c matters. A difference of 0.5% may look inconsequential at the first glance but reducing HbA1c by 0.5% in a real-world setting may mean use of more drugs, higher drug dosage, more adverse effects, and increased cost of care. The classic teaching about the blood glucose has been—the lower-the better but is there any evidence to support the less stricter glycemic control against the intensive glycemic control? The ACP authors looked for evidence from five major Treat-to-Target Trials.

ACCORD (Action to Control Cardiovascular Risk in Diabetes) Trial: In the ACCORD trial, participants had a mean age of 62.2 years and median baseline HbA1c of 8.1% and it compared the effect of intensive glycemic control (HbA1c < 6%) with standard glycemic control (HbA1c 7–7.9%).[10] The trial was terminated prematurely because there was an increase in all-cause mortality [hazard ratio (HR 1.22)], CV death (HR 1.35), and frequency of hypoglycemia requiring assistance in the intensive treatment group. Intensive treatment leads to a small absolute reduction in onset of albuminuria but no clinically significant reduction in renal failure and doubling of serum creatinine. Similarly intensive treatment did not lead to decrease in visual impairment, photocoagulation for retinopathy and neuropathy. Intensive glycemic control leads to fewer incidences of non-fatal MI but no reduction in major adverse CV outcomes such as fatal MI, fatal or non-fatal stroke, fatal or non-fatal congestive heart failure was found. Intensive arm also reported a weight gain of more than 10 kg and clinically significant fluid retention.

ADVANCE (Action in Diabetes and Vascular Disease: Preterax and Diamicron Modified Release Controlled Evaluation) Trial: ADVANCE is another treat-to-target landmark trial in which the average age of participants was 66 years and the mean baseline HbA1c level was 7.5%. The intensive treatment arm target HbA1c was 6.5%. In ADVANCE trial there was no reduction in major CV events, all-cause mortality, and CV death over a median of 5 years.[11] Intensive treatment did show a reduction in macrovascular and microvascular events and this reflected small absolute reduction in the incidence of nephropathy. However, again as in ACCORD, intensive treatment did not affect doubling of serum creatinine, neuropathy, retinopathy, or visual impairment. Intensive treatment also leads to more frequent symptomatic as well as asymptomatic hypoglycemia and hospitalizations.

UKPDS trials: The UKPDS has shown that there exists a continuous relationship between glycemic control and microvascular complications, and microvascular complications reduced by 25% if HbA1c was less than 7%. It was UKPDS which suggested that 1% decrease in HbA1c reduces the risk of microvascular complications by 35%; however, there is no glycemic threshold below which the risk of microvascular complications does not exist.[1] The UKPDS has also taught us that glycemic control had minimal impact on macrovascular complications of diabetes. The STENO 2 study leads the way by convincingly establishing that a multifactorial approach that deals with conventional CV risk factors such as dyslipidemia, hypertension, and smoking along with glycemic control can cause a decrease in all-cause mortality and actually add years to life of patients with diabetes.

VADT (Veterans Affairs Diabetes Trial): In this treat-to-target trial, the median baseline HbA1c was 9.4% and the mean age of participants was 60 years. The median achieved HbA1c was 6.9% in the intensive treatment group and 8.4% in the standard treatment group. This trial again could not find any reduction in major CV events, death, or microvascular events, except for any increase in albuminuria in the intensive arm. There was a small absolute decrease in CV events over an extended follow-up of about 12 years in the intensively treated patients; however, there was no reduction in all-cause mortality or CV-related deaths. There were more frequent hypoglycemic events in intensively treated arm than the standard treatment arm.[12]

So most of these trials had not shown any benefit in terms of all-cause mortality in intensively treated patients with targets less than 7% against those with less strict control with targets around 8%. Contrary to this intensive glucose control was associated with substantial harm, including but not limited to hypoglycemic events. The authors of the ACP guidelines believe that efforts to achieve A1c target less than 7% can lead to increased risk of weight gain, hypoglycemia, other adverse effects, and even death. The above-discussed landmark trials have shown reduction in microvascular complications. The authors favoring relaxed target contest that there is inconsistent evidence for intensive glycemic control. Another key issue highlighted is that there was an improvement in surrogate microvascular endpoints, but this could not translate into reductions in actual clinical events (e.g. reduction in albuminuria could not translate into decrease in creatinine doubling time).

HbA1c: The target itself is not a gold standard target. So, it is pertinent to ask if we are chasing the right target.

Has it been so, why we are not seeing any benefits with intensive glycemic control? A1c measurements can have variability. Any condition that reduces the lifespan of red blood cells (RBCs) or any condition that reduces the mean erythrocyte age will give a falsely low value of HbA1c. HbA1c levels can be affected by drugs, hemoglobinopathies, and various disease states giving rise to falsely low or high HbA1c values. What is important to understand is that linking everything to HbA1c may not be in the best interest of the patient. There is no doubt that diabetes is a dangerous disease with serious consequences. HbA1c is a marker of glycemic control but it is not the true reflection of the underlying disease process and long-term metabolic consequences of diabetes. Any benefit from intensive glucose control will require several years to show clinical benefits if any; hence, it may be appropriate for young individuals with a life expectancy of 15 years or more.

The third ACP guidance states: "Clinicians should consider deintensifying pharmacologic therapy in patients with type 2 diabetes who achieve HbA1c levels less than 6.5%." This statement is the one which cannot be accepted as it is. As stated earlier, HbA1c is not a reflection of disease state, so deintensifying therapy in a patient who is doing well on intensive control is not welcomed at all. There is no disagreement that the target should be individualized in every patient based on his or her personal characteristics (i.e. duration of diabetes, comorbidities, life expectancy, risk of hypoglycemia, education and support available, cost effectiveness, advanced diabetes complications), but it cannot be agreed to universally de-intensify therapy in each and every patient without individual considerations.

DISCUSSION

The A1c confusion demonstrates that there is insufficient evidence to convincingly favor or refute any one recommendation or guideline.[13] All the guidelines collectively support a less aggressive glycemic control with A1c between 7% and 8% in patients with limited life expectancy, extensive comorbid conditions such as end-stage renal disease or liver disease, a history of severe hypoglycemia requiring assistance, cognitive impairment, malignancies, or any medical conditions where risk benefit analysis does not favor intensive glycemic control. Likewise, A1c target of 7–8% for all diabetes patients cannot be generalized. DCCT (Diabetes Control and Complication Trial) and UKPDS have shown the extended benefit of good glycemic control over the years due to metabolic memory. The ACP guidance overlooked the fact that it took more than 10 years in UKPDS and 15 years in DCCT to demonstrate that early intensive glycemic control led to a decrease in both macrovascular and microvascular complications including death.[14] The UKPDS has established a risk relationship for HbA1c levels; for every 1% rise in A1c, there is a 37% increase in severe microvascular complications, a 21% increase in deaths related to diabetes, and 14% increase in MI.

CONCLUSION

The HbA1c target must be individualized considering various factors as discussed earlier. An HbA1c target of 7–8% may be recommended for a certain group of patients as part of individualization for valid reasons. A lower HbA1c, if can be achieved safely, must not be discouraged. Deintensification of treatment in a patient who is well controlled with HbA1c less than 7% and no adverse effects is not recommended and supported by evidence.[15]

REFERENCES

1. UK Prospective Diabetes Study (UKPDS) Group. Intensive blood-glucose control with sulphonylureas or insulin compared with conventional treatment and risk of complications in patients with type 2 diabetes (UKPDS 33). Lancet. 1998;352(9131):837-53.
2. Gæde P, Oellgaard J, Carstensen B, et al. Years of life gained by multifactorial intervention in patients with type 2 diabetes mellitus and microalbuminuria: 21 years follow-up on the Steno-2 randomised trial. Diabetologia. 2016;59(11):2298-307.
3. Qaseem A, Wilt TJ, Kansagara D, et al. Hemoglobin A1c targets for glycemic control with pharmacologic therapy for nonpregnant adults with type 2 diabetes mellitus: a guidance statement updates from the American College of Physicians. Ann Int Med. 2018;168(8):569-76.
4. Garber AJ, Abrahamson MJ, Barzilay JI, et al. Consensus statement by the American Association of Clinical endocrinologists and American college of endocrinology on the comprehensive type 2 diabetes management algorithm–2019 executive summary. Endocr Pract. 2019;25(1):69-100.
5. American Diabetes Association. Glycemic targets: standards of medical care in diabetes—2019. Diabetes Care. 2019;42(Suppl 1):S61-70.
6. Internal Clinical Guidelines Team. Type 2 Diabetes in Adults: Management. London: National Institute for Health and Care Excellence (UK); 2015.
7. Scottish Intercollegiate Guidelines Network. Scottish Intercollegiate Guidelines Network Management of Diabetes: A National Clinical Guideline. SIGN Publication no. 116. Edinburgh, Scotland; 2013.
8. Redmon B, Caccamo D, Flavin P, et al. Institute for Clinical Systems Improvement Diagnosis and Management of Type 2 Diabetes Mellitus in Adults, 16th edition. Bloomington, MN: Institute for Clinical Systems Improvement; 2014.
9. The Management of Type 2 Diabetes Mellitus in Primary Care Work Group. (2017). VA/DoD clinical practice guideline for the management of type 2 diabetes mellitus in primary care. Version 5.0. [online] Available from www.healthquality.va.gov/guidelines/CD/diabetes/VADoDDMCPGFinal508.pdf. [Last accessed September, 2019].

10. Action to Control Cardiovascular Risk in Diabetes Study Group. Effects of intensive glucose lowering in type 2 diabetes. N Engl J Med. 2008;358(24):2545-59.
11. ADVANCE Collaborative Group. Intensive blood glucose control and vascular outcomes in patients with type 2 diabetes. N Engl J Med. 2008;358(24):2560-72.
12. Duckworth W, Abraira C, Moritz T, et al. Glucose control and vascular complications in veterans with type 2 diabetes. N Engl J Med. 2009;360(2):129-39.
13. Maggi D, Montecucco F, Adami G, et al. Glycosylated haemoglobin (A1c) best values for type 2 diabetes in the battlefield much ado about nothing? (apparently). Diabetol Metab Syndr. 2019;11(1):48.
14. Nathan DM, Bayless M, Cleary P, et al. Diabetes control and complications trial/epidemiology of diabetes interventions and complications study at 30 years: advances and contributions. Diabetes. 2013;62(12): 3976-86.
15. Draznin B, Nathan DM, Korytkowski MT, et al. Guidelines versus guidelines: What's best for the patient? Ann Intern Med. 2018;169(3):186-7.

12 SECTION Diabetes and Education

84 CHAPTER Apps for Educating Patients

Shriram V Kulkarni, Sagar Sinha, Priyanka Jadhav, Chitra S Kulkarni, Sayali S Devlalkar, Aditya S Kulkarni

INTRODUCTION

In this era of patient-centered medicine, virtually everybody is connected to technology. A smartphone remains a massively underutilized tool which provides answers for both prophylactic and therapeutic aspects of healthcare. A holistic solution for health lies at the heart of this foundation.

Besides practical aspects and implications for medical practice, smartphone technology has made massive applications in the world of patient-centered care. What has markedly compounded the situation, is the "Google" factor (wherein patients have access to information at their finger-tips) and the meteoric rise of the gray world of social media. However, it is time for the medical world to rise up to the challenge and use this very system to our advantage.

The chapter will aim to cover the various types of mobile and smartphone technology available for patient-centered care including apps for educating patients.

TEXT MESSAGING-BASED PLATFORMS

According to the Telecom Regulatory Authority of India (TRAI), India has been acclaimed as an upcoming super power in the world telecommunication sector marked by enhanced mobile connectivity and Internet and smartphones usage at a reasonable cost. There is patching up of urban rural divide and the growth rate is quite noteworthy.[1] Despite growing access to smartphones and data packs, many rural patients at least have access to text messaging services.

Remarkable work has been done in this field in this decade. Identification of the problems like long-term adherence, secondary prevention challenges, and psychosocial barriers was done early.[2–4]

Multifaceted professional interventions including the first application of technology (like centralized tracking) were identified as potential solutions at the start of century itself.[5] Early work on text messaging systems showed promising progress in supporting young people with diabetes, wherein scheduled and tailored text messaging was associated with improved self-efficacy and adherence.[6]

At the start of this decade, a Cochrane review identified the potential benefit of mobile phone messaging interventions for self-management of long-term illnesses.[7] In a public health-focused text message program targeting type 2 diabetes, the participants too had positive perceptions of the program, which led to positive behavior change.[8] Even early Indian experience found these systems effective and acceptable toward lifestyle modification and primary prevention.[9]

The CHAT-DM (Cardiovascular Health and Texting-Diabetes Mellitus) study that included 502 patients with both coronary heart disease and diabetes mellitus—participants in the intervention arm—received six text messages per week for 6 months in addition to usual care, which were theory driven and culturally tailored to provide educational and motivational information on glucose monitoring, blood pressure control, medication adherence, physical activity, and lifestyle, resulted in better glycemic control.[10]

In 2016, India's Ministry of Health and Family Welfare (WHO partnered) launched the mDiabetes initiative to harnesses the power and potential of the vast mobile telephony network via missed call to 011-22901701 or web access on www.mdiabetes.nhp.gov.in.[11] A commissioned study with over a 100,000 respondents tested the feasibility and demonstrated its acceptability to disseminate knowledge regarding diabetes and healthy lifestyle, and to improve health-seeking behavior.[12]

SOCIAL MEDIA-BASED INTERVENTIONS

With the advent of Digital 2.0, we are living in a virtual world. Our online presence is now an accepted part of our lives. This facet which once was only used by the next generation is now spread across all age groups transcending geographic borders and socioeconomic divides. Although it can be a distraction with many pitfalls, it can be used to do a lot of good!

Online groups and communities are a source of disease information and experience. However, these require a structured platform by health care providers to adjust and correct the information posted by patients, if needed. Recommendations for healthcare providers on how to use social media are available too.[13]

The first Facebook study to evaluate it as a tool to improve diabetes control in patients with type 1 diabetes using insulin pumps with glucose sensors had the following interesting results:[14]

- Allowed patients to gain knowledge and interact for their daily insulin adjustments
- Helped patients cope better with their daily life
- Suggested that patients prefer to communicate with healthcare providers using social media
- Facebook and Skype can improve diabetes control similar to regular clinic visits.

A recent review for social media use in diabetes found 13 publications reporting significant HbA1c reductions and general satisfaction, however mixed results were reported when it came to quality of life or empowerment.[15]

Types of social media interventions for patient education:

- *Social networking* (e.g. WhatsApp, Facebook, and LinkedIn):
  - Easy group creation
  - Wide user base
  - Two-way communication which can be personalized
  - Privacy and encryption improving.
- *Blogging* (e.g. Wordpress, Twitter, and Tumbler):
  - Dynamic and concise form of information exchange.
- *Media* (e.g. YouTube and Vimeo):
  - Physician instructions videos (like insulin injection techniques)
  - Modules for education.

Risks and disadvantages of Social Media:

- Possible poor quality of information dissemination
- Potential damage to personal image (in case of dispute or mudslinging)
- Potential patient privacy breaches
- Legal issues
- Physician personal and professional lives intersection.

There is a lot of progress to be made in this area, especially with accuracy of information. Besides the risk of data theft, it also poses a significant question of the crucial element of a physical patient-doctor interaction. This can be very dangerous in the long term, however it needs to be adapted proactively with integration into the current system of care. Social media interventions should be used as an adjunct to and not a replacement for the doctor. Self-regulation by healthcare providers is a must in this area.

Principles:

- *Content credibility*: Share information from credible sources only and refute inaccurate one.
- *Outreach*: Avoid asking patients to join your network (let them request to join).
- *Communication*: Create a secure zone with best privacy settings.
- *Care*: Do not provide specific medical advice to non-patients.
- *Legal*:
  - Make appropriate disclosures and disclaimers
  - Do not make false claims
  - Respect copyright laws
  - Patient privacy is paramount.

APPS FOR DIABETES MANAGEMENT AND PATIENT EDUCATION

The objective of using smartphone apps is to efficiently manage diabetes by improving glycemic control and eventually, preventing or further delaying complications of diabetes.[16] These apps have essential logging features. Additionally, they contain a comprehensive database, which includes nutritional information on thousands of food items. Most apps would even provide features such as explicit nutritional content, which can effortlessly be saved into a favorites section, making it more suitable for users to log the foods they frequently eat. Besides, these give access to everyone in the healthcare platform. Price, features, and usability are the primary determinants whether the app is suited to a particular individual. Warnings for hypo- or hyperglycemia, weight and activity tracking, food database, interactive graphs, and integration are desirable.

OneTouch Verio Sync *Reveal* mobile app makes it easy to see at a glance a 14-day summary that shows glycemic range. Results populate the 90-day logbook on its own. Glooko's *MeterSync* devices permit patients with diabetes to monitor their blood glucose (BG) levels. The users can also download their data directly to their smartphone. Their glucose reports can be emailed, printed or faxed by the patients to their physicians. *Diabetes WaveSense* helps to track carbohydrate intake, BG levels, and insulin doses. A notes section for users with results is also included that can be shared with doctors.

Blood glucose levels, carbohydrate intake, insulin doses, and exercise can be tracked by the *dLife app*. A food database and notes section have also been included. Specification for exercises and insulin type is also allowed. It also has a Q&A section that is linked to an online support community. *Gather health* is a similar diabetes care app. Tracking of BG levels, HbA1c levels, nutrition, medication, weight, and analyzing blood pressure are provided by *Diabetes Pal*. It works with the Telcare meter with no additional effort. *My Glucose Buddy* app can monitor BG levels, medicines, food, and physical activity; though the drawback is that it has more pop-ups than the typical app, which may be irritating for users. However, it has additional benefits of weight and blood pressure tracking.

For seamless BG monitoring, the new *Contour* app syncs with the smart meter. This easy-to-use app can provide patients with a better understanding of how their daily activities can affect BG results and thus helps managing their diabetes. For diabetic patients on polytherapy, a hypoglycemia detector like *Hypoband*, which is a simple device detects cold sweat induced by hypoglycemia and sends an alert.

Medisafe is an app designed to allow people keep track of their medications. This is enabled by creating reminders and alerting family members if the user has not taken their medication. People with diabetes embody the major group of users on Medisafe, followed by people who have been using hypertension and cholesterol medications. *MedSimple* searches for cost-saving medications. It also has medication reminder and emails reports. *MedCoach* refills prescriptions online with most pharmacies, provides medication, and gives reminders as well.

The *American Association of Diabetes Educators (AADE) Diabetes Goal Tracker* allows users to set, share, and track their goals in seven varied areas of diabetes management—healthy eating, being physically active, blood glucose monitoring, taking medicines, problem solving, healthy coping, and risk reduction. Also, it contains information and resources about diabetes and self-management. *Diabetes Buddy, Diabetes Log* and *Diabetes Pilot* are other examples of such apps.

CONCLUSION

There are innumerable apps depending on the subject and the content desired by the user. Many cross-platform apps, systems, and peripherals have therapeutic applications as well. It is important for the treating physician to discuss with the patient the requirement and need of the desired technology. At the community and national level, social media and text message platforms have an opportunity to revolutionize patient-centered care.

REFERENCES

1. Telecom Regulatory Authority of India. (2018). The Indian Telecom Services Performance Indicators. [Online].. Available from http://www.trai.gov.in/sites/default/files/PIReport27062018_0.pdf. [Last accessed September, 2019].
2. Walsh JM, Sundaram V, McDonald K, et al. Implementing effective hypertension quality improvement strategies: barriers and potential solutions. J Clin Hypertens (Greenwich). 2008;10(4):311-6.
3. Desai NR, Choudhry NK. Impediments to adherence to post myocardial infarction medications. Curr Cardiol Rep. 2013;15(1):322.
4. Peyrot M, Rubin RR, Lauritzen T, et al. Psychosocial problems and barriers to improved diabetes management: results of the Cross-National Diabetes Attitudes, Wishes and Needs (DAWN) Study. Diabet Med. 2005;22(10):1379-85.
5. Renders CM, Valk GD, Griffin S, et al. Interventions to improve the management of diabetes mellitus in primary care, outpatient and community settings. Cochrane Database Syst Rev. 2001;1:CD001481.
6. Franklin VL, Waller A, Pagliari C, et al. A randomized controlled trial of Sweet Talk, a text-messaging system to support young people with diabetes. Diabet Med. 2006;23(12):1332-8.
7. de Jongh T, Gurol-Urganci I, Vodopivec-Jamsek V, et al. Mobile phone messaging for facilitating self-management of long-term illnesses. Cochrane Database of Syst Rev. 2012;12: CD007459.
8. Buis LR, Hirzel L, Turske SA, et al. Use of a text message program to raise type 2 diabetes risk awareness and promote health behavior change (part II): assessment of participants' perceptions on efficacy. J Med Internet Res. 2013;15(12):e282.
9. Ramachandran A, Snehalatha C, Ram J, et al. Effectiveness of mobile phone messaging in prevention of type 2 diabetes by lifestyle modification in men in India: a prospective, parallel-group, randomised controlled trial. Lancet Diabetes Endocrinol. 2013;1(3):191-8.
10. Huo X, Spatz ES, Ding Q, et al. Design and rationale of the Cardiovascular Health and Text Messaging (CHAT) Study and the CHAT-Diabetes Mellitus (CHAT-DM) Study: two randomised controlled trials of text messaging to improve secondary prevention for coronary heart disease and diabetes. BMJ Open. 2017;7(12):e018302.
11. Press Information Bureau, Government of India, Ministry of Health and Family Welfare. (2016). Highlights the importance of Healthy Living and

awareness in prevention and control of Non-communicable Diseases. [Online]. Available from https://pib.gov.in/newsite/PrintRelease.aspx?relid=146417. [Last accessed September, 2019].

12. Ramachandran A, Kumar R, Nanditha A, et al. mDiabetes initiative using text messages to improve lifestyle and health-seeking behaviour in India. BMJ Innovations. 2018;4(4):155-62.
13. Centers for Disease Control and Prevention. (2011). The health communicator's social media toolkit. [Online]. Available from http://www.cdc.gov/healthcommunication/ToolsTemplates/SocialMediaToolkit_BM.pdf. [Last accessed September, 2019].
14. Petrovski G, Zivkovic M, Stratrova SS. Social media and diabetes: can Facebook and Skype improve glucose control in patients with type 1 diabetes on pump therapy? One-year experience. Diabetes Care. 2015;38(4):e51-2.
15. Gabarron E, Årsand E, Wynn R. Social media use in interventions for diabetes: Rapid evidence-based review. J Medical Internet Res. 2018;20(8):e10303.
16. Rao A, Hou P, Golnik T, et al. Evolution of data management tools for managing self-monitoring of blood glucose results: a survey of iPhone applications. J Diabetes Sci Technol. 2010;4(4):949-57.

85 CHAPTER Insulin Injection Techniques: Do's or Don'ts

Swati Srivastava, Yadvendra Gupta, Sonam Gupta

Laughter is the best medicine unless you're diabetic, then insulin comes pretty high on the list.

Jasper Carrott

INTRODUCTION

The discovery of insulin by Banting and Best in 1921 is the major breakthrough in medicine of the 20th century.[1] It gave a new lease of life to millions of people with diabetes all over the world but had also created some new problems in its wake. Among all therapeutic advances seen in the last few years, insulin remains the pillar of treatment. The first person to receive insulin injection was Leonard Thompson in January 1922.[2] But still the art of injecting the insulin is rocket science for patients. With the development of newer insulin delivery devices, acceptance for insulin is increasing day by day.

JOURNEY OF INSULIN: FROM HUMAN INSULIN TO INSULIN ANALOG

The first insulin was animal insulin, bovine and porcine, manufactured from beef and pork respectively. After this, human insulin was produced by genetic engineering using *Escherichia coli* and yeast in 1960. But since the conventional human insulins [regular, neutral protamine Hagedorn (NPH), Lente] have certain drawbacks, so newer insulin analogs are made by altering the amino acid sequence of human insulin to modify the onset or duration of action.

Analog insulins can be either rapid acting or long acting. Premixed combinations of analog insulin are also available (Table 1).[3]

Long-acting insulins Glargine and Detemir are also called peakless insulins with a long duration of action of about 24 hours.

Degludec is an ultralong-acting peakless insulin.

The inhaled insulin has an onset of action within 12–15 minutes, peaking at 30 minutes and duration of 3 hours.

Do's and Don'ts about Insulin Mixing

Mixtures of insulin can be sometimes combined in the same syringe, for example, intermediate-, rapid-, or short-acting insulin. Not all insulin can be mixed together.

For convenience and ease of use, premixed combinations of rapid-acting and intermediate-acting insulins are available. The onset of action of insulin will be of the fastest-acting insulin in the combination. It will peak when each type of insulin typically peaks, and it will last as long as the longest-acting insulin.

Do's: While mixing, the regular insulin should be drawn first into the syringe followed by longer acting insulin.

Don'ts: Insulin glargine has an acidic pH and cannot be mixed with any other insulin.

HOW TO CALCULATE INSULIN DOSE?

Facts to know about insulin:

- *Basal insulin*: Approximately 40–50% of the total daily insulin dose is to replace insulin overnight, when you are fasting, and between meals. This is called background or basal insulin replacement. The basal insulin dose is mostly constant.
- *Bolus insulin*: The other 50–60% of the total daily insulin dose is for carbohydrate coverage (food) and

TABLE 1: Types of insulin.[3]

Insulin type (trade name)	Onset	Peak	Duration
Bolus (prandial) insulins			
Rapid-acting insulin analogs (clear):			
• Insulin aspart	10–15 min	1–1.5 hr	3–5 hr
• Insulin glulisine	10–15 min	1–1.5 hr	3–5 hr
• Insulin lispro	10–15 min	1–2 hr	3.5–4.75 hr
Short-acting insulins (clear): • Insulin regular	30 min	2–3 hr	6.5 h
Basal insulins			
Intermediate-acting insulins (cloudy): • Insulin NPH	1–3 hr	5–8 hr	Up to 18 hr
Long-acting basal insulin analogs (clear) • Insulin detemir • Insulin glargine • Insulin degludec	90 min	Not applicable	Up to 24 hr glargine 24 hr, detemir 16–24 hr
Premixed insulins			
Premixed regular insulin—NPH (cloudy): • 30% insulin regular/70% insulin NPH • 50% insulin regular/50% insulin NPH	A single vial or cartridge contains a fixed ratio of insulin (ratio of rapid-insulin to intermediate-acting insulin)		
Premixed insulin analogs (cloudy): • 30% insulin aspart/70% insulin aspart protamine crystals • 25% insulin lispro/75% insulin lispro protamine • 50% insulin lispro/50% insulin lispro protamine			

(NPH: neutral protamine Hagedorn)

high blood sugar correction. This is called the bolus insulin replacement.

The bolus dose required for the meal intake is calculated as insulin-to-carbohydrate ratio. The insulin-to-carbohydrate ratio indicates how many grams of carbohydrate are metabolized by each unit of insulin. If your insulin-to-carbohydrate ratio is 1:10, then 1 unit of insulin will cover 10 g of carbohydrate.

CORRECTION FACTOR

A correction factor means the amount of reduction in blood glucose by each unit of rapid-acting insulin.

To calculate correction factor:

1. Sum up entire insulin daily intake in 24 hours (long acting and rapid acting). This is called your total daily dose (TDD).
2. Divide 100 by your TDD. The result is your correction factor. Example: 100/50 units (TDD) = 2.0. In this example, 1 unit will lower your blood sugar by 2 mmol/L. If your blood sugar is 10 mmol/L, then 1 unit will lower it to 8 mmol/L and 2 units will lower it to 6 mmol/L.

Total daily insulin requirement:

Calculation for the body's daily insulin requirement usually is:

Total daily insulin requirement (in units of insulin) = 0.55 × Total weight (in kg)

Basal/background insulin dose:

Basal/background insulin dose = 40–50% of total daily insulin dose[4]

When to start insulin:[5]

- *Absolute use*:
  - Type 1 diabetes mellitus (DM)
  - Type 2 DM with oral hypoglycemic agent failure—primary or secondary
  - Gestational diabetes mellitus (GDM).
- *Intermittent use*: In type 2 DM with

- Acute infections
- Surgery
- Acute MI
- Stroke
- Fever
- Acute emergencies—hyperosmolar hyperglycemic state (HHS), diabetic ketoacidosis (DKA)
- Pregnancy
- Microvascular complication—Retinopathy, neuropathy, nephropathy
- Preoperative control.

INSULIN DELIVERY DEVICES (FIG. 1)

- *Insulin syringe*: Usually, two strengths are available in India—U-100 (100 U/mL) and U-40 (40 U/mL). Now U-500 is also available.
- *Insulin pens*: The benefits of insulin pumps are as follows
  - More accurate dosing mechanism
  - Better compliance
  - More convenient and easier than syringes.
- Insulin pump (continuous subcutaneous insulin infusion pump)
  - Advantages
    - Improved quality of life
    - Less hypo- or hyperglycemia excursions
    - Programmable insulin delivery possible.
  - Disadvantages
    - Patient education and motivation is required.
    - High cost
    - Mechanical failure leads to complications and type 1 DM.

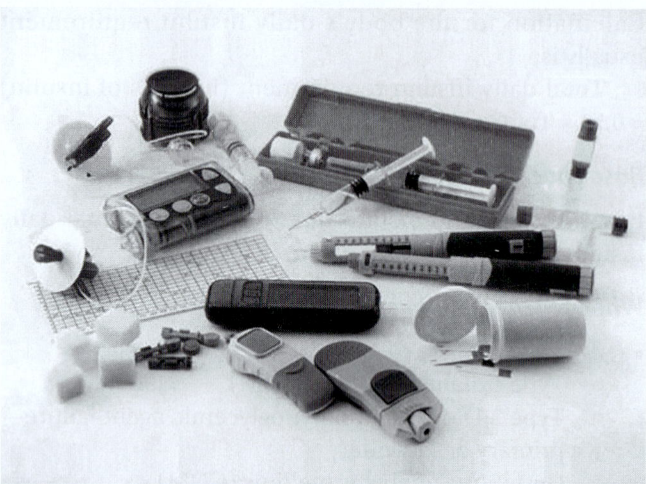

Figure 1 Insulin delivery devices.

INSULIN IN PREGNANCY[6]

Insulin detemir, lispro, and NPH are safe in pregnancy (category B). Insulin glulisine and degludec are pregnancy category C.

Sick Day Guidelines

Sick days refer to periods of minor intercurrent illness and usually last for 1–4 days that need changes in usual diabetes management practices.

When you are sick, there are chances of both hyperglycemia (due to stress hormone) and hypoglycemia (due to poor oral intake) which can lead to further complications such as DKA and HHS.[7]

Sick day management is tailored to the individual needs of the patients and is started with the first sign of illness. Try to eat your normal type and amount of food and to drink extra fluid. Continue your diabetic medications even if you are sick. If you are still not able to take orally, then call your doctor to adjust insulin dose. Never discontinue taking insulin, especially basal insulin. In case of dehydration or renal impairment, metformin should be avoided. Check your blood sugar levels at least 3–4 hourly, even through night. The patient on insulin should test for ketones.

In Pregnant Women

Diabetic ketoacidosis during pregnancy occurs more often in type 1 DM than type 2 DM or GDM. Diabetic ketoacidosis is more likely to occur in second and third trimesters because of increased insulin resistance, relative insulin deficiency, and starvation leading to increased free fatty acids which are then converted to ketones in liver. Prompt care and hospitalization should occur when there is hyperglycemia and/or emesis and/or ketosis and/or other concurrent illness in pregnant women.

Insulin Injection Techniques (Fig. 2)

Do's

- Insulin vials should be refrigerated when not in use.
- Before injecting the insulin, it should be brought to room temperature to avoid pain.
- Gently roll the vial between the palms of the hand before injecting.
- Wash your hands and clean the skin.

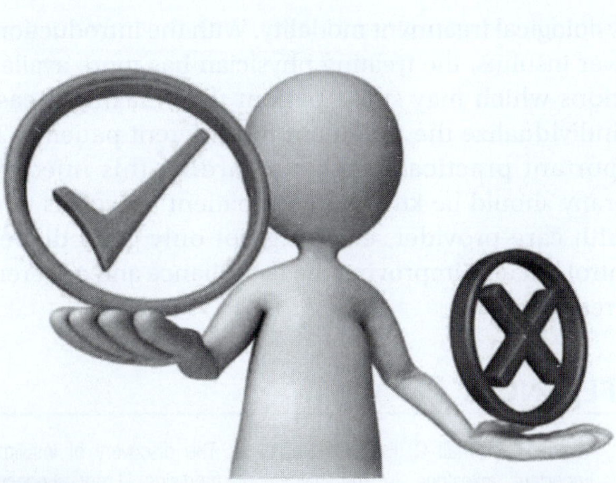

Figure 2 Insulin injection techniques.

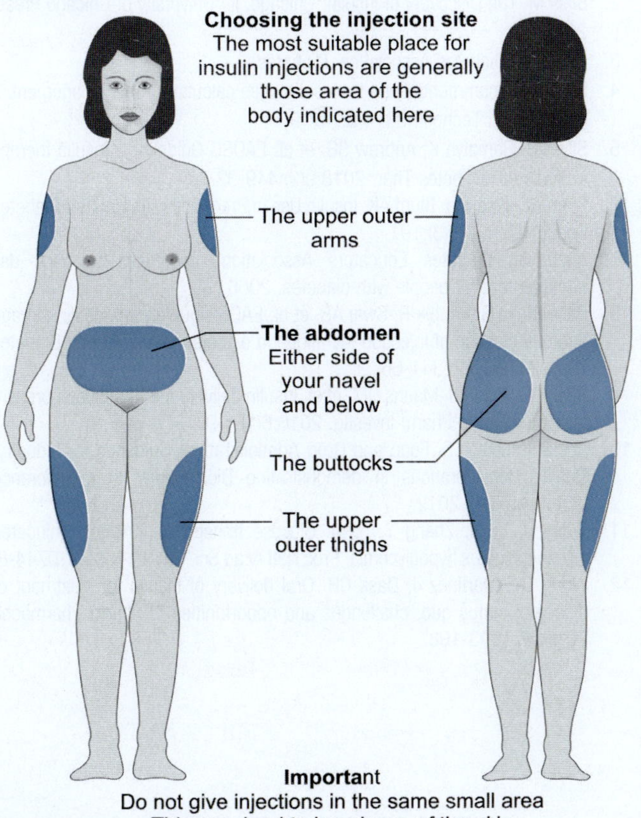

Figure 3 Injection sites.

- Remove air bubbles from the syringe because air displaces insulin and alters the dose.
- Injection sites—the abdomen, the upper arms, the anterior or lateral aspect of thighs, or the hips or buttocks. The abdomen is the preferred site because of fastest and less variable absorption. Injection should be avoided 5 cm around the umbilicus (Fig. 3).
- For better absorption and to minimize lipodystrophy, follow a pattern to rotate injection site within one anatomical area such as abdomen.
- Pinch up the skin fold and inject at 90° to skin surface. For thin patient use 45° angle to avoid intramuscular (IM) injection.
- Insulin syringe or pen needle should be replaced after three to four pricks.[8,9]

Don'ts

- Insulin pen should not refrigerated.
- Do not use insulin that appears clumped or granular or sticks to the side of the vial.
- Should not inject too intramuscular.

BARRIERS OF INSULIN THERAPY

- Psychological insulin resistance, from patients and treating doctor
- Pain and needle phobia
- Inconvenience
- False belief that insulin is only for "serious" cases
- Fear of hypoglycemia
- Need to monitor the sugar more frequently.

WHAT IS NEW IN INSULIN?

Biosimilar insulins: They are designed to be highly similar to the original, reference, insulin product described in a patent.[10] Biosimilar insulins are analog to the generic version and are manufactured by similar techniques but are not identical to the patent. So, the patent and biosimilar insulin have the same amino acid sequence but differ slightly in molecular characteristics and clinical profiles. The primary target by manufacturers of biosimilar insulin is expected to be insulin Glargine. The introduction of biosimilars into the insulin market will have significant impact on diabetes management cost, accessibility of insulin, number of choices, insulin available, and market competition. But the manufacturers have to face major challenges on regulatory, ethical, commercial, and competitive fronts.

NEW SMART INSULIN: BRING LIGHT TO DARK SIDE OF INSULIN

Smart insulin is a next-generation insulin that would revolutionize the treatment of diabetes as it automatically responds to changing blood glucose levels. The more the blood sugar, the more the insulin release. So, it is also known as GRI (glucose response insulin) or i-insulin. In the body, insulin behaves as a "key" to assist glucose enter into cells from the blood. When insulin attaches to a cell's surface, it activates glucose transporter, a protein inside the cell which allows glucose to enter the cell.

A molecule is added to create this new smart insulin. The glucose transporter inhibitor, which is the added one, blocks the glucose transporter molecule that has come to the surface chemically. It does not inhibit all glucose from entering nor does it permanently block the transporter molecules. On the other hand, it is a dynamic process that relies on how many inhibitor and glucose molecules are present keeping blood sugar at normal levels and reducing the risk of hypoglycemia.[11]

Oral Insulins

They are a much-awaited form of insulin delivery because of inconvenience and poor compliance with injections. Oral insulin is claimed to be better than subcutaneous administration as it mimics the physiology of endogenous insulin secreted by pancreas. After oral ingestion, it reaches the liver through the portal system.[12] Also, it has the potential to protect pancreatic B-cells from autoimmune destruction. The major problem with oral insulin is to overcome several physiological barriers which lead to low bioavailability. So, many manufacturers are actively pursuing to develop oral insulin.

CONCLUSION

Insulin treatment, which is offered to millions of people with diabetes, has undergone radical developments in the last decades providing a pure, less antigenic, and more physiological treatment modality. With the introduction of newer insulins, the treating physician has more available options which may suit a patient thus making it easier to individualize the treatment for different patients. The important practical aspects regarding this injectable therapy should be known to the patient as well as to the health care provider, ensuring not only good diabetes control but also improving the compliance and adherence to treatment.

REFERENCES

1. Vecchio I, Tornali C, Bragazzi NL, et al. The discovery of insulin: An important milestone in the history of medicine. Front. Endocrinol. 2018;9:613.
2. Bliss M. The Discovery of Insulin. Chicago, IL: University of Chicago Press; 2007.
3. Canadian Diabetes Association. Diabetes.
4. Rees C. Recommendations for insulin dose calculator risk management. J Diabetes Sci Technol. 2014;8:142-9.
5. Silver B, Ramaiya K, Andrew SB, et al. EADSG Guidelines: Insulin therapy in diabetes. Diabetes Ther. 2018;9(2):449-92.
6. Blum AK. Erratum: Blum AK. Insulin Use in Pregnancy: An Update. Diabetes Spectr. 2016;;29(3):191.
7. Australian Diabetes Educators Association. Guidelines for sick day management for people with diabetes. 2006.
8. Bahendeka S, Kauhik R, Swai AB, et al. EADSG guidelines: insulin storage and optimisation of injection technique in diabetes management. Diabetes Ther. 2019;10(2):341-66.
9. Shah RB, Patel M, Maahs DM, et al. Insulin delivery methods: past, present and future. Int J Pharm Investig. 2016;6(1):1-9.
10. Rockville MD. U.S. Food and Drug Administration: Guidance for industry: Quality Considerations in demonstrating Biosimilarity to a Reference protein product 2012.
11. Wang J, Yu J, Zhang Y, et al. Glucose transporter inhibitor-conjugated insulin mitigates hypoglycemia. Proc Natl Acad Sci. 2019;116(22):10744-8.
12. Wong CY, Martinez J, Dass CR. Oral delivery of insulin for treatment of diabetes: status quo, challenges and opportunities. J Pharm Pharmacol. 2016;68:1093-108.

CHAPTER 86 Managing Diabetes during Travel and Sick Days

Meenaxi Sharda, Nitesh Kumar Bauddh

"The impulse to travel is one of the hopeful symptoms of life"
and
"Sickness is mankind's greatest defect"

INTRODUCTION

Travel as well as sickness often leads to drastic departure in daily routine and may cause problems in diabetic patient by predisposing to hyper- and hypoglycemia, therefore demanding special care on part of patients and treating physicians. This chapter summarizes practical points for managing diabetes during travel and sickness.

MANAGING DIABETES DURING TRAVEL

Travelling poses challenges in diabetes management due to:

- Less or more physical activity than usual
- Skipped/delayed meals/overeating
- Crossing time zones in overseas travel
- Infections and trauma (especially foot) during leisure and religious activities
- Limited access to healthcare facilities.

General advice for patients:

- Visit doctor at least 3–4 weeks prior to major travel[1-3] (>2–3 days or overseas travel)
- Gets a physician's prescription mentioning disease, treatment details, complications, specific things to be carried during travel, and contact details of treating doctor. Get information about the local doctors and healthcare facilities of travel area[1,2]
- Get information about timings of arrival and departure, mode and duration of travel, weather information, specific diets of the place, and leisure activities to be done. Choose "diabetic meal" option in airline, if available
- Get information about prevalent endemic and communicable diseases in visiting area to receive chemoprophylaxis and vaccines accordingly
- Pack baggage wisely, especially in case of major or international travel (Box 1)[1-3]
- Patients on insulin should monitor blood sugar (BS) frequently (4–6 hourly), especially while experiencing symptoms of hypoglycemia.[1-3] Check BS before high-risk activities (long driving, surfing, rafting, trekking, bungee jumping, and paragliding)
- Patients on oral hypoglycemic agents (OHA) with good glycemic control prior to travel can check BS as and when needed, as regular monitoring is not necessary for them

BOX 1 Things to be packed.

- Physician's prescription, insurance papers, and diabetic identification card with contact numbers in case of emergency
- Double quantity of medicines, insulin, and syringes in two different bags and preferably carry them in cabin luggage
- Pump users should carry insulin and syringes as an alternative option in case of pump malfunction
- Glucometer with extra batteries, glucose and ketone strips, and lancets
- Keep a first aid kit and medicines for common ailments
- Snacks (dry fruits, nuts, roasted peas, biscuits) to avoid hypoglycemia in case of delayed meals.
- Rescue medicines for hypoglycemia—glucose tablets, candies, and glucagon injection

TABLE 1: Management of diabetes during overseas travel.

Travel → ↓ Basal insulin	Eastward	Westward
Once daily	Take reduced dose# on usual time, follow normal schedule thereafter	On day of travel, take half of usual dose when due, then change watch to arrival time zone and take the 2nd half dose when due, according to arrival time zone. Follow normal schedule thereafter
Twice daily	Reduce# first dose encountered after departure and take as per departure time. Then set watch to arrival time zone and follow normal schedule thereafter	Take half of first encountered dose during travel when due according to departure time, then change watch to arrival time zone and take the second half dose when due. Follow normal schedule thereafter

#Reduced dose = Normal Dose $\times \left(0.9 - \frac{\text{Number of time zones crossed}}{\text{Hours between basal dose}}\right)$

- Keep yourself well hydrated during travel. Eat frequent, light homemade meals, fresh fruits, and vegetables while avoiding unhygienic street food
- Wear comfortable clothes and proper fitting footwear. Avoid walking barefoot in religious premises, gardens, and beaches. Inspect your foot daily for any blisters or ulcerations

Advice for healthcare providers:
- Thorough checkup of patient including routine laboratory tests as required
- Any change in treatment regimen should be done well in advance of departure
- Vaccinate for influenza and pneumonia as per guidelines
- It is safe to keep slightly high BS levels then causing hypoglycemia, especially in elders
- Explain symptoms of hypoglycemia to patient and educate accompanying persons about detection and management of hypoglycemia[1,2]

Management during overseas travel:
Traveling north and south needs no dose adjustment, however adjustments are needed in drug dosages and timings, if more than three time zones are crossed during eastward or westward travel as travelling east shortens day while travelling west lengthens it causing risk of hypo- and hyperglycemia, respectively.[1-3]
- *Adjustment Of OHA:*[1,3]
  - *Non-sulfonylurea OHAs*: Continue unadjusted
  - *Sulfonylurea*:
    - *Westward travel*: Continue unadjusted, but hold, if meals missed.
    - *Eastward travel*: Immediate release—skip evening dose on day of travel.
    - *Extended release*: Hold on day of travel
- *Adjustment of insulin*:[1,3] Regimen should be changed to basal bolus and use of insulin pens should be encouraged:
  - *Bolus insulin*: Analogs are preferred over regular insulin:
    - Continue unadjusted and take insulin before each meal
    - Interval between two doses should be at least 3–4 hours for analog and 6 hours for regular insulin.
  - *Basal insulin*: Change needed while crossing >3 time zones (Table 1):
    - Eastward travel requires reduction in basal insulin dose.
    - Westward travel needs either extending or adding additional coverage of insulin.

MANAGING DIABETES DURING SICK DAYS

Medical and surgical illnesses cause derangements in hormonal milieu of body with increase in counter regulatory hormones (glucagon, cortisol, norepinephrine, and growth hormone) and various cytokines.[4,5] This leads to a relative insulin resistant state, increased production of glucose from liver, and decreased peripheral utilization causing hyperglycemia.[4,5] Recurrent vomiting, decreased appetite, and severe sepsis can lead to hypoglycemia. Thus managing diabetes and hyperglycemia in sick patients is a challenge for treating physicians.

Outpatient management:
Patients with minor illness and stable blood sugars can be managed on OPD basis with following advice:
- Do not take any over the counter medicines without doctor's advice
- Keep yourself well hydrated and take medicines as earlier, even if you are eating less

- Patients on insulin should monitor their BS frequently and should do urine ketone test, if blood sugar >250 mg/dL
- Contact your doctor or emergency department if blood sugars are low, or persistently high, or if warning symptoms of ketoacidosis are present (recurrent vomiting, abdominal pain, and breathlessness).

Inpatient management:

- In hospitalized patients, both hypoglycemia (BS <70 mg/dL) and hyperglycemia (BS >140 mg/dL) are associated with poor outcomes including prolonged hospital stay, more severe illness, infections, disability after hospital discharge, and death[4-7]
- In-hospital management depends on various factors—type of diabetes, nature and severity of illness, baseline BS, glycated hemoglobin (HbA1c) (to differentiate stress hyperglycemia from undiagnosed diabetes), insulin sensitivity, feeding pattern [oral, enteral, parenteral, or nil per oral (NPO)], associated comorbidities (renal/liver failure, elderly or terminally ill) and risk of hypoglycemia.[4-7]

Noncritically ill patients:

- HbA1c should be done in all patients, if not done in last 3 months
- Target blood sugar is 140–180 mg/dL as per the American Diabetes Association (ADA),[6]
    - Premeal <140 mg/dL and post meal <180 mg/dL as per RSSDI[7]
- Initiate insulin when blood sugar is more than 180 mg/dL and follow regimen (Table 2) depending on oral intake of patient.

Critically Ill/intensive care unit (ICU) patients:

- *Target blood sugar*: 140–180 mg/dL[6,7]
- *Frequency* of sugar monitoring: 1–2 hourly
- *Insulin regimen:* Continuous intravenous (IV) infusion of regular insulin through an accurate infusion pump using validated protocols.[6]
- *Infusion rate*—initial IV bolus dose of 0.1 unit/kg, if blood sugar >300 mg/dL
    - Initial infusion rate/hour = Blood sugar ÷ 100
    - Further adjustments tailored as per trend of blood sugar till target of 140–180 mg/dL is achieved. Once a stable BS (two consecutive target readings) is achieved, monitoring of BS can be done 2–3 hourly.

Management of hyperglycemia in surgical patients:

- Target blood sugar during perioperative period is 80–180 mg/dL[8,9]

TABLE 2: Noncritically ill patients.[6,7]

Adequate oral intake	Poor oral intake/NPO
• *BS monitoring*: Premeals and at bedtime • *Regimen*: Basal bolus *Basal insulin*: (NPH–12 hourly, Detemir 12–24 hourly or glargine 24 hourly) • Starting dose—0.2–0.3 u/kg/day or 30–50% of total daily dose (TDD)* • Adjust 10–20% every 2–3 days *Bolus insulin*: (Regular, aspart, lispro, glulisine) before meals • *Prandial or nutritional insulin:* ○ Dose—0.05–0.1 u/kg/meal or ○ 50% of TDD divided in three parts + • *Correctional insulin:* ○ For blood sugar >150, add graded scale of 1–4 units for each increment of 50 mg/dL as per insulin sensitivity *TDD = 0.3–0.5 u/kg/day body weight Consider starting with 0.1–0.3 u/kg/day for patients with renal and hepatic impairment and geriatric patients.	*BS monitoring*: 4–6 hourly **Bolus enteral feeds** • *Regimen*: Basal + correctional + nutritional • *Basal insulin*: (NPH–12 hourly, Detemir 12–24 hourly or glargine 24 hourly) ○ Starting Dose—0.2–0.3 u/kg/day or ○ Adjust 10–20% every 2–3 days. • *Correctional insulin*: Regular insulin 6 hourly OR analog insulin 4 hourly • For blood sugar >150, add graded scale of 1–4 units for each increment of 50 mg/dL as per insulin sensitivity • *Nutritional insulin*: Add 1 unit insulin for each 10–15 g carbohydrate in feeds. **Continuous enteral feeds** • *Regimen*: basal + correctional (as above) **Total parenteral nutrition (TPN):** • *Regimen*: Basal + correctional (as above) + *Nutritional insulin*: Add 1 unit insulin for each 10 g dextrose in TPN

(BS: blood sugar; NPH: neutral protamine Hagedorn; NPO: nil per oral)

TABLE 3: Preoperative adjustment of OHA.

Day before surgery	On day of surgery (normal oral intake anticipated on same day)	On day of surgery (reduced oral intake anticipated)
Continue all OHAs, except SGLT2 inhibitors	Withhold SU and SGLT2 inhibitors Others can be taken	Withhold all OHAs, except DPP4 inhibitors

(OHA: oral hypoglycemic agents; SU: sulfonylurea; SGLT2: sodium-glucose cotransporter 2; DPP4: dipeptidyl peptidase-4)

- Adjustment of OHA depends on the nature of surgery and anticipated oral intake thereafter[8,9] (Table 3)
- Insulin adjustment depends on the type of insulin being taken by patient[8,9] (Table 4)
- Irrespective of preoperative mode of treatment or need of surgery (emergency/elective), insulin is given for intra- and postoperative management of hyperglycemia when BS >180 mg/dL (Table 5).

Transition from intravenous to subcutaneous insulin:
- Start when patient resumes adequate oral intake
- Calculate TDD based on insulin infusion rate over last 8 hours
- Give 50–70% of TDD as basal insulin and 30–50% as prandial bolus insulin divided in 3 doses
- Stop insulin infusion 2–4 hours after giving basal insulin dose.

Transition from hospital to home:
- Patients with mild hyperglycemia or those with HbA1c <7–8% can be restarted on preadmission regimen at the time of discharge with close follow-up.
- Critically ill patients, patients with marked hyperglycemia, high HbA1c (>8–9%), and comorbidities may be continued on insulin (basal bolus or premixed) at discharge for few more months and additionally OHA can be started (if not contraindicated) as per patients glycemic status. In author's view and experience, teneligliptin [dipeptidyl peptidase-4 (DPP4) inhibitor] is cheaper and safe option in combination with insulin and metformin or as monotherapy.

TABLE 4: Preoperative adjustment of insulin.[8,9]

Insulin used	Day before surgery		Day of surgery
	AM dose	*PM dose*	*AM dose*
Glargine/Detemir	As usual	75–80%	50–80% of usual
NPH/Premixed	As usual	75–80%	50% if BS >120, otherwise hold it
Short-acting	As usual	As usual	HOLD

(NPH: neutral protamine Hagedorn)

TABLE 5: Intra- and postoperative management.[8,9]

Intraoperatively	Postoperatively
• Intravenous insulin infusion OR subcutaneous insulin (if duration of surgery <4 hours) • Use scale as per critically ill patients with sugar monitoring 1–2 hourly.	• Reduced oral intake: ○ Basal + correctional insulin • Adequate oral intake: ○ Basal + nutritional + correctional insulin.

CONCLUSION

Undue fear of dealing with diabetes medications, especially insulin should not prevent people with diabetes from traveling for work or recreation. Caution and vigilance on patient's part and simple specific individualized advice from physicians along with diabetes education and protocol based in-hospital management can help in maintaining euglycemia in special situation of travel and sickness.

REFERENCES

1. Pavela J, Suresh R, Blue RS, et al. Management of diabetes during air travel: a systematic literature review of current recommendations and their supporting evidence. Endocr pract. 2018;24(2):205-19.
2. Chandran M, Edelman SV. Have Insulin, Will Fly: Diabetes management during air travel and time zone adjustment strategies. Clinical Diabetes. 2003;21(2):82-5.
3. Pinsker JE, Becker E, Mahnke CB, et al. Extensive clinical experience: a simple guide to basal insulin adjustments for long-distance travel. J Diabetes Metab Disord. 2013;12(1):59.
4. Umpierrez G, Pasquel FJ. Management of inpatient hyperglycemia and diabetes in older adults. diabetes care. 2017;40(4):509-17.
5. Corsino L, Dhatariya K, Umpierrez G. (2017). Management of diabetes and hyperglycemia in hospitalized patients. [Online]. Available from https://www.ncbi.nlm.nih.gov/books/NBK279093. [Last accessed October, 2019].
6. American Diabetes Association. Diabetes Care in the Hospital:Standards of Medical Care in Diabetes—2019. Diabetes Care. 2019;42(Suppl 1):S173-81.
7. Panikar V, Sosale A, Agarwal S, et al. RSSDI clinical practice recommendations for management of In-hospital hyperglycaemia. Int J Diabetes Dev Ctries. 2016;36:S1-21.
8. Duggan EW, Carlson K, Umpierrez GE. Perioperative Hyperglycemia Management: An Update. Anesthesiology. 2017;126(3):547-60.
9. Simha V, Shah P. Perioperative Glucose Control in Patients With Diabetes Undergoing Elective Surgery. JAMA. 2019;321(4):399-400.

87 CHAPTER Quality of Life: An Important Parameter in Diabetes Management

Ashok K Taneja, Akshat Taneja, Divya Taneja

INTRODUCTION

The quality of life is more important than Life itself.

Alexis Carrel

Good quality life is the one which has perfect balance between the healthy status of mind, body, and soul. It has all the elements of the body working in perfect harmony to create peace, happiness, healthy, and ultimately the longevity. By having good quality of life, the individual is healthy, comfortable, and able to participate in or enjoy life events. Quality of life is highly subjective. Whereas one person may define quality of life according to wealth, another person may define it in terms of capabilities. Our life is guided by the values, goals, and sociocultural, economic situations with the balancing of negative and positive features leading to healthy body with healthy mind. Happiness or good quality life cannot be measured on any scale; however, an index is made for reference only.

How to measure quality index:

- GDP or standard of living
- Human development index
- Happiness index
- Life index—disease free
- Civil index of society.

In the field of healthcare, quality of life is often regarded in terms of how a certain ailment affects a patient on an individual level or at family level. There may be a debilitating weakness that is not life-threatening; life-threatening illness that is not terminal; or terminal illness which may bring doom to the family.

There are many factors which influence the quality of life:

- Disease
- Economic
- Family disharmony
- Society conflict
- Psychosocial mismatch

Diabetes is a chronic illness requiring medication lifelong. It may require simple and basic treatment or may require advanced treatment like laser therapy for retinopathy, amputations or even organ transplants as in chronic kidney disease (CKD), chronic lung disease (CLD) etc. However the good quality of life in diabetics can be achieved in the following ways:

Dictum of good quality of life in diabetics is— "Maintain healthy weight, proper nutritious diet, regular exercise, and good psychosocial well-being with tight control of blood sugar levels."

We postulate ten commandants for wholesome wellbeing of mind-body-soul, i.e. improving quality of life in diabetics:

- Diet
- Salt
- Sweeteners
- Micronutrients
- Exercise
- Psychosocial management like sleep, yoga, music, meditation
- Sex
- Tobacco
- Alcohol
- Pollution—air/water/earth.

DIET

Food exhibits a direct effect on blood glucose levels. Certain food items raise blood glucose more than others. Thus, knowing what and how much to eat, and following an eating plan that not only fits your lifestyle but also helps to control blood glucose forms an important part of diabetes management. The three major nutrients found in foods are carbohydrates (carbs), proteins, and fats. The ideal diet in diabetics (normal weight) should be:

- *Normal weight*: 50% carbohydrates—30% proteins, 20% fats
- *Diabetic obese*: 30–40% carbohydrates, 40–50% proteins, and 10–15% fats.

The dictum is "Increase proteins to around 40% of calorie intake".

Carbohydrates

Carbohydrates are the starches, sugar, and fiber found in the foods, for example, grains, fruits, vegetables, milk products, and sweets. They lead to a rapid and higher rise in blood glucose values than other nutrients in foods. It is very important to know which foods contain carbohydrates and in how much quantity. Choosing carbohydrates from healthy sources like vegetables, fruits, and whole grains (high fiber) is preferred. Addition of sugar to any diet and sugar-added beverages are to be strictly avoided.

Proteins

Proteins are a necessary part of a balanced diet and help in controlling satiety. They do not directly raise blood glucose like carbohydrates. Rather, they build the body muscles and liver functionality to store glycogen. In type 2 diabetics, protein makes insulin to work faster, so treating low blood sugar with protein shakes or mixes may not be a good idea.

Fats

Fats are necessary part of a balanced diet, especially healthy fats from fatty fish, nuts, and seeds. They do not raise blood glucose but are high in calories. Intake in higher quantities can cause weight gain and hence, poor diabetic control.

Dictum for diabesity:
Have balanced diet and calories as per your body's need with 30–40% intake of proteins and <30% of carbohydrates.

SALT

Guyton's physiologic concept, that the role of the kidney in managing sodium is the key to the long-term regulation of blood pressure, is now usually accepted. Restriction on dietary sodium is strongly advocated as a lifestyle change for preventing and treating hypertension and as a result, cardiovascular morbidity and mortality. More so, in diabetics those are suffering from end-stage renal disease (ESRD) or diabetes mellitus (DM) with stroke/PVDs. The WHO strongly recommends restricting the daily sodium intake to less than 2,000 mg, while the American Heart Association (AHA) advises lesser than 1,500 mg sodium per day.

Tips for reducing your salt intake:

- Decrease the amount you use in cooking and determine what you put in instead of just shaking the salt cellar over the pan! As your taste buds get adapted to less salt intake, set a target to cut it out completely.
- Do not buy processed food as they are high in salt and fat contents. For packed foods, first read the label, and how much salt it contains?
- Avoid fast foods like burgers/fried potato wedges/samosa/vadas etc.
- Add flavor to your food with herbs and spices instead of using the salt shaker. We end up often sprinkling salt on food out of habit more than need.
- Instead of salt, use paprika, ground white or black pepper, mild chili powder, lemon, ginger, chopped coriander thyme, rosemary or oregano on salads, fish, egg and other foods.
- Use more of fruits, fresh raw vegetables, and sprouts on your dining table.

SWEETENERS: WHICH SUGAR TO TAKE?

Sweeteners are the ingredients that are added to food to bring sweetness. They can be grouped as sugar or sugar substitutes, or they can be grouped as—nutritive or nonnutritive.

Nutritive Sweeteners

Nutritive sweeteners are those sugars which contain carbohydrates and provide calories. There are different types of nutritive sweeteners which can be natural, like in fruits/vegetables or nonnatural which are synthesized from natural sources and are added as sweeteners like sugar and jaggery.

Natural sugars are glucose, fructose, sucrose, maltose, honey, polyols, etc. Nonnatural or synthetic sugars are sugar, jaggery, khaand, etc.

Polyols: One class of nutritive sweeteners is polyols, which are sugar alcohols. It includes erythritol, isomalt, mannitol, sorbitol, maltitol, and xylitol. Polyols contain carbohydrates and calories, but the calories are fewer and have minimal effects on the blood glucose levels. They can be natural or artificially produced. Polyols are generally used in products being marketed as "diabetic" or "suitable for diabetics". However occasionally, these products may contain high levels of fats and calories as the standard products. Large amounts of polyols can exert a laxative effect and may cause bloating, flatulence, and diarrhea. Their use is not recommended by the Diabetes UK and the European Commission Regulations.

Nonnutritive or Artificial Sweeteners

Nonnutritive sweeteners are used to reduce overall carbohydrate and calories intake. They are added as artificial sweeteners and are usually found in "sugar-free" or "diet" foods and drinks, fizzy drinks, fruit juices, jellies, yogurts, chewing gums, etc.

There are various artificial sweeteners licensed for use like—aspartame, saccharin, sucralose, acesulfame potassium (acesulfame-K), and cyclamate. Some products are combination of two artificial sweeteners also. A new group of nonnutritive, calorie-free sweeteners is made from the stevia plant, e.g. Truvia and Stevia. They are 200–300 times sweeter than sucrose (sugar) and are heat stable, so can be used in cooking and baking.

Which sweetener to use?

- *Natural*: The most naturally sweet foods are dates. Dried fruits, such as cherries, raisins, apricots and figs are also naturally sweet. Fresh fruits such as grapes, bananas, and melon can also impart sweet flavor to your food. Fresh and dried fruits can be added to several dishes like kheer, custard, yoghurt, raita or milk shakes—smoothies, cereals, and muffins in diced or puree form.
- *Artificial sweeteners*:
  - *Stevia*: Naturally derived from plant, it makes a good artificial sweetener. It has a bitter aftertaste that may bother some people. For this reason, some manufacturers add other sugars and ingredients for balancing the taste, which decreases the nutritional benefit of pure stevia. Some people have reported nausea, bloating, and stomach upset after using stevia. According to the FDA, the acceptable daily intake (ADI) of stevia is 4 mg/kg of body weight.
  - *Tagatose*: This is a form of fructose that is around 90% sweeter than sucrose. Though it is rare, some fruits, like apples, oranges, and pineapples, naturally provide tagatose. This has been used by manufacturers in foods as a low-calorie sweetener, texturizer, and stabilizer. Not only do the FDA class tagatose as GRAS (Generally Recognized As Safe), but scientists are also researching its potential to facilitate type 2 diabetes management.

    Some studies signify that tagatose has a low glycemic index (GI). It may thus support the treatment of obesity.
  - *Sucralose*: It is available under the brand name Splenda and an artificial sweetener made out of sucrose. This sweetener is about 600 times sweeter than table sugar but contains very less calories. This is heat-stable and thus a popular choice for sugar-free baking and sweetening hot drinks.

    Sucralose has been approved by the FDA as a general-purpose sweetener and set an ADI of 5 mg/kg of body weight. A 2016 study found that male mice that consumed sucralose were more likely to develop malignant tumors. However, more studies are required to confirm sucralose safety.
  - *Aspartame*: Aspartame has been available in the US since the 1980s and is a very common artificial sweetener. It is around 200 times sweeter than sugar and added to a wide variety of food products, including diet soda by the manufacturers. Aspartame breaks down at high temperatures, so generally can only be used as a table top sweetener. The FDA considers aspartame to be safe at an ADI of 50 mg/kg of body weight.
  - *Acesulfame potassium*: Acesulfame potassium is also known as acesulfame K and Ace-K. This is around 200 times sweeter than sugar. To combat its bitter aftertaste, manufacturers often combine acesulfame potassium with other sweeteners. The recommended use is 15 mg/kg of body weight. Acesulfame potassium is highly recommended by the FDA as a low-calorie sweetener after the results of more than 90 studies to support its safety.
  - *Saccharin*: This is a zero-calorie sweetener that is 200–700 times sweeter than table sugar. Concern had been raised about its association with bladder cancer in rats. However, its safety has been supported by more than 30 human studies and the National Institutes of Health no longer consider this as potential carcinogen. The ADI of saccharin as determined by the FDI is 15 mg/kg of body weight.
  - *Neotame:* Neotame is a low-calorie artificial sweetener. This is about 7,000–13,000 times sweeter

than table sugar. This sweetener can withstand high temperatures, rendering it suitable for baking. It is available under the brand name Newtame. It was approved by the FDA in 2002 as a general-purpose sweetener and flavor enhancer for all foods except for meat and poultry. It has been stated that more than 113 animal and human studies support the safety of neotame. The set ADI for neotame is 0.3 mg/kg of body weight.

MICRONUTRIENTS

Although use of micronutrients as nutrition therapy is a cornerstone of the management of diabetes, but uncertainty prevails in its guidelines. Whether the micronutrients are causative agents of diabetes or its complications or just innocent bystanders, is yet to be established. However, people with uncontrolled hyperglycemia are prone to develop deficiencies of some minerals like potassium, magnesium, zinc, chromium which may predispose to carbohydrate intolerance and insulin resistance. It has been postulated that some micronutrients have potent antioxidant properties. These include alpha-lipoic acid, carotenoids, vitamins E and C, selenium, and some of the B vitamins, notably folate, pyridoxine, and cyanocobalamin. *Their use as adjuvant in diet therapy helps in controlling diabetes and its complications.*

EXERCISE

Regular moderate exercise utilizes glucose and thus reduces blood sugar to reduce diabetes-related complications. Furthermore, it prevents development and progression of atherosclerosis, hence cardiovascular disease (CVD)-related mortality. Researchers have estimated (Framingham Study) that exercise increases longevity by 1.5 years in moderate and 3.5 years in vigorous exercise individuals. Results include reduction of triglycerides (TGs) (9.5%), low-density lipoprotein (LDL) (13.7%) and increase of high-density lipoprotein (HDL) (9.6%). American College of Sports Medicine and AHA current recommendation for exercise is:

- *30 minutes of moderate exercise (5–6 scale*, i.e. Mild increase in heart rate and breathing)—5 days a week.*
- *20 minutes of vigorous exercise (7–8 scale, i.e. noticeable change in heart rate breathing)—5 days a week.*
- *In addition, resistance training (weight training × 10 minutes) daily. All major muscle groups should be involved using 8–10 repetitions.*

10 point scale: Sitting is 0 scale and all-out effort is 10.

WHO has recommended 10,000 steps to walk daily. Those who cannot walk should do sitting exercises as per AHA scale.

YOGA AND MEDITATION

Reduce stress hormones and catecholamines. Lifestyle Heart Trial—Pranayama, Surya namaskar, Vajrasana asanas; meditation; group support sessions; and music therapy all lead to correction of glycosylated HbA1c levels, dyslipidemias with reversal of atherosclerotic plaques.

Meditation, sound sleep for 6–7 hours, listening to music, and dancing, all lead to reduction of stress hormones and relaxation of mind and body. This results in improving good quality of life.

SEX

Studies show that men with diabetes often have reduced testosterone levels, which can affect their sex drive. Moreover diabetes damages the blood vessels, which affect blood flow to the penis leading to erectile dysfunction. This is mediated by lower levels of nitrous oxide and hardening of vessels. Diabetes can also lead to nerve damage and compounds the problem further. Similarly in women also, there is reduced libido and decreased vaginal lubrication. Treatment is control of glycemia, vasodilators like sildenafil or vacuum pumps.

Tips for better sex in diabetics are:

- Approach sex like exercise with full emotional support.
- Use a lubricant. If you are a woman with vaginal dryness, a vaginal lubricant can make sex feel better.
- Creativity is sexy. If you have trouble getting aroused, stretch beyond your go-to bedroom moves. Watch erotica or porn together. Try out new positions or sex toys. Explore different ways to climax.
- Limit alcohol. A little alcohol may boost your desire, but drinking can also make your blood sugar level drop quickly.
- Get help for emotional issues. Depression, anxiety, poor self-image, and other emotional concerns can hurt your sex life.
- Relax—be confident and be relaxed. Do not try to force yourself. Be active.
- Use sildenafil or tadalafil, if erectile dysfunction (ED) is the problem.

TOBACCO

Chewing or smoking tobacco lowers HDL cholesterol with direct effect on endothelial lining of blood vessels hence more thrombogenic plaque formation. This results in enhanced diabetic complications. It induces insulin resistance also.

Complete cessation is the answer.

ALCOHOL

Mild level of alcohol intake lowers the risk of blood clots due to decreased inflammation markers and increased HDL levels. Moderate-to-heavy drinking increases CVD-related mortality due to increased LDL, TGs, blood pressure, and increased inflammatory markers with the result of increased insulin resistance. There is increased incidence of cardiomyopathy, ventricular arrhythmias, and endothelial dysfunction. There is also increased incidence of cirrhosis of liver, cancers, and most importantly, accidents.

What is the safe limit?

One Standard Drink is 10 g of pure ethyl alcohol. This amounts to 375 mL of beer (5% alcohol), 150 mL of wine (12% alcohol), and 45 mL of whiskey (40% alcohol). This is considered safe limit in a day for men. For women, it is 75% of above values. Red wine offers better protection due to presence of plant sterol—resveratrol.

Caution: No alcohol is the best option

POLLUTION

Air Pollution

According to the World Health Organization (WHO), air pollution can lead to lung cancer, respiratory infection, stroke, and even heart disease. Researchers at Washington University School of Medicine in St. Louis, MO, in collaboration with the Veterans Affairs St. Louis Health Care System in Missouri, found a strong link between air pollution and diabetes. The exact mechanism behind the relationship between air pollution and diabetes has not yet been proven. However increased exposure to levels of carbon monoxide, lead, and nitrogen dioxide with depletion of ozone may result in enhanced incidence of diabetes.

Water Pollution

Contaminants, especially arsenic, lead, cadmium, aniline dyes, and high levels of dissolved salts are suspected to contribute to higher incidence of type 1 diabetes, but may affect adults also due to increased incidence of hypertension and insulin resistance.

Earth Pollution

Use of pesticides, insecticides, and overuse of chemical fertilizers has shown the increased incidence of diabetes. Agricultural Health Study (AHS) project in the USA, a large cohort study of 33,457 pesticide applicators, reported an association between diabetes and seven organochlorine pesticides, including aldrin, chlordane, heptachlor, dichlorvos, trichlorfon, alachlor, and cyanazine.

SUGGESTED READING

1. Gregory D, Johnston R, Pratt G, Watts M, Whatmore S (Eds). The Dictionary of Human Geography, 5th edition. Oxford: Wiley-Blackwell; 2009.
2. UN General Assembly (65th sess.: 2010–2011). UN DAG Repository. (2011). Happiness: towards a holistic approach to development: resolution/ adopted by the General Assembly.
3. National Institutes of Health, Office of Dietary Supplements. (2011). Dietary supplements: what you need to know. [Online] Available from https://ods.od.nih.gov/HealthInformation/DS_WhatYouNeedToKnow.aspx [Last accessed October, 2019].
4. Campbell A. Joslin Diabetes Center. Common Food Myths for People with Diabetes Debunked.
5. Guerrero-Wyss M, Durán Agüero S, Angarita Dávila L. D-Tagatose is a promising sweetener to control glycaemia: A new functional food. Biomed Res Int. 2018;2018
6. Colberg SR, Sigal RJ, Yardley JE, et al. Physical activity/exercise and diabetes: a position statement of the American Diabetes Association. Diabetes Care. 2016;39(11):2065-79.
7. Chehade JM, Sheikh-Ali M, Mooradian AD. The role of micronutrients in managing diabetes. Diabetes Spectrum. 2009;22(4):214-8.
8. Centers for Disease Control and Prevention. (2017). Diabetes Public Health Resource: Prevent Diabetes.
9. American Diabetes Association. (2014). Erectile dysfunction. [Online] Available from http://www.diabetes.org/living-with-diabetes/treatment-and-care/men/erectile-dysfunction.html [Last accessed October, 2019].
10. Warshaw HS. Diabetes Meal Planning Made Easy, 4th edition. American Diabetes Association; 2017.
11. Inzucchi SE, Bergenstal RM, Buse JB, et al. Management of hyperglycemia in type 2 diabetes, 2015: a patient-centered approach: update to a position statement of the American Diabetes Association and the European Association for the Study of Diabetes. Diabetes Care. 2015;38:140-9.
12. Lawrence AM, Abraira C. New modalities in diabetes treatment. Am J Med. 1988;85(5A):153-8.
13. Steven S, Hollingsworth KG, Ar-Mrabeh A, et al. Very-low-calorie diet and 6 months of weight stability in type 2 diabetes: pathophysiologic changes in responders and nonresponders. Diabetes Care. 2016;39(5):808-15.
14. O'Donovan G, Cadena C. Air pollution and diabetes: it's time to get active!; Lancet. 2018;2(7):PE287-E288.
15. Longnecker MP, Daniels JL. Environmental contaminants as etiologic factors for diabetes. Environ Health Perspect. 2001;109(Suppl 6):871-6.
16. Montgomery MP, Kamel F, Saldana TM, et al. Incident diabetes and pesticide exposure among licensed pesticide applicators: agricultural health study, 1993-2003. Am J Epidemiol. 2008;167(10):1235-46.

13 SECTION

Diabetes and Technology

88 CHAPTER

Merits and Demerits of Insulin Pump and Continuous Glucose Monitoring

Jothydev Kesavadev

INTRODUCTION

Diabetes is regarded as a leading noncommunicable disease (NCD) that contributes substantially to morbidity and mortality. Expensive medical technologies are currently used for the treatment of complications associated with diabetes, such as coronary artery disease, diabetic foot, retinopathy, nephropathy, sexual dysfunction, etc. Though insulin pumps have been commercially available for more than four decades, they are seldom popular. The same is true with continuous glucose monitoring (CGM) technologies, which have been launched in India in the year 2004. The limited use of technologies could be attributed to a variety of reasons such as lack of knowledge among healthcare providers, need for extra time to convince the patients, paucity of a supporting diabetes care team, and prohibitively high cost. However, there is evidence from clinical trials and real-world experience on the prevention of microvascular and macrovascular complications, and significant reduction in the cost of care with the use of insulin pumps and CGM.

Insulin pumps and CGM are two technologies, which can be used together or separately for the optimal management of glycemia beyond aiming for conventional glycated hemoglobin (HbA1c), so as to reach "personalized time in target". This chapter briefly discusses the advantages of insulin pump therapy (IPT) and CGM, along with their limitations.

WHY IS TECHNOLOGY A BLESSING IN DIABETES?

Clinicians always face the challenge of addressing discrepancies between glucose values recorded by patients and their HbA1c values. Technology plays a vital role in efficiently managing such ambiguous situations.[1] However, in the past, glucose monitoring was considered a tedious task and involved several ambiguities. Benefits of intensive glucose management in type 2 diabetes were evident after the success of the landmark clinical trial, the United Kingdom Prospective Diabetes Study (UKPDS). Despite the practice of blood glucose monitoring, patients were not able to achieve desired outcomes. Thus, the idea of complementing technology took root.[1]

Diabetes technology has rapidly evolved in the past decade. Technological advances have mostly focused on the use of continuous glucose monitoring systems (CGMS) and continuous subcutaneous insulin infusions (CSII or insulin pump) for the management of patients with type 1 diabetes (T1D) and type 2 diabetes (T2D).[2] Insulin pumps have been found beneficial not only in all stages and types of diabetes but also in patients requiring insulin.[1]

CONTINUOUS GLUCOSE MONITORING AND INSULIN PUMPS FOR DIABETES MANAGEMENT

Maintenance of glycemic control within a very narrow range is of paramount priority in diabetes management. Measurement and management of the volatility or variability in glucose excursions is therefore extremely important. Advent of CGM has made it feasible. Development of CGM devices can be traced back to mid-1970s. Followed by CGM devices, sensor technology and implantable glucose sensors were developed in early 1980s. The technology became commercially available in 1999, when MiniMed continuous glucose monitoring system, CGMS Gold (Medtronic MiniMed, CA, USA) received the Food and Drug Administration (FDA) approval.[3] Now, several CGMS are available, which can provide information on the glycemic status—either real-time or retrospective.[4] According to the intended use, CGMS are classified as professional CGMS (P-CGM) (that give retrospective glucose data to a healthcare professional) and personal CGMS (that give real-time glucose data to the user himself). They can retrieve glucose data over a particular time period, usually ranging from 6 days (e.g. iPro2, G5 Mobile CGM) to 14 days (FreeStyle Libre/FreeStyle Libre Pro).[5]

Currently available CGMS are of two types, namely real-time CGM (rtCGM) and intermittently scanned (isCGM). Real-time CGM brings about automatic transmission of a continuous stream of glucose data to the user. It can provide alerts, active alarms, and transmit glucose data (trend and numerical) in real time to a receiver, smart watch, or smartphone. Same type of glucose data is provided by isCGM system; however, the information is sent to the user upon scanning the sensor. The user does not get any alerts and alarms. The only isCGM system available currently is the FreeStyle Libre Flash Glucose Monitoring System. On the other hand, five rtCGM sensors are available or being evaluated currently by the USFDA. They include Medtronic Enlite and Medtronic Guardian 3 sensors, Dexcom G5 and Dexcom G6 sensors, and the Eversense sensor. G6 sensor has been approved by the FDA for use as an integrated CGM (iCGM) system that is compatible with other medical devices and electronic interfaces. Compatible medical devices include automated insulin dosing systems (e.g. bolus calculators), insulin pumps, blood glucose meters, and other diabetes management devices.[6]

Continuous glucose monitoring system can provide complete glycemic picture of an individual, as it can record the sugar levels at daytime as well as at night. Thus, it can detect even the unnoticed glycemic patterns like nocturnal hypoglycemia, Dawn phenomenon, postprandial hyperglycemia, etc. and thereby assist in the management of diabetes therapies.[7] This is possible even without confining the patient to the hospital.[8] A typical CGMS consists of a glucose oxidase-based electrochemical sensor inserted through the skin using a needle introducer, a transmitter that is fixed onto the sensor, and a receiver that picks up the interstitial fluid (ISF) signal. The oxidation of ISF glucose by the sensor generates an electrical current. The electrical current data are filtered and cleared from background noise by the transmitter and sent to the receiver which provides an approximation of the blood glucose level.[3]

Insulin Pump Therapy

Insulin pump therapy is also an important advanced technology in diabetes management. It is a small computerized device which can be worn externally, and it provides continuous infusion of rapid-acting insulin. The device has the potential to mimic the insulin release pattern of a normal healthy pancreas. Since its commercialization in 1970s, it has evolved from a large bulky device that could deliver at a single basal rate and needed manual calculation of the bolus doses to the present-day, pager-sized devices having sophisticated technology. Insulin pumps are of two types—one with infusion set, also known as durable or tethered pumps, and the other without infusion set or patch pumps.[9]

Insulin pump therapy is rapidly evolving as a lifesaving indication in selected subjects with type 1 and type 2 diabetes.[10] Insulin pump has an insulin reservoir connected to the insulin delivery line, which is connected to a subcutaneous cannula used for delivering insulin to the patient. The amount of insulin to be delivered is calculated on the basis of patient's daily dose of injected insulin.[10] Major advantages of CSII include better glycemic control, lower hypoglycemic episodes, improved psychosocial functioning, and better quality of life.[8] Insulin pump therapy is not a new therapy, but it is an alternative delivery mechanism for insulin, which is superior to conventional syringes and pens. This property makes insulin pumps unique compared to other devices. Success of the long-term insulin pump therapy is dependent on several factors including patient's willingness, cost of the pump and consumables, extensive education, motivation and implementation of sophisticated programs.[11] International Diabetes Federation guidelines (2009) recommend insulin pump therapy only at the comprehensive care level and to stringently selected subjects with T2DM.[11]

A combination of these two technologies seems to have a huge potential. Intensive research has been conducted in last 10 years on approaches to automatically tune insulin dosing based on CGM measurements. Academic research groups and companies have investigated algorithms to automatically attenuate or suspend basal insulin infusion based on CGM measurements as a first step toward the development of a fully closed-loop system, also called artificial pancreas. Basal insulin attenuation algorithms

TABLE 1: Advantages and disadvantages of insulin pump therapy.

Advantages	Disadvantages
Predictable and precise insulin delivery[13]	Risk of skin infections at the catheter site [13]
Reduction in variation in insulin absorption and treatment-related burden	Risk of diabetic ketoacidosis (DKA) from pump malfunction or absorption problems [13]
Ability to accurately deliver 1/10th of a unit of insulin [13]	Pumps are expensive and the users have to incur the continuing cost of supplies[13]
Reducing wide fluctuations in blood glucose[14]	Checking blood glucose regularly[13]
Tighter blood glucose control, while reducing the risk of hypoglycemia[13]	The discomfort of a device attachment[9]
Reducing episodes of severe hypoglycemia[13]	Letting others know that you have diabetes[13]
Reduction in the need for hospitalization and the cost of care[2]	Improper use of insulin boluses leading to insulin stacking[5]
Helping manage the "dawn phenomenon"[13]	Necessitates patient education on pump use and assistance from a technician[11]
Varying the basal insulin delivery to meet anticipated changes in insulin needs[15]	
Increased flexibility, normalization of lifestyle and sense of well-being[13,14]	
Suitable in patients with chronic kidney disease[11]	
Useful for the treatment of recalcitrant diabetes. Also improves sexual function[11]	
Better patient compliance due to less frequent change of pump infusion site[11]	

are thus a promising approach for reducing the risk of hypoglycemia in sensor-augmented pump (SAP) therapy and they are the first step in the direction of a fully closed-loop system.[12]

Advantages and Disadvantages of Insulin Pump Therapy

Insulin pump therapy is the most physiological way of insulin delivery amongst the various methodologies available for insulin delivery. However, the diabetes care provider and the patient with diabetes need to make choices, and the choice needs to be individualized based on the pros and cons of treatment options. The advantages and disadvantages of insulin pump therapy are summarized in Table 1.

Advantages and Disadvantages of Continuous Glucose Monitoring

Glucose monitoring is the prerequisite of diabetes management. Treatment of hyperglycemia with insulin pumps is based on the blood glucose profile of the patient. Blood glucose monitoring using CGM is found to be advantageous over self-monitoring of blood glucose (SMBG). However, CGM has its own set of advantages and disadvantages, which must be considered before adapting the technology. These are summarized in Table 2.

CONCLUSION

Ever-increasing threat of diabetes epidemic could be reduced with the aid of technology. Timely diagnosis is not sufficient for controlling and treating the disease; but understanding the disease progression is crucial for appropriate management. Advent of continuous glucose monitoring is a major milestone in addressing glycemic variability. It allows real time as well as flash monitoring of blood glucose, and aids in understanding the patient-specific pattern of variation in blood glucose. This can be highly advantageous for physicians in therapy decision-making. Insulin pump is another such pathbreaking technology, which closely resembles the natural way of insulin secretion and thus reduces the disadvantages associated with treatment of hyperglycemia. Understanding the merits and demerits of these technologies will improve their usage in diabetes management and will create an opportunity for advancement of these technologies for future use.

TABLE 2: Advantages and disadvantages of continuous glucose monitoring.

Advantages	Disadvantages
Provides better glycemic picture and improved quality of life compared to SBGM	Use of CGM is time consuming owing to a lot of time required for analysis and interpretation of the huge data
Provision of continuous glucose profile over a particular time period aids in optimum therapeutic decision and interventions	Continuous glucose monitoring systems measure glucose in interstitial fluid and not in the blood and thus are not completely reliable for deciding the treatment, particularly in case of prominent glucose fluctuations
Vast information provided by CGM assists in optimization of therapeutic decisions and interventions	Associated with biocompatibility problems like biofouling, passivation of electrodes, and degeneration which leads to signal drifting over time
Can be integrated with insulin pumps and determine insulin doses under different conditions	Continuously wearing the CGM sensor may cause inconvenience to the patients
Most useful diagnostic tool which can be used for preventing hypoglycemia, hypoglycemic unawareness, etc.	Displacement of sensor needle, which is less common with advanced CGM systems, could be scary for the patient
Provides better clinical outcomes in terms of reduction in HbA1c, glycemic variability and reduced risk of hypoglycemia, in T1DM as well as T2DM patients and improved quality of life.[16,17]	The systems are costly compared to SMBG
Beneficial in people on either MDI or IPT	
Improves understanding of patients as well as healthcare professionals about effect of diet, exercise and lifestyle on glucose levels	Efficacy is not yet established in pediatric population[18]
Can be used for tight glycemic control in conditions like pregnancy	

(CGM: continuous glucose monitoring; SBGM: self-monitoring of blood glucose; T1DM: type 1 diabetes mellitus; T2DM: type 2 diabetes mellitus; MDI: multiple daily injections; IPT: insulin pump therapy)

REFERENCES

1. Danne T, De Vries H, Doyle FJ, et al. The Official Journal of ATTD Advanced Technologies & Treatments for Diabetes Conference Austria, Vienna—February 14–17, 2018. Diabetes Technol Ther. 2018;20(S1):A1-52.
2. Umpierrez GE, Klonoff DC. Diabetes technology update: use of insulin pumps and continuous glucose monitoring in the hospital. Diabetes Care. 2018;41(8):1579-89.
3. Cengiz E, Sherr JL, Weinzimer SA, et al. New-generation diabetes management: glucose sensor-augmented insulin pump therapy. Expert Rev Med Devices. 2011;8(4):449-58.
4. Zisser H, Lane JE, Shivers JP. Continuous glucose monitoring: professional and real time. InTechnological Advances in the Treatment of Type 1 Diabetes. 2015;24 :81-98.
5. American Diabetes Association. (2018). Role of continuous glucose monitoring in diabetes treatment. [Online]. Available from https://professional.diabetes.org/sites/professional.diabetes.org/files/media/final_ada-abbott_cgm_compendium_final.pdf. [Last accessed September, 2019].
6. Edelman SV, Argento NB, et al. Clinical implications of real-time and intermittently scanned continuous glucose monitoring. Diabetes Care. 2018;41(11):2265-74.
7. Klonoff DC, Buckingham B, Christiansen JS, et al. Continuous glucose monitoring: an endocrine society clinical practice guideline. J Clin Endocrinol Metab. 2011;96(10):2968-79.
8. Kesavadev J, Jain SM, Muruganathan A, et al. Consensus evidence-based guidelines for use of insulin pump therapy in the management of diabetes as per Indian clinical practice. J Assoc Physicians India. 2014;62(Suppl7):34-41.
9. Kesavadev J, Krishnan G. From Insulin Pumps to Artificial Pancreas: Indian Experience over 12 years. Kerala Medical Journal. 2016;9(3):106.
10. Paldus B, Lee MH, O'Neal DN. Insulin pumps in general practice. Austr Prescr. 2018;41(6):186-90.
11. Kesavadev J, Das AK, Unnikrishnan R, et al. Use of insulin pumps in India: suggested guidelines based on experience and cultural differences. Diabetes Technol Ther. 2010;12(10):823-31.
12. Vettoretti M, Facchinetti A. Combining continuous glucose monitoring and insulin pumps to automatically tune the basal insulin infusion in diabetes therapy: a review. Biomed Eng Online. 2019;18(1):37.
13. Joslin Diabetes Center. The Advantages and Disadvantages of an Insulin Pump. [Online]. Available fromhttps://www.joslin.org/info/the_advantages_and_disadvantages_of_an_insulin_pump.html. [Last accessed September, 2019].
14. Kozlova IV. The features of insulin pump therapy for treatment of diabetes mellitus. The Pharma Innovation. 2017;6(6):36-9.
15. Schade DS, Valentine V. To pump or not to pump. Diabetes Care. 2002;25(11):2100-2.
16. Juvenile Diabetes Research Foundation Continuous Glucose Monitoring Study Group, Tamborlane WV, Beck RW, et al. Continuous glucose monitoring and intensive treatment of type 1 diabetes. N Engl JMed. 2008;359(14):1464-76.
17. Vigersky RA, Fonda SJ, Chellappa M, et al. Short-and long-term effects of real-time continuous glucose monitoring in patients with type 2 diabetes. Diabetes Care. 2012;35(1):32-8.
18. Maiorino MI, Petrizzo M, Bellastella G, et al. Continuous glucose monitoring for patients with type 1 diabetes on multiple daily injections of insulin: pros and cons. Endocrine. 2018;59(1):62-5.

89 CHAPTER

Digital Diabetes: From Now to Future

Rakesh M Parikh, Avani Verma

INTRODUCTION

International Diabetes Federation (IDF) states that there are currently 425 million people with diabetes worldwide in 2017 and the number will increase to 629 million by the year 2045.[1] In parallel to the rising prevalence of diabetes, technology is getting advanced and is being used more and more in the healthcare system. Digital healthcare and technology is unlikely to replace the multidisciplinary medical team in near future but it will provide a meaningful individual and family support in between the clinic visits and largely will help the population health management for diabetes.[2] However, we are still in the early days of digital healthcare, the future can even be better, with the world moving toward smartphone apps, connected devices, internet of things, social media, telemedicine and e-health. This can completely change the landscape of diabetes management.[3,4]

Technology has penetrated various aspects and has touched upon various stakeholders involved in the management of a diabetic patient. For the sake of convenience we would divide digital diabetes into desktop- and web-based application, mobile applications, gadgets, digital data, and artificial intelligence in this chapter.

DESKTOP- AND WEB-BASED APPLICATIONS

Desktop applications run on desktops and laptops and do not need internet connections, while those dependent on internet are called web-based applications. These are largely used for maintaining electronic medical records (EMRs). In the management of diabetic patients, it is very important to have their chronological database. Most of practitioners are used to maintaining the medical records of their patients in hardcopies. Maintaining that database on a desktop or laptop makes the data quite handy to retrieve at the time of patient visit and to analyze the data in bulk, though digital data comes at a risk of losing it if secured well. With the use of web-based application the risk of data loss is minimized but it comes at a cost of data leakage. There are several desktop- and web-based applications, a few specially designed for diabetic patients. Most of the senior physicians being used to traditional pen- and paper-based methodology, a few products have been launched that would capture data from physicians pen and would upload it to the application.

The desktop- and web-based application are very useful in maintaining the database of patients, retrieving it during patient visits, providing printed prescriptions and analysis of data. There are a few applications that are offering chat, audio- and video-based consultations, which are very useful for follow-up visits of patients. The patients do not any more need to travel long distances for a follow-up visit. With all their advantages desktop- and web-based applications are still limited in terms of mobility.

MOBILE-BASED APPLICATIONS

With the advent of smartphone and tablets mobile-based applications have conquered the limitation of mobility. Most of the features of desktop and web-based applications are available on mobile-based applications. Several applications like Practo are becoming popular among physicians for providing tele-consultations to their patients on the go.

There are several other aspects of patient management for which specialized mobile applications are available. Be it for maintaining their self-monitored glycemic profile, dietary intake records, calorie burning data or insulin doses calculation; there are numerous mobile-based applications in market.

Example of such a free technology solution is the widely popular diabetes mobile app, mySugr. It wirelessly connects with compatible glucose meters, creates graphs and trends, provides insulin carb ratio, insulin sensitivity factor and has got the entire list of medications in it. Structured self-monitoring of blood glucose (SMBG), telemedicine, and iPDM (Integrated Personalized Diabetes Management) are all proven to reduce A1c significantly with minimal chance of hypoglycemia.[5] In fact, a latest meta-analysis reported an average benefit of 0.49% in levels of glycated hemoglobin (HbA1c) for individuals who use mobile apps for management of T2D as compared to controls.[6] But these studies are done in underpowered small-to-moderate sample populations, hence there is need to conduct large scale real life studies.[7]

Multiple mobile apps also provide the feature of personalized nutrition plans adapted to the person's glycemic profile but there is still need to standardize and validate these apps.[8]

GADGETS

Glucose monitoring devises, insulin injection devises and insulin pumps have been in market for long time. All these gadgets are getting digitally improvised with the help of involving technology and artificial intelligence. Abbot has launched its Libre Pro sensor which is very small in size and captures glucose readings at 15 minute interval for a span of 14 days. It has significantly brought down the cost of continuous glucose monitoring compared to conventional continuous glucose monitoring devises.

Newer gadgets like noninvasive glucose sensors and smart socks that are supposed to monitor foot temperature, mini electrocardiograms to track cardiovascular health are being developed.

With the ongoing advancement in technology, currently there is increased adoption of smart devices. In the present time, changing lifestyle habits such as physical activity and sleep are considered as a priority for affecting trends in chronic disease evolution and improving health-related QoL.[9] As per one landmark paper published in 2015, wearable devices were described as "facilitators, not drivers, of health behavior change".[10] Currently available lifestyle modification devices play a key role in lifestyle interventions, key to the initial management of diabetes mellitus throughout life.[11]

The insulin pump technology has advanced to a great extent, providing better efficacy and safety. Insulin pumps are now giving way to the concept of artificial pancreas.[12] The artificial pancreas is a closed loop of blood glucose measurement and insulin delivery combined in a single system, using a glucose sensor, a control algorithm and an insulin pump.[13] The effectiveness and safety of the in-home use of a hybrid closed-loop (HCL) system, which automatically enhances, reduces, and suspends insulin delivery in response to continuous monitoring of glucose were examined and showed good glycemic control without much hypoglycemia or ketoacidosis.[12] This dream of closed loop system became a reality with the FDA approval of hybrid CL SYSTEM the 670G for type 1 diabetes treatment, where pump would increase insulin delivery when glucose is going high and decrease insulin delivery when glucose is going low, users still have to take bolus doses for meals.[14]

The next step in development is MiniMed 780G, the MiniMed 780G automated insulin delivery system will bring several exciting updates to the existing 670G: automated correction boluses for high blood sugars, Bluetooth connectivity, and remote monitoring (for caregivers) and software updates. The automated correction boluses are particularly exciting, as they should improve time-in-range and reduce user burden. Early feasibility studies of the 780G show a time-in-range (70–180 mg/dL) of around 80%, up by two hours per day from the 70% time-in-range seen in real-world 670G user data and the pivotal study. Also expected is that the MiniMed 780G system will also upgrade the Guardian Sensor 3 continuous glucose monitor (CGM) for "non-adjunctive use", enabling bolus insulin dosing without a confirmatory fingerstick.[15] Another hybrid closed loop system "DBLG1" comprises an android controller, the Dexcom G6 CGM, and the Kaleido insulin pump.[16] In Europe, it is the second approved hybrid closed loop for adults having type 1 diabetes.

Another advancement in insulin pumps is the development of Alternate Controller Enabled Infusion Pump (ACE pump). It is an interoperable pump, which means that it can be used along with different components that constitute the diabetes therapy systems. These diabetes therapy systems may include an ACE insulin pump as well as other compatible medical devices, comprising continuous glucose monitors, automated insulin dosing systems, other electronic devices, or blood glucose meters that are used for management of diabetes. FDA has granted marketing clearance for t:Slim X2 insulin pump, the first in new alternate controller enabled infusion pumps (ACE pumps) category.[17]

Another artificial pancreas in development, Beta Bionics iLet Gen 4 showed that iLet bionic pancreas (BP) significantly increased the percentage of time adults with type 1 diabetes (T1D) had glucose levels between 70 mg/dL and 180 mg/dL, when compared to usual care (UC) therapy of either multiple daily insulin injections (MDI) or continuous subcutaneous insulin infusion (CSII).[18]

Advancement in CGM includes EVERSENSE CGM system. The Eversense CGM System measures glucose from interstitial fluid below the skin surface on the basis of innovative fluorescence technology that is implanted in a tiny sensor. The sensor sends data of glucose wirelessly to the smart transmitter, which is worn on the upper arm above insertion site of the sensor. The smart transmitter calculates the current glucose value with the direction it is headed, how fast, and whether levels of glucose are anticipated to go beyond preset low and high targets. Simultaneously, alerts and data are sent to the smartphone app, which gives real-time tracking, intuitive displays to assist define patterns and information to assist you to remain within range.[19]

Another great social media movement impacting diabetes is "#We Are Not Waiting". A movement started at Stanford University in 2013 by advocates Lane Desborough and Howard Look while attempting to sum up the sentiments of the diabetes do-it-yourselfers and entrepreneurs taking charge. Hashtag # We Are Not Waiting is the rally cry of individuals of the diabetes community who take matters into their own hands. They develop platforms and applications and cloud-based solutions, and reverse engineering current products when required to assist individuals with diabetes better use equipment and health information for better results.

Digitosomes

With the advent of these gadgets and applications, large amount of data is being generated. A new term digitosomes is coined for this collective digital information. A few ongoing studies are looking at the correlation of these digitosomes with risk of complications. Artificial intelligence is being incorporated to develop algorithms that can predict the risk of complications based on information gathered in the form of digitosomes. Artificial intelligence is also being used in newer fundus cameras that can diagnose diabetic retinopathy. This is bypassing the need for an ophthalmologist consultation to a large extent.

FUTURE OF DIGITAL DIABETES

Future of digital diabetes will be an amalgamation and advancement at various avenues like but not limited to—mobile apps, social media and communities, internet, continuous/flash glucose monitoring with closed loop systems and artificial intelligence based algorithms. Future challenges will be to identify new digital markers based on data generated by continuous glucose monitoring/hybrid close loop systems, activity trackers and other connected devices. This is likely to profoundly change the diabetes landscape from an individualized approach of HbA1c monitoring to personalized diabetes management.[20,21] With the availability of more and more of data from connected devices and electronic health records, the role of artificial intelligence will suffice, there will be development of more accurate risk prediction models for diabetes and its complications.[22] This will boost our goal of personalized management and will lead to the advancement of precision medicine in diabetes.[23] Lastly, advancement of digital diabetes will serve to overcome social inequities and removing barriers for socially disadvantaged people and getting them early access to innovations.[24] For this it is important to expand the diversity of participants and reach out to hard-to-reach populations in epidemiological and clinical studies.[25] If we can achieve this than we can proudly say that the "future is bright".

REFERENCES

1. International Diabetes Federation. IDF Diabetes Atlas, 8th edition. Brussels, Belgium: International Diabetes Federation; 2017.
2. Kerr D, Axelrod C, Hoppe C, et al. Diabetes and technology in 2030: a utopian or dystopian future? Diabet Med. 2018;35:498-503.
3. Cameron JD, Ramaprasad A, Syn T. An ontology of and roadmap for mHealth research. Int J Med Inform. 2017;100:16-25.
4. Boogerd EA, Arts T, Engelen LJ, et al. "What Is eHealth": Time for An Update? JMIR Res Protoc. 2015;4:e29.
5. Kulzer B, Daenschel W, Daenschel I, et al. Integrated personalized diabetes management improves glycemic control in patients with insulin-treated type 2 diabetes: Results of the PDM-ProValue study program. Diabetes Res Clin Prac. 2018;144:200-12.
6. Hou C, Carter B, Hewitt J, et al. Do mobile phone applications improve glycemic control (HbA1c) in the self-management of diabetes? A systematic review, meta-analysis, and GRADE of 14 randomized trials. Diabetes Care. 2016;39:2089-95.
7. Shah VN, Garg SK. Managing diabetes in the digital age. Clin Diabetes Endocrinol. 2015;1:16.
8. Zeevi D, Korem T, Zmora N, et al. Personalized nutrition by prediction of glycemic responses. Cell. 2015;163:1079-94.
9. Block G, Sternfeld B, Block CH, et al. Development of Alive! (A Lifestyle Intervention Via Email), and its effect on health-related quality of life, presenteeism, and other behavioral outcomes: randomized controlled trial. J Med Internet Res. 2008;10:e43.

10. Patel MS, Asch DA, Volpp KG. Wearable devices as facilitators, not drivers, of health behavior change. JAMA. 2015;313:459-60.
11. Lentferink AJ, Oldenhuis HK, de Groot M, et al. Key components in eHealth interventions combining self-tracking and persuasive eCoaching to promote a healthier lifestyle: a scoping review. J Med Internet Res. 2017;19:e277.
12. Garg SK, Weinzimer SA, Tamborlane WV, et al. Glucose outcomes with the in-home use of a hybrid closed-loop insulin delivery system in adolescents and adults with type 1 diabetes. Diabetes Technol Ther. 2017;19:155-63.
13. Cobelli C, Renard E, Kovatchev B. Artificial pancreas: past, present, future. Diabetes. 2011;60:2672-82.
14. U.S. Food and Drug Administration. (2018). Minimed 670G System—P160017/S031. [online]. Available from https://www.accessdata.fda.gov/cdrh_docs/pdf16/P160017S031a.pdf [Last accessed, October, 2019].
15. Clinicaltrials.gov. (2019). Safety Evaluation of the Advanced Hybrid Closed Loop (AHCL) System. [online] Available from https://clinicaltrials.gov/ct2/show/NCT03959423 [Last accessed October, 2019].
16. Benhamou PY, Franc S, Reznik Y, et al. Closed-loop insulin delivery in adults with type 1 diabetes in real-life conditions: a 12-week multicentre, open-label randomised controlled crossover trial. The Lancet Digital Health. 2019 May 1;1(1):e17-25.
17. U.S. Food and Drug Administration. (2019). [online] t:Slim X2 insulin pump with interoperable technology. Available from https://www.accessdata.fda.gov/cdrh_docs/pdf18/DEN180058.pdf [Last accessed October, 2019].
18. American Diabetes Association. (2019). The iLet Bionic Pancreas Increased Time in Range for Adults with Type 1 Diabetes. [online]. Available from https://www.diabetes.org/newsroom/press-releases/2019/the-ilet-bionic-pancreas [Last accessed October, 2019].
19. Cappon G, Acciaroli G, Vettoretti M, et al. Wearable continuous glucose monitoring sensors: a revolution in diabetes treatment. Electronics. 2017;6(3):65.
20. Draznin B, Nathan DM, Korytkowski MT, et al. Guidelines versus guidelines: what's best for the patient? Ann Intern Med. 2018;169:186-7.
21. Wright LA, Hirsch IB. Metrics beyond hemoglobin A1C in diabetes management: time in range, hypoglycemia, and other parameters. Diabetes Technol Ther. 2017;19:S16-26.
22. Miotto R, Li L, Kidd BA, et al. Deep patient: an unsupervised representation to predict the future of patients from the electronic health records. Sci Rep. 2016;6:26094.
23. Dagliati A, Marini S, Sacchi L, et al. Machine learning methods to predict diabetes complications. J Diabetes Sci Technol. 2018;12: 295-302.
24. Buch V, Varughese G, Maruthappu M. Artificial intelligence in diabetes care. Diabet Med. 2018;35:495-7.
25. Char DS, Shah NH, Magnus D. Implementing machine learning in health care—addressing ethical challenges. N Engl J Med. 2018;378: 981-3.

14 SECTION Diabetes Prevention

90 CHAPTER Is it Possible for Prevention of Diabetes in Typical Indian Phenotype?

A Nanditha, K Satheesh, R Arun

INTRODUCTION

Diabetes mellitus is the most common metabolic disease and is prevalent in all parts of the world. The prevalence of diabetes is increasing globally in alarming numbers. About 79% of patients with diabetes live in low- and middle-income countries.[1] It is estimated that globally, there were 424.9 million adults with diabetes in 2017. The number is likely to rise to 628.6 million by the year 2045.[1] India has the 2nd largest number of people with diabetes (72.9 million), which is expected to increase further to 134.3 million by 2045.[1] India also has a large number of adults with impaired glucose tolerance (IGT) (24.0 million in 2017), and an increase in this number to 41.0 million is likely to occur by 2045.[1] The proportion of undiagnosed diabetes patient is also in a higher mark (57.9% in 2017). Undiagnosed diabetes and IGT can considerably increase the incident cases of diabetes.[1] To decrease the incidence of diabetes, prevention strategies have to be implemented in the early stage of diabetes to prevent persons with prediabetes and undiagnosed to convert to diabetes.

THE INDIAN PHENOTYPE

Indians and South Asians, in general, have strong racial and genetic predisposition to develop diabetes. Genetic predisposition is triggered in younger age in South Asians compared to the western population by weight gain, unhealthy diet, and sedentary behavior. Prevalence of obesity particularly abdominal obesity has increased among Asian countries.[2] The other peculiarities observed in Asian Indians are younger age of onset, lower BMI threshold with higher insulin resistance, and a higher percentage of body fat that mainly contribute to a higher predisposition to develop diabetes.[3]

There is a strong relationship between body mass index (BMI) ≥23 kg/m^2 and glucose intolerance in Asian Indians. The World Health Organization (WHO) has recommended that a BMI of 18.5–22 kg/m^2 is ideal for Asians as compared to 18.5–24.9 kg/m^2 for other ethnic population.[4] Studies have shown that when compared with European and American population, Asian Indians have insulin resistance without increased intraperitoneal fat mass and have a higher amount of truncal fat and low glucose disposal rate.[5]

SCOPE FOR PRIMARY PREVENTION OF TYPE 2 DIABETES

Several studies in India[6] and in migrant Asian Indians in Western countries[7] have shown the presence of hyperinsulinemia to combat higher insulin resistance. In Asian Indians, there is a delay in the diagnosis of type 2 diabetes (T2D) for various reasons; in such a scenario, hyperinsulinemia may be prolonged and cause deterioration of the beta-cell function. Various pathogenic mechanisms lead to insulin resistance, which leads to exhaustion of the beta-cell function.

In Asian Indians, to reduce the burden of diabetes, primary prevention should be started in the early part of life. By reducing the incidence of diabetes, many complications associated with diabetes, such as cardiovascular, renal, and neurological complications, can be prevented. Urbanization has led to changes in lifestyle habits, including consumption of energy-rich food, reduced physical activity, changing pattern in leisure activities, longer working hours, and decreasing sleep hours.

Modifiable risk factors such as obesity, sedentary habits, dietary factors, and smoking can be addressed in primary prevention strategies. Modifying these factors will reduce insulin resistance and increase beta-cell function

Many prevention studies done in the USA, Finland, China, India, and Japan[8] have proved primary prevention as the most potential and effective strategy to combat the rising epidemic of T2D, both in developed and developing countries.

Different methods to change the lifestyle were used through education and motivation such as personalized trainer, group education, telephonic contact, and mobile text messages. Sustained weight loss attributed to lifestyle modification (LSM) in the white population, but in Asian Indians, even without weight reduction, there was a reduction in the incidence of T2D.[8] Changes in the diet habits had beneficial effects on the improved insulin metabolism in the Indian population.[9]

PRIMARY PREVENTION STUDIES IN ASIAN INDIANS

Indian Diabetes Prevention Programme-1

Indian Diabetes Prevention Programme-1 (IDPP-1)[10] was a prospective randomized control trial that included persons with a mean age of 45 years and BMI 25.7 kg/m^2. Persons who had IGT on two oral glucose tolerance test (OGTT) were randomized into control, LSM, Metformin, and LSM + Metformin group. Control group received advise about healthy LSM at baseline only, LSM group received periodic motivation about healthy LSM, metformin group received 500 mg/day, and LSM + metformin group received both healthy LSM and metformin 500 mg/day. Use of these intervention strategies significantly reduced the conversion to diabetes to a similar extent. In control group, there was a 55% conversion to diabetes, 39.3% in LSM group, 40.5% in metformin group, and 39.5% in LSM + metformin group. The relative risk reduction (RRR) was 28.5% with LSM, 26.4% with metformin, and 28.2% with LSM + metformin, as compared with the control group. To prevent one incidence case of diabetes, the number needed to treat (NNT) was 6.4 for LSM, 6.9 for metformin, and 6.5 for LSM + metformin.[10] This study showed the effectiveness of LSM in preventing T2D in Indians with IGT. The reduction in incidence was not associated with weight in this study group. There was no significant weight reduction observed in the groups during the study period. In western prevention studies such as Diabetes Prevention Program (DPP) in the USA[9] and the Finnish Diabetes Prevention Study (DPS),[9] the beneficial changes were associated with weight reduction.

This study has proven that prevention strategies have beneficial effects in typical Asian Indian phenotypes such as younger age, lean body mass, and abdominal obesity. There was improved insulin sensitivity in persons who reversed from IGT to normoglycemia and deterioration in beta-cell function in people with persistent IGT (PIGT).[6]

Indian Diabetes Prevention Programme-2

Indian Diabetes Prevention Programme-2 (IDPP-2)[11] was a prospective randomized control trial that included persons with a mean age of 45 years and mean BMI 25.9 kg/m^2. Persons who had IGT on two OGTT randomized into LSM + placebo and pioglitazone + LSM group. LSM + placebo group received periodic motivation about healthy LSM and pioglitazone + LSM group received both healthy LSM and pioglitazone 30 mg/day. The cumulative incidence of diabetes with pioglitazone was 29.8%, and with LSM + placebo was 31.6%. Normoglycemia was achieved in 40.9% and 32.3% of participants receiving pioglitazone and LSM + placebo, respectively.[11] At the end of 2 years of study, we noted that the addition of pioglitazone did not enhance the effectiveness of LSM.[11]

Community-based Intervention Study

Adults and youth aged 10–92 years were provided educational intervention using trained trainers for 7 months. The crude prevalence of diabetes and prediabetes among adults were 5.1% and 13.5%, respectively. The intervention helped to reduce fasting blood glucose levels of persons with prediabetes by 16% and 25% in persons with T2D. The intervention also improved dietary intake and obesity parameters. The educational intervention was successful in reducing some of the obesity parameters and improving dietary patterns of individuals with prediabetes and diabetes.[12]

Diabetes Community Lifestyle Improvement Program

Diabetes Community Lifestyle Improvement Program (DCLIP) study[13] was a randomized control trial involving isolated impaired glucose tolerance (iIGT), isolated impaired fasting glucose (iIFG), and IFG + IGT. Individuals were randomized into two groups, the control group received standard care advice, and the intervention group received aggressive LSM training through once-weekly classes regarding diet and exercise modeled based on DPP study. If there is no significant improvement in blood glucose level during the 4th month, metformin 500 mg twice daily was added for participants at highest risk of conversion to diabetes. The RRR was 32%, the NNT to prevent one case of diabetes was 9.8, and 34.9% of control and 25.7% of intervention participants developed diabetes. The RRR varied by the type of prediabetes. Stepwise diabetes prevention in people with prediabetes was thus found to be effective in reducing diabetes incidence. Most participants (72%) required metformin in addition to lifestyle.

Indian SMS Study

The four above studies and western studies were labor-intensive, costly, and required trained personnel to conduct the programme. Ramachandran et al. in 2009[14] implemented a prevention programme on larger scales, to motivate people about healthy lifestyle modification using text messaging service via mobile phones. Text messaging is a cost-effective tool, does not require trained personnel, and is accessible to all individuals in the remote parts of the country.

Indian SMS study[14] was a prospective randomized control trial that included persons with age 35–55 years. Persons who had IGT on two OGTT were randomized into standard care and mobile phone messaging group. Standard care group received motivation about healthy lifestyle modification at baseline only, and mobile phone messaging group received motivational text messages on LSM through mobile phones at least three times a week. The cumulative incidence of T2D was lower in those who received mobile phone messages (18%) than in controls (27%). The NNT to prevent one case of type 2 diabetes was 11.[14] Absolute risk reduction (ARR) was 9%, and the RRR was 36% which was highly significant, and improvement in high-density lipoprotein cholesterol (HDL-c) was noted.[14]

At the end of 2 years of study, we noted that mobile phone messaging was an effective and acceptable method to deliver LSM advice to prevent T2D. Beta-cell function showed significant improvement in persons who reversed to normoglycemia from IGT.[15] The reduction in the incidence of diabetes was associated with improved dietary adherence which helped to increase the secretion of insulin and improvement in tissue insulin sensitivity.[9] The persons with hypertriglyceridemia (fasting serum triglycerides ≥150 mg/dL) and waist circumference (WC) (≥90 cm in men) had a relatively higher risk of 49% of developing incident diabetes in 2 years.

The same set of the population was followed up after 3 years of the final visit of the study. The conversion rate to diabetes in 5 years in the same population was significantly lower among transient IGT (TIGT) than among PIGT. PIGT had a higher rate of risk factors for diabetes than TIGT. The risk of conversion to diabetes was 80% lower in TIGT than in PIGT.[16]

mHealth Intervention Study

A large study by Pfammatter and coworkers[17] addressed the utility of mHealth intervention to improve diabetes risk behaviors using text messaging among one million Indian adults. mDiabetes participants received 56 text messages in the choice of native languages for over 6 months, and control participants received no contact. Participants receiving the messages showed a definite improvement in health behavior scores compared with those who received no messages. The study showed that text messaging intervention was feasible and was useful in assessing diabetes-related health behaviors in a low-/middle-income country.[17]

Long-term Effects of LSM

The long-term prevention studies conducted in the USA,[18] China,[19] Finland,[20] and India[16] have shown that the effect of lifestyle intervention persists for many years even after the withdrawal of active intervention. It has also shown a delay in micro and macrovascular incidence and increased life expectancy.[19]

CONCLUSION

Indian Diabetes Prevention Programmes proved that young, nonobese Indians with IGT respond to LSM. Diabetes could be prevented or postponed by moderate LSM without significant reduction in weight. Mobile phone messaging could be a practical and affordable way to deliver lifestyle advice to delay or prevent the onset of T2D. Early improvement in glucose tolerance (normoglycemia in 6 months) significantly reduces the risk of development of diabetes.[15] Although the effectiveness is lower than in the western population (~30% vs. 50%), practice of LSM appears to be consistently effective. Strategies have to be formulated considering the cultural, socioeconomic aspects and structure of the healthcare system. The advent of mobile technology has provided a cost-effective prevention tool. It has shown that the use of information and communication technology such as computer, mobile phones, and communication satellites help to reach a vast number of participants at a low cost. It can also be used for education and motivation and regular contact with the participants in the prevention programmes.

REFERENCES

1. International Diabetes Federation. IDF Diabetes Atlas, 8th edn. Brussels, Belgium: International Diabetes Federation, 2017. http://www.diabetesatlas.org [Last assessed September 2019]
2. Yoon KH, Lee JH, Kim JW, et al. Epidemic obesity and type 2 diabetes in Asia. Lancet. 2006;368(9558):1681-8.
3. Ramachandran A, Snehalatha C, Vijay V, et al. Derivation and validation of diabetes risk score for urban Asian Indians. Diabetes Res Clin Pract. 2005;70(1):63-70.
4. WHO Expert Consultation. Appropriate body-mass index for Asian populations and its implications for policy and intervention strategies. Lancet. 2004(9403);363:157-63.
5. Ramachandran A, Ma RC, Snehalatha C. Diabetes in Asia. Lancet. 2010;375(9712):408-18.
6. Snehalatha C, Mary S, Selvam S, et al. Changes in insulin secretion and insulin sensitivity in relation to the glycemic outcomes in subjects with impaired glucose tolerance in the Indian Diabetes Prevention Programme-1. Diabetes Care. 2009;32(10):1796-1801.
7. Abate N, Chandalia M, Snell PG, et al. Adipose tissue metabolites and insulin resistance in nondiabetic Asian Indian men. J Clin Endocrinol Metab. 2004;89(6):2750-5.
8. Ramachandran A, Snehalatha C, Shetty SA, et al. Primary Prevention Trials in Type 2 Diabetes. Chapter 4. In: Bergman M (Ed). Global Health Perspectives in Prediabetes and Diabetes Prevention. Singapore: World Scientific Publication; 2014. pp. 49-74.
9. Ram J, Selvam S, Snehalatha C, et al. Improvement in diet habits, independent of physical activity helps to reduce incident diabetes among prediabetic Asian Indian men. Diabetes Res Clin Pract. 2014;106(3):491-5.
10. Ramachandran A, Snehalatha C, Mary S, et al.; Indian Diabetes Prevention Programme (IDPP). The Indian Diabetes Prevention Programme shows that lifestyle modification and metformin prevent type 2 diabetes in Asian Indian subjects with impaired glucose tolerance (IDPP-1). Diabetologia. 2006;49(2):289-97.
11. Ramachandran A, Snehalatha C, Mary S, et al. Pioglitazone does not enhance effectiveness of life style modification in preventing conversion of impaired glucose tolerance to diabetes in Asian Indians—Results of Indian Diabetes Prevention Programme- (IDPP-2). Diabetologia. 2009;52(6):1019-26.
12. Balagopal P, Kamalamma N, Patel TG, et al. A community-based diabetes prevention and management education program in a rural village in India. Diabetes Care. 2008;31(6):1097-104.
13. Weber MB, Ranjani H, Meyers GC, et al. A model of translational research for diabetes prevention in low and middle-income countries: The Diabetes Community Lifestyle Improvement Program (D-CLIP) trial. Prim Care Diabetes. 2012;6(1):3-9.
14. Ramachandran A, Snehalatha C, Ram J, et al. Effectiveness of mobile phone messaging in prevention of type 2 diabetes by lifestyle modification in men in India: a prospective, parallel-group, randomised controlled trial. Lancet Diabetes Endocrinol. 2013;1(3):191-8.
15. Nanditha A, Ram J, Snehalatha C, et al. Early improvement predicts reduced risk of incident diabetes and improved cardiovascular risk in prediabetic Asian Indian men participating in a 2-year lifestyle intervention program. Diabet Care. 2014;37(11):3009-15.
16. Pfammatter A, Spring B, Saligram N, et al. mHealth Intervention to Improve Diabetes Risk Behaviors in India: A Prospective, Parallel Group Cohort Study. J Med Internet Res. 2016;18(8):e207.
17. Knowler WC, Fowler SE, Hamman RF, et al. 10-Year follow-up of diabetes incidence and weight loss in the Diabetes Prevention Program Outcomes Study. Lancet. 2009;374(9702):1677-86.
18. Lindström J, Peltonen M, Eriksson JG, et al.; Finnish Diabetes Prevention Study (DPS). Improved lifestyle and decreased diabetes risk over 13 years: long-term follow-up of the randomised Finnish Diabetes Prevention Study (DPS). Diabetologia. 2013;56(2):284-93.
19. Nanditha A, Snehalatha C, Raghavan A, et al. The post-trial analysis of the Indian SMS diabetes prevention study shows persistent beneficial effects of lifestyle intervention. Diabetes Res Clin Pract. 2018;142:213-21.
20. Gong Q, Zhang P, Wang J, et al. Morbidity and mortality after lifestyle intervention for people with impaired glucose tolerance: 30-year results of the Da Qing Diabetes Prevention Outcome Study. Lancet Diabetes Endocrinol. 2019;7(6):452-61.

15 SECTION

Research Methodology

91 CHAPTER

Microvascular and Macrovascular Complications in Diabetes Mellitus: Distinct or Continuum?*

Aastha Chawla, Rajeev Chawla, Shalini Jaggi

INTRODUCTION

Diabetes mellitus (DM) has routinely been described as a metabolic disorder characterized by hyperglycemia that develops as a consequence of defects in insulin secretion, insulin action, or both. Type 2 diabetes encompasses individuals who have insulin resistance (IR) and usually relative (rather than absolute) insulin deficiency.[1] The pathologic hallmark of DM involves the vasculature leading to both microvascular and macrovascular complications.[2] Chronicity of hyperglycemia is associated with long-term damage and failure of various organ systems, mainly affecting the eyes, nerves, kidneys, and heart.[1]

According to diabetes atlas (7th edition), the global prevalence of diabetes is estimated at 415 million (8.8%), which is predicted to rise to 642 million in the next 25 years.[3] In India, there are about 69.2 million people with diabetes and are expected to cross 123.5 million by 2040.[3] Moreover, worldwide approximately 193 million diabetics remain undiagnosed predisposing them to the development of several long-term complications of untreated chronic hyperglycemia.[3] Although intensive glycemic control lowers the incidence and progression of microvascular complications, the morbidity associated with these complications is still increasing.[4] Several landmark studies such as the United Kingdom Prospective Diabetes Study (UKPDS) have demonstrated that strict glycemic control does limit microvascular disease while attempts to improve macrovascular outcomes through glucose-lowering interventions still remain shrouded with controversy. A relative risk (RR) reduction in myocardial infarction (MI) ($P = 0.052$) has been observed in the 10 years of post-trial follow-up of UKPDS.[5] Similarly, the risk of cardiovascular mortality, nonfatal MI, and stroke reduced with pioglitazone in the Prospective Pioglitazone Clinical Trial in Macrovascular Events as compared to placebo group.[6] The action in diabetes and vascular disease: Preterax and Diamicron MR Controlled Evaluation and the Veterans Affairs Diabetes Trial failed to show any significant improvement in cardiovascular risk with the intensification of diabetes therapy.[7,8] To further complicate matters, in the Action to Control Cardiovascular Risk in Diabetes trial, the use of intensive therapy for 3.5 years increased mortality but did not significantly reduce major cardiovascular events.[9]

In recent years, much attention has been focused on the management of macrovascular complications such as stroke and acute coronary syndromes. It is well recognized that vascular complications in a given tissue are often accompanied by evidence of pathology in other vascular territories. A linear relationship between microvascular complications and duration of disease was established by the authors where they documented the presence of microvasculopathy across different age groups in their study in 25–40% of diabetic patients aged >25 years with more than 5 years' duration of diabetes.[10] Researchers such as Krentz et al. and Al-Wakeel et al. have observed that both microvascular and macrovascular complications develop simultaneously in diabetes.[11,12] On the contrary,

*Chawla A, Chawla R, Jaggi S. Microvasular and macrovascular complications in diabetes mellitus: Distinct or continuum? Indian J Endocr Metab. 2016;20:546-53.

Matheus and Gomes described the case report of type 1 DM (T1DM) patient with early and aggressive coronary artery disease (CAD) without evidence of nephropathy, retinopathy, or classical risk factors for CAD.[13] Thus, there is not much clarity over whether microvascular complication precedes macrovascular complications or they progress simultaneously.

The present review attempts an insight into this delicate relationship between microvascular and macrovascular complications of diabetes to understand whether they are discrete entities or in continuum with each other. We propose a unique continuum bridging the microvascular and the macrovascular risk which is based on our evidence-based studies consistently over a decade.

PATHOPHYSIOLOGICAL BASIS OF MICRO- VERSUS MACROVASCULAR COMPLICATIONS

Patients with DM and associated microvascular complications appear particularly at higher risk of accelerated atherosclerosis which ultimately culminates in cerebrovascular and cardiovascular events and premature death.[14] Microvessels are the basic functional unit of the cardiovascular system comprising arterioles, capillaries, and venules.[2] They differ from macrovessels in both their architecture and cellular components. In contrast to macrovessels supplying blood to organs, microvessels play important roles in maintaining blood pressure and proper nutrient delivery.[2] The microcirculation also has regulatory systems controlling vascular permeability and myogenic responses that can adapt blood flow according to local metabolic needs. Alteration in microvascular function may arise even before overt hyperglycemia and vascular pathologic changes manifest. Diabetes induces pathognomonic changes in the microvasculature, affecting the capillary basement membrane including arterioles in the glomeruli, retina, myocardium, skin, and muscle, by increasing their thickness, leading to the development of diabetic microangiopathy. This thickening eventually leads to abnormality in vessel function, inducing multiple clinical problems such as hypertension, delayed wound healing, and tissue hypoxia. Similarly, neovascularization arising from the vasa vasorum may interconnect macro- and microangiopathy, predict platelet rupture, and promote atherosclerosis. The role of microvascular pathology in systemic diabetic complications, including macrovascular atherosclerosis, remains a subject for further debate.[2]

INTERSECTION OF MICROVASCULAR AND MACROVASCULAR COMPLICATIONS OF DIABETES: EVIDENCE-BASED PROOF OF CONCEPT

Diabetic Retinopathy

The risk of development of diabetic retinopathy (DR) in patients with (T2DM) has been found to be related to both severities of hyperglycemia and presence of hypertension. Fong et al. attributed approximately 10,000 new cases of blindness to DR in the United States.[15] In India, The Chennai Urban Rural Epidemiology Study (CURES) reported an overall DR prevalence of 17.6% [confidence interval (95% CI): 15.8–19.5] in the diabetic population.[16] More recently, the Sankara Nethralaya DR Epidemiology and Molecular Genetic Study has estimated an urban prevalence of 18.0% (95% CI: 16.0–20.1) and a rural prevalence of 10.3% (95% CI: 8.53–11.97%) of DR in South India.[17,18] Similar to this, the Aravind Comprehensive Eye Study has reported 10.5% prevalence of DR (in self-reported subjects with diabetes) in the rural South Indian population.[19] A DR prevalence of 21.2% has been reported by Chawla et al. in their cohort of North Indian patients. This study also found a significant association between HbA1c, body mass index, duration of diabetes, and microalbuminuria in the development of DR ($P = 0.001$).[20]

Several studies have explored the association between DR and macrovascular complications. As retinal microvasculature shares embryologic and anatomic characteristics with that of cerebral circulation, researchers have studied retinal abnormalities to provide clues to understand the underlying pathophysiology of different cerebrovascular diseases.[21] In the World Health Organization Multinational Study of Vascular Disease in Diabetes, retinopathy was related to the incidence of MI and death from cardiovascular disease (CVD).[22] In the Atherosclerosis Risk in Communities study, increased incidence of clinical stroke was associated with retinal microvascular abnormalities and generalized arteriolar narrowing.[23] Furthermore, retinopathy was significantly associated with combined stroke events (RR 1.7, 95% CI: 1.0–2.8) in persons without diabetes after controlling for age, sex, and systolic blood pressure. This association was stronger in those with two or more retinal microvascular signs (RR 2.7, CI: 1.5–5.2).[24] Targher et al. followed up 2103 T2DM outpatients for 7 years and found a remarkably increased risk of incident CVD in patients with proliferative/laser-treated retinopathy [hazard ratio 2.08 (1.02–3.7) for men and 2.41 (1.05–3.9) for women], after adjustment of hypertension and advanced nephropathy.[25] Contrary to this, Matheus and Gomes have reported cardiovascular events without any presence of retinopathy.[13]

Diabetic Nephropathy

Proteinuria occurs in 15–40% of patients with type 1 diabetes while it ranges from 5 to 20% in patients with T2DM.[26] According to the European Diabetes Prospective Complications Study, the cumulative incidence of microalbuminuria was 12.6% over 7.3 years in patients with T1DM.[26] However, 18 years follow-up study from Denmark reported a prevalence rate of 33% in the T1DM population.[27]Similarly, in the UKPDS, T2DM patients showed a 2.0% incidence of microalbuminuria per year, which reached up to 25% in 10 years postdiagnosis.[28] The prevalence of diabetic nephropathy was higher in African Americans, Asians, and Native Americans than Caucasians.[26] In India, CURES 45 reported a prevalence of 2.2% for overt diabetic nephropathy and 26.9% for microalbuminuria.[29]

The association of intense control with reduced microvascular complication, as reported by the Diabetes Control and Complications Trial, has emerged as a strong proof of concept for hyperglycemia, it being an important modifiable risk factor for diabetic nephropathy. A reduction in 10 mm Hg of systolic blood pressure is associated with a 13% decrease in the microvascular complications with minimal risk in patient with a systolic pressure < 120 mm Hg.[30] Dyslipidemia with increased low density lipoprotein (LDL) cholesterol and triglycerides is independently associated with diabetic kidney disease.[31]

The pathogenic mechanisms underlying diabetic nephropathy involve generation of reactive oxygen species (ROS), accumulation of advanced glycation end product (AGE), and activation of intracellular signaling molecules such as protein kinase C (PKC).[32,33] A strong association between diabetic nephropathy and retinopathy was demonstrated by Arora et al. in 2004–2005 in 50 newly diagnosed patients with diabetes.[34] The direct association between the presence of microalbuminuria and macrovascular complications has also been well established in many studies.[35] In an observational study, Hägg et al. (2013) reported the increased incidence of both cerebral infarction and cerebral hemorrhage in patients with severe DR (SDR) and advanced diabetic nephropathy in 4083 patients with T1DM with 36,680 person-years of follow-up. Both nephropathy and SDR were found to be independently increasing the risk for all subtypes of stroke.[36] The increased incidence of stroke in diabetic nephropathy has also been reiterated in the Pittsburgh Epidemiology of Diabetes Complications study, where overt nephropathy increases the risk of ischemic stroke 4.4-fold (but not the risk for hemorrhagic stroke, probably due to the insufficient number of samples).[36] Retinopathy and macroalbuminuria produce higher rates of cardiovascular events among Chinese patients.[37]

Diabetic Neuropathy

Diabetic neuropathy, a life-threatening complication involves both peripheral and autonomic nerves, affecting almost half of the diabetic population.[38] The risk of development of diabetic neuropathy is directly proportional to both the duration and the magnitude of hyperglycemia. In addition, some individuals may also possess genetic facets that influence their predisposition in developing such complications.[35] The prevalence of diabetic neuropathy varies from country to country. In India, a high prevalence (29.2%) of diabetic peripheral neuropathy was reported among the North Indian population.[39] Further studies in the North Indian region (Lucknow) and North-eastern region (Imphal) revealed a prevalence of 29.2% and 29.0%, respectively, among newly diagnosed diabetic patients (duration < 6 months).[40,41] Chawla et al. reported the prevalence of 15.3% in their study involving 720 North Indian patients from New Delhi.[20]

Although the precise nature of the injury to the peripheral nerves from hyperglycemia is not yet certain, the mechanisms of hyperglycemia-induced polyol pathway, injury from AGEs, and enhanced oxidative stress have been implicated in its pathogenesis. The damage to peripheral nerves may be mediated by effects on nerve tissue or by endothelial injury or vascular dysfunction.[2] Peripheral neuropathy in diabetes appears in several forms depending on the site, manifesting as sensory, focal/multifocal, and autonomic neuropathies. Diabetic neuropathy has resulted in more than 80% amputations after foot ulceration or injury.[35]

A study conducted by Miguel et al. demonstrated a significant correlation between diabetic neuropathy and the existence of one or more macrovascular complications showing that diabetic patients with peripheral neuropathy presented with significantly higher rates of cardiac events and peripheral vascular disease

(PVD) than diabetic patients without neuropathy. Strokes were also numerically higher in the neuropathy group.[42] Chawla et al. in 2011–2012 demonstrated an association between diabetic neuropathy and development of DR and microalbuminuria in 855 patients.[43] Diabetic cardiac autonomic neuropathy has been found to have a strong co-association with DR (22% vs. 14.3%), diabetic neuropathy (14% vs. 6.8%), and poor glycemic control.

Hence, it is recommended to evaluate autonomic nervous system function at the time of T2DM diagnosis and annually thereafter.[44] Chawla et al. established a positive correlation between autonomic neuropathy and peripheral neuropathy ($P = 0.00014$); however, the further association between autonomic neuropathy and PVD failed to reach statistical significance.[45] In addition, a direct relationship of lower extremity arterial disease (LEAD) with T2DM was also documented by Chawla et al. They found symptoms of peripheral vascular insufficiency or weak peripheral vessels in 13.8% of patients with foot Doppler confirming the prevalence of LEAD in 7.4% of patients.[46] The authors validated and advocated the use of neuropathy symptoms score and neuropathy disability score in the clinical and bedside diagnosis of peripheral neuropathy.[47]

COMMON PATHWAYS FOR DEVELOPMENT OF BOTH MICRO-AND MACROVASCULAR COMPLICATIONS

Advanced Glycation Products

Advanced glycation end products are a heterogeneous group of molecules formed by the nonenzymatic glycation of plasma proteins causing a disruption in their normal functioning by altering their molecular conformation, disrupting enzyme activity, and interfering with receptor functioning. AGEs accumulate in different types of cells and affect their extracellular and intracellular structure and function by cross-linking not only with proteins but also with lipids and nucleic acids contributing to a variety of diabetic complications.[48] AGEs crosslink with plasma membrane-localized receptors for AGEs (RAGE) leading to up-regulation of transcription factors such as nuclear factor-κB and its target genes, release of pro-inflammatory molecules and free radicals. Soluble AGEs activate monocytes, and AGEs in the basement membrane inhibit monocyte migration. AGE-bound RAGE increases endothelial permeability to macromolecules. AGEs block nitric oxide activity in the endothelium and cause the production of ROS.[49]

Further, AGEs modify LDL particles and together with vascular damage accelerate atherosclerosis.[50] Kalousová et al. found significant elevation of AGE in patients with T2DM as compared to both healthy ($5.11 \pm 1.15 \times 103$ AU/g vs. $4.08 \pm 0.71 \times 103$ AU/g, $P < 0.001$) as well as T1DM patients ($4.14 \pm 0.86 \times 103$ AU/g, $P < 0.005$).[51] Kilhovd et al. demonstrated a significant increase in the levels of AGEs in patients with T2DM compared with nondiabetic control subjects [7.4 (4.4–10.9) vs. 4.2 (1.6–6.4) U/mL, $P < 0.0001$]. Besides, they also found elevated levels of AGE in patients with coronary heart disease (CHD) than in those without CHD [8.1 (6.4–10.9) vs. 7.1 (3.5–9.8) U/mL, $P = 0.03$] in patients with T2DM.[52]

Oxidative Stress

Oxidative stress, caused by the overproduction of ROS, plays an important role in the activation of other pathogenic pathways involved in diabetic complications, including elevated polyol pathway activity, nonenzymatic glycation, and PKC levels which in turn lead to the development of micro- and macrovascular complications.[53] It also inactivates two critical antiatherosclerotic enzymes—endothelial nitric oxide synthase and prostacyclin synthase.[54] Hyperglycemia promotes the formation of ROS, which interacts with both deoxyribonucleic acid (DNA) and proteins, causing cellular damage, especially targeting mitochondrial DNA. A study on the human retinal endothelial cell (EC) demonstrated very early mitochondrial DNA damage with hyperglycemia-induced overproduction of ROS.[55] ROS-mediated cellular damage may be a form of pathologic "memory" in the microvasculature that persists even after glucose normalization. Several experimental evidences point to mitochondrial superoxide overproduction as the major culprit in the development of metabolic abnormalities in diabetics.[56] IR induces mitochondrial ROS production from free fatty acids and inhibits antiatherosclerotic enzymes causing atherosclerosis and cardiomyopathy in T2DM patients. In subjects without diabetes or impaired glucose tolerance, those in the highest quintile of IR had a 2.0-fold increase in CVD risk compared to those in the lowest quintile after adjusting several known cardiovascular risk factors, including LDL, triglycerides, high-density lipoprotein, systolic blood pressure, and smoking.[57]

The other pathways implicated in diabetic complications such as AGE formation, PKC activation, increased polyol flux, and hexosamine formation are also linked to oxidative stress in promoting macrovascular complications through multiple mechanisms. Increased glucose

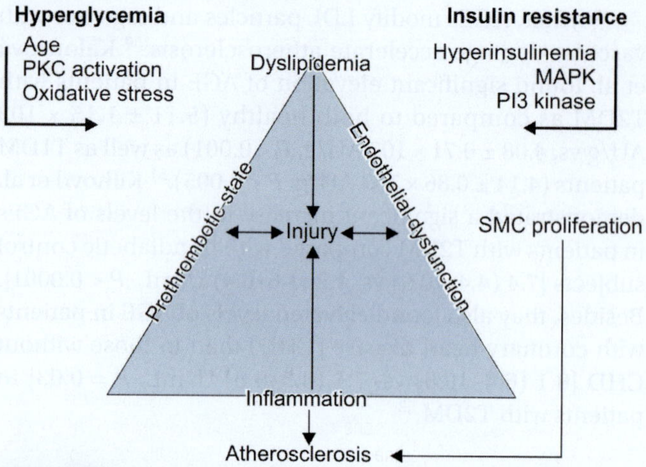

Figure 1 Insulin resistance and hyperglycemia drive the atherosclerotic process.

concentrations can activate nuclear factor-κB, a key mediator that regulates multiple pro-inflammatory and pro-atherosclerotic target genes in vascular smooth muscle cells (VSMCs), ECs, and macrophages.[55] Hyperglycemia itself stimulates oxidative stress, which indeed acts as a driving force in accelerated atherosclerosis.

Low-grade Inflammation

Inflammation has been recognized as one of the potent risk factors in both atherosclerosis and T2DM. Vascular cells encounter many early pathologic changes in response to hyperglycemia, causing a loss of nonadhesive property and adhesion of monocyte to ECs, which is an early step in atherogenesis. Hyperglycemia has been reported to provoke monocyte adhesion to arterial ECs.[58] The association between hyperglycemia and AGEs with oxidative stress is manifested as both can stimulate EC production of superoxide (Fig. 1). Glucose also activates matrix-degrading enzyme metalloproteinase which causes plaque rupture and arterial remodeling as well as VSMC proliferation, migration, and altered activity. The role of increased level of tumor necrosis factor alpha in the development of IR is well documented. IR itself has inflammatory action as described above. The levels of several other inflammatory markers such as C-reactive protein, fibrinogen, plasminogen activator inhibitor I, and interleukine 6 have been shown to increase with the onset of diabetes. Monocyte activation has been documented in the presence of high glucose with induction of inflammatory mediators such as PKC and nuclear factor κB promoting oxidative stress.[59]

Neovascularization of Vasa Vasorum

The proliferation of vasa vasorum is associated with increased plaque burden, which subsequently promotes atherosclerosis.[60] Many cellular processes such as inflammation, plaque perfusion, and concomitant intraplaque hemorrhage are critical during the development of atherosclerotic plaques and are linked with vasa vasorum proliferation. Neovascularization develops by the growth from both adventitial layer (outward) and arterial lumen (inward) toward the intima.[61] In T2DM, plaque rupture is associated with increased angiogenesis, and diabetic atherosclerosis is further accelerated by neovasculature microangiopathy.[62] The initial angiogenic response in the adventitial vasa vasorum, an important component of homeostatic mechanisms, appears to be stimulated by hypoxia through identification of increased hypoxia-inducible factor and vascular endothelial growth factor (VEGF) action.[63]

VEGF, a multifunctional cytokine, also contributes to microvascular complications by increasing the vascular permeability to macromolecules, monocyte chemotaxis, and tissue factor production.[64] Up-regulation of VEGF is also reported in experimental diabetic kidney disease models. However, contrary to this, VEGF treatment has been shown to restore microcirculation in the vasa nervorum and limit diabetic neuropathy as demonstrated by rodent VEGF gene transfer experiment.[2] In the eye, a neurotropic factor-pigment epithelium-derived factor (PEDF) may offset VEGF action by its potent angiogenic inhibition.[65] PEDF level is decreased in proliferative DR, whereas VEGF levels are increased. Decreased PEDF levels may also likely contribute to diabetic nephropathy. Other growth factors such as insulin-like growth factor 1, basic fibroblast growth factor, and hepatocyte growth factor may foster proliferative retinopathy.[66]

MICROVASCULAR AND MACROVASCULAR COMPLICATIONS—CONTINUUM OR SEPARATE: THE DEBATE CONTINUES (FIG. 2)

Heart involvement in diabetes may not be only a macrovascular disease where there is Orchestra of contributing factors to the development of diabetic cardiomyopathy concerning fatty acid and glucose complex structural macrovascular derangements such as hypertrophy and loss of function due to glycation but also a microvascular involvement following "common soil" hypothesis of diabetes complications. Atherosclerosis in

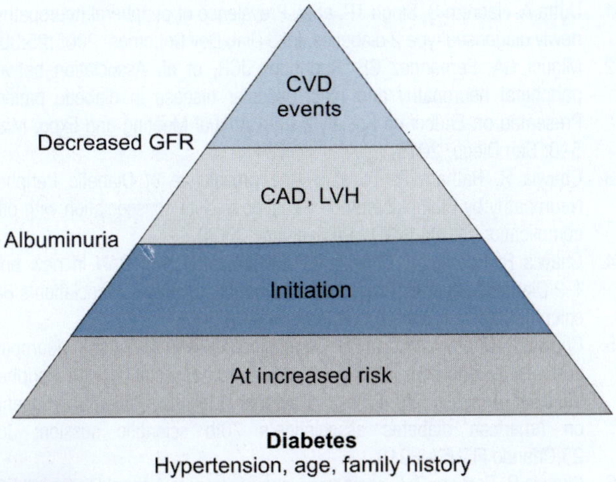

Figure 2 The diabetes continuum.

large arteries as well as cardiomyopathy in diabetes as microvascular component may go hand in hand.[67]

Therefore, changes in small arteries and capillaries are not responsible for only microvascular long-term complications in patients with diabetes (retinopathy, nephropathy, and neuropathy) but also for other manifestations of heart disease in diabetes.

This review highlights the need for implementing programs for early detection, screening, and awareness to mitigate the burden of managing the complications.

Good blood glucose control improves microvascular disease and should be implemented early and maintained for the optimum length of time. Appropriate controls of blood pressure as well as dyslipidemia are extremely important in macrovascular disease prevention besides glycemic control. Patients with microvascular complications appear particularly prone to accelerated atherosclerosis and premature death. Neovascularization arising from the vasa vasorum may interconnect macro- and microangiopathy.

A clearer picture on differing responses to therapeutic interventions could lead to better management and improve T2DM outcomes regarding not only microvascular but also macrovascular complications as well. Further systematic research on the above interlinking hypothesis will help us get more clarity whether microvascular complications precede macrovascular complications or they are two ends of the same spectrum of disease existing in continuum.

Conflict of Interest

All authors declare no conflict of interest.

REFERENCES

1. Standards of medical care in diabetes-2016: Summary of revisions. Diabetes Care. 2016;39(Suppl 1):S4-5.
2. Orasanu G, Plutzky J. The pathologic continuum of diabetic vascular disease. J Am Coll Cardiol. 2009;53(5 Suppl):S35-42.
3. International Diabetes Federation. IDF Atlas. 7th edition. [online] Available from: http://www.diabetesatlas.org. [Last accessed on October, 2019].
4. ADVANCE Collaborative Group, Patel A, MacMahon S, Chalmers J, et al. Intensive blood glucose control and vascular outcomes in patients with type 2 diabetes. N Engl J Med. 2008;358:2560-72.
5. Holman RR, Paul SK, Bethel MA, et al. A 10-year follow-up of intensive glucose control in type 2 diabetes. N Engl J Med. 2008;359:1577-89.
6. Charbonnel B, Dormandy J, Erdmann E, et al. PROactive Study Group. The prospective pioglitazone clinical trial in macrovascular events (PROactive): Can pioglitazone reduce cardiovascular events in diabetes? Study design and baseline characteristics of 5238 patients. Diabetes Care. 2004;27:1647-53.
7. Duckworth W, Abraira C, Moritz T, et al. Glucose control and vascular complications in veterans with type 2 diabetes. N Engl J Med. 2009;360:129-39.
8. Patel A, Chalmers J, Poulter N. ADVANCE: Action in diabetes and vascular disease. J Hum Hypertens. 2005;19(Suppl 1):S27-32.
9. Action to Control Cardiovascular Risk in Diabetes Study Group, Gerstein HC, Miller ME, Byington RP, et al. Effects of intensive glucose lowering in type 2 diabetes. N Engl J Med. 2008;358:2545-59.
10. Chawla A, Chawla R, Bhasin GK, et al. Profile of adolescent diabetics in North Indian population. J Clin Diabetol. 2014;1:1-3.
11. Krentz AJ, Clough G, Byrne CD. Interactions between microvascular and macrovascular disease in diabetes: Pathophysiology and therapeutic implications. Diabetes Obes Metab. 2007;9:781-91.
12. Al-Wakeel JS, Hammad D, Al Suwaida A, et al. Microvascular and macrovascular complications in diabetic nephropathy patients referred to nephrology clinic. Saudi J Kidney Dis Transpl. 2009;20:77-85.
13. Matheus AS, Gomes MB. Early aggressive macrovascular disease and type 1 diabetes mellitus without chronic complications: A case report. BMC Res Notes. 2013;6:222.
14. Kalofoutis C, Piperi C, Kalofoutis A, et al. Type II diabetes mellitus and cardiovascular risk factors: Current therapeutic approaches. Exp Clin Cardiol 2007;12:17-28.
15. Fong DS, Aiello LP, Ferris FL 3rd, et al. Diabetic retinopathy. Diabetes Care. 2004;27:2540-53.
16. Rema M, Premkumar S, Anitha B, et al. Prevalence of diabetic retinopathy in urban India: The Chennai Urban Rural Epidemiology Study (CURES) eye study, I. Invest Ophthalmol Vis Sci. 2005;46:2328-33.
17. Raman R, Rani PK, Reddi Rachepalle S, et al. Prevalence of diabetic retinopathy in India: Sankara Nethralaya Diabetic Retinopathy Epidemiology and Molecular Genetics Study report 2. Ophthalmology. 2009;116:311-8.
18. Raman R, Ganesan S, Pal SS, et al. Prevalence and risk factors for diabetic retinopathy in rural India. Sankara Nethralaya Diabetic Retinopathy Epidemiology and Molecular Genetic Study III (SN-DREAMS III), report no 2. BMJ Open Diabetes Res Care. 2014;2:e000005.
19. Nirmalan PK, Tielsch JM, Katz J, , et al. Relationship between vision impairment and eye disease to vision-specific quality of life and function in rural India: The Aravind Comprehensive Eye Survey. Invest Ophthalmol Vis Sci. 2005;46:2308-12.
20. Chawla A, Chawla R, Chawla A. Correlation Between Retinopathy Microalbuminuria and Other Modifiable Risk Factors. Presented on American Diabetes Association's 75th Scientific Session; June 5-9; Boston, Massachusetts; 2015.

21. Wong TY, Klein R, Couper DJ, et al. Retinal microvascular abnormalities and incident stroke: The atherosclerosis risk in communities study. Lancet. 2001;358:1134-40.
22. Fuller JH, Stevens LK, Wang SL. Risk factors for cardiovascular mortality and morbidity: The WHO mutinational study of vascular disease in diabetes. Diabetologia. 2001;44(Suppl 2):S54-64.
23. Yatsuya H, Folsom AR, Wong TY, et al. Retinal microvascular abnormalities and risk of lacunar stroke: Atherosclerosis Risk in Communities Study. Stroke. 2010;41:1349-55.
24. Mitchell P, Wang JJ, Wong TY, et al. Retinal microvascular signs and risk of stroke and stroke mortality. Neurology. 2005;65:1005-9.
25. Targher G, Bertolini L, Zenari L, Lippi G, Pichiri I, Zoppini G, et al. Diabetic retinopathy is associated with an increased incidence of cardiovascular events in Type 2 diabetic patients. Diabet Med. 2008;25:45-50.
26. Gross JL, de Azevedo MJ, Silveiro SP, et al. Diabetic nephropathy: diagnosis, prevention, and treatment. Diabetes Care. 2005;28:164-76.
27. Soedamah-Muthu SS, Chaturvedi N, Witte DR, , et al. Relationship between risk factors and mortality in type 1 diabetic patients in Europe: the EURODIAB Prospective Complications Study (PCS). Diabetes Care. 2008;31:1360-6.
28. Hovind P, Tarnow L, Rossing P, et al. Predictors for the development of microalbuminuria and macroalbuminuria in patients with type 1 diabetes: inception cohort study. Bmj. 2004;328:1105.
29. Adler AI, Stevens RJ, Manley SE, et al. Development and progression of nephropathy in type 2 diabetes: the United Kingdom Prospective Diabetes Study (UKPDS 64). Kidney Int. 2003;63:225-32.
30. Unnikrishnan RI, Rema M, Pradeepa R, et al. Prevalence and risk factors of diabetic nephropathy in an urban South Indian population: the Chennai Urban Rural Epidemiology Study (CURES 45). Diabetes Care. 2007;30:2019-24.
31. Adler AI, Stratton IM, Neil HA, et al. Association of systolic blood pressure with macrovascular and microvascular complications of type 2 diabetes (UKPDS 36): prospective observational study. Bmj. 2000;321:412-9.
32. Trevisan R, Dodesini AR, Lepore G. Lipids and renal disease. J Am Soc Nephrol. 2006;17:S145-7.
33. Cade WT. Diabetes-related microvascular and macrovascular diseases in the physical therapy setting. Phys Ther. 2008;88:1322-35.
34. Arora GS, Chawla R, Ahuja CP. To evaluate the clinical profile and determine the prevalence of complications in newly detected type-2 diabetes patients. Presented on Research society for the study of diabetes in India's (RSSDI) 33rd annual conference; September 23rd–25th, Bangalore.2005.
35. Fowler MJ. Microvascular and macrovascular complications of diabetes. Clinical diabetes. 2008;26:77-82.
36. Hagg S, Thorn LM, Putaala J, et al. Incidence of stroke according to presence of diabetic nephropathy and severe diabetic retinopathy in patients with type 1 diabetes. Diabetes Care. 2013;36:4140-6.
37. Lloyd CE, Klein R, Maser RE, et al. The progression of retinopathy over 2 years: the Pittsburgh Epidemiology of Diabetes Complications (EDC) Study. J Diabetes Complications. 1995;9:140-8.
38. Tong PC, Kong AP, So WY, et al. Hematocrit, independent of chronic kidney disease, predicts adverse cardiovascular outcomes in chinese patients with type 2 diabetes. Diabetes Care. 2006;29:2439-44.
39. Tapp R, Shaw J. Epidemiology of diabetic neuropathy. In: Boulton STaA (Ed). Diabetic Neuropathy. New York: Oxford University Press; 2009. Recent Advances in Diabetes 102
40. Bansal D, Gudala K, Muthyala H, et al. Prevalence and risk factors of development of peripheral diabetic neuropathy in type 2 diabetes mellitus in a tertiary care setting. Journal of diabetes investigation. 2014;5: 714-21.
41. Dutta A, Naorem S, Singh TP, et al. Prevalence of peripheral neuropathy in newly diagnosed type 2 diabetics. Int J Diab Dev Countries. 2005;25:30-3.
42. Miguel GA, Fernández GE, Rodríguez JCR, et al. Association between peripheral neuropathy and macrovascular disease in diabetic patients. Presented on Endocrine Society's 97th Annual Meeting and Expo; March 5–8; San Diego. 2015.
43. Chawla R, Rathore P. To study the prevalence of Diabetic Peripheral Neuropathy by Biothesiometric evaluation and its coassociation with other complications 2004 (NNDU Proceedings 2004).
44. Chawla R, Poddar A, Chawla R. High prevalence of CAN in new onset T-2 Diabetes patients. Presented on American diabetes association's 68th scientific session; June 8;San Francisco,CA.2008.
45. Chawla R, Gupta S, Punyani H. Correlation between Autonomic Neuropathy and Distal Peripheral Neuropathy and its co-association with Peripheral Vascular Disease in Type-2 Diabetes Mellitus Patients. Presented on American diabetes association's 70th scientific session; June 25;Orlando,FL,USA.2010.
46. Chawla R, Rathore P. Evaluation of lower Extremity Arterial Disease (LEAD/ PVD) in Type-2 diabetics and its co association with other macro vascular complications. Presented on annual conference of Diabetic foot society of India's scientific session; September 4-5;Bhopal,India. 2004.
47. Chawla A, Bhasin GK, Chawla R. Validation of Neuropathy Symptoms Score (NSS) and Neuropathy Disability Score (NDS) in the Clinical Diagnosis of Peripheral Neuropathy in Middle Aged People with Diabetes. Int J Fam Pract. 2013;12(1).
48. Singh VP, Bali A, Singh N, et al. Advanced Glycation End Products and Diabetic Complications. The Korean Journal of Physiology and Pharmacology: Official Journal of the Korean Physiological Society and the Korean Society of Pharmacology. 2014;18:1-14.
49. Schmidt AM, Hori O, Brett J, et al. Cellular receptors for advanced glycation end products. Implications for induction of oxidant stress and cellular dysfunction in the pathogenesis of vascular lesions. Arterioscler Thromb. 1994;14:1521-8.
50. Goldin A, Beckman JA, Schmidt AM, et al. Advanced glycation end products: sparking the development of diabetic vascular injury. Circulation. 2006;114:597-605.
51. Kalousova M, Skrha J, Zima T. Advanced glycation end-products and advanced oxidation protein products in patients with diabetes mellitus. Physiological research/Academia Scientiarum Bohemoslovaca. 2002;51:597-604.
52. Kilhovd BK, Berg TJ, Birkeland KI, et al. Serum levels of advanced glycation end products are increased in patients with type 2 diabetes and coronary heart disease. Diabetes care. 1999;22:1543-8.
53. Jakus V, Rietbrock N. Advanced glycation end-products and the progress of diabetic vascular complications. Physiological research/Academia Scientiarum Bohemoslovaca. 2004;53:131-42.
54. Folli F, Corradi D, Fanti P, et al. The role of oxidative stress in the pathogenesis of type 2 diabetes mellitus micro- and macrovascular complications: avenues for a mechanistic-based therapeutic approach. Curr diabetes rev. 2011;7:313-24.
55. Giacco F, Brownlee M. Oxidative stress and diabetic complications. Circ res. 2010;107:1058-70.
56. Xie L, Zhu X, Hu Y, et al. Mitochondrial DNA oxidative damage triggering mitochondrial dysfunction and apoptosis in high glucose-induced HRECs. Investigative ophthalmology and visual science. 2008;49:4203-9.
57. Duncan JG. Mitochondrial dysfunction in diabetic cardiomyopathy. Biochimica et biophysica acta. 2011;1813:1351-9.
58. Syed Ikmal SI, Zaman Huri H, Vethakkan SR, et al. Potential biomarkers of insulin resistance and atherosclerosis in type 2 diabetes mellitus patients with coronary artery disease. Inter j endocrinol. 2013;2013:698567.

59. Otsuka A, Azuma K, Iesaki T, et al. Temporary hyperglycaemia provokes monocyte adhesion to endothelial cells in rat thoracic aorta. Diabetologia. 2005;48:2667-74.
60. Tian J, Hu S, Sun Y, et al. Vasa vasorum and plaque progression, and responses to atorvastatin in a rabbit model of atherosclerosis: contrast-enhanced ultrasound imaging and intravascular ultrasound study. Heart (British Cardiac Society). 2013;99:48-54.
61. Hayden MR, Tyagi SC. Vasa vasorum in plaque angiogenesis, metabolic syndrome, type 2 diabetes mellitus, and atheroscleropathy: a malignant transformation. Cardiovas diabetol. 2004;3:1.
62. Patel A. Does the Role of Angiogenesis play a Role in Atherosclerosis and Plaque Instability? Anat Physiol. 2014;4:2161-0940.
63. Xu J, Lu X, Shi GP. Vasa vasorum in atherosclerosis and clinical significance. Inter j mol sci. 2015;16:11574-608.
64. Bonnefond A, Saulnier PJ, Stathopoulou MG, et al. What is the contribution of two genetic variants regulating VEGF levels to type 2 diabetes risk and to microvascular complications. PLoS One. 2013;8:e55921.
65. Schratzberger P, Walter DH, Rittig K, et al. Reversal of experimental diabetic neuropathy by VEGF gene transfer. J clin invest. 2001;107:1083-92.
66. Gao G, Li Y, Zhang D, et al. Unbalanced expression of VEGF and PEDF in ischemia-induced retinal neovascularization. FEBS letters. 2001;489:270-6.
67. Laakso M. Heart in diabetes: a microvascular disease. Diabetes care. 2011;34 (Suppl 2):S145-9.